BONE METASTASIS

CANCER DRUG DISCOVERY AND DEVELOPMENT

BEVERLY A. TEICHER, SERIES EDITOR

BONE METASTASIS

EXPERIMENTAL AND CLINICAL THERAPEUTICS

Edited by

GURMIT SINGH, PhD

Department of Pathology and Molecular Medicine
Juravinski Cancer Centre, McMaster University
Hamilton, Ontario, Canada

SHAFAAT A. RABBANI, MD

Calcium Research Laboratory
McGill University Health Centre
Montreal, Quebec, Canada

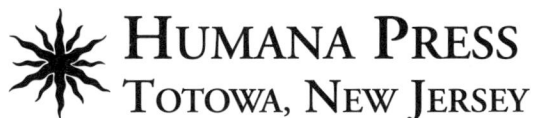

HUMANA PRESS
TOTOWA, NEW JERSEY

Production Editor: Nicole E. Furia
Cover design by Patricia F. Cleary
Cover illustration:Figure 1 from Chapter 1, "Overview," by Sadmeet Singh and Gurmit Singh and Figure 4 from Chapter 10, "PTHrP and Cancer: *Prostate and Lung*," by Leonard J. Deftos, D. W. Burton, and Randolph H. Hastings.

This publication is printed on acid-free paper. ∞
ANSI Z39.48-1984 (American National Standards Institute)
Permanence of Paper for Printed Library Materials

For additional copies, pricing for bulk purchases, and/or information about other Humana titles,
contact Humana at the above address or at any of the following numbers: Tel.:973-256-1699;
Fax: 973-256-8341; Email: humana@humanapr.com; or visit our Website: http://humanapress.com.

Printed in the United States of America. 10 9 8 7 6 5 4 3 2 1

eISBN 1-59259-892-7

Library of Congress Cataloging-in-Publication Data
Bone metastasis : experimental and clinical therapeutics / edited by Gurmit
Singh, Shafaat A. Rabbani.
     p. ; cm.
 Includes bibliographical references and index.
 ISBN 1-58829-403-X (hardcover : alk. paper)
 1. Bone metastasis.
 [DNLM: 1. Bone Neoplasms—secondary. 2. Neoplasm Metastasis. WE 258
B7107 2005] I. Singh, Gurmit. II. Rabbani, Shafaat A.
 RC280.B6B645 2005
 616.99'471—dc22
                          2004014785

DEDICATION

This text is dedicated to all the graduate students, postdoctoral fellows, and technical staff who tirelessly commit their energy and time to improve the lives of cancer patients.

PREFACE

Bone Metastasis: Experimental and Clinical Therapeutics is intended as an introduction to the molecular underpinnings of bone metastasis. Contributions from internationally recognized authorities on the fundamental concepts, current treatment approaches, and future therapeutic strategies provide a synopsis of bone metastasis. Our insights into the molecular mechanisms underlying the pathophysiology of bone metastasis are still evolving. These advances are driving the application of new therapeutic strategies directed at recently discovered molecular targets.

The first 11 chapters in *Bone Metastasis: Experimental and Clinical Therapeutics* focus on fundamental concepts associated with the process of metastasis. The roles of the various autocrine, paracrine, and immunological factors are intimately involved in the progression and establishment of bone metastases. Understanding these concepts has led to and will continue to provide novel approaches to their treatment. Chapters 12–19 discuss various strategies that appear to have promise and that are currently deployed in treatment or are at the experimental stage. Understanding of the physiological process that leads to bone degradation, pain, angiogenesis, and dysregulation of bone turnover by the tumor is critical. Thus, the treatment of bone metastases may need to be individualized, employing a combination of surgical, radiation, and/or pharmacological maneuvers. Further understanding of various pharmacogenomic parameters and tissue environmental factors is essential for progress beyond the current standard approaches of using radiation and/or bisphosphonates for palliation.

The editors would like to express their gratitude to all the authors for their scholarly contributions, which have summarized current literature in their field. We would also like to thank Dr. Beverly Teicher for inviting us to edit this book for the *Cancer Drug Discovery and Development* series. We would like to acknowledge the persistence and encouragement from Paul Dolgert, Editorial Director at Humana Press. Finally, the support and assistance of Ms. Heather Blackborow is greatly appreciated.

Gurmit Singh, PhD
Shafaat A. Rabbani, MD

CONTENTS

CONTRIBUTORS

ALISON L. ALLAN, PhD • *Departments of Oncology and Pathology, London Regional Cancer Program/University of Western Ontario, London, Ontario, Canada*

MARCEL B. BALLY, PhD • *Department of Pathology and Laboratory Medicine and British Columbia Cancer Research Centre, University of British Columbia, Vancouver, British Columbia, Canada*

ELIZABETH TONI BARNES, MD, FRCPC • *Department of Radiation Oncology, Toronto Sunnybrook Regional Cancer Centre, University of Toronto, Toronto, Ontario, Canada*

GWYN BEBB, BMBCh, PhD • *British Columbia Cancer Agency, Department of Medical Oncology and British Columbia Cancer Research Centre, Vancouver, British Columbia, Canada*

VIVIEN H. C. BRAMWELL, PhD, MBBS, FRCPC • *Department of Oncology/Medicine, Tom Baker Cancer Centre, University of Calgary, Calgary, Alberta, Canada*

SHANE BURCH, MD • *Sunnybrook and Women's College Health Centres and Division of Orthopaedic Surgery, University of Toronto, Toronto, Ontario, Canada*

D. W. BURTON, BSc • *Department of Medicine, University of California, San Diego, La Jolla, CA*

MARTIN K. BUTCHER, Hon.BSc • *Department of Pathology and Molecular Medicine, McMaster University, Hamilton, Ontario, Canada*

ANN F. CHAMBERS, PhD • *Departments of Oncology and Pathology, London Regional Cancer Program/University of Western Ontario, London, Ontario, Canada*

KIM CHI, MD • *Department of Advanced Therapeutics and Systemic Therapy Program, British Columbia Cancer Agency, British Columbia, Canada*

EDWARD CHOW, MBBS, FRCPC • *Department of Radiation Oncology, Toronto Sunnybrook Regional Cancer Centre, University of Toronto, Toronto, Ontario, Canada*

LELAND W. K. CHUNG, PhD • *Department of Urology, Emory University School of Medicine, Atlanta, GA*

NIGEL COLTERJOHN, MD • *Department of Orthopedic Surgery, Hamilton Health Sciences, Hamilton, Ontario, Canada*

RICHARD J. COOK, PhD • *Department of Statistics and Actuarial Science, University of Waterloo, Waterloo, Ontario, Canada*

LEONARD J. DEFTOS, MD, JD • *Department of Medicine, University of California, La Jolla, CA*

FERNANDO DOÑATE, PhD • *Attenuon, LLC, San Diego, CA*

LINCOLN EDWARDS, BSc • *Department of Pathology and Laboratory Medicine, University of British Columbia and British Columbia Cancer Research Centre, Vancouver, British Columbia, Canada*

KAREN FANG, BSc • *Department of Pathology and Laboratory Medicine, University of British Columbia and British Columbia Cancer Research Centre, Vancouver, British Columbia, Canada*

ERIN GILES, BSc • *McMaster University/Juravinski Cancer Centre, Hamilton, Ontario, Canada*

MARTIN GLEAVE, MD • *Vancouver General Hospital, Prostate Centre, Vancouver, British Columbia, Canada*

DAVID GOLTZMAN, MD • *Department of Medicine, McGill University, Montreal, Quebec, Canada*

RANDOLPH H. HASTINGS, MD, PhD • *Department of Anesthesiology, University of California, La Jolla, CA*

WEN-CHIN HUANG, PhD • *Department of Urology, Emory University School of Medicine, Atlanta, GA*

ARIF HUSSAIN, MD • *Greenebaum Cancer Centre, University of Maryland, School of Medicine, Baltimore, MD*

RICHARD KREMER, MD • *Royal Victoria Hospital, McGill University Health Centre, Montreal, Quebec, Canada*

PIERRE P. MAJOR, MD, FRCPC • *Department of Medical Oncology, Juravinski Cancer Centre, Hamilton, Ontario, Canada*

ANDREW P. MAZAR, PhD • *Attenuon, LLC, San Diego, CA*

LAURIE A. MCDUFFEE, PhD, DVM, DACVS • *Department of Health Management, Atlantic Veterinary College, Charlottetown, Prince Edward Island, Canada*

SHAKER A. MOUSA, PhD, MBA, FACC, FACB • *Department of Basic and Pharmaceutical Sciences, Albany College of Pharmacy & Pharmaceutical Research Institute, Albany, NY*

VALERIE ODERO-MARAH, PhD • *Department of Urology, Emory University School of Medicine, Atlanta, GA*

GRAHAM C. PARRY, PhD • *Attenuon, LLC, San Diego, CA*

SUJATA PERSAD, PhD • *Department of Research, Juravinski Cancer Centre, Hamilton, Ontario, Canada*

STEVEN PIRIE-SHEPHERD, PhD • *Attenuon, LLC, San Diego, CA*

MARIAN L. PLUNKETT, PhD • *Attenuon, LLC, San Diego, CA*

SHAFAAT A. RABBANI, MD • *Calcium Research Laboratory, McGill University Health Centre, Montreal, Quebec, Canada*

FRED SAAD, MD, FRCS • *Department of Urology, University of Montreal, Montreal, Quebec, Canada*

ZEINA SAIKALI, PhD • *Juravinski Cancer Centre, McMaster University, Hamilton, Ontario, Canada*

ERIC SEIDLITZ, MSc • *Juravinski Cancer Centre, McMaster University, Hamilton, Ontario, Canada*

STEPHEN G. SHAUGHNESSY, PhD • *Department of Pathology and Molecular Medicine, McMaster University/ Henderson Research Centre, Hamilton, Ontario, Canada*

DAVID E. SHAW, PhD • *D. E. Shaw Research and Development, LLC, New York, NY*

RYAN R. SIMON, MSc • *Department of Pathology and Molecular Medicine, McMaster University, Hamilton, Ontario, Canada*

GURMIT SINGH, PhD • *Department of Pathology and Molecular Medicine/Juravinski Cancer Centre, McMaster University, Hamilton, Ontario, Canada*

SADMEET SINGH, BM, BS, FRCS • *Department of Research, Juravinski Cancer Centre, Hamilton, Ontario, Canada*

KRISTINA A. SZABO, MSc • *Department of Pathology and Molecular Medicine, McMaster University, Hamilton, Ontario, Canada*

ALAN B. TUCK, MD, PhD • *London Regional Cancer Program/University of Western Ontario, Departments of Oncology and Pathology, London Health Sciences Centre, London, Ontario, Canada*

THEODORE A. VANDENBERG, MD • *Department of Oncology, London Regional Cancer Program/University of Western Ontario, London, Ontario, Canada*

ELLEN K. WASAN, RPh, PhD • *Department of Advanced Therapeutics, British Columbia Cancer Research Centre, Vancouver, British Columbia, Canada*

ERIC W. WINQUIST, MSc, MD • *Department of Oncology, London Regional Cancer Program/University of Western Ontario, London, Ontario, Canada*

JACKSON WU, MD, FRCPC • *Department of Radiation Oncology, Tom Baker Cancer Centre, University of Calgary, Calgary, Alberta, Canada*

ALBERT J. M. YEE, MD • *Sunnybrook and Women's College Health Centres and Division of Orthopaedic Surgery, University of Toronto, Toronto, Ontario, Canada*

I FUNDAMENTAL CONCEPTS

1 Overview

Sadmeet Singh, BM, BS, FRCS,
and Gurmit Singh, PhD

CONTENTS

1. INTRODUCTION

Metastases rather than primary tumors are responsible for the lion's share of the morbidity and mortality arising from malignant disease. Patients with advanced breast or prostate cancers usually develop bone metastases and usually harbor the bulk of their tumor burden in the bone at the time of death. Although it is difficult to quantify the prevalence of bone metastases, natural history and autopsy studies give an indication of the scope of the problem. In breast cancer, the skeleton is the most common site for metastasis and first distant relapse, and median survival following detection is more than 20 mo *(1)*. At their presentation with prostate cancer, 8% of white American males and 14% of African-American males have bone metastases *(2)*, whereas the mean incidence of bone metastasis in an analysis of autopsy studies of prostate cancer is 70% *(3)*. It is clear, therefore, that bone metastases are both a common manifestation in patients with breast and prostate cancer and often a prolonged one. Given these considerations and the fact that bone metastases are not usually clinically silent, their importance in the context of the overall suffering and management associated with these malignancies is evident. Clinically, the lesions behave somewhat differently in the two cancers, with pathological fractures being relatively more common in breast cancer and severe, often intractable pain a classic feature of metastases in patients with advanced prostate cancer *(4)*. Spinal cord compression as a result of vertebral metastasis is perhaps the most devastating complication of skeletal involvement with hypercalcemia and leukoerythroblastic anemia being the commonest systemic sequelae.

From: *Cancer Drug Discovery and Development*
Bone Metastasis: Experimental and Clinical Therapeutics
Edited by: G. Singh and S. A. Rabbani © Humana Press Inc., Totowa, NJ

2. HOW TUMOR CELLS GET TO THE BONE

The principles underlying the dissemination of a primary tumor and the development of metastasis involve a series of steps that are the same for bone metastases as for hematogenous spread to other sites *(5)*. Tumor cells from the primary lesion must first invade into the normal surrounding tissue, which they accomplish by producing proteolytic enzymes. This gives the tumor cells access to the microvasculature of the surrounding tissue, but they also make use of the neovascularization that the primary tumour induces, a process termed "angiogenesis" *(6)*. Cancer cells then have to survive in the circulation and travel to distant sites where, once arrested, they have to cross from the vascular network back into normal tissue. In order for a metastasis to be established, the cells need to be able to survive in the new environment. In the case of bone metastases, tumor cells entering the sinusoidal vascular channels of the bone marrow cavity have to traverse the sinusoidal wall in order to invade the marrow stroma. Angiogenesis is then required for the cells to form a macroscopic tumor at the endosteal surface of the bone. It is well known that this sequence of events is inefficient; a very small proportion of the tumour cells that enter the circulation eventually end up as clinically detectable metastases *(7)*. Recent data from experimental models of metastasis suggest that the initial steps of the metastasis cascade are completed highly efficiently and that the inefficiency of the process is apparent from the point at which tumor cells extravasate from the circulation at secondary sites *(8,9)*.

A "homing" mechanism for cancer cells to specific organs has recently been proposed in experiments with breast cancer cells. Investigators showed that lung and bone stromal cells secrete a chemokine, CXCL12, and that breast cancer cells express high levels of a specific receptor, CXCR4. Using neutralizing antibodies to the receptor, they were able to block pulmonary metastasis. There has long been a search for such mechanisms and this finding offers exciting prospects for targeting bone metastases *(10)*.

3. THE BONE MICROENVIRONMENT: OSTEOLYTIC AND OSTEOBLASTIC METASTASES

The relationship between the tumor cells and the host tissue is a major factor in their ability to develop into macroscopic metastases. This is often referred to as the "seed" (the tumor cells) and "soil" (the metastatic site) hypothesis of metastasis after Paget's paper of 1889 discussing the distribution of metastases in breast cancer *(11)*. The unravelling of the molecular mechanisms involved in the interaction between the host microenvironment and tumor cell is seen as a key to the development of new therapies to deal with metastases.

It has been traditional to consider bone metastases arising from breast cancer as osteolytic and those from prostate cancer to be osteoblastic. This difference between the two diseases is evident in the radiological appearances of the bone metastases, but the classification is an oversimplification of the mechanisms involved. Here, the molecular crosstalk between the tumor cells and the bone microenvironment play a large part in determining the nature of the lesions. Osteolytic and osteoblastic lesions are two extremes, with the metastases of breast and prostate cancers usually containing elements of both in different proportions.

3.1. Parathyroid Hormone-Related Peptide

The damage caused to the skeleton by bony metastases is usually in excess of what would be expected by the presence and volume of the tumor cells alone, particularly in the clinically lytic lesions of breast cancer. The osteolysis that causes this damage is a result of the activation of osteoclasts, specialized bone-resorbing cells that are derived from monocytes. The principle mediator of this osteoclast activation is parathyroid hormone-related peptide (PTHrP) *(12)*. PTHrP was initially discovered during the search for a peptide sharing amino-terminal homology with parathyroid hormone from tumors associated with hypercalcemia *(13)* PTHrP plays a central role in the hypercalcemia of malignant disease by acting on the parathyroid hormone receptor to cause increased renal absorption and bone release of calcium *(14)*. It is worth emphasizing here that although bone destruction is an important etiological factor in the development of hypercalcemia in malignancy, the role of renal mechanisms has tended to be underestimated.

Parathyroid hormone-related peptide is undetectable in health, but it is present in most patients with breast cancer and its levels are higher in bone metastases than in either soft tissue secondaries or in primary tumors *(15)*. Osteoclastic bone resorption resulting from bone-induced tumor cell overproduction of PTHrP causes the release of active growth factors. A "vicious cycle" of bone loss is then established because the growth factors lead to proliferation of tumor cells, which, in turn, continue to produce osteolysis-promoting PTHrP *(16)*. The expression of PTHrP in the biopsies of bone metastases from patients with untreated prostate cancer has recently been shown in an immunohistochemical study *(17)*. This finding is consistent with our understanding that osteoclast activation occurs in prostate cancer, although the role of PTHrP in the pathogenesis of skeletal disease in this malignancy requires further investigation.

3.2. The RANK-RANKL System and Bone Metastasis

Following from the discovery of the role of PTHrP in the etiology of osteolytic bone metastasis has been the identification and characterization of a new cytokine system capable of regulating the proliferation, differentiation, activation and apoptosis of osteoclasts *(18)*. This cytokine system is comprised of receptor activator of nuclear factor $\kappa\beta$ ligand (RANKL), its receptor (RANK), and its "decoy receptor," osteoprotegrin (OPG). The exogenous administration of RANKL to normal mice has been shown to increase the number and activity of osteoclasts and promote the development of severe osteoporosis and lethal humoral hypercalcemia. Recently, it has been shown that PTHrP-producing breast cancer cells led to bone erosion and the expression of RANKL when injected into the periosteum of mice skulls, whereas non-PTHrP-producing cells did not lead to destructive bone lesions *(19)*. OPG acts as a endogenous receptor antagonist able to neutralize the biological effects of RANKL. A variety of both in vitro and in vivo data have demonstrated the antiosteoclastic effects and bone-protective actions of OPG as recently reviewed by Hofbauer et al. *(20)*.

3.3. Growth Factors

Interactions between members of a number of growth factor families secreted by breast and prostate cancer tumors and the bone have been observed. Members of the transforming growth factor-β (TGF-β) family have been implicated in the development of bone metastases in breast and prostate cancers at many levels. They are powerful in vivo stimulators of new bone and their involvement in the development of osteoblastic lesions in prostate cancer has been shown by a number of investigators *(20)*. Recent evidence also suggests that TGF-β is involved in PTHrP-induced osteolytic metastases *(21)* and the RANKL system *(22)*.

Prostate cancers secrete large amounts of acidic and basic fibroblast growth factors (FGFs). These have been shown to stimulate bone formation in vivo and thus act as mediators for osteoblastic metastases *(23)*. Endothelin-1 is another growth factor shown to be associated with the development of metastases in prostate cancer. It is found at increased levels in patients with prostate cancer, and bone metastases *(24)* and prostate cancer cells have been shown to stimulate osteoblast activity by secreting it *(25)*.

4. MATRIX METALLOPROTEINASES AND BONE METASTASIS

The matrix metalloproteinase (MMP) family comprises over 20 zinc-dependent proteases that, collectively, are able to degrade all of the components of the extracellular matrix. As experience has accumulated with MMPs, so has the discovery that their substrates include a wide variety of extracellular proteins such as other proteinases, proteinase inhibitors, chemotactic molecules, cell surface receptors, and adhesion molecules *(26)*. MMPs play a role in the physiological remodeling of bone: They are involved in osteoclast recruitment to sites of remodeling *(27)* and are among the enzymes that degrade the mineralized bone matrix *(28)*. Increased MMP expression has been documented in nearly all epithelial tumors. In prostate cancer, MMP-2 expression has been found to be a marker for tumor vs normal tissue and to be correlated with tumor grade *(29)* and the presence of metastasis *(30)*. Similarly, a wide variety of MMPs have been implicated in the pathogenesis and metastasis of breast cancer *(31)*. MMP activity seems to be particularly relevant in the development of bone metastases as a result of the abundance of the extracellular matrix and its resistance to degradation.

5. THERAPEUTIC APPROACHES

The above-discussed molecular mechanisms all present opportunities for therapeutic intervention. The successful use of bisphosphonates for metastatic bone disease is an example of application of the understanding of these mechanisms for therapeutic purposes. They and some of the approaches, which will hopefully yield benefit in the future, are discussed in the following subsections. A schematic diagram of some of the mechanisms involved, the sites, and the modes of intervention discussed is shown in Fig. 1.

5.1. Bisphosphonates

These drugs are already indicated for the treatment of metastatic bone pain in breast and prostate cancer as well as for the prevention of skeletal-related events in breast cancer. In addition, they are a highly effective therapy for the treatment of hypercalcemia in patients with all tumor types, in the presence or absence of bone metastases, and are used for the treatment/prevention of osteoporosis in women.

All bisphosphonates have a central P-C-P-containing structure, which is able to bind to mineralized bone matrix, and a variable side chain that determines the potency, side effects, and precise mechanism of action. The rationale for the use of bisphosphonates

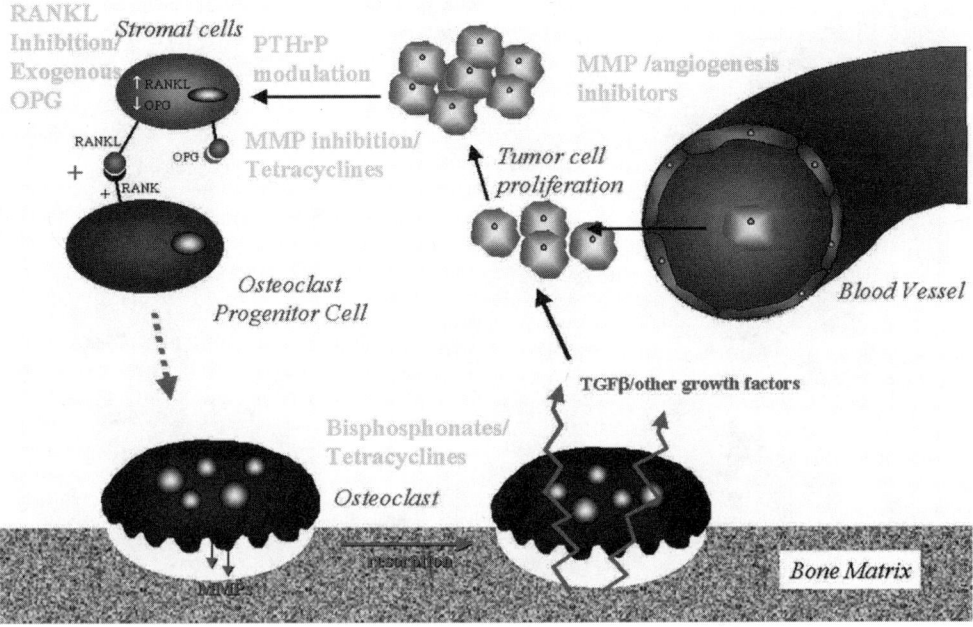

Fig. 1. Schematic showing some of the steps involved in the development of bone metastases along with sites and modes of current and proposed intervention.

in metastatic bone disease lies in their inhibitory action against osteoclasts enabling them to diminish bone resorption. Bisphosphonates bind avidly to exposed bone matrix around resorbing osteoclasts, reaching very high concentrations at these sites. Once released from the bone surface, they are taken up by osteoclasts, where they disrupt the biochemical processes involved in bone resorption. Bisphosphonates also cause osteoclast apoptosis and recent data suggest that they might be directly apoptotic to tumor cells *(32)*, although the molecular targets for these actions remain unknown.

The antiosteolytic action of these drugs and their proven efficacy in decreasing the burden of bone metastasis in breast cancer *(33)* has led to the evaluation of their use in the management of skeletal disease in prostate cancer. This is based on the realization that osteolysis occurs in bone lesions from prostate cancer, but it occurs in the background of an intense osteoblastic reaction *(16,34)*. However, data have been unconvincing. The most encouraging results have recently been published in a randomized controlled clinical trial assessing the efficacy of zoledronic acid (the most powerful bisphosphonate currently used) in patients with hormone-refractory metastatic prostate cancer *(35)*. Some of the end points measured (skeletal related events and time to first skeletal-related event) demonstrated significant benefit in favor of the treatment arm. A review of the results, however, did not recommend the routine use of the drug in patients with metastatic prostate cancer on the basis of the lack of demonstration of net benefit and probable cost implications *(36)*.

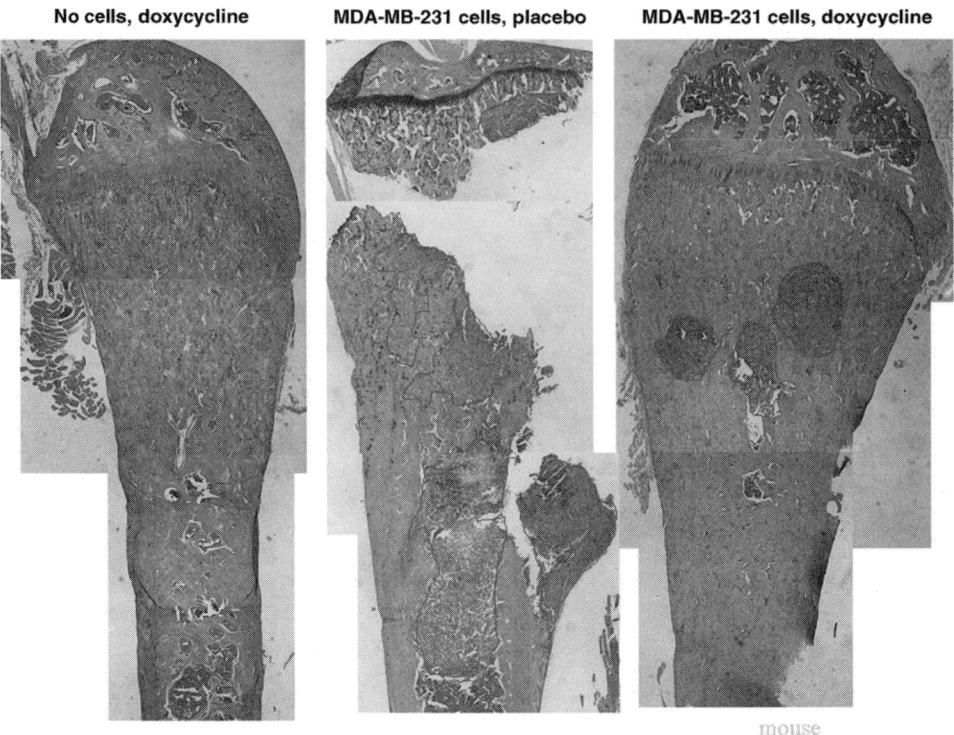

Fig. 2. Examples of femurs harvested from mouse bone metastasis model. The left-hand panel shows a control animal in which no tumor cells were injected and no drug was given. In the middle panel is a femur in which the animal received breast cancer cells. There is widespread destruction of the bone with metastatic tumour shown by the outline. The third femur is from an animal injected with tumor cells and treated with doxycycline. There is a dramatic decrease in tumor burden compared with the untreated animal.

5.2. Other Approaches Targeting Osteolytic and Osteoblastic Factors

The elucidation of some of the molecular mechanisms involved in bone metastasis discussed earlier have opened new avenues for targeting of therapies. The endogenous decoy receptor to RANK, OPG, has been shown to effectively inhibit osteolysis and bone metastasis burden in murine models *(37)*. RANK-Fc is molecule that acts in the same way as OPG and, again, has shown very promising results in suppressing bone resorption in an animal model of tumor-induced osteolysis *(38)*. PTHrP has also been used as a therapeutic target. Using antibodies to PTHrP in bone metastases from breast cancer cells implanted into nude mice, investigators were able to show abrogation of osteolytic lesions *(12)*. It is thought that these strategies might be more effective than using bisphosphonates both decreasing bone resorption and treating hypercalcemia.

5.3. MMP Inhibitors

Inhibition of MMPs is conceptually a very good aim in the management of metastatic disease. MMPs are produced largely by stromal tissue in response to tumor cells, so therapy targeted here theoretically avoids the problem of tumor resistance. Tumor cells do, however, utilize their own MMP production *(39)* in order to intravasate from their primary site and extravasate at the site of metastasis *(40)*. Therefore, therapy is potentially active at multiple levels; against primary tumor cells, at the site of metastasis, and in the stroma. Following successful in vitro and in vivo studies, a number of MMP inhibitors have been tested in clinical trials for a variety of tumors, although not specifically for bone metastasis. Unfortunately, the results of phase III trials have been disappointing with little evidence of clinical efficacy; indeed, two trials were terminated early because of poorer survival in the treatment arms *(41)*.

Encouraging preclinical data have recently shown MMP inhibitors to be effective against bone metastases in animal models of breast and prostate cancer. One group has demonstrated that an MMP inhibitor can decrease bone tumor burden and increase survival in a mouse model of metastatic breast cancer *(42)*. Another *(43)* has provided in vivo confirmation of in vitro results from our laboratory *(44)* that prostate cancer cells produce MMPs when introduced to the bone environment. Using a model in which human prostate cancer cells are injected into human bone implanted within a mouse, they observed that an MMP inhibitor prevented bone degradation and reduced tumor cell proliferation. Both of these recent studies have highlighted and exploited the relationship of the skeleton with the prostate to show a beneficial effect of MMP inhibition in bone metastasis.

5.4. Tetracyclines and Bone Metastasis

The use of the tetracycline family of antibiotics for the treatment and prevention of bone metastasis from breast and prostate cancer is a particular research interest in our laboratory. Tetracyclines are broad-spectrum antibiotics indicated in a wide range of Gram-negative and Gram-positive infections. The finding that led to the interest in the use of tetracyclines in metastatic bone disease was the discovery that they inhibited connective tissue breakdown by a nonantimicrobial mechanisms *(45)*. It has since been determined that the principle mechanism by which tetracyclines achieve this is MMP inhibition. This is thought to be a result of their ability to chelate zinc ions on which MMP activity is dependent *(46)*. Tetracyclines also inhibit the production and activation of MMP proenzymes—the latent form that MMPs are secreted before activation by endogenous proteases *(47)*. Tetracyclines have also been shown to directly inhibit the proliferation of human tumor cell lines, including breast and prostate in vitro *(48,49)*. Chemically modified tetracyclines that possess MMP inhibition activity but do not have antibacterial activity have recently been developed and these have been shown to successfully decrease bone loss in models of osteoporosis *(50)*. The use of tetracycline to prevent bone loss has been given further support by the finding that tetracyclines induce apoptosis in osteoclasts *(51)*. The final, but perhaps most compelling, rationale for the use of tetracyclines in the treatment or prevention of bone metastasis is the high concentrations they achieve in bone. They are quickly cleared from the bloodstream but accumulate in the skeleton, where their maximum therapeutic benefit is proposed *(48)*.

REFERENCES

1. Coleman RE, Rubens RD. The clinical course of bone metastases from breast cancer. *Br J Cancer* 1987; 55(1):61–66.
2. Landis SH, Murray T, Bolden S, Wingo PA. Cancer statistics, 1999. *CA Cancer J Clin* 1999, 49(1):8–31.
3. Bova GA, Chan-Tack KM, LeCates WW. Lethal metastatic human prostate cancer. In: Prostate cance: biologym genetics, and new therapeutics. Chung, LW (ed.) Totowa, NJ: Humana, 2001:39–60.

4. Body JJ, Mancini I. Bisphosphonates for cancer patients: why, how, and when? *Support Care Cancer* 2002; 10(5):399–407.

5. Chambers AF, Naumov GN, Varghese HJ, Nadkarni KV, MacDonald IC, Groom AC. Critical steps in hematogenous metastasis: an overview. *Surg Oncol Clin N Am* 2001; 10(2):243–55.

6. Folkman J. The role of angiogenesis in tumor growth. *Semin Cancer Biol* 1992; 3(2):65–71.

7. Weiss L. Metastatic inefficiency. *Adv Cancer Res* 1990; 54:159–211.

8. Luzzi KJ, MacDonald IC, Schmidt EE, Kerkvliet N, Morris VL, Chambers AF, et al. Multistep nature of metastatic inefficiency: dormancy of solitary cells after successful extravasation and limited survival of early micrometastases. *Am J Pathol* 1998; 153(3):865–873.

9. Cameron MD, Schmidt EE, Kerkvliet N, Nadkarni KV, Morris VL, Groom AC, et al. Temporal progression of metastasis in lung: cell survival, dormancy, and location dependence of metastatic inefficiency. *Cancer Res* 2000; 60(9):2541–2546.

10. Muller A, Homey B, Soto H, Ge N, Catron D, Buchanan ME. Involvement of chemokine receptors in breast cancer metastasis. *Nature* 2001; 410:50–56.

11. Paget S. The distribution of secondary growths in cancer of the breast. *Lancet* 1889; 1:571–573.

12. Guise TA, Yin JJ, Taylor SD, Kumagai Y, Dallas M, Boyce BF, et al. Evidence for a causal role of parathyroid hormone-related protein in the pathogenesis of human breast cancer-mediated osteolysis. *J Clin Invest* 1996; 98(7):1544–1549.

13. Moseley JM, Kubota M, Diefenbach-Jagger H, Wettenhall RE, Kemp BE, Suva LJ, et al. Parathyroid hormone-related protein purified from a human lung cancer cell line. *Proc Natl Acad Sci USA* 1987; 84(14):5048–5052.

14. Yates AJ, Gutierrez GE, Smolens P, Travis PS, Katz MS, Aufdemorte TB, et al. Effects of a synthetic peptide of a parathyroid hormone-related protein on calcium homeostasis, renal tubular calcium reabsorption, and bone metabolism in vivo and in vitro in rodents. *J Clin Invest* 1988; 81(3):932–938.

15. Powell GJ, Southby J, Danks JA, Stillwell RG, Hayman JA, Henderson MA, et al. Localization of parathyroid hormone-related protein in breast cancer metastases: increased incidence in bone compared with other sites. *Cancer Res* 1991; 51(11):3059–3061.

16. Roodman GD. Biology of osteoclast activation in cancer. *J Clin Oncol* 2001; 19(15):3562–3571.

17. Bryden AA, Hoyland JA, Freemont AJ, Clarke NW, George NJ. Parathyroid hormone related peptide and receptor expression in paired primary prostate cancer and bone metastases. *Br J Cancer* 2002; 86(3): 322–325.

18. Hofbauer LC, Neubauer A, Heufelder AE. Receptor activator of nuclear factor-kappaB ligand and osteoprotegerin: potential implications for the pathogenesis and treatment of malignant bone diseases. *Cancer* 2001; 92(3):460–470.

19. Kitazawa S, Kitazawa R. RANK ligand is a prerequisite for cancer-associated osteolytic lesions. *J Pathol* 2002; 198(2):228–236.

20. Ritchie CK, Andrews LR, Thomas KG, Tindall DJ, Fitzpatrick LA. The effects of growth factors associated with osteoblasts on prostate carcinoma proliferation and chemotaxis: implications for the development of metastatic disease. *Endocrinology* 1997; 138(3):1145–1150.

21. Kakonen SM, Selander KS, Chirgwin JM, Yin JJ, Burns S, Rankin WA, et al. Transforming growth factor-beta stimulates parathyroid hormone-related protein and osteolytic metastases via Smad and mitogen-activated protein kinase signaling pathways. *J Biol Chem* 2002; 277(27):24,571–24,578.

22. Ishida A, Fujita N, Kitazawa R, Tsuruo T. Transforming growth factor-beta induces expression of receptor activator of NF-kappa B ligand in vascular endothelial cells derived from bone. *J Biol Chem* 2002; 277(29):26,217–26,224.

23. Dunstan CR, Boyce R, Boyce BF, Garrett IR, Izbicka E, Burgess WH et al. Systemic administration of acidic fibroblast growth factor (FGF-1) prevents bone loss and increases new bone formation in ovariectomized rats. *J Bone Miner Res* 1999; 14(6):953–959.

24. Nelson JB, Hedican SP, George DJ, Reddi AH, Piantadosi S, Eisenberger MA et al. Identification of endothelin-1 in the pathophysiology of metastatic adenocarcinoma of the prostate. *Nat Med* 1995; 1(9): 944–949.

25. Chiao JW, Moonga BS, Yang YM, Kancherla R, Mittelman A, Wu-Wong JR, et al. Endothelin-1 from prostate cancer cells is enhanced by bone contact which blocks osteoclastic bone resorption. *Br J Cancer* 2000; 83(3):360–365.

26. McCawley LJ, Matrisian LM. Matrix metalloproteinases: they're not just for matrix anymore! *Curr Opin Cell Biol* 2001; 13(5):534–540.

27 Sato T, Foged NT, Delaisse JM. The migration of purified osteoclasts through collagen is inhibited by matrix metalloproteinase inhibitors. *J Bone Miner Res* 1998; 13(1):59–66.

28. Everts V, Delaisse JM, Korper W, Beertsen W. Cysteine proteinases and matrix metalloproteinases play distinct roles in the subosteoclastic resorption zone. *J Bone Miner Res* 1998; 13(9):1420–1430.

29. Stearns M, Stearns ME. Evidence for increased activated metalloproteinase 2 (MMP-2a) expression associated with human prostate cancer progression. *Oncol Res* 1996; 8(2):69–75.

30. Gohji K, Fujimoto N, Hara I, Fujii A, Gotoh A, Okada H, et al. Serum matrix metalloproteinase-2 and its density in men with prostate cancer as a new predictor of disease extension. *Int J Cancer* 1998; 79(1): 96–101.

31. Sternlicht MD, Bissell MJ, Werb Z. The matrix metalloproteinase stromelysin-1 acts as a natural mammary tumor promoter. *Oncogene* 2000; 19(8):1102–1113.

32. Jagdev SP, Coleman RE, Shipman CM, Rostami H, Croucher PI. The bisphosphonate, zoledronic acid, induces apoptosis of breast cancer cells: evidence for synergy with paclitaxel. *Br J Cancer* 2001; 84(8): 1126–1134.

33. Diel IJ, Solomayer EF, Costa SD, Gollan C, Goerner R, Wallwiener D, et al. Reduction in new metastases in breast cancer with adjuvant clodronate treatment. *N Engl J Med* 1998; 339(6):357–363.

34. Adami S. Bisphosphonates in prostate carcinoma. *Cancer* 1997; 80(8 Suppl):1674–1679.

35. Saad F, Gleason DM, Murray R, Tchekmedyian S, Venner P, Lacombe L, et al. A randomized, placebo-controlled trial of zoledronic Acid in patients with hormone-refractory metastatic prostate carcinoma. *J Natl Cancer Inst* 2002; 94(19):1458–1468.

36. Canil CM, Tannock IF. Should bisphosphonates be used routinely in patients with prostate cancer metastatic to bone? *J Natl Cancer Inst* 2002; 94(19):1422–1432.

37. Morony S, Capparelli C, Sarosi I, Lacey DL, Dunstan CR, Kostenuik PJ. Osteoprotegerin inhibits osteolysis and decreases skeletal tumor burden in syngeneic and nude mouse models of experimental bone metastasis. *Cancer Res* 2001; 61(11):4432–4436.

38. Oyajobi BO, Anderson DM, Traianedes K, Williams PJ, Yoneda T, Mundy GR. Therapeutic efficacy of a soluble receptor activator of nuclear factor kappaB-IgG Fc fusion protein in suppressing bone resorption and hypercalcemia in a model of humoral hypercalcemia of malignancy. *Cancer Res* 2001; 61(6):2572–2578.

39. Lhotak S, Elavathil LJ, Vukmirovic-Popovic S, Duivenvoorden WC, Tozer RG, Singh G. Immunolocalization of matrix metalloproteinases and their inhibitors in clinical specimens of bone metastasis from breast carcinoma. *Clin Exp Metastasis* 2000; 18(6):463–470.

40. John A, Tuszynski G. The role of matrix metalloproteinases in tumor angiogenesis and tumor metastasis. *Pathol Oncol Res* 2001; 7(1):14–23.

41. Coussens LM, Fingleton B, Matrisian LM. Matrix metalloproteinase inhibitors and cancer: trials and tribulations. *Science* 2002; 295(5564):2387–2392.

42. Winding B, NicAmhlaoibh R, Misander H, Hoegh-Andersen P, Andersen TL, Holst-Hansen C, et al. Synthetic matrix metalloproteinase inhibitors inhibit growth of established breast cancer osteolytic lesions and prolong survival in mice. *Clin Cancer Res* 2002; 8(6):1932–1939.

43. Nemeth JA, Yousif R, Herzog M, Che M, Upadhyay J, Shekarriz B, et al. Matrix metalloproteinase activity, bone matrix turnover, and tumor cell proliferation in prostate cancer bone metastasis. *J Natl Cancer Inst* 2002; 94(1):17–25.

44. Sanchez-Sweatman OH, Orr FW, Singh G. Human metastatic prostate PC3 cell lines degrade bone using matrix metalloproteinases. *Invasion Metastasis* 1998; 18(5-6):297–305.

45. Golub LM, Lee HM, Lehrer G, Nemiroff A, McNamara TF, Kaplan R et al. Minocycline reduces gingival collagenolytic activity during diabetes. Preliminary observations and a proposed new mechanism of action. *J Periodontal Res* 1983; 18(5):516–526.

46. Golub LM, Ramamurthy NS, McNamara TF, Greenwald RA, Rifkin BR. Tetracyclines inhibit connective tissue breakdown: new therapeutic implications for an old family of drugs. *Crit Rev Oral Biol Med* 1991; 2(3):297–321.

47. Smith GN, Jr., Brandt KD, Hasty KA. Activation of recombinant human neutrophil procollagenase in the presence of doxycycline results in fragmentation of the enzyme and loss of enzyme activity. *Arthritis Rheum* 1996; 39(2):235–244.

48. Duivenvoorden WC, Hirte HW, Singh G. Use of tetracycline as an inhibitor of matrix metalloproteinase activity secreted by human bone-metastasizing cancer cells. *Invasion Metastasis* 1997; 17(6):312–322.

49. Fife RS, Sledge GW, Jr. Effects of doxycycline on in vitro growth, migration, and gelatinase activity of breast carcinoma cells. *J Lab Clin Med* 1995; 125(3):407–411.

50. Golub LM, Ramamurthy NS, Llavaneras A, Ryan ME, Lee HM, Liu Y, et al. A chemically modified nonantimicrobial tetracycline (CMT-8) inhibits gingival matrix metalloproteinases, periodontal break- down, and extra- oral bone loss in ovariectomized rats. *Ann NY Acad Sci* 1999; 878:290–310.
51. Bettany JT, Peet NM, Wolowacz RG, Skerry TM, Grabowski PS. Tetracyclines induce apoptosis in osteoclasts. *Bone* 2000; 27(1):75–80.
52. Duivenvoorden WC, Popovic SV, Lhotak S, Seidlitz E, Hirte HW, Tozer RG, et al. Doxycycline decreases tumor burden in a bone metastasis model of human breast cancer. *Cancer Res* 2002; 62(6):1588–1591.

2

Parathyroid Hormone-Related Peptide and Malignancy

David Goltzman, MD

CONTENTS

1. INTRODUCTION

Parathyroid hormone-related peptide (PTHrP) was originally isolated as a causal factor for hypercalcemia of malignancy (HM), one of the most frequent paraneoplastic syndromes. The association of hypercalcemia with malignancy was originally assumed to be the result of tumor invasion of bone with resultant osteolysis *(1,2)*, but subsequent studies demonstrated an association of hypercalcemia with cancer, even when the tumor had not metastasized to bone. In a careful clinical analysis of a case of renal cell carcinoma with metastases, it was noted that hypercalcemia was associated with hypophosphatemia *(3)*. It was therefore postulated, because lysis of bone should liberate both calcium and phosphate, that the tumor was producing a factor that was both hypercalcemic and phosphaturic, analogous to parathyroid hormone (PTH) *(3)*. The concept arose that tumors might "ectopically" produce PTH, which is normally expressed only in the parathyroid gland. The term "pseudohypoparathyroidism" was therefore employed to describe a syndrome in which cancers had not metastasized to bone, but were associated with hypercalcemia and other PTH-like biochemical abnormalities *(4)*. Certain biochemical alterations were, however, found to differ in primary hyperparathyroidism and "pseudohyperparathyroidism," including a higher level of serum calcium in the latter and a tendency in the latter toward an alkalosis rather than an acidosis. The development of sensitive bioassays for PTH-like bioactivity confirmed the presence of PTH-like material

From: *Cancer Drug Discovery and Development*
Bone Metastasis: Experimental and Clinical Therapeutics
Edited by: G. Singh and S. A. Rabbani © Humana Press Inc., Totowa, NJ

in the tumors and serum of patients with pseudohyperparathyroidism *(5)*. Although analyses of tumors for PTH-protein *(6)* and mRNA-encoding PTH *(7)* failed to detect PTH in this syndrome, a PTH-like substance was subsequently isolated and cloned from several tumors *(8–10)*. This material was referred to initially as both PTH-like peptide and PTH-related peptide and is now known by the term "PTH-related peptide" (PTHrP).

2. MOLECULAR CHARACTERISTICS OF PTHrP AND ITS GENE EXPRESSION AND REGULATION

Parathyroid hormone-related peptide is a member of a gene family, which encompasses PTH, PTHrP, and a hypothalamic peptide, tuberoinfundibular peptide 39 or TIP39 *(11)* (Fig. 1). The human gene encoding PTHrP is assigned to the short arm of chromosome 12, whereas that for PTH is located on the short arm of chromosome 11. Chromosomes 11 and 12 carry other functionally related genes and are thought to have arisen from a common ancestral gene. Similarities in the structural organization of the PTH and PTHrP genes exist in that corresponding exons encode similar functional domains. Furthermore, PTH and PTHrP share limited but biologically important amino-acid-sequence homology in their NH_2-terminal domains, where most of the best documented bioactivity is believed to reside. Both PTH-like and PTHrP-like peptides have been found in many species as far back as teleosts *(13)*.

The human PTHrP gene spans more than 14 kb of DNA and contains a minimum of 7 exons and 3 promoters. Alternative promoter usage and/or different splicing patterns account for heterogeneous PTHrP mRNA species. These species encode secretory proteins with mature isoforms up to 139, 141, and 173 amino acids. Consequently, amino acid identity exists in all three forms of position 139 *(13)*. The significance of the carboxyl heterogeneity remains uncertain because there is no consistent evidence that tissue-specific or developmental splicing patterns occur. Tumor-specific promoter utilization has been suggested as a possible explanation of why many malignancies express PTHrP mRNA and protein but only a subset of cancer patients in fact secrete PTHrP in sufficient quantity to develop hypercalcemia *(14)*. In some studies, a general increase in transcription has been suggested rather than enhanced single-promoter usage with alternative splicing to account for PTHrP overproduction in cancer. Region-specific promoter demethylation *(15)* and gene amplification *(16)* have also been noted to enhance PTHrP expression in certain malignancies. A number of studies have examined the molecular regulation of PTHrP gene expression. A variety of growth factors, including epidermal growth factor (EGF) *(17)*, insulin-like growth factor (IGF)-1 *(18)*, and transforming growth factor (TGF)-β *(19)* have been shown to stimulate PTHrP expression, whereas 1,25-dihydroxyvitamin D [1,25(OH)D] and androgens have been shown to inhibit its expression *(20,21)* (Fig. 2). Growth factors produced in a paracrine/autocrine mode by a PTHrP-producing neoplasm or released from surrounding host cells when tumors invade the skeleton or soft tissues might play an important role in enhancing PTHrP production by the tumor cells *(19)* (Fig. 3).

3. PTHrP ACTIONS

3.1. PTHrP as a Polyhormone

Parathyroid hormone-related peptide has been postulated to be a polyhormone and diverse biological actions have been ascribed to its amino (NH_2)-terminal, midregion,

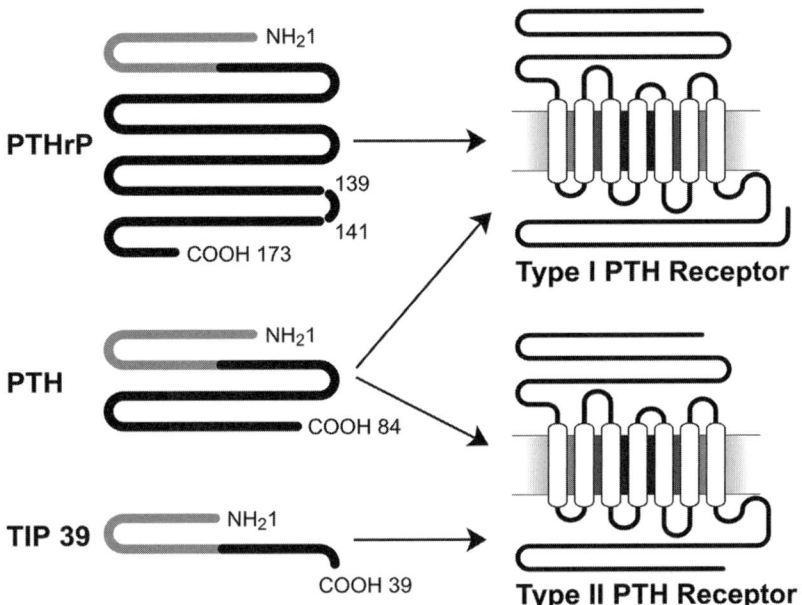

Fig. 1. PTH ligand and PTH receptor families. PTHrP is a member of a gene family that includes parathyroid hormone (PTH) and tuberoinfundibular peptide (TIP39). Amino acid sequence homology is restricted to the amino-terminal domains (shaded regions) of these hormones. Human PTHrP can occur as isoforms of 139, 141, or 173 amino acids, whereas PTH is an 84-amino-acid peptide. The plasma membrane target tissue receptors for these peptides are two G-protein-coupled receptors that are also members of a single gene family. PTHrP and PTH interact with the Type I PTH receptor, and PTH and TIP39 interact with the Type II receptor.

and carboxyl regions. The carboxyl region has been shown, in some studies, to exert an osteoclast inhibitory role *(22)*. A mid-region domain has been demonstrated to contain a nuclear localization sequence that might direct the molecule *(23)*, via the use of the importin B system *(24)*, into the nucleus and then to the nucleolus, where it might alter cell growth, differentiation, and/or apoptosis. Indeed, several studies have demonstrated the presence of intranuclear PTHrP both in tissues in vitro and in vivo. Since nascent PTHrP contains a leader sequence *(25)* that ordinarily would direct the molecule into the secretory pathway, several cellular routes have been reported that could lead to the presence of PTHrP in the cytoplasm and enable its nuclear import. These pathways include the use of an alternate translational start site that would exclude expression of the leader sequence *(25)*, internalization of secreted PTHrP *(26)*, and back-transport of PTHrP from the secretory system to the cytoplasm, where it could be available for nuclear import or degraded by the ubiquitin–proteosome pathway *(27)*. Future studies employing "knock-in" technology might be useful for understanding the role of the midregion and carboxyl regions of PTHrP to its biological functions in vivo. The majority of the well-documented bioactivity of PTHrP is present within its NH_2-terminal domain so that, in analogy with synthetic PTH (1–34), synthetic PTHrP (1–34), or synthetic PTHrP (1–36) appear to mimic many of the effects of the full-length PTHrP molecule. Sequence homology between PTH and PTHrP is restricted to 8 of the first 13 amino acids at the NH_2-

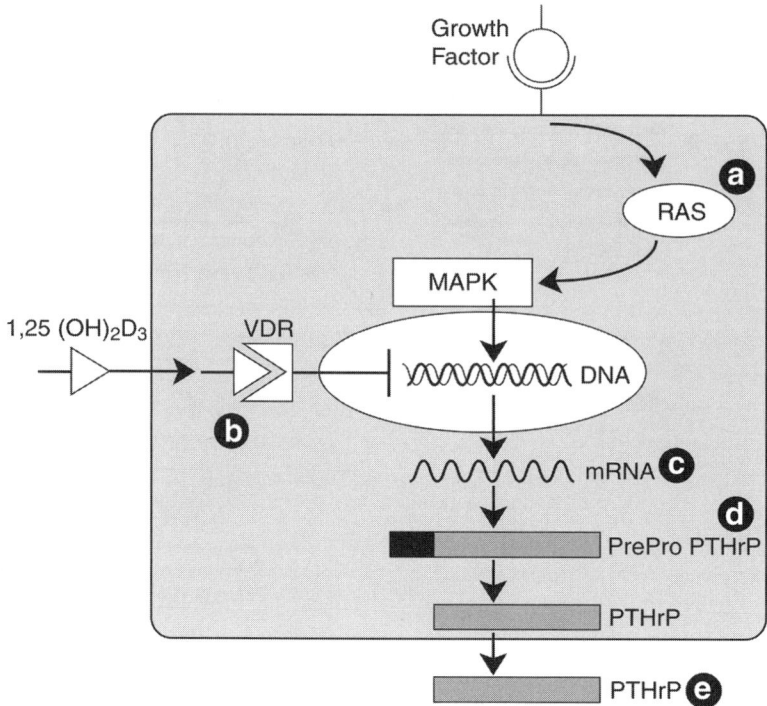

Fig. 2. Regulation of PTHrP production. Growth factors might stimulate PTHrP production by increasing gene transcription via the RAS–mitogen-activated protein kinase (MAPK) pathway whereas 1,25-dihydroxyvitamin D3 [1,25 (OH)2 D3] might act via the vitamin D receptor (VDR) to inhibit PTHrP gene transcription. The mRNA translation product, Pre Pro PTHrP, must first be processed by a furin-like enzyme to remove a "leader" or "pre pro" amino acid sequence, and the mature PTHrP molecule can then be secreted. Sites of potential inhibition of PTHrP include (a) RAS inactivation (via farnesyl transferase inhibitors), (b) use of low calcemic vitamin D analogs to inhibit PTHrP gene transcription, (c) use of antisense RNA to reduce PTHrP translation, (d) use of furin antagonists to inhibit PTHrP processing, and (e) use of inhibitors or antibodies to interfere with PTHrP action.

terminus including those at positions 1 and 2, which are critical for the activation of adenylate cyclase. This limited homology, as well as conformational similarities in the nonhomologous 14–34 sequence permits the 1–34 domain of PTHrP and of PTH to bind to a common receptor with equal affinity (Fig. 1). To date, no receptor for domains other than the NH_2-terminal domain have been identified for PTHrP.

3.2. PTHrP Receptor and Postreceptor Signaling

The NH_2-terminal domains of PTHrP and of PTH bind to a common seven-transmembranc-spanning receptor that is linked by G proteins to both the adenylate cyclase and phospholipase C signaling pathways (28,29). With the discovery of a second receptor which binds PTH, the receptor common to both PTH and PTHrP has been termed the type I PTH/PTHrP receptor (PTR). The second (type II) receptor has weak affinity for PTHrP but binds PTH and TIP39 (30) (Fig. 1). In view of its primary expression in the brain and

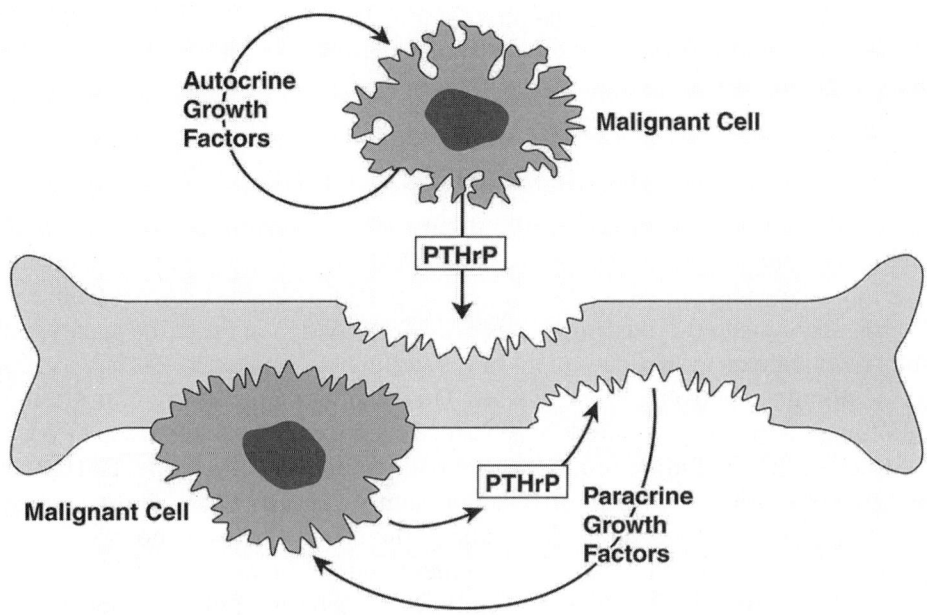

Fig. 3. Endocrine and paracrine effects of PTHrP on tumor-induced bone resorption. Growth factors released by malignant cells that have not metastasized to bone might stimulate PTHrP production and secretion in an autocrine mode; PTHrP might then function in an endocrine manner to resorb bone. Alternatively, PTHrP that is released by malignant cells that have colonized bone can locally resorb bone and release growth factors that can act in a paracrine mode to enhance PTHrP production.

outside of calcium-regulating tissues, it appears to be the primary receptor for TIP39 and its role, if any, in calcium and skeletal homeostasis remains to be determined.

In addition to the traditional signaling molecules cAMP/protein kinase A and calcium/diacylglycerol/protein kinase C, increasing work in recent years has identified other signaling molecules, presumably linked directly or via crosstalk to the PTR, including phospholipase D *(31)*, MAP kinase *(32)*, and, possibly, nitric oxide *(33)*.

3.3. Physiologic Roles of PTHrP

Parathyroid hormone-related peptide effects on cell growth and differentiation and the Type I PTR are expressed in a variety of cells and tissues beginning in early embryogenesis. In vitro and in vivo studies in animals have shown that PTHrP can alter the growth, differentiation, and differentiated functions of a variety of different normal cells and tissues, including, for example, keratinocytes *(34)*, mammary cells *(35)*, brain cells *(36)*, smooth muscle cells *(37)*, respiratory epithelial cells *(38)*, renal cells *(39)*, and pancreatic β cells *(40)*. In some tumor situations, PTHrP has also been shown to exert growth-promoting effects. However, a profound physiologic effect of PTHrP has been demonstrated, via studies of targeted gene ablation, on endochondral bone formation. Normal growth and differentiation of the cartilaginous growth plate appears critically dependent on the action of PTHrP *(41)*. In studies of postnatal animals, PTHrP appears important for normal bone formation *(42)*. The physiologic effects of PTHrP are almost certainly subserved through local paracrine/autocrine effects. When PTHrP is overproduced in neoplasia and enters the circulation, its endocrine role in HM largely mimics the effects of circulating PTH on the kidney and on bone *(43)*.

3.4. Renal Effects of PTHrP

In view of its prominent effect on stimulating adenylate cyclase in the kidney, PTHrP, as with PTH, enhances renal cell intracellular cAMP, a fraction of which enters the renal tubular lumen and is excreted as a nephrogenous portion of urinary cAMP. Consequently, in PTHrP-associated HM, nephrogenous cAMP (NcAMP) in the urine is elevated *(44)*. Cyclic AMP appears to mediate many of the cellular responses to PTHrP, as it does to PTH, including the phosphaturic response. This response appears to occur via enhanced protein kinase A but also protein kinase C-mediated internalization of the (Type II) Na/PO_4 cotransporter leading to diminished phosphate reabsorption *(45)*. PTHrP-induced stimulation of calcium reabsorption, predominantly via active transcellular transport in the ascending limb of the loop of Henle and in the distal tubule, is another critical renal effect that seems important for the development and maintenance of the hypercalcemia in HM *(46)*. Mobilization of calcium from bone resorption might be responsible of the episodes of severe hypercalcemia observed in more advanced stages of the disease.

A third major effect of PTHrP in the kidney is its effect on the renal 1α hydroxylase enzyme. Intravenous administration of NH_2-termal fragments of PTH or PTHrP both in animals *(47)* and humans results in an elevation in serum $1,25(OH)_2D$. Additionally, it has been suggested that a positive correlation might also exist between $1,25(OH)_2D$ and PTHrP in the early stages of HM *(48)*. Nevertheless, serum $1,25(OH)_2D$ concentrations are often suppressed in the terminal stages of HM, when the patient is severely hypercalcemic *(44)*. It is possible that non-NH_2-terminal domains of PTHrP could be inhibitory on the renal 1α hydroxylase enzyme, that additional inhibitory materials might be cosecreted with PTHrP by the tumor, or that severe hypercalcemia *per se* might inhibit the enzyme. These possibilities remain to be definitively explored. Finally, whether HCO_3 reabsorption by the kidney can be handled differently by PTHrP and by PTH leading to a mild metabolic akalosis in HM vs a mild metabolic acidosis in primary hyperparathyroidism also remains to be clarified. To date, few major differences have been observed in PTHrP and PTH effects of the kidney in controlled animal studies or in humans, suggesting that other mechanisms might converge to modulate kidney function in the patient with HM and advanced neoplasia.

3.5. Skeletal Actions of PTHrP

Both PTHrP and PTH bind in vivo to cells of the osteoblastic phenotype *(49)*, which express the Type I PTR. Each peptide can enhance both osteoblastic bone formation and osteoclastic bone resorption through this interaction. The mechanism of osteoclastic bone resorption involves the enhancement of expression, in osteoblastic stromal cells, of the cytokine, receptor activator of nuclear factor-$\kappa\beta$ (RANK) ligand (RANKL), which can then bind to its cognate receptor RANK on cells of the hematopoietic lineage (Fig. 4) *(50)*. RANKL is a member of the tumor necrosis factor (TNF) family of cytokines and RANK transduces the RANKL signal via second messengers such as TRAF6. This interaction then promotes differentiation and fusion of mononuclear

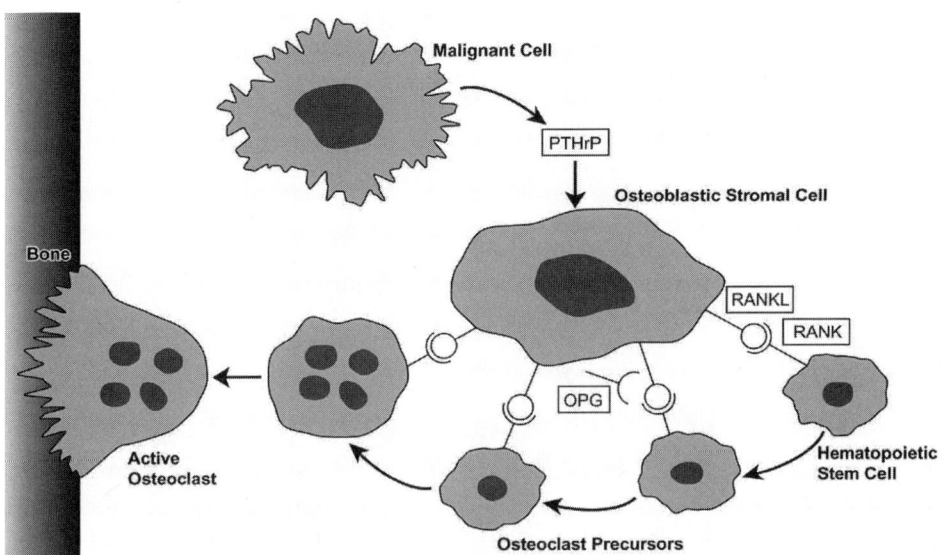

Fig. 4. Role of the RANKL–RANK–OPG system in PTHrP-induced osteoclastogenesis. PTHrP secreted from malignant cells can interact with an osteoblastic stromal cell, causing increased production of RANKL and decreased production of OPG. RANKL binds to its cognate receptor RANK in osteoclast precursor cells, which are of the hematopoietic lineage, causing them to differentiate and fuse to form multinucleated cells that are then activated to form bone-resorbing osteoclasts.

osteoclast precursors to multinucleated cells and then activation of the multinucleated osteoclasts to resorb bone *(51,52)*. Simultaneously, PTHrP (and PTH) can reduce the expression of a soluble decoy receptor for RANKL termed "osteoprotegerin" (OPG) *(53)* and thereby enhance the capacity of RANKL to interact with RANK (Fig. 4). In HM, PTHrP clearly enhances osteoclastic bone resorption to an extent that exceeds osteoblastic bone formation, thereby causing a net mobilization of calcium from bone and contributing to hypercalcemia.

When PTHrP is released from a tumor that has not yet invaded bone, this might cause diffuse osteopenia, but even when neoplasms such as breast cancer have metastasized to bone, locally released PTHrP might also contribute to local osteolysis in the microenvironment adjacent to the tumor metastasis (Fig. 3). This localized resorption around skeletal metastatic lesions might or might not result in hypercalcemia probably depending on the extent of the metastasis and the capacity of the kidney to clear the increased filtered load of calcium. Just as autocrine growth factors can stimulate PTHrP production in a tumor that has not yet metastasized to bone, growth factors released from bone such as TGF-β can stimulate PTHrP production locally in a paracrine mode (Fig. 3). Although, in animal models of HM, bone formation appears to accompany the accelerated resorption caused by PTHrP, this might not always occur in humans with HM, such that "uncoupled" resorption might occur *(54)*. Whether other tumor products or the extent of hypercalcemia play a role in this discordance remains to be clarified.

Table 1
Causes of Hypercalcemia of Malignancy (HM)

HM with overproduction of PTHrP
    Humoral Hypercalcemia of Malignancy (HHM)
    Solid tumors with skeletal metastases
    Hematopoietic malignancies
HM with overproduction of other factors
    Lymphomas with overproduction of 1,25-dihydroxyvitamin D
    Malignancies with overproduction of other cytokines
    Ectopic hyperparathyroidism

3.6. Spectrum of Tumors Associated With PTHrP Overproduction

In contrast to PTH, whose expression is virtually restricted to the parathyroid gland, PTHrP is widely expressed in a variety of normal fetal and adult tissues. Consequently, it is likely that overproduction of PTHrP by a broad spectrum of tumors likely represents eutopic overexpression, as malignant transformation of these tissues occurs, rather than ectopic expression. However, true ectopic overexpression of PTH as a cause of HM has been documented in a small number of tumors.

The syndrome of HM in the absence of skeletal metastasis (humoral hypercalcemia of malignancy or HHM) has classically been associated with renal cell carcinomas and squamous cell carcinomas derived from a variety of primary sites (Table 1). Once it was demonstrated that PTHrP infusion could induce the biochemical and skeletal abnormalities of HM it was believed that PTHrP overproduction would only be associated with such tumors. With the introduction of molecular biological and immunological techniques to detect PTHrP, it became clear that overexpression of PTHrP and elevated circulating concentrations of this peptide can occur with a much broader histological spectrum of tumors than was originally envisioned. Thus, breast cancers produce PTHrP (55), as do a variety of other tumors, including endometrial (56) and colon cancers and even mesotheliomas (57). A variety of endocrine tumors have also been shown to produce PTHrP (58), including pleochromocytomas (59), insulinomas (60), parathyroid adenomas (61), pituitary tumors (62), and thyroid cancers (63). Furthermore, increased circulating concentrations of PTHrP have been detected in some patients with hematological malignancies, especially those with advanced-stage lymphomas (64). In contrast, PTHrP overproduction in multiple myeloma seems less frequent than in other hematologic malignancies. PTHrP can contribute to HM in patients with lymphomas whose hypercalcemia in the past was attributed solely to excess $1,25(OH)_2D$. Although not all tumors that show increased expression of PTHrP secrete sufficient PTHrP so that it is detectable in the serum, even with such tumors (e.g., breast cancer), PTHrP released locally can induce osteolysis around metastases and contribute to the localized bone resorption.

4. HYPERCALCEMIA OF MALIGNANCY: CLINICAL CONSIDERATIONS

4.1. Clinical Manifestations of HM

Hypercalcemia is usually a manifestation of advanced malignancy, as compared with early stages of malignancy. Gastrointestinal manifestations of anorexia, nausea, and vomiting are common in association with hypercalcemia and could lead to dehydration.

Renal involvement, manifested by polyuria and evidence of azotemia caused by dehydration, can also occur. Finally, central nervous system manifestations of weakness progressing toward psychoses, stupor, and coma can ultimately ensue. The acuteness and severity of the hypercalcemia can, therefore, lead to life-threatening consequences if left untreated.

4.2. Diagnosis of PTHrP-Associated HM

The biochemical abnormalities observed with PTHrP-associated HM are similar, but usually more severe than those seen with primary hyperparathyroidism. In particular, the hypercalcemia is generally more pronounced. Its onset is generally acute and the elevation quite marked, with serum calcium concentrations not infrequently greater than 12 mg/dL or 3 mmol/L. Hypophosphatemia, reduced renal phosphate threshold, and increased renal tubular reabsorption of calcium are all seen, as is increased NcAMP excretion. In view of the high filtered load of calcium resulting from bone resorption, urinary calcium excretion might be increased.

Biochemical markers of bone resorption such as Type I collagen crosslinked N-telopeptides and C-telopeptides or pyridinium crosslinks might also be increased (65). In contrast, indices of bone formation such as bone-specific alkaline phosphatase and osteocalcin might not be elevated in HM because of the suppression of formation, whereas these indices are generally elevated in patients with primary hyperparathyroidism in whom formation and resorption are coupled. The most significant biochemical difference between HM and primary hyperparathyroidism, however, and a highly useful diagnostic tool is the concentration of circulating PTH, which is elevated in hyperparathyroidism but suppressed in HM because of hypercalcemia-induced suppression of the parathyroid gland. This is particularly helpful as a tool for differential diagnosis because of the high specificity and sensitivity of modern two-site immunoradiometric PTH assays.

Although occasional cases of true ectopic hyperparathyroidism have been reported, and some tumors might cause HM via overproduction of 1,25-dihydroxyvitamin D or of bone-resorbing cytokines (Table 1), the majority of cases of HM are associated with increased PTHrP production. The use of PTHrP immunoassays should be the most definitive method of diagnosing HM, because most cases of HM will be associated with excess PTHrP secretion. However, the three isoforms of PTHrP appear to undergo complicated posttranslational processing in the tumor cell of origin (66,67) and secreted metabolites may undergo differential metabolic clearance once secreted. As a result of the complexity of this process, multiple forms of bioactive PTHrP have been identified in the plasma of hypercalcemic cancer patients, and the precise character of circulating forms remains to be determined in order to maximize the sensitivity and specificity of PTHrP immunoassays.

In view of the fact the PTHrP bioactivity resides within the NH_2-terminal domain, initial efforts were developed using antisera directed against epitopes in this region. NH_2-terminal immunoassays measured elevated PTHrP not only in the majority of patients with HM but also in some normocalcemic cancer patients, although mean levels in the normocalcemic subjects were lower than in the hypercalcemic (68,69). This could reflect the capacity of such assays to measure bioinactive as well as bioactive NH_2 terminal fragments or the capacity to measure lower concentrations of PTHrP that are insufficient to cause hypercalcemia.

Immunoassays detecting primarily midregion and carboxyl-terminal epitopes of PTHrP have proven to be of less value clinically in the differential diagnosis of HM *(70)*. Assays that recognize carboxyl-terminal fragments might show elevated levels in patients with renal insufficiency probably reflecting the renal clearance of such fragments rather than their hypersecretion by tumors.

The most prevalent and useful PTHrP assays appear to be two-site immunoradiometric assays that employ one antibody recognizing an NH_2-terminal epitope and a second antibody recognizing a more carboxyl epitope (although generally within the PTHrP [1–86] sequence) *(71,72)*. These tend to be the most sensitive and specific assays for diagnosis and for monitoring therapy. The presence of an elevated concentration of PTHrP with malignancy has however been reported to portend a poor prognosis *(73)*.

4.3. Treatment of HM

The most urgent treatment of HM generally involves treatment of severe, acute hypercalcemia. Because dehydration is an inevitable consequence of the hypercalcemia, treatment should initially begin with rehydration via the use of intravenous saline. Saline infusion will expand the intravascular volume, improve the glomerular filtration rate, and reduce proximal tubular sodium-linked calcium reabsorption. Once the patient is adequately hydrated, therapy can be directed to inhibit bone resorption. Intravenous bisphosphonates (zoledronic acid or pamidronate), which inhibit osteoclastic activity, are currently the most potent antiresorptive agents and the resultant reduction in serum calcium can last for several days to weeks *(74)*. Nevertheless, because the onset of calcium lowering might be delayed for 1 or 2 d, parenteral calcitonin can be concomitantly administered. This peptide hormone will also directly inhibit osteoclastic action but has a peak response at 2–4 h after administration *(75)*.

However, tachyphylaxis could occur after repeated doses of calcitonin. An additional approach, to rapidly reduce the serum calcium once the patient is adequately hydrated, is to administer in moderation, a loop diuretic such as furosemide to inhibit renal calcium reabsorption and promote calciuresis. Consequently, a treatment regimen involving initial rehydration followed by administration of calcitonin and/or furosemide (for rapidity) and intravenous bisphosphonate (for potency) would be most efficacious in correcting hypercalcemia.

Once the hypercalcemia has been corrected, efforts should be directed at reducing tumor burden or at least at inhibiting PTHrP production and action. A variety of approaches have been used with reasonable success to inhibit PTHrP production in animal models, including farnesyl transferase inhibitors to diminish growth factor mediated production *(76)*, furin inhibitors to diminish PTHrP processing from its inert prohormone form to the mature bioactive form *(77)*, and low calcemic vitamin D analogs to suppress PTHrP gene expression *(78)* (Fig. 2). None of these approaches have yet reached the clinic for application in humans. Antibodies to PTHrP have also been used in animal models with success *(46,79)* and have undergone early clinical trials in humans *(80)*. Finally, because the RANKL–RANK pathway represents a final common pathway for bone resorption induced by PTHrP as well as by other stimulators of osteoclastogenesis that might be released by tumors (including a variety of cytokines), considerable attention is being paid to the development of inhibitors of this system *(81)*, including OPG analogs,

RANKL production inhibitors, RANK antagonists, and inhibitors of the RANK signaling pathway.

Even when hypercalcemia has not occurred, in view of the apparent role of PTHrP in stimulating ostoeclastic bone resorption adjacent to some skeletal metastases, considerable attention is being paid to inhibiting osteoclast production and activity *(80)*, both by antagonizing PTHrP *(81)* and by employing bisphosphonates *(82)* or components of the RANKL–RANK–OPG pathway. This approach to altering the bone microenvironment appears to reduce the number of metastases and the untoward events related to metastases and is being assessed in virtually all skeletal metastatic disease. Indeed, it has become the standard of care in metastatic breast cancer.

5. CONCLUSION

The discovery of PTHrP has led to improved understanding of the molecular basis of HM—particularly HM occurring in the absence of significant skeletal metastasis but also HM induced by some tumors metastasizing to bone. This has led to improved ability to diagnose this condition and could ultimately lead to effective therapies to reduce PTHrP production and action both to prevent hypercalcemia and to control malignancies where PTHrP might play a growth-promoting role.

ACKNOWLEDGMENTS

The author gratefully acknowledge the National Cancer Institute of Canada and the Canadian Institutes for Health Research for their grant support.

REFERENCES

1. Zondek H, Petrow H, Siebert W. Die bedeutung der calcium-bestimmung in blute fur die diagnose der nierrenin-siffizientz. *Z Clin Med* 1923; 99:129–132.
2. Gutman AB, Tyson TL, Gutman EB. Serum calcium, inorganic phosphorus and phosphatase activity in hyperparathyroidism, Paget's disease, multiple myeloma and neoplastic disease of the bones. *Arch Intern Med* 1936; 57:379–413.
3. Albright F. Case records of the Massachusetts General Hospital (case 27461). *N Engl J Med* 1941; 225: 789–791.
4. Lafferty FW. Pseudohyperparathyroidism. *Medicine* 1966; 45:247–260.
5. Goltzman D, Stewart AF, Broadus AE. Malignancy associated hypercalcemia: evaluation with cytochemical bioassay for parathyroid hormone. *J Clin Endocrinol Metab* 1981; 53:899–904.
6. Sherwood LM, O'Riordan JLH, Aurbach GD, Potts JT. Production of parathyroid hormone by nonparathyroid tumors. *J Clin Endocrinol Metab* 1967; 27:140–144.
7. Simpson EL, Mundy GR, D'Souza SM, Ibbotson KJ, Bockman MD, Jacobs JW. Absence of parathyroid hormone messenger RNA in non-parathyroid tumors associated with hypercalcemia. *N Engl J Med* 1983; 309(6):325–330.
8. Suva LJ, Winslow GA, Wettenhall RE, Hammonds RG, Moseley JM, Diefenbach-Jagger H, Rodda CP, et al. A parathyroid hormone-related protein implicated in malignant hypercalcemia: cloning and expression. *Science* 1987; 237(4817):893–896.
9. Burtis WJ, Wu J, Bunch CM, Wysolmerski TJ, Jusogna KL, Weir EC, et al. Identification of a novel 17,000-dalton parathyroid hormone-like adenylate cyclase-stimulating protein from a tumor associated with humoral hypercalcemia of malignancy. *J Biol Chem* 1987; 262:7151–7156.
10. Strewler GJ, Stern PH, Jacobs JW, Eveloff J, Klein RF, Leung SC, et al. Parathyroid hormonelike protein from human renal carcinoma cells. Structural and functional homology with parathyroid hormone. *J Clin Invest* 1987; 80:1803–1807.
11. Usdin TB, Hoare SR, Wang T, Mezey E, Kowalak JA. TIP39: a new neuropeptide and PTH2-receptor agonist from hypothalamus. *Nat Neurosci* 1999; 2(11):941–943.

13. Goltzman D, Hendy GN, Banville D. Parathyroid hormone-like peptide: molecular characterization and biological properties. *Trends Endocrinol Metab* 1989; 1:39–44.

12. Gensure RC, Ponugoti B, Gunes Y, Papasani MR, Lanske B, Bastepe M, et al. Identification and characterization of two PTH-like molecules in zebrafish. *Endocrinology* 2003; 145:1634–1639.

14. Southby J, O'Keefe LM, Martin TJ, Gillespie MT. Alternative promoter usage and mRNA splicing pathways for parathyroid hormone-related protein in normal tissues and tumours. *Br J Cancer* 1995; 72:702–707.

15. Holt EH, Vasavada RC, Bander NH, Broadus AE, Philbrick WM. Region-specific methylation of the parathyroid hormone-related peptide gene determines its expression in human renal carcinoma cell lines. *J Biol Chem* 1993; 268:20,639–20,645.

16. Sidler B, Alpert L, Henderson JE, Deckelbaum R, Amizuka N, Silva JE, et al. Amplification of the parathyroid hormone-related peptide (PTHrP) gene in a colonic carcinoma. *J Clin Endocrinol Metab* 1996; 81:2841–2847.

17. Kremer R, Karaplis AC, Henderson JE, Gulliver W, Banville D, Hendy GN, et al. Regulation of parathyroid hormone-like peptide in cultured normal human keratinocytes. *J Clin Invest* 1991; 87:884–893.

18. Sebag M, Henderson JE, Goltzman D, Kremer R. Regulation of parathyroid hormone-related peptide production in normal human mammary epithelial cells in vitro. *Am J Physiol* 1994; 267:C723–C730.

19. Kakonen SM, Selander KS, Chirgwin JM, Yin JJ, Burns S, Rankin WA, Grubbs BG, et al. Transforming growth factor-beta stimulates parathyroid hormone-related protein and osteolytic metastases via Smad and mitogen-activated protein kinase signaling pathways. *J Biol Chem* 2002; 277(27):24,571–24,578.

20. Haq M, Kremer R, Goltzman D, Rabbani SA. A vitamin D analogue (EB1089) inhibits parathyroid hormone-related peptide production and prevents the development of malignancy-associated hypercalcemia in vivo. *J Clin Invest* 1993; 91:2416–2422.

21. Pizzi H, Gladu J, Carpio L, Miao D, Goltzman D, Rabbani SA. Androgen regulation of parathyroid hormone-related peptide production in human prostate cancer cells. *Endocrinology* 2003; 144(3):858–867.

22. Cornish J, Callon KE, Lin C, Xiao C, Moseley JM, Reid IR. Stimulation of osteoblast proliferation by C-terminal fragments of parathyroid hormone-related protein. *J Bone Miner Res* 1999; 14(6):915–922.

23. Henderson JE, Amizuka N, Warshawsky H, Biasotto D, Lanske BMK, Goltzman D, et al. Nucleolar targeting of PTHrP enhances survival of chondrocytes under conditions that promote cell death by apoptosis. *Mol Cell Biol* 1995; 15:4064–4075.

24. Lam MH, Briggs LJ, Hu W, Martin TJ, Gillespie MT, Jans DA. Importin beta recognizes parathyroid hormone-related protein with high affinity and mediates its nuclear import in the absence of importin alpha. *J Biol Chem* 1999; 274:7391–7380.

25. Nguyen M, He B, Karaplis A. Nuclear forms of parathyroid hormone-related peptide are translated from non-AUG start sites downstream from the initiator methionine. *Endocrinology* 2001; 142(2):694–703.

26. Aarts MM, Rix A, Guo J, Bringhurst R, Henderson JE. The nucleolar targeting signal (NTS) of parathyroid hormone related protein mediates endocytosis and nucleolar translocation. *J Bone Miner Res* 1999; 14:1493–1503.

27. Meerovitch K, Wing S, Goltzman D. Proparathyroid hormone-related protein is associated with the chaperone protein BiP and undergoes proteasome-mediated degradation. *J Biol Chem* 1998; 273(33): 21,025–21,030.

28. Juppner H, Abou-Samra A-B, Freeman M, Kong XF, Schipani E, Richards J, et al. A G protein-linked receptor for parathyroid hormone and parathyroid hormone-related peptide. *Science* 1991; 254:1024–1026.

29. Abou-Samra AB, Juppner H, Force T, Freeman MW, Kong XF, Schipani E, et al. Expression cloning of a common receptor for parathyroid hormone and parathyroid hormone-related peptide from rat osteoblast-like cells: A single receptor stimulates intracellular accumulation of both cAMP and inositol trisphosphates and increases intracellular free calcium. *Proc Natl Acad Sci USA* 1992; 89:2732–2736.

30. Usdin TB, Gruber C, Bonner TI. Identification and functional expression of a receptor selectively recognizing parathyroid hormone, the PTH2 receptor. *J Biol Chem* 1995; 270(26): 15,455–15,458.

31. Radeff JM, Singh AT, Stern PH. Role of protein kinase A, phospholipase C and phospholipase D in parathyroid hormone receptor regulation of protein kinase Calpha and interleukin-6 in UMR-106 osteoblastic cells. *Cell Signal* 2004; 16(1):105-114.

32. Miao D, Tong XK, Chan GK, Panda D, McPherson PS, Goltzman D. Parathyroid hormone-related peptide stimulates osteogenic cell proliferation through protein kinase C activation of the Ras/mitogen-activated protein kinase signaling pathway. *J Biol Chem* 2001; 276(34):32,204–32,213.

33. Kalinowski L, Dobrucki LW, Malinski T. Nitric oxide as a second messenger in parathyroid hormone-related protein signaling. *J Endocrinol* 2001; 170(2):433–440.

34. Kaiser SM, Laneuville P, Bernier SM, Rhim JS, Kremer R, Goltzman D. Enhanced growth of a human keratinocyte cell line induced by antisense RNA for parathyroid hormone-related peptide. *J Biol Chem* 1992; 267(19):13,623–13,628.

35. VanHouten JN, Dann P, Stewart AF, Watson CJ, Pollak M, Karaplis AC, et al. Mammary-specific deletion of parathyroid hormone-related protein preserves bone mass during lactation. *J Clin Invest* 2003; 112(9):1429–1436.

36. Macica CM, Broadus AE. PTHrP regulates cerebral blood flow and is neuroprotective. *Am J Physiol Regul Integr Comp Physiol* 2003; 284(4):R1019,1020.

37. Stuart WD, Maeda S, Khera P, Fagin JA, Clemens TL. Parathyroid hormone-related protein induces G1 phase growth arrest of vascular smooth muscle cells. *Am J Physiol Endocrinol Metab* 2000; 279(1): E60–E67.

38. Hastings RH, Quintana RA, Sandoval R, Duey D, Rascon Y, Burton DW, Deftos LJ. Proapoptotic effects of parathyroid hormone-related protein in type II pneumocytes. *Am J Respir Cell Mol Biol* 2003; 29(6): 733–742.

39. Aya K, Tanaka H, Ichinose Y, Kobayashi M, Seino Y. Expression of parathyroid hormone-related peptide messenger ribonucleic acid in developing kidney. *Kidney Int* 1999; 55(5):1696–1703.

40. Cebrian A, Garcia-Ocana A, Takane KK, Sipula D, Stewart AF, Vasavada RC. Overexpression of parathyroid hormone-related protein inhibits pancreatic beta-cell death in vivo and in vitro. *Diabetes* 2002; 51(10):3003–3013.

41. Amizuka N, Warshawsky H, Henderson JE, Goltzman D, Karaplis AC. Parathyroid hormone-related peptide-depleted mice show abnormal epiphyseal cartilage development and altered endochondral bone formation. *J Cell Biol* 1994; 126(6):1611–1623.

42. Amizuka N, Karaplis AC, Henderson JE, Warshawsky H, Lipman ML, Matsuki Y, et al. Haploin-sufficiency of parathyroid hormone-related peptide (PTHrP) results in abnormal postnatal bone development. *Dev Biol* 1996; 175(1):166–176.

43. Fraher LJ, Avram R, Watson PH, Hendy GN, Henderson JE, Chong KL, et al. Comparison of the biochemical responses to human parathyroid hormone-(1-31)NH2 and hPTH-(1-34) in healthy humans. *J Clin Endocrinol Metab* 1999; 84(8):2739–2743.

44. Stewart AF, Horst R, Deftos LJ, Cadman EC, Lang R, Broadus AE. Biochemical evaluation of patients with cancer-associated hypercalcemia. Evidence for humoral and non-humoral groups. *N Engl J Med* 1980; 303:1377–1381.

45. Murer H, Hernando N, Forster I, Biber J. Regulation of Na/Pi transporter in the proximal tubule. *Annu Rev Physiol* 2003; 65:531–542.

46. Henderson J, Bernier S, D'Amour P, Goltzman D. Effects of passive immunization against parathyroid hormone (PTH)-like peptide and PTH in hypercalcemic tumor-bearing rats and normocalcemic controls. *Endocrinology* 1990; 127(3):1310–1318.

47. Horiuchi N, Caulfield MP, Fisher JE, Goldman ME, McKee RL, Reagan JE, et al. Similarity of synthetic peptide from human tumor to parathyroid hormone in vivo and in vitro. *Science* 1987; 238: 1566–1568.

48. Schweitzer DH, Hamdy NA, Frolich M, Zwinderman AH, Papapoulos SE. Malignancy-associated hypercalcemia: resolution of controversies over vitamin D metabolism by a pathophysiological approach to the problem. *Clin Endocrinol* 1994; 41:251–256.

49. Rouleau MF, Mitchell J, Goltzman D. Characterization of the major parathyroid hormone target cell in the endosteal metaphysis of rat long bones. *J Bone Miner Res* 1990; 5(10):1043–1053.

50. Wong BR, Rho J, Arron J, Robinson E, Orlinick J, Chao M, et al. TRANCE is a novel ligand of the tumor necrosis factor receptor family that activates c-Jun N-terminal kinase in T-cells. *J Biol Chem* 1997; 272: 25,190–25,194.

51. Yasuda H, Shima N, Nakagawa N, Yamaguchi K, Kinosaki M, Mochizuki S-I, et al. Osteoclast differentiation factor is a ligand for osteoprotegerin/osteoclastogenesis inhibitory factor and identical to TRANCE/RANKL. *Proc Natl Acad Sci USA* 1998; 95:3597–3602.

52. Lacey DM, Timms E, Tan H-L, Kelley MJ, Dunstan CR, Burgess T, et al. Osteoprotegerin ligand is a cytokine that regulates osteoclast differentiation and activation. *Cell* 1998; 93:165–176.

53. Simonet WS, Lacey DL, Dunstan CR, Kelley M, Chang MS, Luthy R, et al. Osteoprotegerin: a novel secreted protein involved in the regulation of bone density. *Cell* 1997; 89:309–319.

54. Stewart AF, Vignery A, Silvergate A, Ravin ND, LiVolsi V, Broadus AE, et al. Quantitative bone histomorphometry in humoral hypercalcemia malignancy: uncoupling of bone cell activity. *J Clin Endocrinol Metab* 1982; 55:219–227.
55. Powell GJ, Southby J, Danks JA, Stilwell RG, Haymen JA, Henderson MA, Bennett RC, et al. Localization of parathyroid hormone-related protein in breast cancer metastases: increased incidence in bone compared with other sites. *Cancer Res* 1991; 51:3059–3601.
56. Sachmechi I, Kalra J, Molho L, Chawla K. Paraneoplastic hypercalcemia associated with uterine papillary serous carcinoma. *Gynecol Oncol* 1995; 58:378–382.
57. McAuley P, Asa SL, Chiu B, Henderson JE, Goltzman D, Drucker DJ. Parathyroid hormone-like peptide in normal and neoplastic mesothelial cells. *Cancer* 1990; 66:1975–1979.
58. Asa SL, Henderson JE, Goltzman D, Drucker DJ. Parathyroid hormone-like peptide in normal and neoplastic human endocrine tissues. *J Clin Endocrinol Metab* 1990; 71:1112–1118.
59. Kimura S, Nishimura Y, Yamaguchi K, Nagaski K, Shimada K, Uchida H. A case of pheochromocytoma producing parathyroid hormone-related protein and presenting with hypercalcemia. *J Clin Endocrinol Metab* 1990; 70:1559–1563.
60. Drucker DJ, Asa SL, Henderson JE, Goltzman D. The parathyroid hormone-like peptide gene is expressed in the normal and neoplastic human endocrine pancreas. *Mol Endocrinol* 1988; 3:1589–1595.
61. Ikeda K, Arnold A, Magin M, Kinder B, Vydelingum NA, Brennan MR, et al. Expression of transcripts encoding a parathyroid hormone-related peptide in abnormal human parathyroid tissues. *J Clin Endocrinol Metab* 1989; 69:1240–1248.
62. Ito M, Enomoto H, Usa T, Villadolid MC, Ohtsuru A, Namba H, et al. Expression of parathyroid hormone-related peptide in human pituitary tumors. *J Clin Pathol* 1993; 46:682,683.
63. Nakashima M, Ohtsuru A, Luo WT, Nakayama T, Enomoto H, Usa T, et al. Expression of parathyroid hormone-related peptide in human thyroid tumors. *J Pathol* 1995; 175:227–236.
64. Kremer R, Shustik C, Tabak T, Papavasiliou V, Goltzman D. Parathyroid hormone-related peptide (PTHrP) in hematological malignancies. *Am J Med* 1996; 100:406–411.
65. Body JJ, Delmas PD. Urinary pyridinium cross-links as markers of bone resorption in tumor-associated hypercalcemia. *J Clin Endocrinol Metab* 1992; 74:471–475.
66. Rabbani SA, Haq M, Goltzman D. Biosynthesis and processing of endogenous parathyroid hormone-related peptide (PTHrP) by the rat Leydig cell tumor H-500. *Biochemistry* 1993; 32:4931–4937.
67. Yang KH, dePapp AE, Soifer NE, Dreyer BE, Wu TL, Porter SE, et al. Parathyroid hormone-related protein: Evidence for isoform and tissue-specific post-translational processing. *Biochemistry* 1994; 33:7460–7469.
68. Budayr AA, Nissenson RA, Klein RF, Pun KK Clark OH, Diep D, Arnaud CD, Strewler GJ. Increased serum levels of a parathyroid hormone-like protein in malignancy-associated hypercalcemia. *Ann Intern Med* 1989; 111:807–812.
69. Henderson JE, Shustik C, Kremer R, Rabbani SA, Hendy GN, Goltzman D. Circulating concentrations of parathyroid hormone-like peptide in malignancy and hyperparathroidism. *J Bone Miner Res* 1990; 5:105–113.
70. Burtis WJ, Dann P, Gaich GA, Soifer NE. A high abundance midregion species of parathyroid hormone-related protein: immunological and chromatographic characterization in plasma. *J Clin Endrocinol Metab* 1994; 78:317–322.
71. Burtis WJ, Brady TG, Orloff JJ, Ersbak JB, Warrell RP, Olson BR, et al. Immunochemical characterization of circulating parathyroid hormone-related protein in patients with humoral hypercalcemia of cancer. *N Engl J Med* 1990; 322:1106–1112.
72. Ratcliffe WA, Norbury S, Stott RA, Heath DA, Ratcliffe JG. Immunoreactivity of plasma parathyrin-related peptide: three region-specific radioimmunoassays and a two-site immunoradiometric assay compared. *Clin Chem* 1991; 37:1781–1787.
73. Truong NU, deB Edwardes MD, Papavasiliou V, Goltzman D, Kremer R. Parathyroid hormone-related peptide and survival patients with cancer and hypercalcemia. *AM J Med* 2003; 115(2):115–121.
74. Body JJ. Hypercalcemia of malignancy. *Semin Nephrol* 2004; 24(1):48–54.
75. Sexton PM, Findlay DM, Martin TJ. Calcitonin. *Curr Med Chem* 1999; 6(11):1067–1093.
76. Aklilu F, Park M, Goltzman D, Rabbini SA. Induction of parathyroid hormone-related peptide by the Ras oncogene: role of Ras farnesylation inhibitors as potential therapeutic agents for hypercalcemia of malignancy. *Cancer Res* 1997; 57(20):4517–4522.

77. Liu B, Amizuka N, Goltzman D, Rabbani SA. Inhibition of processing of parathyroid hormone-related peptide by antisense furin; Effect in vitro and in vivo on rat Leydig (H-500) tumor cells. *Int J Cancer* 1995; 63:1–6.

78. Yu J, Papavasiliou V, Rhim J, Goltzman D, Kremer R. Vitamin D analogs: new therapeutic agents for the treatment of squamous cancer and its associated hypercalcemia. *Anti Cancer Drugs* 1995; 6:101–108.

79. Kukreja SC, Shevrin DH, Wimbiscus SA, Ebeling PR, Danks JA, Rodda CP, et al. Antibodies to parathyroid hormone-related protein lower serum calcium in athymic mouse models of malignancy-associated hypercalcemia due to human tumors. *J Clin Invest* 1988; 82:1798–1802.

80. Sato K, Onuma E, Yocum RC, Ogata E. Treatment of malignancy-associated hypercalcemia and cachexia with humanized anti-parathyroid hormone-related protein antibody. *Semin Oncol* 2003; 30(5);167–173.

81. Hofbauer LC, Neubauer A, Heufelder AE. Receptor activator of nuclear factor-kappaB ligand and osteoprotegerin: potential implications for the pathogenesis and treatment of malignant bone diseases. *Cancer* 2001; 92(3):460–470.

82. Lipton A. Bisphosphonate therapy in the oncology setting. *Expert Opin Emerg Drugs* 2003; 8(2):469–488.

3

Vitamin D and Vitamin D Analogs in Cancer Progression and Metastasis

Richard Kremer, MD and Shafaat A. Rabbani, MD

CONTENTS

1. INTRODUCTION

Vitamin D is a pro-hormone with a wide variety of biological actions once converted to its biologically active compound 1,25-dihydroxyvitamin D_3 [$1,25(OH)_2D_3$]. Its classical effect in the prevention and treatment of rickets has been known for over a century *(1)*. More recently, nonclassical actions of vitamin D have been recognized and, in particular, its potent action on the proliferation and differentiation of a variety of cells, including normal and malignant cells *(2)*. In this chapter, we first review the biological effects of vitamin D. We then describe the structure and functions of a variety of vitamin D analogs. Finally, we give a detailed description of the many studies that investigated the activity and the mechanism of the effect of vitamin D analogs in tumor growth and metastasis.

2. BIOLOGICAL ACTIONS OF VITAMIN D

2.1. Synthesis, Transport, and Metabolism

1,25-Dihydroxyvitamin D_3, the biologically active metabolite of vitamin D_3, is a fat-soluble secosteroid molecule generated nonenzymatically from 7-dehydrocholesterol in the human epidermis by radiation with ultraviolet (UV) light *(3)*. Vitamin D_3 is biologically inert in vitro, and requires a series of successive hydroxylations to be active in vivo *(4)*. Vitamin D_3 circulating in the blood is either taken up immediately by adipose tissue for storage or by the liver for metabolism. The initial step in the activation of vitamin D_3 is hydroxylation at C-25 to produce 25-hydroxyvitamin D_3 [$25(OH)D_3$].

From: *Cancer Drug Discovery and Development*
Bone Metastasis: Experimental and Clinical Therapeutics
Edited by: G. Singh and S. A. Rabbani © Humana Press Inc., Totowa, NJ

$25(OH)D_3$ is the most abundant metabolite of vitamin D_3 and its levels fluctuate with the seasons, the highest during the summer months. Vitamin D_3 25-hydroxylase activity is present in the mitochondrial fractions of the liver, the principal site of 25-hydroxylation in vivo *(5)*. The $25(OH)D_3$ 1α-hydroxylase represents the most important enzyme in determining the level of $1,25(OH)_2D_3$. This enzyme catalyzes the hydroxylation of $25(OH)D_3$ on the 1α-position to produce the biologically active $1,25(OH)_2D_3$. The major site of 1α-hydroxylation is the renal proximal tubule *(6)*. However, 1α-hydroxylase activity has also been detected at several extrarenal sites, most notably in keratinocytes and activated macrophages *(7)*. 1α-Hydroxylase activity is downregulated by $1,25(OH)_2D_3$, a mechanism that prevents its overproduction and, potentially, vitamin D intoxication.

In humans, the normal circulating concentration of $1,25(OH)_2D_3$ is approx 1000-fold less than $25(OH)D_3$ *(8)*. Vitamin D in the circulation is complexed with a 55-kDa α-globulin synthesized in the liver, known as the vitamin D-binding protein or transcalciferin (DBP). This transport protein has a single, high-affinity site that binds vitamin D and all of its metabolites; however, it has a higher affinity for $25(OH)D_3$ and $24,25(OH)_2D_3$ than for $1,25(OH)_2D_3$ *(9)*. This strong affinity of $25(OH)D_3$ for the DBP in the blood might also facilitate access of the biologically active $1,25(OH)_2D_3$ into target cells *(10)*. Under normal conditions, only 5% of the vitamin D-binding sites on DBP are occupied because the concentration of the protein in the plasma is in large excess of the concentration of vitamin D and its metabolites *(11)*.

Both $25(OH)D_3$ and $1,25(OH)_2D_3$ are subject to hydroxylation at C-24, producing $24,25(OH)_2D_3$ and $1,24,25(OH)_3D_3$, respectively. $24,25(OH)_2D_3$ is the second most abundant circulating metabolite of vitamin D_3, and under normal circumstances in humans, its serum concentration is approx 10-fold less than $25(OH)D_3$ *(12)*. The principal site of 24-hydroxylation is the renal tubular cells; however, 24-hydroxylase activity is not confined to the kidney. Extrarenal locations of 24-hydroxylase activity include the intestine and bone *(13–15)*. Introduction of a hydroxyl group at C-24 renders the molecules susceptible to side-chain cleavage and oxidation, indicating that 24-hydroxylation initiates a pathway for the degradation and elimination of vitamin D_3 and its metabolites *(16)*. The activity of 24-hydroxylase was found to be upregulated by $1,25(OH)_2D_3$, a feedback mechanism that could prevent $1,25(OH)_2D_3$ intoxication *(17)*.

Other vitamin D metabolites include 25,26-dihydroxyvitamin D_3, $25(OH)D_3$-26,23-lactone, and 23-oxo-$1,25(OH)_2D_3$ *(18)*. The physiological role, if any, of these metabolites remains uncertain.

2.2. Physiological Actions of $1,25(OH)_2D_3$

The traditional action of $1,25(OH)_2D_3$ is to maintain calcium and phosphate homeostasis to ensure the deposition of bone mineral. The plasma calcium concentration is tightly controlled in humans *(19)* and $1,25(OH)_2D_3$ plays an important role in mammalian calcium homeostasis mainly through its actions on the skeleton and the intestine. $1,25(OH)_2D_3$ stimulates intestinal calcium and phosphate absorption, bone calcium and phosphate resorption, and renal calcium and phosphate reabsorption, thus increasing the serum calcium and phosphate ion concentration.

In addition to the classic actions of $1,25(OH)_2D_3$ on mineral homeostasis, this hormone also has the ability to regulate the growth and differentiation of several cell types. $1,25(OH)_2D_3$ induces differentiation of HL-60 cells, a human leukemia cell line, into macrophage-like cells *(20)*. $1,25(OH)_2D_3$ also stimulates the progression of basal epidermal keratinocytes into mature keratinocytes and is important in the formation of the multinucleated osteoclast in bone marrow cultures *(21,22)*.

Some of the most interesting targets for $1,25(OH)_2D_3$ action are the immune system and skin. This hormone functions to suppress the immune system, especially T-cell-mediated immune responses such as delayed hypersensitivity *(23)*. This has led to the suggestion that vitamin D might have a therapeutic potential in organ transplants or the treatment of autoimmune disorders, including multiple sclerosis, lupus erythematosis, autoimmune thyroiditis, and autoimmune diabetes *(24–27)*.

Recent experiments have identified human keratinocytes as an interesting alternate source for $1,25(OH)_2D_3$ production. In addition to producing previtamin D_3 from 7-dehydrocholesterol, keratinocytes are also able to produce the biologically active metabolite, $1,25(OH)_2D_3$ *(28)*. Furthermore, the skin is well established as a target tissue for $1,25(OH)_2D_3$ because it expresses the vitamin D receptor *(29)*. Recently, it was shown that this steroid, therefore, has the potential to act on epidermal cells in an autocrine manner *(30)*. Keratinocytes respond to $1,25(OH)_2D_3$ by changes in proliferation and differentiation. When cultured human keratinocytes are incubated with $1,25(OH)_2D_3$, this hormone inhibits their proliferation and induces them to terminally differentiate *(31,32)*. Cultured normal keratinocytes respond to concentrations of $1,25(OH)_2D_3$ as low as $10^{-10}\,M$, a range that is physiologically relevant *(32)*.

c-*myc* is one of the key players in the control of cell proliferation and is required for normal cell growth *(33)*. In fact, the addition of growth factors to quiescent cells in culture results in the immediate induction of c-*myc* mRNA and, therefore, cell proliferation *(34)*. However, treatment of human keratinocytes with $1,25(OH)_2D_3$ results in growth inhibition preceded by a marked inhibition of c-*myc* mRNA *(35,36)*. Therefore, $1,25(OH)_2D_3$ is an important negative regulator of keratinocyte cell growth.

Calcium has been shown to attenuate cell proliferation and stimulate differentiation. In culture, keratinocytes in low calcium concentrations (0.03 m*M*) do not differentiate and resemble basal epidermal cells. Increasing the extracellular calcium concentration above 0.1 m*M* induces keratinocyte differentiation *(37)*. Keratinocytes in culture in the presence of high calcium concentrations for several days begin to express proteins necessary for differentiation, such as transglutaminase, the calcium-dependent enzyme responsible for crosslinking the proteins of the cornified envelope to form a structure containing keratin fibers *(38)*, and involucrin, a marker of keratinocyte differentiation *(39)*. These effects are supported by the in vivo finding that there is a gradient of increasing intracellular calcium concentration from the basal layers of the epidermis to the progressively differentiated outer layers (40).

Several studies indicate that $1,25(OH)_2D_3$ potentiates the effect of calcium on keratinocyte proliferation and differentiation. At low calcium concentration, $1,25(OH)_2D_3$ exerts a growth-inhibitory action in normal human keratinocytes. However, 1.0 m*M* Ca^{2+} in combination with $1,25(OH)_2D_3$ produces a synergistic effect and completely abolishes cell division *(31)*. Both calcium and $1,25(OH)_2D_3$ enhance the formation of morphological features associated with terminal differentiation of epidermal keratinocytes in culture *(32)*. Involucrin mRNA expression is an excellent marker of keratinocyte differentiation, and both calcium and $1,25(OH)_2D_3$ strongly stimulate involucrin expression in keratinocytes in culture *(31,41)*. The stimulation of involucrin mRNA levels is potentiated within the first 24 h of exposure of the keratinocytes to $1,25(OH)_2D_3$ and an increase in the calcium concentration *(42)*. Hence, $1,25(OH)_2D_3$ and calcium act in concert to control the cell growth and differentiation of normal human epidermal keratinocytes.

2.3. Mechanism of Action of Vitamin D

Most of the actions induced by $1,25(OH)_2D_3$ are mediated through the nuclear vitamin D receptor, which binds to vitamin D response elements in the regulatory regions of $1,25(OH)_2D_3$ target genes. Activation of genomic pathways after $1,25(OH)_2D_3$ binding to its nuclear receptor leads to the modulation of gene expression as either an increase or decrease of a target gene product (Fig. 1). These genomic effects include the majority, if not all, of the known effects of $1,25(OH)_2D_3$.

In addition to its effect on gene regulation through the nuclear vitamin D receptor (VDR), it has become evident that $1,25(OH)_2D_3$ can also exert its action on target cells through nongenomic mechanisms *(43)*. The genomic pathways mediated by nuclear hormone receptors are relatively slow, occurring in hours or days, whereas in the case of a nongenomic effect, a physiological response can be observed in milliseconds to minutes following administration of the hormone. The non-genomic effects of $1,25(OH)_2D_3$ include the stimulation of calcium influx through voltage-sensitive Ca^{2+} channels, release of calcium from intracellular stores, induction of phosphorylation cascades, and phospholipids turnover leading to the release of calcium *(44)*.

VDR is a member of the nuclear receptor superfamily, a large family of transcriptional regulators that mediate development, differentiation, and physiological responses to lipophilic hormones, including steroids, thyroid hormones, retinoids, and vitamin D_3 *(45)*. These hormones easily traverse the cell membrane and bind to their specific intra-cellular nuclear receptors, which function by recognizing specific DNA sequences in the promoter elements of target genes known as response elements. Nuclear receptors function to modulate the transcription of target genes *(46)*. Activation of nuclear receptor target genes requires binding of the receptor to specific DNA response elements. The core motif of a nuclear receptor response element is a 6-basepair (bp) recognition sequence, or half-site, arranged into direct or inverted repeats *(47)*. Furthermore, the spacing of the two half-sites of the DNA response element is important for the specificity of nuclear receptor binding.

The nuclear receptors have been divided into several subfamilies *(48)*: the steroid receptors, which function as homodimers and bind the DNA response elements in the form of pseudopalindromic inverted repeats; the nonsteroid receptors such as the VDR, which function as heterodimers with the retinoid X receptor (RXR) and bind to DNA response elements in the form of direct repeats; the orphan receptors, which are receptors with no known ligands and bind to DNA as heterodimers with the RXR or as monomers. The DNA response elements reflect the manner of receptor interaction as heterodimers, homodimers, or monomers.

The nuclear receptor superfamily exhibits a conserved structure with several domains (Fig. 2) *(49)*. The amino-terminal A/B region is greatly variable among the nuclear receptors. The function of this region is not yet fully elucidated; however, it often possesses a ligand-independent transactivation function, called AF-1. The C region is responsible for DNA recognition and binding and is the most highly conserved region

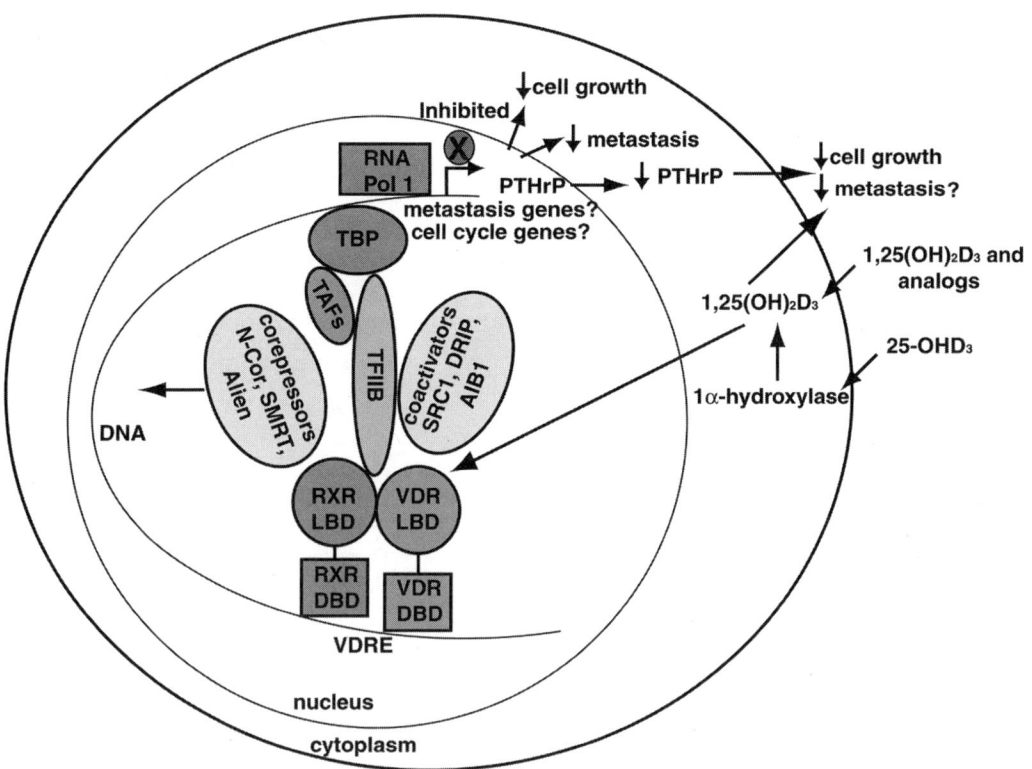

Fig. 1. Mechanism of action of 1,25(OH)$_2$D$_3$ and analogs and targeting of cell growth and parathyroid hormone-related peptide (PTHrP) expression. Following the delivery of 1,25(OH)$_2$D$_3$ or its analogs to target cells, binding to the vitamin D receptor (VDR) occurs and induces conformational changes and heterodimerization with retinoid X receptor (RXR). The heterodimeric complex binds to the promoter regions of target genes through discrete elements called vitamin D responsive elements (VDREs). This process triggers the release of corepressor(s) and the binding of coactivator(s) to the complex and activates or represses the transcriptional machinery. Vitamin D response can be elicited by the active form of vitamin D (1,25(OH)$_2$D$_3$) or 1α-hydroxylated analogs but also by the local conversion of 25OHD$_3$ to 1,25(OH)$_2$D$_3$ regulated by intracellular activation of 1α-hydroxylase. Shown are the downstream targets of 1,25(OH)$_2$D$_3$ or analogs such as cell cycle regulators and the malignancy-associated hypercalcemia mediator, PTHrP.

among the nuclear receptors. The hinge region, or D domain, whose function remains unclear, is highly variable between the different nuclear receptors, whereas the highly conserved E domain is responsible for ligand binding, dimerization, and transactivation *(50)*. Furthermore, the E region contains the ligand-dependent activation function called AF-2, which has been shown to be essential for interaction with coactivators, a bridge to the transcriptional machinery *(50)*. The function of the hypervariable F region, if any, remains elusive *(51)*.

In addition to the VDR, the nonsteroid receptors that heterodimerize to bind to DNA include the thyroid hormone receptor (TR), retinoic acid receptor (RAR), and the peroxisome proliferator-activated receptor (PPAR). It has been shown that RXR binds to the 5' half-site of the DNA response element and the other nuclear receptors that heterodimerize

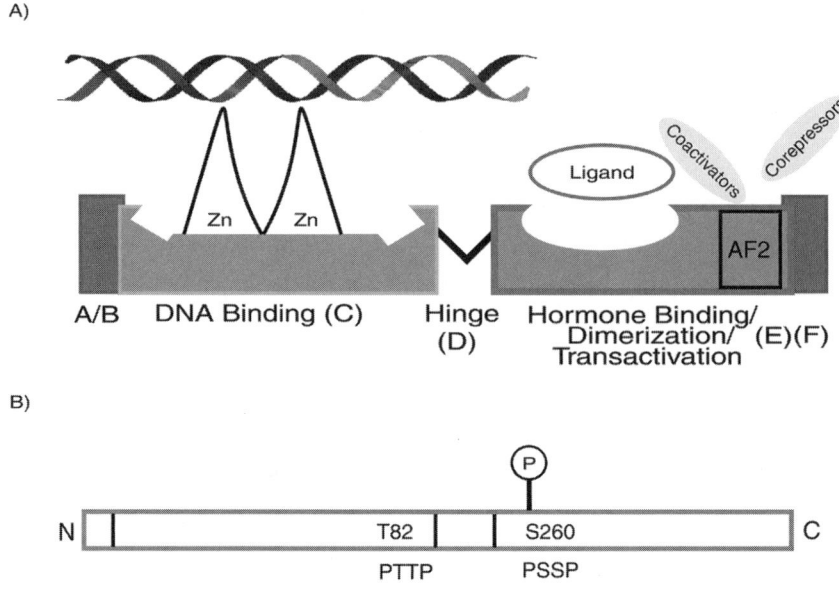

Fig. 2. Molecular structure of nuclear receptors and MAPK consensus sequences and phosphorylation of the RXR. The nuclear receptor superfamily structure is shown in **(A)**. The aminoterminal region A/B is highly variable among nuclear receptors. The C region is responsible for DNA recognition and binding and is the most highly conserved among receptors. The hinge region, or D domain, is highly variable between receptors and its function unclear. The highly conserved E domain is responsible for ligand binding, dimerization, and transactivation and contains the ligand-dependent activation function AF-2, which is essential for coactivator interaction. The F domain is highly variable and its function is largely unknown. **(B)** Localization of MAPK consensus sequences within the RXR and the phosphorylation site at ser260 located in the E domain in close proximity to coactivators interaction.

with RXR are able to recognize and interact with unique DNA response elements. Protein dimerization results in the formation of novel heterodimeric complexes that cooperatively bind to DNA with precise target sequence specificity. Subtle differences in the six nucleotide consensus half-site and the spacing between the half-sites confers response element discrimination. The DNA response elements for RXR heterodimers with the PPAR, RAR, VDR, and TR are composed of direct repeats spaced by one, two, three, or four nucleotides, respectively. The RXR-RAR heterodimer is also able to bind to a direct repeat (DR) spaced by five nucleotides *(52–56)*.

The human vitamin D receptor is a 427-amino acid protein organized into several domains, like the other members of the nuclear receptor superfamily *(57)*. The 20-amino acid A/B domain is truncated and no function has been attributed to this region in the VDR *(45)*. The E domain is responsible for high-affinity ligand binding as well as coactivator interaction and heterodimerization with RXR. Heterodimerization with RXR is required in order for the VDR to efficiently bind DNA *(58)*. The E domain of VDR contains nine hydrophobic heptad repeats critical for this heterodimerization *(59)*. Experiments have demonstrated that mutations within the fourth heptad repeat (amino acids 325–332) and the ninth heptad repeat (amino acids 392–402) of the VDR abrogate VDR-RXR complex formation *(60)*.

Three isoforms of RXR have been identified: RXRα, RXRβ, and RXRγ *(61)*. VDR is capable of forming heterodimers with each RXR isoform, and each heterodimer can subsequently bind vitamin D response elements in DNA. However, only RXRα and RXRγ are capable of mediating VDR-induced transactivation *(62)*. The three RXR isoforms are present in both unique and overlapping expression patterns. Tissue distribution of both RXRα and RXRβ expression is widespread, including the liver, kidney, lung, and spleen. Distribution of RXRγ is much more restricted with strong expression in the heart and muscle. The adult human epidermis and keratinocytes express high levels of only the RXRα isoform *(61)*.

2.3.1. VITAMIN D RESPONSE ELEMENTS AND TRANSCRIPTION

Activation of vitamin D_3 target genes requires that the VDR–RXR heterodimerization complex binds to specific DNA sequences called vitamin D response elements (VDREs) in the promoter regions of these genes. Binding of the heterodimers to the response element induces a bend in the DNA of the promoter *(63)*. It is thought that this DNA bending facilitates and stabilizes the recruitment of the various components of the pre-initiation complex by positioning the receptor complex in the proximity of other transcription factors. However, the precise role of DNA bending in the regulation of transcription remains elusive.

Several positive and negative VDREs have been identified in $1,25(OH)_2D_3$ target genes that mediate transcriptional stimulation or repression, respectively. Genes known to be transcriptionally activated by $1,25(OH)_2D_3$ include rat and human osteoclacin, mouse osteopontin, and rat 24-hydroxylase *(54,64–66)*. The positive recognition site in the DNA of $1,25(OH)_2D_3$ responsive genes is a DR3 which interacts with the VDR–RXR complex where the 5'-half-site is occupied by RXR *(67)*. In contrast, some genes are negatively controlled at the level of transcription by $1,25(OH)_2D_3$, including mouse osteoclacin, human parathyroid hormone (PTH), and rat PTHrP *(68,69)*. The functional features of the VDRE that dictate whether it mediates transactivation or transrepression are still elusive.

The natural ligand for RXR, 9-*cis* retinoic acid, represents an additional level of control over RXR-containing heterodimers. Combination studies of 9-*cis* retinoic acid and $1,25(OH)_2D_3$ have produced a myriad of results, including antagonistic, additive, and synergistic effects. The antagonistic effect was demonstrated through the attenuation of $1,25(OH)_2D_3$-induced activation of the rat osteocalcin gene by 9-*cis* retinoic acid. Furthermore, this study established that 9-*cis* retinoic acid inhibited DNA binding of the VDR–RXR heterodimer, as well as transcription from a vitamin D response element-containing reporter construct *(70)*. The mechanism of antagonism by 9-*cis* retinoic acid in this rat osteocalcin system is thought to involve the diversion of RXR favoring the formation of retinoid-occupied RXR homodimers *(71)*. The additive effect of 9-*cis* retinoic acid on the growth inhibitory action of $1,25(OH)_2D_3$ has been demonstrated in human pancreatic carcinoma (Capan) cells and colon carcinoma (Caco-2) cells *(72,73)*. The synergistic effect of the combination of these ligands was demonstrated through the enhanced accumulation of 24-hydroxylase mRNA in human skin *(74)*, as well as the growth inhibition of LNCaP prostate cancer cells *(75)*.

2.3.2. COACTIVATORS AND COREPRESSORS

The mechanism by which nuclear receptors activate or repress gene transcription is quickly coming into focus. Considerable evidence has shown that nuclear receptors work through complexing with proteins known as nuclear receptor coactivators and corepressors. Initial evidence for the existence of such proteins came from experiments where different receptors interfered with each other's transactivation capacity by competing for essential, limiting factors *(76)*.

Recently, numerous coactivators and corepressors have been cloned and characterized that interact with the nuclear receptors and enhance their capacity to modulate target genes. Several classes of coactivator have been described that capable of interacting with the VDR (Fig. 1) and include SRC/p160, NCOA-62/Ski interacting protein (SKIP) and vitamin D receptor interacting protein (DRIP). Among SRC/p160 coactivators, steroid receptor coactivator (SRC-1) was identified through the use of the yeast two-hybrid system using the progesterone receptor as bait *(77)*. SRC-1 enhances ligand-dependent transactivaton by the GR, ER, RXR, VDR, and TR by up to 10-fold *(77)*. Most coactivators, including SRC-1, interact with nuclear receptors via the highly conserved activation function (AF-2) domain, an amphipathic α-helix identified in the C-terminal region E of transcriptionally active members of the nuclear receptor superfamily *(78–80)*. Other SRC/p160 coactivators include SRC-2 and are also known as TIF2 or GRIP-1 and SRC-3 also known as PCIP or ACTR.

Binding of the ligand to a nuclear receptor induces a conformational change in the AF-2 domain, allowing it to interact with SRC-1 and other coactivators, which form a bridge to other components of the transcriptional machinery *(81)*. Experiments have shown that the AF-2 domain of VDR is critical for $1,25(OH)_2D_3$-dependent transactivation and $1,25(OH)_2D_3$-dependent coactivator interaction. VDR mutants lacking the C-terminal AF-2 domain were transcriptionally inactive and unable to bind SRC-1 *(81)*. Furthermore, deletion of the AF-2 domain of RAR, ER, or TR abolishes ligand-dependent transcription *(78,79,82)*. SRC/p160 coactivators possess intrinsic histone acetyl transferase (HAT) activity, which remodels chromatin.

In contrast to SRC/p160, SKIP does not interact with AF-2 but, instead, forms a ternary complex with VDR and SRC/p160 coactivators *(83)*. SKIP does not have intrinsic HAT activity. The DRIP complex was recently described as a new class of coactivators and binds VDR in a ligand-dependent manner at the AF domain in the ligand-binding region *(84)*. Among the DRIP subunits, DRIP205 seems to play a critical role in VDR transactivation by allowing the recruitment of the basal transcriptional machinery following chromatin remodeling by HAT *(85)*.

Two transcriptional corepressors have been identified that associate with unliganded receptors, leading to the suppression of basal transcription, the silencing mediator for retinoid and thyroid hormone receptors (SMRT) and the nuclear receptor corepressor (N-CoR) *(86,87)*. Hormone binding causes the dissociation of corepressors, allowing for the recruitment of positive factors and transactivation *(88,89)*.

Although $1,25(OH)_2D_3$ is a potent calcemic agent capable of the correction of hypocalcemia and bone abnormalities resulting from vitamin D deficiency, the therapeutic potential of this hormone is limited because of hypercalcemic side effects thought to be mediated via these nongenomic pathways *(90)*.

3. VITAMIN D ANALOGS

The emergence of neoclassical functions of vitamin D, such as its role in controlling cell proliferation and differentiation, led to the indication that patients with psoriasis and other hyperproliferative disorders could benefit from biologically active vitamin D preparations. Analogs that activate or block specific genomic effects of $1,25(OH)_2D_3$ with less calcemic effects could offer improved therapeutic potential over $1,25(OH)_2D_3$ by causing fewer undesirable side effects, such as hypercalcemia and hypercalciuria *(91)*. Consequently, the chemical synthesis of new analogs of $1,25(OH)_2D_3$ where the calcemic properties could be separated from the antiproliferative cell-differentiating properties has been an intensive area of investigation in recent years *(90)*.

3.1. Structure

Structural modification of the parent hormone $1,25(OH)_2D_3$ include (1) modification of the A-ring, (2) modification of the side chain, and (3) deletion of the C- and D-rings (nonsteroidal analogs).

3.1.1. MODIFICATION OF THE A-RING

The A-ring plays a critical role in vitamin D action because of the presence of two crucial hydroxyl sites at positions 1 and 3. Modifications of the A-ring at position 2 lead to substantial changes in biological properties of vitamin D. Addition of a 2α-(3-hydroxypropyl) group enhances both VDR binding and the antiproliferative action of this compound at the expense of a sharp fivefold increase in its calcemic activity *(92)*. In contrast, the 2α-(3-hydroxypropyl) analog has a reduced binding to the VDR, a reduced antiproliferative effect, and a 100-fold reduction in calcemic activity *(92)*.

3.1.2. MODIFICATION OF THE SIDE CHAIN

1. Gemini Analogs: RO27-2310 is a $1,25(OH)_2D_3$ analog with two identical side chains attached to carbon 20 and is 100-fold more potent than $1,25(OH)_2D_3$ in inhibiting cell growth of several cancer cell lines *(93)*. A closely related analog, RO27-5646 or 19 non-Gemini, is at least 400-fold more potent than the parent Gemini analog as assessed by growth inhibition of leukemic cells *(94)*.
2. 20 epi Analogs: EB1213 and GS1500 are characterized by an aromatic ring in the side chain at position 20, and because of a strong antiproliferative effect on keratinocytes, they might find future applications in the treatment of psoriasis *(95)*. KH1060 is another 20 epi analog with potent immunosuppressive effect with antirejection properties on skin and renal allografts *(96,97)*. Additionally, the combination of 2α-methyl and 20-epimerization results in very potent differentiating effect on leukemic cells *(98)*.
3. 19 Nor-analogs: These are characterized by modifications of the B-ring and the side chain. TX522 [19-non-14-epi-23-yne-1α25(OH)₂D₃] and TX527 [19-non-14,20-bisepi-23-yne-1α25(OH)₂D₃] are 10–60 times more potent than $1,25(OH)_2D_3$ in inhibiting tumor growth in vitro and in vivo while having less or comparable calcemic activity, making them potentially interesting compounds in the treatment of cancer (99).
4. Other Side Chain Analogs: EB1089 possesses dimethyl groups and two double bonds at positions 26 and 27 and possesses strong antitumor effects both in vitro *(100)* and in vivo *(101–104)*, including an inhibitory effect on the metastatic spread in lungs *(101,105)*. 22-oxa 1α,25(OH)₂D₃ is also a potent antiproliferative agent both in vitro *(106,107)* and in vivo in breast cancer models *(108)* and pancreatic cancer *(109)*.

3.3.3. Deletion of the C- and D-Rings and Other Nonsteroidal Analogs

The first class of these nonsteroidal analogs are characterized by the absence of normal C- and D-rings, which are replaced by a five-membered ring called the E-ring. Belonging to this group are the KS and CD analogs *(110)*. KS291 is equipotent to $1,25(OH)_2D_3$ in inhibiting cell growth but has at least 100-fold less calcemic activity than $1,25(OH)_2D_3$.

Other nonsteroidal analogs were discovered by screening combinatorial chemistry libraries and belong to a group known as bis-phenyl derivatives or LG analogs. They are characterized by low calcemic activities and potent antitumor effects both in vitro and in vivo *(111,112)*. Interestingly, despite their nonsteroidal structure, they bind with high affinity and specificity to the VDR but have very low affinity for the DBP.

3.2. Mechanism of Action of Vitamin D Analogs

The precise mechanism(s) of action of vitamin D analogs is not yet fully understood but likely involves a combination of actions targeting the vitamin D signaling pathway. First, several studies indicate that most of these analogs bind to the DBP (Fig. 1) with less affinity than the parent molecule $1,25(OH)_2D_3$ *(113)*, thus increasing the bioavailability of the free form in target tissues. The analog then enters the cell, activates a number of key elements, and is also metabolized into inactive compounds *(114,115)*. Several studies indicate that upon binding to the VDR, these vitamin D analogs enhance the stability of the VDR *(116)* and perhaps that of the VDR–RXR complex better than the parent compound $1,25(OH)_2D_3$, resulting in an increased transactivating activity on target genes. Interestingly, this improved transactivating capacity seems independent of the binding affinity of the analogs to the VDR because the majority of these compounds bind with less affinity to the VDR than $1,25(OH)_2D_3$ *(117,118)*. Finally, recent studies *(118,119)* indicate that the biological activity of several 20-epi analogs correlates well with the recruitment of the coactivator DRIP205 *(85)* or, alternatively, the 22-oxa $1\alpha,25(OH)_2D_3$ selectively induces the recruitment of TIF-2 *(120)*, indicating that selective recruitment of coactivators might direct the biological potency of these compounds.

4. VITAMIN D, VITAMIN D ANALOGS, AND CANCER

The relationship between the vitamin D system and cancer was first noted in studies showing the induction of differentiation and suppression of growth of leukemia cells by vitamin D *(121)*. Since then, many studies have tried to determine a pathophysiological link between vitamin D and several types of cancer as well as evaluating the potency of $1,25(OH)_2D_3$, its precursors, or its analogs in a wide variety of cancer types.

Perhaps one of the most intriguing and still unresolved aspects of this relationship between vitamin D and cancer is the result of several epidemiological studies linking vitamin D directly or indirectly to cancer development and/or survival. Earlier studies suggested an association between endogenous vitamin D production and carcinogenesis after discovering an inverse relationship between average sunlight exposure and the incidence/mortality of breast, colon, and prostate cancer in the United States, Canada, and the former Soviet Union *(122–125)*. These studies suggested that vitamin D deficiency or a low vitamin D status was a major determinant in cancer risk/mortality in areas where a decrease of UV exposure is found, because UV is necessary to the synthesis of vitamin D by the skin. This hypothesis was supported by some but not all prospective studies aimed at determining an association between vitamin D levels in the blood of individuals and cancer risk *(126–129)*. Interestingly, in several studies, levels of the precursor 25(OH)D$_3$ had a better predictive value on cancer risk than the active metabolite 1,25(OH)$_2$D$_3$ *(130,131)* suggesting that other metabolites or local conversion of 25(OH)D$_3$ to 1,25(OH)$_2$D$_3$ might play a major role in cancer development. Indeed, we have recently shown that 1α-hydroxylase activity in *ras*–transformed human keratinocyte contributes to tumor growth inhibition in vivo via a unique autocrine system in which tumor cells supply their own 1,25(OH)$_2$D$_3$ active metabolite from its inactive precursor 25(OH)D$_3$ (Fig. 1) *(132)*.

The potent antiproliferative effect of 1,25(OH)$_2$D$_3$ was demonstrated in many cancer cell types in vitro, including breast, prostate, colon, skin, leukemia, and melanoma *(36,104,121,133–137)* and its antitumoral effect in a number of in vivo models (Table 1). However, the clinical usefulness of using 1,25(OH)$_2$D$_3$ in human subjects is severely limited by its well-known hypercalcemic and hypercalciuric side effects *(138)*. Furthermore, malignancy is often associated with hypercalcemia and, therefore, could preclude the use of 1,25(OH)$_2$D$_3$ in this setting *(139)*. Consequently, the search of potent vitamin D analogs with lesser calcemic/calciuric side effects but with superior antiproliferative and prodifferentiating activities has been very active and resulted in the synthesis of many compounds that have antitumoral effecting in animal models representing various types of cancer (Table 1).

4.1. Mechanism of Vitamin D Antitumor Effect: Genomic vs Nongenomic Effects

It is likely that most of the effect observed with 1,25(OH)$_2$D$_3$ and its analogs are VDR-mediated. Mammalian VDRs have been located in numerous tissues, including the intestine, kidney, skin, bone, hematopoietic cells, brain, and breast *(164)*. VDRs have equally been found in various malignant cell lines *(165)*. The presence of VDR in malignant tissue may be a prognostic indicator in patients with breast cancer, as VDR-positive breast cancer patients have a better prognosis than patients with VDR-negative tumors *(166)*. VDR expression/concentration is also regulated by a number of factors through transcriptional regulation in its promoter regions and by 1,25(OH)$_2$D$_3$-dependent stabilization of the ligand–receptor complex *(167,168)*. Furthermore, VDR activity itself depends on phosphorylation at specific sites, which results in either upregulation or downregulation of its activity *(169)*. Adding to the complexity of the regulatory process is the recent discovery of a new isoform of the VDR that might have specific biological actions *(170)*.

As indicated earlier (Section 2.3.), the VDR transcriptional activation occurs following its binding to RXR and it is the 1,25(OH)$_2$D$_3$–VDR–RXR heterodimer complex, which acts as the signal transducer of vitamin D actions. RXR ligands can, therefore, add another level of control to this transcriptional machinery. Indeed, it has been shown that specific RXR ligands, also called retinoids, have a synergistic effect on 1,25(OH)$_2$D$_3$ mediated transcription *(171)*. In contrast, 9-*cis* retinoic acid, which can bind both RAR and RXR tends to inhibit 1,25(OH)$_2$D$_3$-mediated transactivation by scavenging RXR receptors from the VDR–RXR complex to the RAR–RXR complex *(172)*. In addition, several isoforms of RXR exist (α, β, and γ) and can interact with the VDR to further refine the regulation of VDR signaling. RXRα has been implicated in directing VDR-mediated hair follicle and keratinocyte growth and differentiation *(173)*, whereas RXRγ appears to be essential for VDR-mediated growth plate development *(174)*.

Table 1
Anticancer Effect of $1,25(OH)_2D_3$ and Its Analogs
in Various Animal Models

Effect	Type of cancer (ref.)
$1,25(OH)_2D_3$	
Tumor growth	Breast (140)
Prostate (141)	
Renal (142)	
Squamous (skin) (143)	
Metastasis	Prostate (lung) (141)
Survival	Myeloid leukemia (144)
	Renal (142)
Analogs	
$1\alpha OHD_3$	
Tumor growth	Renal (142)
Metastasis	Hepatoma (145)
Survival	Renal (142)
EB1089	
Tumor growth	Breast (146,147)
	Colon (102,148)
	Leydig tumor (149)
	Melanoma (104)
	Pancreatic (156)
	Prostate (151)
	Squamous (skin) (152)
Metastasis	Breast (skeletal) (105)
	Prostate (lung) (101)
Survival	Breast (105)
	Leydig tumor (149)
RO 23-7553	
Tumor growth	Prostate (153)
	Retinoblastoma (153)
	Squamous (skin) (155)
Survival	Leukemia (156)
RO 25-6760	
Tumor growth	Colon (157)
	Prostate (141)
RO 24-5531	
Tumor growth	Breast (158)
	Colon (159)
	Prostate (160)
OCT [22-oxa-$1,25(OH)_3D_3$]	
Tumor growth	Colon (161)
	Pancreatic (109)
$25OHD_3$	
Tumor growth	Prostate (162,163)
	Squamous (skin) (132)

As indicated earlier (Section 2.3.), the transcriptional machinery is activated/repressed following binding of the ligand(s)–VDR–RXR complex to small sequences of DNA in the promoter region of target genes called vitamin D responsive elements (VDREs) (Fig. 1) *(175)*. Several types of VDRE exist, including a direct repeat-3 spacing nucleotide (DR3) *(176,177)*, DR4, DR6, and an inverted palindrome-9 spacing nucleotides (IP9). $1,25(OH)_2D_3$ can trigger interaction with any of these VDREs *(178)*, whereas the vitamin D analog EB1089 preferentially triggers VDR–RXR binding to an IP-9 VDRE *(179)* and other analogs preferentially stimulate the interaction with DR3–VDREs *(180)*. $1,25(OH)_2D_3$ trans-repression of the cancer-associated hypercalcemic gene PTHrP also occurs through VDRE interaction, but its mechanism might be more complex because the putative $1,25(OH)_2D_3$-mediated repression sequence overlaps with a growth-factor-mediated stimulatory sequence identified in the rat PTHrP promoter *(181)*. Furthermore, the human PTHrP VDRE *(182)* recognizes a VDR homodimer complex similar to PTH–VDRE *(183)* in contrast to the rat PTHrP VDRE, which recognizes a classical DR3 VDR-RXR complex *(68)*.

Coactivators/corepressors interacting with the VDR–RXR complex might also modulate $1,25(OH)_2D_3$ and its analogs activity in cancer cells. Indeed, it has been reported that coactivators/corepressors are either underexpressed or overexpressed in certain cancer cell types *(184–188)* and it remains to be determined if such alterations affect vitamin D action in certain types of cancer. In this case, analogs that promote specific coactivator interaction such as 20-epi analogs *(119)* could be selected to target specific cancer types.

Finally $1,25(OH)_2D_3$ and its analogs might affect cancer cells by mechanism(s) independent of transcription, the so-called rapid nongenomic effects. Such effects appear to be mediated either by a new membrane receptor for $1,25(OH)_2D_3$ *(189)* or by the VDR itself localized near or on the cell membrane *(190)*. Interestingly, these nongenomic effects include the opening of calcium and chloride channels and the activation of intracellular signaling molecules such as protein kinase C and the Ras–Raf–MAPKinase pathway *(191)*. $1,25(OH)_2D_3$ can also inhibit the JNK signaling pathway probably through a nongenomic effect *(192)*.

4.2. Vitamin D Resistance

Drug resistance is a common occurrence in many cancer therapeutic strategies and is known to occur with $1,25(OH)_2D_3$. Ras-transformed keratinocytes are not only resistant to the growth inhibitory effect of $1,25(OH)_2D_3$ and its analogs *(36,136)* but also to $1,25(OH)_2D_3$/analogs-mediated PTHrP repression *(136,193)*. Unlike normal human keratinocytes, ras-transformed keratinocytes are partially resistant to the growth inhibitory action of $1,25(OH)_2D_3$ or its analogs secondary to phosphorylation of hRXRα on ser260 (Fig. 2) *(194,195)*. Phosphorylation of hRXRα in ras-transformed keratinocytes is mediated through overexpression of the ras oncoprotein, leading to activation of the Ras–Raf–MAPKinase cascade. Because RXR heterodimerizes with other nuclear receptors other than VDR, including RAR, TR, PPAR, and RXR itself, the possibility that RXR phosphorylation at ser260 could also affect transcriptional and biological activity of these heterodimeric partners was also investigated. It was demonstrated that in addition to the inhibition of vitamin D signaling, phosphorylation of hRXRα or ser260 caused a similar resistance to the growth inhibitory effect of LG1069, an RXR-specific ligand *(194)*, transretinoic acid, and 9-*cis* retinoic acid (Fig. 3) *(196)*.

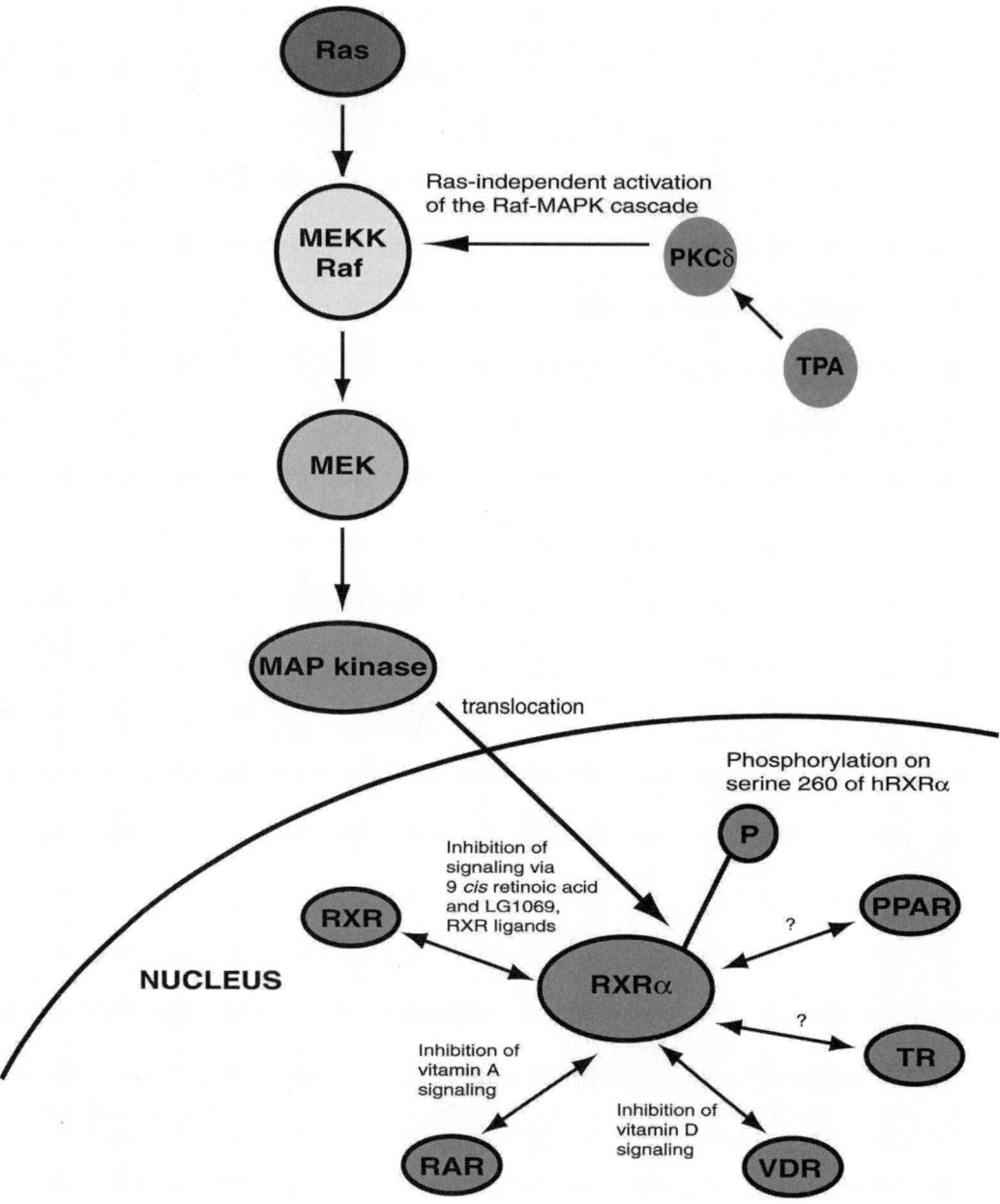

Fig. 3. Ras–Raf–MAPKinase pathway activation and downstream effect of RXR interaction with its heterodimeric partners. Ras targets Raf, which then phosphorylates and activates MAPKinase, a dual-specification kinase directly responsible for the phosphorylation and activation of MAPKinase. MAPKinase then translocates to the nucleus and phosphorylates a variety of substrates, including h RXRα on ser260. This phosphorylation event could affect signal transduction through the many members of the nuclear receptor superfamily in addition to the VDR. The MAPKinase pathway can also be activated in a ras-independent manner via protein kinase C δ (PKC 5), a target of 12-0-tetradecanolyphorbel-13-actate (TPA).

Furthermore, this "resistance" could be reversed by treating the cells with a nonphosphorylable ALA260 mutant hRXRα, a strategy that may find potential clinical applications in cancer therapy in combination with specific ligands for the VDR or other partners of the RXR *(194)*. Vitamin D resistance could also occur through intracellular catabolism of $1,25(OH)_2D_3$ or its analogs. The key enzyme that directs $1,25(OH)_2D_3$ catabolism in target cells is a 24hydroxylase (CYP24) leading to the production of calcitroic acid in target cells *(16,197)*. Interestingly, CYP24 activity was found to be overexpressed in ras-transformed keratinocytes as compared to the parent immortalized nontransformed keratinocyte cell line *(114)* as well as other cancer cell lines, indicating that this mechanism could lead to early deactivation of $1,25(OH)_2D_3$ or its analogs in certain cancer cell types. Targeting CYP24 using specific inhibitors can, therefore, represent an additional therapeutic strategy in cancer given in combination with $1,25(OH)_2D_3$ or its analogs. Several inhibitors of CYP24 have been investigated and include ketoconazole *(198)*, liarazole *(199)*, as well as more powerful and selective inhibitors named VID-400 and SDZ89-443 *(200)*.

4.3. Effect of Vitamin D on PTHrP and on Bone Metastasis

Parathyroid hormone-related protein (PTHrP) has long been known as a paraneoplastic hypercalcemic mediator produced by many types of cancer, especially solid tumors *(201)*. In addition, PTHrP produced by cancer cells exhibits growth factor-like properties that could promote tumor growth *(202–205)*. Furthermore, in normocalcemic cancer patients PTHrP enhances the ability of cancer to invade bone *(206)* and is associated with a shorter survival in hypercalcemic cancer patients *(207)*.

As indicated earlier, a major negative regulator of PTHrP production *in vitro* is $1,25(OH)_2D_3$ (Fig. 1) *(136,181,208,209)*. Vitamin D analogs also inhibit PTHrP production in vitro *(136,209,210)*. This regulation, which occurs through a $1,25(OH)_2D_3$ responsive repressor sequence located upstream of the PTHrP gene *(68)* is altered in ras-transformed keratinocytes secondary to the vitamin D resistance phenomenon described in Section 3.2. It is possible but has not yet been proven that this vitamin D resistance leads to overproduction of PTHrP in vivo and, consequently, severely limits the clinical usefulness of $1,25(OH)_2D_3$ in this setting. An alternative strategy, therefore, would be to use low-calcemic vitamin D analogs to block PTHrP production without worsening hypercalcemia. This strategy might be beneficial when used alone or in combination with bisphosphonates in hypercalcemic cancer patients. Indeed, release of PTHrP by tumors contributes to hypercalcemia by both a skeletal and renal mechanism *(149)*. The effect of PTHrP is to enhance renal calcium reabsorption and, therefore, constitutes an important contribution to the development of hypercalcemia in malignant states. Currently, the mainstay of treatment in malignancy-associated hypercalcemia is bisphosphonate therapy, which is bone-specific and has no effect on renal calcium reabsorption. This bone-specific effect of bisphosphonates could account for the resistance to the antihypercalcemic effect of bisphosphonates in patients with elevated circulating PTHrP levels *(211)*, likely through its renal effect. Consequently, vitamin D analogs could be interesting adjuncts in the therapeutic arsenal against malignancy-associated hypercalcemia (MAH) by blocking PTHrP production in this setting. We have used the vitamin D analog, EB1089, in two hypercalcemic animal cancer models to test its efficacy as an inhibitor of both PTHrP and hypercalcemia. In the first study, EB1089 was administered to Fisher rats implanted with

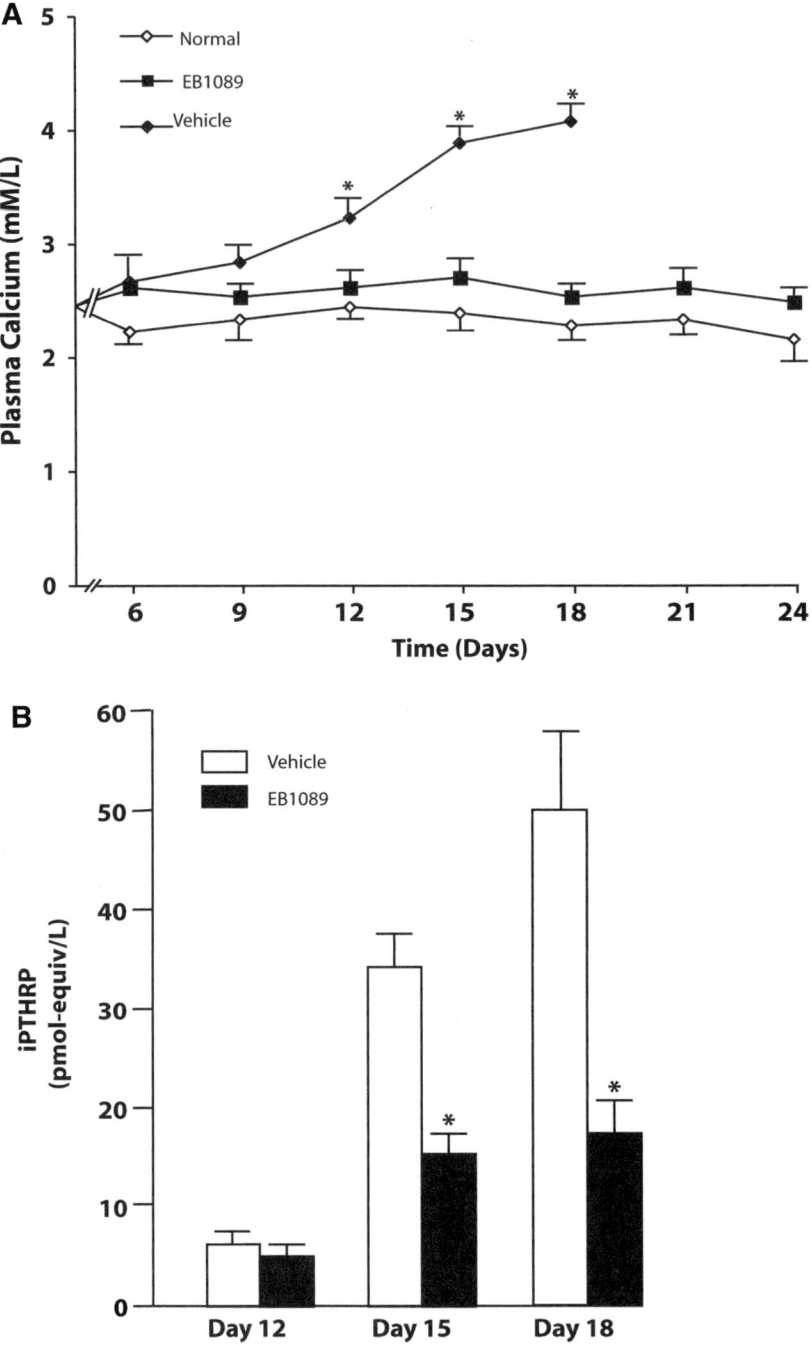

Fig. 4. Effect of EB 1089 on plasma calcium and PTHrP in H-500 tumor animals. Male Copenhagen rats were inoculated with rat Leydig tumor cells H500 via subcutaneous route into the flank. Tumor-bearing animals were infused with vehicle alone or EB1089 (200 pmol/24 h) via osmotic minipumps. Plasma calcium (**A**) and immunoreactive (i) PTHrP (**B**) was determined at timed intervals. Results represent ± SEM of six starting animals in each group in four different experiments. Significant differences from central tumor-bearing animals at each timepoint is shown by an asterisk ($p < 0.05$).

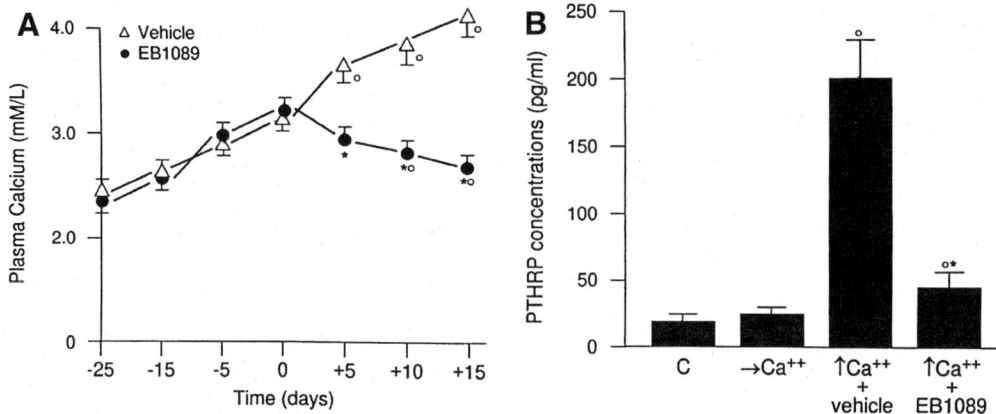

Fig. 5. Effect of the vitamin D analog EB1089 or hypercalcemia and PTHrP production in a nude mice model of malignancy associated hypercalcemia (MAH). Animals were implanted with HPKIA ras cells and received a constant infusion of EB1089 or vehicle via osmotic minipumps when blood calcium levels reached 3 mmol/L (time 0). (**A**) Plasma calcium continued to rise in mice treated with vehicle, whereas they returned to near normal levels in animals treated with a constant infusion of EB1089 for 15 d. (**B**) Plasma PTHrP concentrations were measured at sacrifice in vehicle-treated ($\uparrow$Ca^{2+}, vehicle), EB1089 treated ($\uparrow$Ca^{2+}, EB1089) as well as in normocalcemic tumor-transplanted mice ($\rightarrow$ Ca^{2+}) and control non-tumor-bearing animals (**C**). Note the significant elevation of circulating PTHrP concentrations in vehicle-treated animals and their subsequent reduction in EB1089 treated animals.

the H500 Leydig tumor, which results in hypercalcemia consistently 2 wk after tumor implantation and death occurs approx 1 wk later. In this model, EB1089 was administered in a preventative fashion at the time of tumor implantation and was shown to inhibit the development of hypercalcemia *(149)*. Furthermore, PTHrP production, which increased progressively over the course of tumor development in untreated animals, was inhibited by EB1089 and the animals survived significantly longer (Fig. 4). Overall this study demonstrated that EB1089 inhibits PTHrP production by tumor cells, which, in turn, causes a reduction in circulating calcium levels. However, this model, although useful from the mechanistic standpoint did not reflect the clinical setting or the type of tumors seen in hypercalcemic cancer patients. Consequently, additional studies were needed to determine the effect of the vitamin D analog in a human tumor model once hypercalcemia was achieved. For this purpose, a nude mouse model was established in which PTHrP producing squamous cancer cells were implanted and EB1089 treatment was introduced following the establishment of the hypercalcemic state *(152)*. Animals treated with vehicle had worsening of hypercalcemia, whereas animals treated with EB1089 had a significant decrease in both PTHrP and circulating calcium levels over time (Fig. 5). These studies, therefore, indicated that the vitamin D analog EB1089 had the potential to be used clinically in two distinct situations (1) in patients with an established diagnosis of cancer but prior to the development of hypercalcemia and (2) in cancer patients diagnosed with MAH combined with an elevation of circulating levels of PTHrP.

In addition, vitamin D analogs might be useful in targeting PTHrP-producing tumors with high avidity for bone such as breast cancer. Indeed, over 90% of skeletal metastatic

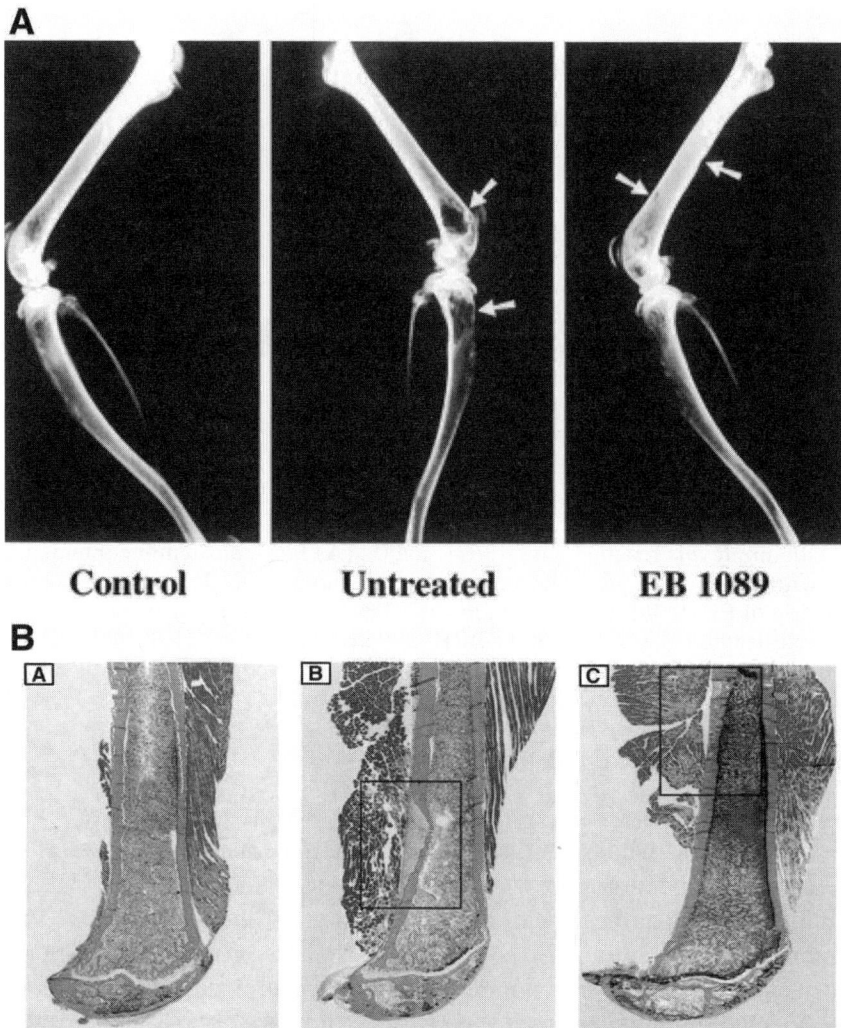

Fig. 6. Effect of EB1089 on skeletal metastasis. Female BALB/C/nu.nu mice were inoculated with MDA-231 cells via the left cardiac ventricle. Animals were treated with vehicle alone or EB1089 (14 μpm/24 h) via osmotic minipumps implanted the same day of tumor cells injections. Representative radiographs of normal animals (control) and animals receiving vehicle (untreated) or EB1089 are shown. Area of osteolytic legions in the tibia and femur are marked by arrows (upper panel). **Lower panel:** Histolgic analysis of the femora from a normal animal treated with EB1089 alone **(A)**. Osteolytic lesions of animals treated with vehicle alone **(B)** and osteolytic metastases in animals treated with EB1089 as assessed by Goldner-trichrome staining **(C)** (magnification, ×20).

breast cancer lesions have been reported to overexpress PTHrP *(212,213)* and it has been suggested that PTHrP influences the establishment/development of osteolytic lesions in breast cancer *(212,214)*. Several models of osteolytic metastases have been developed in both mice and rats *(105,215,216)* using intracardiac injection of tumor cells. In these models, animals rapidly develop osteolytic bone metastasis visible by radiologic examination used to monitor tumor progression and the effects of potential therapeutic agents.

Interestingly, bone lesions often occur without hypercalcemia but, nevertheless, lead to the death of the animals in just a few weeks *(105,117)*. We designed a preventative protocol using EB1089 in nude mice injected in the left cardiac ventricle with the human breast cancer cell line MDA-MB231 *(105)*. The development of bone metastasis in animals treated with either EB1089 or vehicle was assessed radiologically and by histomorphometric analysis of tumor volume within bones. Bone X-rays taken 5.5 wk following intracardiac injection of cancer cells showed a very significant reduction in the number and surface area of osteolytic lesions in EB1089-treated animals as compared to vehicle-treated mice (Fig. 6A). Furthermore, histomorphometric tumor volume evaluation showed large tumors invading both cortical and trabecular bone extending into the bone marrow cavity in untreated animals. In contrast, EB1089-treated mice had smaller lesions with minimal invasion of trabecular bone and the marrow cavity (Fig. 6B). Finally, EB1089-treated animals had less hindlimb paralysis (a measure of metastatic lesions impinging on the spinal cord) and survive much longer than nontreated mice. Although PTHrP expression was not measured in bone lesions, it was hypothesized that EB1089 suppressed tumor growth directly as well as indirectly through PTHrP suppression. More recently, we devised another strategy to block PTHrP production using its inactive precursor 25OHD$_3$ (Fig. 1). Here, we demonstrated that local conversion of 25(OH)D$_3$ to 1,25(OH)$_2$D$_3$ by the A375 PTHrP-producing melanoma cell line resulted in a strong inhibition of PTHrP production *(205)*. It remains to be established if this strategy could work in vivo.

In summary, our studies suggest that inhibition of PTHrP production with low-calcemic vitamin D analogs could be beneficial in both PTHrP-induced MAH and osteolytic bone metastasis with a substantial benefit on the patient's survival.

5. CONCLUSIONS

The new nonclassical actions of vitamin D have triggered considerable interest of this simple nutrient. The potent effect of 1,25(OH)$_2$D$_3$ in many cancer systems has led to the development of more potent and potentially suitable vitamin D analogs in cancer treatment. Many challenges remain in this novel field and, in particular, a need for a rational design of these analogs based on their mechanism of action. It is likely that some of the current analogs or even more potent and selective analogs will soon be part of our armamentorium in the fight against cancer.

ACKNOWLEDGMENTS

This work was supported by CIHR grants MOP-10839, MOP-64204, and the Dairy Farmers of Canada to Richard Kremer and CIHR grants MOP-10630 and MOP-12609 to Shafaat A. Rabbani. We thank Michael Macoritto, Cindy Solomon, Michael Sebag, Khadija El Abdaimi, and Dao Huang for their contributions and Connie Annett and Pat Hales for secretarial assistance.

REFERENCES

1. DeLuca HF. The vitamin D story: a collaborative effort of basic science and clinical medicine. *FASEB J* 1988;2(3):224–236.
2. Holick MF. Noncalcemic actions of 1,25-dihydroxyvitamin D3 and clinical applications. *Bone* 1995; 17(2 Suppl):107S–111S.

3. Bell PA. The chemistry of the vitamin D. In: Lawson DEM, ed. *Vitamin D*. New York, NY: Academic, 1978:1–50.

4. Holick MF, DeLuca HF. A new chromatographic system for vitamin D_3 and its metabolites; resolution of a new vitamin D_3 metabolite. *J Lipid Res* 1971; 12:460–465.

5. Masumoto O, Ohyama Y, Okuda K. Purification and characterization of vitamin D 25-hydroxylase from rat liver mitochondria. *J Biol Chem* 1988; 263:14,256–14,260.

6. Kawashima H, Jorika S, Kurokawa K. Localization of 25-hydroxyvitamin D_3-1α-hydroxylase and 24-hydroxylase along the rat nephron. *Proc Natl Acad Sci USA* 1981; 78:1199–1203.

7. Bell NH. Renal and non-renal 25-hydroxyvitamin D-1α-hydroxylases and their clinical significance. *J Bone Miner Res* 1998; 13:350–353.

8. Markestad T. Plasma concentrations of 1,25-dihydroxyvitamin D, 24,25-dihydroxyvitamin D, and 25,26-dihydroxyvitamin D in the first year of life. *J Clin Endocrinol Metab* 1983; 57:755–759.

9. Belsey R, Clark MB, Bernat M, Glowacki J, Holick MF, DeLuca HF, et al. The physiologic significance of plasma transport of vigtamin D and metabolites. *Am J Med* 1974; 57:50–56.

10. Cooke NC, Haddad JG. Vitamin D binding protein. In: Pike JW ed. *Vitamin D*. San Diego, CA: Academic, 1997:87–101.

11. Bouillon R, Van Baelen H, DeMoor P. The measurement of vitamin D-binding protein in human serum. *J Clin Endocrinol Metab* 1977; 45:225–231.

12. Jones G, Kung M, Kano D. The isolation and identification of two new metabolites of 25-hydroxyvitamin D_3 produced in the kidney. *J Biol Chem* 1983; 258:12,920–12,929.

13. Ohyama Y, Okuda K. Isolation and characterization of a cytochrome P-450 from rat kidney mitochondria that catalyzes the 24-hydroxylation of 25-hydroxyvitamin D_3. *J Biol Chem* 1991; 266:8690–8695.

14. Kumar R. Metabolism of 1,25-dihydroxyvitamin D_3. *Physiol Rev* 1984; 64:478–504.

15. Turner RT, Puzas JE, Forte MD, Lester GE, Gray TK, Howard GA, et al. In vitro synthesis of 1α,25-dihydroxycholecalciferol and 24,25-dihydroxycholecalciferol by isolated calvarial cells. *Proc Natl Acad Sci USA* 1980; 77:5720–5724.

16. Makin G, Lohnes D, Byford V, Ray R, Jones G. Target cell metabolism of 1,25-dihydroxyvitamin D_3 to calcitroic acid. Evidence for a pathway in kidney and bone involving 24-oxidation. *Biochem J* 1989; 262:173–180.

17. Tanaka Y, Lorenc RS, DeLuca HF. The role of 1,25-dihydroxyvitamin D_3 and parathyroid hormone in the regulation of chick renal 25-dihydroxyvitamin D_3-24-hydroxylase. *Arch Biochem Biophys* 1975; 171:521–526.

18. DeLuca HF. Metabolism and mechanism of action of vitamin D. In: Peck WA, ed. *Bone and Mineral Research Annual 1*. Princeton, NJ: Excerpta Medica, 1983:7–73.

19. Rasmussen H, DeLuca HF. Calcium homeostasis. *Ergebnisse der Physiol* 1963; 53:107–173.

20. Suda T, Miyaura C, Abe E. Modulation of cell differentiation, immune responses and tumor promotion by vitamin D compounds. In: Peck WA ed. *Bone and Mineral Research. Vol. 4*. New York, NY: Elsevier, 1986:1–48.

21. Hosomi J, Hosoi J, Abe E, Suda T, Kuroki T. Regulation of terminal differentiation of cultured mouse epidermal cells by 1α,25-dihydroxyvitamin D_3. *Endocrinology* 1983; 113:1950–1957.

22. Takahashi N, Akatsu T, Sakasi T. Induction of calcitonin receptors by 1,25-dihydroxyvitamin D_3 in osteoclast-like multinucleated cells formed in mouse bone marrow cells. *Endocrinology* 1988; 123:1504–1510.

23. Yang S, Smith C, DeLuca HF. 1α,25-dihydroxyvitamin D_3 and 19-nor-1α,25-dihydroxyvitamin D_2 suppress immunoglobulin production and thymic lymphocyte proliferation in vivo. *Biochem Biophys Acta* 1993; 1158:269–286.

24. Lemire JM, Archer DC. 1,25-dihydroxyvitamin D_3 prevents the in vivo induction of murine experimental autoimmune encephalomyelitis. *J Clin Invest* 1991; 87:1103–1107.

25. Abe J, Nakamura K, Takita Y, Nakano T, Irie H, Nishii Y. Prevention of immunological disorders in MRL/I mice a new synthetic analogue of vitamin D3: 22-oxa-1 alpha,25-dihydroxyvitamin D3. *J Nutr Sci Vitaminol* 1990; 36:21–31.

26. Fournier G, Gepner P, Sadouk M, Charreire J. In vivo beneficial effects of cyclosporin A and 1,25-dihydroxyvitamin D3 on the induction of experimental autoimmune thyroiditis. *Clin Immunol Immunopathol* 1990; 54:53–63.

27. Casteels KM, Mathieu C, Waer M, Valckx D, Overbergh L, Laureys JM, Bouillou R. Prevention of type I diabetes in nonobese diabetic mice by late intervention with nonhypercalcemic analogs or 1,25-

dihydroxyvitamin D_3 in combination with a short induction course of cyclosporin A. *Endocrinology* 1998; 139:95–102.

28. Bikle DD, Nemanic MK, Whitney JO, Elias PW. Neonatal human foreskin keratinocytes produce 1,25-dihydroxyvitamin D_3. *Biochemistry* 1986; 25:1545–1548.

29. Feldman D, Chen T, Hirst M, Colston K, Karasek M, Cone C. Demonstration of 1,25-dihydroxyvitamin D_3 receptors in human skin biopsies. *J Clin Endocrinol Metab* 1980; 52:1463–1465.

30. Huang DC, Papavasiliou V, Rhim J, Kremer R. Targeted disruption of the 25-hydroxyvitamin D_3 1α-hydroxylase gene in a *ras*–transformed human keratinocyte cell line: evidence for an autocrine growth regulatory function of 1α,25-dihydroxyvitamin D_3 *in vitro* and *in vivo*. *J Bone Miner Res* 1999; S141 (abstract 1033).

31. Sebag M, Gulliver W, Kremer R. Effects of 1,25-dihydroxyvitamin D_3 and calcium on growth and differentiation and on c-*fos* and p53 gene expression in normal human keratinocytes. *J Invest Dermatol* 1994; 103:323–329.

32. Smith EL, Walworth NC, Holick MF. Effect of 1_,25-dihydroxyvitamin D_3 on the morphologic and biochemical differentiation of cultured human epidermal keratinocytes grown in serum-free conditions. *J Invest Dermatol* 1986; 86:709–714.

33. Meichle A, Philipp A, Eilers M. The functions of Myc proteins. *Biochem Biophys Acta* 1992; 1114:129–146.

34. Almendral JM, Sommer D, Macdonald-Bravo H, Burckhardt J, Perera J, Bravo R. Complexity of the early genetic response to growth factors in mouse fibroblasts. *Mol Cell Biol* 1988; 8:2140–2148.

35. Matsumoto K, Hashimoto K, Nishida Y, Hashiro M, Yoshikawa K. Growth-inhibitory effects of 1,25-dihydroxyvitamin D_3 on human keratinocytes cultured in serum-free medium. *Biochem Biophys Res Commun* 1990; 166:916–923.

36. Sebag M, Henderson J, Rhim J, Kremer R. Relative resistance to 1,25-dihydroxyvitamin D_3 in a keratinocyte model of tumor progression. *J Biol Chem* 1992; 267:12,162–12,167.

37. Yuspa SH, Kilkenny AE, Steinert PM, Roop DR. Expression of murine epidermal differentiation markers is regulated by restricted extracellular calcium concentrations in vitro. *J Cell Biol* 1989; 109:1207–1217.

38. Simon M, Green H. Participation of membrane associated proteins in the formation of the cross-linked envelope of the keratinocyte. *Cell* 1984; 36:827–834.

39. Simon M, Green H. Enzymatic cross-linking of involucrin and other proteins by keratinocyte particulates in vitro. *Cell* 1985; 40:677–683.

40. Menon GK, Grayson S, Elias PM. Ionic calcium reservoirs in mammalian epidermis: ultrastructural localization by ionic capture cytochemistry. *J Invest Dermatol* 1985; 84:508–512.

41. Younus J, Gilchrest B. Modulation of mRNA levels during human keratinocyte differentiation. *J Cell Physiol* 1992; 152:232–239.

42. Su M-J, Bikle DD, Mancianti M-L, Pillai S. 1,25-dihydroxyvitamin D_3 potentiates the keratinocyte response to calcium. *J Biol Chem* 1994; 269:14,723–14,729.

43. Norman AW, Nemere I, Zhou L-X, Bishop JE, Lowe KE, Maiyar AC, et al. 1,25(OH)$_2$-vitamin D_3, a steroid hormone that produces biologic effects via both genomic and non-genomic pathways. *J Steroid Biochem Mol Biol* 1992; 41:231–240.

44. Civitelli R, Kim YE, Gunsten SL, Fujimori A, Huskey M, Avioli LV, et al. Nongenomic activation of the calcium message system by vitamin D metabolites in osteoblast-like cells. *Endocrinology* 1990; 127:2253–2262.

45. Evans RM. The steroid and thyroid hormone receptor superfamily. *Science* 1988; 240:889–895.

46. Mangelsdorf DJ, Thummel C, Beato, M, Herrlich P, Schutz G, Umesono K, et al. The nuclear receptor superfamily: the second decade. *Cell* 1995; 83:835–839.

47. Glass CK. Differential recognition of target genes by nuclear receptor monomers, dimers, and heterodimers. *Endocrine Rev* 1994; 15:391–407.

48. Stunnenberg HG. Mechanisms of transactivation of retinoic acid receptors. *Bioessays* 1993; 15:309–315.

49. Leid M, Kastner P, Chambon P. Multiplicity generates diversity in the retinoic acid signaling pathways. *Trends Biochem Sci* 1992; 17:427–433.

50. Chambon P. A decade of molecular biology of retinoic acid receptors. *FASEB J* 1996; 10:940–954.

51. Wahli RL, Martinez E. Superfamily of steroid nuclear receptors: positive and negative regulators of gene expression. *FASEB J* 1991; 7:273–282.

52. Mangelsdorf DJ, Umesono K, Kliewer SA, Borgmeyer Y, Ong ES, Evans RM. A direct repeat in the cellular retinol-binding protein type II gene confers differential regulation by RXR and RAR. *Cell* 1991; 66:555–561.

53. Smith WC, Nakshatri H, Leroy P, Rees J, Chambon P. A retinoic acid response element is present in the mouse cellular retinol binding protein I (mCRMPI) promoter. *EMBO J* 1991; 10:22,223–22,230.

54. Noda M, Vogel R, Craig AM, Prahl J, DeLuca HF, Denhardt D. Identification of a DNA sequence responsible for binding of the 1,25-dihydroxyvitamin D_3 receptor and 1,25-dihydroxyvitamin D_3 enhancement of mouse secreted phosphoprotein 1 (spp-1 or osteopontin) gene expression. *Proc Natl Acad Sci USA* 1990; 87:9995–9999.

55. Hoffman B, Lehmann JM, Zhang XK, Hermann T, Husmann M, Graupner G, et al. A retinoic acid receptor-specific element controls the retinoic acid receptor-beta promoter. *Mol Endocrinol* 1990; 4: 1727–1736.

56. Mangelsdorf DJ, Umesono K, Evans RM. The retinoid receptors. In: *The Retinoids: Biology, Chemistry, and Medicine.* New York: Raven, 1994:319–349.

57. Baker AR, McDonnell M, Hughes M, Crisp TM, Mangelsdorf DJ, Haussler MR, et al. Cloning and expression of full-length cDNA encoding human vitamin D receptor. *Proc Natl Acad Sci USA* 1988; 85:3294–3298.

58. Sone T, Ozono K, Pike JW. A 55-kilodalton accessory factor facilitates vitamin D receptor DNA binding. *Mol Endocrinol* 1991; 5:1578–1586.

59. Forman BM, Samuels HH. Interactions among a subfamily of nuclear hormone receptors: the regulatory zipper model. *Mol Endocrinol* 1990; 4:1293–1301.

60. Nakajima S, Hsieh J-C, MacDonald PN, Galligan MA, Haussler CA, Whitfield GK, Haussler MR. The C-terminal region of the vitamin D receptor is essential to form a complex with a receptor auxiliary factor required for high affinity binding to the vitamin D responsive element. *Mol Endocrinol* 1994; 8:159–172.

61. Mangelsdorf DJ, Borgmeyer U, Heyman RA, Zhou JY, Ong ES, Oro AE, Kakizuka A, Evans RM. Characterization of three RXR genes that mediate the action of 9-*cis* retinoic acid. *Genes Dev* 1992; 86:329–344.

62. Kephart DD, Walfish PG, DeLuca HF, Butt TR. Retinoid X receptor isotype identity directs human vitamin D receptor heterodimer transactivation from the 24-hydroxylase vitamin D response element in yeast. *Mol Endocrinol* 1996; 10:408–419.

63. Kimmel-Jehan C, Darwish HM, Strugnell SA, Jehan F, Wiefling B, DeLuca HF. DNA bending is induced by binding of vitamin D receptor-retinoid X receptor heterodimers to vitamin D response elements. *J Cell Biochem* 1999; 74:220–228.

64. DeMay MB, Gerardi JM, DeLuca HF, Kronenberg HM. DNA sequences in the rat osteocalcin gene that bind the 1,25-dihydroxyvitamin D_3 receptor and confer responsiveness to 1,25-dihydroxyvitamin D_3. *Proc Natl Acad Sci USA* 1990; 87:369–373.

65. Kerner SA, Scott RA, Pike JW. Sequence elements in the human osteocalcin gene confer basal activation and inducible response to hormonal vitamin D3. *Proc Natl Acad Sci USA* 1989; 86:4455–4459.

66. Jurutka PW, Hsieh J-C, Haussler MR. Characterization of a new functional 1,25-dihydroxyvitamin D_3 responsive element in the promoter region of the rat 25-hydroxyvitamin D_3 24-hydroxylase gene. *J Bone Miner Res* 1994; 9(Suppl 1):S160.

67. Darwish HM, DeLuca HF. Analysis of binding of the 1,25-dihydroxyvigtamin D_3 receptor to positive and negative vitamin D response elements. *Arch Biochem Biophys* 1996; 334:223–234.

68. Kremer R, Sebag M, Champigny C, Meerovitch K, Hendy GN, White J, et al. Identification and characterization of 1,25-dihydroxyvitamin D_3-responsive repressor sequences in the rat parathyroid hormone related peptide gene. *J Biol Chem* 1996; 271:16,310–16,316.

69. Lian JB, Shalhoub V, Aslam F, Frenkel B, Green J, Hamrah M, et al. Species-specific glucocorticoid and 1,25-dihydroxyvitamin D responsiveness in mouse MC3T3-E1 osteoblasts: dexamethasone inhibits osteoblast differentiation and vitamin D down-regulates osteocalcin gene expression. *Endocrinology* 1997; 138:2117–2127.

70. MacDonald PN, Dowd DR, Nakajima S, Galligan MA, Reeder MC, Haussler CA, et al. Retinoid X receptor stimulate and 9-*cis* retinoic acid inhibits 1,25-dihydroxyvitamin D_3-activated expression of the rat osteocalcin gene. *Mol Cell Biol* 1993; 13:5907–5917.

71. Haussler MR, Haussler CA, Jurutka PW, Thompson PD, Hsieh J-C, Remus LS, Selznick SH, et al. The vitamin D hormone and its nuclear receptor: molecular actions and disease states. *J Endocrinol* 1997; 154:S57–S73.

72. Zugmaier, Jager R, Grage B, Gottardis MM, Havemann K, Knabbe C. Growth-inhibitory effects of vitamin D analogues and retinoids on human pancreatic cancer cells. *Br J Cancer* 1996; 73(11):1341–1346.

73. Kane KF, Langman MJS, Williams GR. Antiproliferative responses of two human colon cancer cell lines to vitamin D_3 are differentially modified by 9-*cis* retinoic acid. *Cancer Res* 1996; 56:623–632.

74. Kang S, Xiao-Yan L, Duell EA, Voorhees J. The retinoid X receptor agonist 9-*cis* retinoic acid and the 24-hydroxylase inhibitor ketoconazole increase activity of 1,25-dihydroxyvitamin D_3 in human skin *in vivo*. *J Invest Dermatol* 1997; 108:513–518.

75. Blutt SE, Allegretto EA, Pike JW, Weigel JL. 1,25-dihydroxyvitamin D_3 and 9-*cis* retinoic acid act synergistically to inhibit the growth of LNCaP prostate cells and cause accumulation of cells in G_1. *Endocrinology* 1997; 138:1491–1497.

76. Meyer M-E, Gronemeyer H, Turcotte B, Bocquel M-T, Tasset D, Chambon P. Steroid hormone receptors compete for factors that mediate their enhancer function. *Cell* 1989; 57:433–442.

77. Onate K, Tsai SY, Rsai M-J, O'Malley BW. Sequence and characterization of a coactivator for the steroid hormone receptor superfamily. *Science* 1995; 270:1354–1357.

78. Durand B, Saunders M, Gaundon C, Roy B, Losson R, Chambon P. Activation function 2 (AF-2) of retinoic acid receptor and 9-*cis*-retinoic acid receptor: presence of a conserved autonomous constitutive activating domain and influence of the nature of the response element on AF-2 activity. *EMBO J* 1994; 13:5370–5382.

79. Danielian PS, White R, Lees JA, Parker MG. Identification of a conserved region required for hormone dependent transcriptional activation by steroid hormone receptors. *EMBO J* 1992; 11:1025–1033.

80. Barettino D, Ruiz MV, Stunnenberg HG. Characterization of the ligand-dependent transactivation domain of thyroid hormone receptor. *EMBO J* 1994; 13:3039–3049.

81. Masuyama H, Brownfield CM, St-Arnaud R, MacDonald PN. Evidence for ligand-dependent intramolecular folding of the AF-2 domain in vitamin D receptor-activated transcription and coactivator interaction. *Mol Endocrinol* 1997; 11:1507–1517.

82. Tone Y, Collingwood TN, Adams M, Chatterjee VK. Functional analysis of a transactivation domain in the thyroid hormone beta receptor. *J Biol Chem* 1994; 269:31,157–31,161.

83. Zhang C, Baudino TA, Dowd DR, Tokumaru H, Wang W, MacDonald PN. Ternary complexes and cooperative interplay between NCoA-62/Ski-interacting protein and steroid receptor coactivators in vitamin D receptor-mediated transcription. *J Biol Chem* 2001; 276(44):40,614–40,620.

84. Rachez C, Suldan Z, Ward J, Chang CP, Burakov D, Erdjument-Bromage H, et al. A novel protein complex that interacts with the vitamin D3 receptor in a ligand-dependent manner and enhances VDR transactivation in a cell-free system. *Genes Dev* 1998; 12:1787–1800.

85. Rachez C, Lemon BD, Suldan Z, Bromleigh V, Gamble M, Naar AM, et al. Ligand-dependent transcription activation by nuclear receptors requires the DRIP complex. *Nature* 1999; 398(6730):824–828.

86. Chen JD, Evans RM. A transcriptional corepressor that interacts with nuclear hormone receptors. *Nature* 1995; 377:454–457.

87. Horlein AJ, Naar AM, Heinzel T, Torchia J, Gloss B, Kurokawa R, et al. Ligand-independent repression by the thyroid hormone receptor mediated by a nuclear receptor corepressor. *Nature* 1995; 377:397–404.

88. Heinzel T, Lavinsky RM, Mullen T-M, Soderstrom M, Laherty CD, Torchia J, et al. A complex containing N-CoR, mSin3 and histone deacetylase mediates transcriptional repression. *Nature* 1997; 387:43–48.

89. Perlmann T, Vennstrom B. The sound of silence. *Nature* 1995; 377:387–388.

90. Jones G, Calverley MJ. A dialogue on analogues: newer vitamin D drugs for use in bone disease, psoriasis, and cancer. *Trends Endocrinol Metab* 1993; 4:297–303.

91. Farach-Carson MC, Abe J, Nishii Y, Khoury R, Wright GC, Norman AW. 22-oxacalcitriol: dissection of 1,25(OH)$_2$D$_3$ receptor-mediated and Ca^{2+} entry-stimulating pathways. *Am J Physiol* 1993; 265: F705–F711.

92. Tsugawa N, Nakagawa K, Kurobe M, Ono Y, Kubodera N, Ozono K, et ak. In vitro biological activities of a series of 2 beta-substituted analogues of 1 alpha,25-dihydroxyvitamin D3. *Biol Pharm Bull* 2000; 23(1):66–71.

93. Norman AW, Manchand PS, Uskokovic MR, Okamura WH, Takeuchi JA, Bishop JE, et al. Characterization of a novel analogue of 1alpha,25(OH)(2)-vitamin D(3) with two side chains: interaction with its nuclear receptor and cellular actions. *J Med Chem* 2000; 43(14):2719–2730.

94. Hisitake J, O'Kelly J, Uskokovic MR, Tomoyasu S, Koeffler HP. Novel vitamin D(3) analog, 21-(3-methyl-3-hydroxy-butyl)-19-nor D(3), that modulates cell growth, differentiation, apoptosis, cell cycle, and induction of PTEN in leukemic cells. *Blood* 2001; 97:2427–2433.

95. Bury Y, Ruf D, Hansen CM, Kissmeyer AM, Binderup L, Carlberg C. Molecular evaluation of vitamin D3 receptor agonists designed for topical treatment of skin diseases. *J Invest Dermatol* 2001; 116(5): 785–792.

96. Veyron P, Pamphile R, Binderup L, Touraine JL. Two novel vitamin D analogues, KH 1060 and CB 966, prolong skin allograft survival in mice. *Transpl Immunol* 1993; 1(1):72–76.

97. Rewin E, Olgaard K. The in vivo effect of a new, in vitro, extremely potent vitamin D3 analog KH1060 on the suppression of renal allograft rejection in the rat. *Calcif Tissue Int* 1994; 54(2):150–154.

98. Fujishima T, Konno K, Nakagawa K, Kurobe M, Okano T, Takayama H. Efficient synthesis and biological evaluation of all A-ring diastereomers of 1alpha,25-dihydroxyvitamin D3 and its 20-epimer. *Bioorg Med Chem* 2000; 8(1):123–134.

99. Verlinden L, Verstuyf A, Van Camp M, Marcelis S, Sabbe K, Zhao XY, et al. Two novel 14-Epi-analogues of 1,25-dihydroxyvitamin D3 inhibit the growth of human breast cancer cells in vitro and in vivo. *Cancer Res* 2000; 60(10):2673–2679.

100. Colston KW, Mackay AG, James SY, Binderup L, Chander S, Coombes RC. EB1089: a new vitamin D analogue that inhibits the growth of breast cancer cells in vivo and in vitro. *Biochem Pharmacol* 1992; 44(12):2273–2280.

101. Lokeshwar BL, Schwartz GG, Selzer MG, Burnstein KL, Zhuang SH, Block NL, et al. Inhibition of prostate cancer metastasis in vivo: a comparison of 1,23-dihydroxyvitamin D (calcitriol) and EB1089. *Cancer Epidemiol Biomarkers Prev* 1999; 8(3):241–248.

102. Diaz GD, Paraskeva C, Thomas MG, Binderup L, Hague A. Apoptosis is induced by the active metabolite of vitamin D3 and its analogue EB1089 in colorectal adenoma and carcinoma cells: possible implications for prevention and therapy. *Cancer Res* 2000; 60(8):2304–2312.

103. Colston KW, James SY, Ofori-Kuragu EA, Binderup L, Gran AG. Vitamin D receptors and anti-proliferative effects of vitamin D derivatives in human pancreatic carcinoma cells in vivo and in vitro. *Br J Cancer* 1997; 76(8):1017–1020.

104. El Abdaimi K, Papavasiliou V, Goltzman D, Kremer R. Expression and regulation of parathyroid hormone-related peptide in normal and malignant melanocytes. *Am J Physiol Cell Physiol* 2000; 279: C1230–C1238.

105. El Abdaimi K, Dion N, Papavasiliou V, Cardinal P-E, Binderup L, Goltzman D, et al. ARTICLE TITLE MISSING HERE. *Cancer Res* 2000; 60:4412–4418.

106. Oikawa T, Hirotani K, Ogasawara H, Katayama T, Nakamura O, Iwaguchi T, et al. Inhibition of angiogenesis by vitamin D3 analogues. *Eur J Pharmacol* 1990; 178(2):247–250. Erratum: *Eur J Pharmacol* 1990; 182(3):616.

107. Abe J, Nakano T, Nishii Y, Matsumoto T, Ogata E, Ikeda K. A novel vitamin D3 analog, 22-oxa-1,25-dihydroxyvitamin D3, inhibits the growth of human breast cancer in vitro and in vivo without causing hypercalcemia. *Endocrinology* 1991; 129:832–827.

108. Abe Hashimoto J, Kikuchi T, Matsumoto T, Nishii Y, Ogata E, Ikeda K. Antitumor effect of 22-oxa-calcitriol, a noncalcemic analogue of calcitriol, in athymic mice implanted with human breast carcinoma and its synergism with tamoxifen. *Cancer Res* 1993; 53(11):2534–2537.

109. Kawa S, Yoshizawa K, Tokoo M, Imai H, Oguchi H, Kiyosawa K, et al. Inhibitory effect of 220-oxa-1,25-dihydroxyvitamin D3 on the proliferation of pancreatic cancer cell lines. *Gastroenterology* 1996; 110(5):1605–1613.

110. Verstuyf A, Verlinden L, van Etten E, Shi L, Wu Y, D'Halleweyn C, et al. Biological activity of CD-ring modified 1alpha,25-dihydroxyvitamin D analogues: C-ring and five-membered D-ring analogues. *J Bone Miner Res* 2000; 15(2):237–252.

111. Boehm MF, Fitzgerald P, Zou A, Elgort MG, Bischoff ED, Mere L, et al. Novel nonsecosteroidal vitamin D mimics exert VDR-modulating activities with less calcium mobilization than 1,25-dihydroxyvitamin D3. *Chem Biol* 1999; 6(5):265–275.

112. Polek TC, Murthy S, Blutt SE, Boehm MF, Zou A, Weigel NL, et al. Novel nonsecosteroidal vitamin D receptor modulator inhibits the growth of LNCaP xenograft tumors in athymic mice without increased serum calcium. *Prostate* 2001; 49(3):224–233.

113. Bouillon R, Allewaert K, Xiang DZ, Tan BK, van Baelen H. Vitamin D analogs with low affinity for the vitamin D binding protein: enhanced in vitro and decreased in vivo activity. *J Bone Miner Res* 1991; 6(10):1051–1057.

114. Masuda S, Strugnell S, Calverley MJ, Makin HL, Kremer R, Jones G. In vitro metabolism of the anti-psoriatic vitamin D analog, calcipotriol, in two cultured human keratinocyte models. *J Biol Chem* 1994; 269:4794–4803.

115. Masuda S, Byford V, Kremer R, Makin HL, Kubodera N, Nishii Y, et al. In vitro metabolism of the vitamin D analog, 22-oxacalcitriol, using cultured osteosarcoma, hepatoma, and keratinocyte cell. *J Biol Chem* 1996; 271(15):8700–8708.

116. Jaaskelainen T, Ryhanen S, Mahonen A, DeLuca HF, Maenpaa PH. Mechanism of action of superactive vitamin D analogs through regulated receptor degradation. *J Cell Biochem* 2000; 76(4):548-558.

117. Sasaki H, Harada H, Handa Y, Morino H, Suzawa M, Shimpo E, et al. Transcriptional activity of a fluorinated vitamin D analog on VDR-RXR-mediated gene expression. *Biochemistry* 1995; 34(1): 370–377.

118. Cheskis B, Lemon BD, Uskokovic M, Lomedico PT, Freedman LP. Vitamin D3-retinoid X receptor dimerization, DNA binding, and transactivation are differentially affected analogs of 1,25-dihydroxybvitamin D3. *Mol Endo* 1995; 9(12):1814–1824.

119. Yang W, Freedman LP. 20-Epi analogues of 1,25-dihydroxyvitamin D3 are highly potent inducers of DRIP coactivator complex binding to the vitamin D3 receptor. *J Biol Chem* 1999; 274(24):16,838–16,845.

120. Takeyama K, Masuhiro Y, Fuse H, Endoh H, Murayama A, Kitanaka S, et al. Selective interaction of vitamin D receptor with transcriptional coactivators by a vitamin D analog. *Mol Cell Biol* 1999; 19(2): 1049–1055.

121. Abe E, Miyaura C, Sakagami H, Takeda M, Konno K, Yamazaki T, Yoshiki S, Suda T. Differentiation of mouse myeloid leukemia cells induced by 1 alpha,25-dihydroxyvitamin D3. *Proc Natl Acad Sci USA* 1981; 78(8):4990–4994.

122. Garland FC, Garland CF, Gorham ED, Young JF. Geographic variation in breast cancer mortality in the United States: a hypothesis involving exposure to solar radiation. *Prev Med* 1990; 19(6):614–622.

123. Gorham ED, Garland CF, Garland FC. Acid haze air pollution and breast and colon cancer mortality in 20 Canadian cities. *Can J Public Health* 1989; 80(2):96–100.

124. Gorham ED, Garland FC, Garland CF. Sunlight and breast cancer incidence in the USSR. *Int J Epidemiol* 1990; 19(4):820–824.

125. Schwartz GG, Hulka BS. Is vitamin D deficiency a risk factor for prostate cancer? (hypothesis). *Anticancer Res* 1990; 10(5A):1307–1311.

126. Garland C, Shekelle RB, Barrett-Connor E, Criqui MH, Rossof AH, Paul O. Dietary vitamin D and calcium and risk of colorectal cancer: a 19-year prospective study in men. *Lancet* 1985; 1(8424):307–309.

127. Corder EH, Guess HA, Hulka BS, Friedman GD, Sadler M, Vollmer RT, et al. Vitamin D and prostate cancer: a prediagnostic study with stored sera. *Cancer Epidemiol Biomarkers Prev* 1993; 2(5):467–472.

128. Braun MM, Helzlsouer KJ, Hollis BW, Comstock GW. Prostate cancer and prediagnostic levels of serum vitamin D metabolites (Maryland, United States). *Cancer Causes Control* 1995; 6(3):235–239.

129. Nomura AM, Stemmermann GN, Lee J, Kolonel LN, Chen TC, Turner A, et al. Serum vitamin D metabolite levels and the subsequent development of prostate cancer (Hawaii, United States). *Cancer Causes Control* 1998; 9(4):425–432.

130. Ahonen MH, Tenkanen L, Teppo L, Hakama M, Tuohimaa P. Prostate cancer risk and prediagnostic serum 25-hydroxyvitamin D levels. (Finland) *Cancer Causes Control* 2000; 11(9):847–852.

131. Garland FC, Comstock GW, Garland FC, Helsing KJ, Shaw EK, Gorham ED. Serum 25-hydroxyvitamin D and colon cancer: eight-year prospective study. *Lancet* 1989; 2(8673):1176–1178.

132. Huang DC, Papavasiliou V, Rhim JS, Horst RL, Kremer R. Targeted disruption of the 25-hydroxyvitamin D3 1alpha-hydroxylase gene in ras-transformed keratinocytes demonstrates that locally produced 1alpha,25-dihydroxyvitamin D3 suppresses growth an induces differentiation in autocrine fashion. *Mol Cancer Res* 2002; 1(1):56–67.

133. Colston KW, Hansen CM. Mechanisms implicated in the growth regulatory effects of vitamin D in breast cancer [review]. *Endocr Relat Cancer* 2002; 9(1):45–59.

134. Polek TC, Weigel NL. Vitamin D and prostate cancer [review]. *J Androl* 2002; 23(1):9–17.

135. Wargovich MJ, Lointier PH. Calcium and vitamin D modulate mouse colon epithelial proliferation and growth characteristics of a human colon tumor cell line [review]. *Can J Physiol Pharmacol* 1987; 65(3): 472–477.

136. Yu J, Papavasiliou V, Rhim J, Goltzman D, Kremer R. Vitamin D analogs: new therapeutic agents for the treatment of squamous cancer and its associated hypercalcemia. *Anticancer Drugs* 1995; 6(1):101–108.

137. Colston K, Colston MJ, Feldman D. 1,25-dihydroxyvitamin D3 and malignant melanoma: the presence of receptors and inhibition of cell growth in culture. *Endocrinology* 1981; 108(3):1083–1086.

138. Bouillon R, Okamura WH, Norman AW. Bouillon R et al Structure-function relationships in the vitamin D endocrine system [review]. *Endocr Rev* 1995; 16(2):200–257.

139. Kremer R, and Goltzman D. Hypercalcemia due to PTHrP. In: Bilezikian J, Levine M, Marcus R, eds. *The Parathyroids: Basic and Clinical Concepts*, 2nd ed. San Diego, CA: Academic, 2001:671–689.

140. Eisman JA, Barkla DH, Tutton PJ. Suppression of in vivo growth of human cancer solid tumor xenografts by 1,25-dihydroxyvitamin D_3. *Cancer Res* 1987; 47(1):21–25.

141. Getzenberg RH, Light BW, Lapco PE, Konety BR, Nangia AK, Acierno JS, et al. Vitamin D inhibition of prostate adenocarcinoma growth and metastasis in the Dunning rat prostate model system. *Urology* 1997; 50(6):999–1006.

142. Fujioka T, Hasegawa M, Ishikura K, Matsushita Y, Sato M, Tanji S. Inhibition of tumor growth and angiogenesis by vitamin D_3 agents in murine renal cell carcinoma. *J Urol* 1998; 160(1):247–251.

143. Yu WD, McElwain MC, Modzelewski RA, Russell DM, Smith DC, Trump DL, et al. Enhancement of 1,25-dihydroxyvitamin D_3-mediated antitumor activity with dexamethasone. *J Natl Cancer Inst* 1998; 90(2):134–141.

144. Honma Y, Hozumi M, Abe E, Konno K, Fukushima M, Hata S, et al. 1 alpha,25-Dihydroxyvitamin D_3 and 1 alpha-hydroxyvitamin D_3 prolong survival time of mice inoculated with myeloid leukemia cells. *Proc Natl Acad Sci USA* 1983; 80(1):201–204.

145. Sato T, Takusagawa K, Asoo N, Konno K. Effect of 1 alpha-hydroxyvitamin D_3 on metastasis of rat ascites hepatoma K-231. *Br J Cancer* 1984; 50(1):123–125.

146. VanWeelden K, Flanagan L, Binderup L, Tenniswood M, Welsh J. Apoptotic regression of MCF-7 xenografts in nude mice treated with the vitamin D_3 analog, EB1089. *Endocrinology* 1998; 139(4): 2102–2110.

147. James SY, Mercer E, Brady M, Binderup L, Colston KW. EB1089, a synthetic analogue of vitamin D, induces apoptosis in breast cancer cells in vivo and in vitro. *Br J Pharmacol* 1998; 125(5):953–962.

148. Akhter J, Chen X, Bowrey P, Bolton EJ, Morris DL. Vitamin D_3 analog, EB1089, inhibits growth of subcutaneous xenografts of the human colon cancer cell line, LoVo, in a nude mouse model. *Dis Colon Rectum* 1997; 40(3):317–321.

149. Haq M, Kremer R, Goltzman D, Rabbani SA. A vitamin D analogue (EB1089) inhibits parathyroid hormone-related peptide production and prevents the development of malignancy-associagted hypercalcemia in vivo. *J Clin Invest* 1993; 91:2416–2422.

150. Colston KW, James SY, Ofori-Kuragu EA, Binderup L, Grant AG. Vitamin D receptors and antiproliferative effects of vitamin D derivatives in human pancreatic carcinoma cells in vivo and in vitro. *Br J Cancer* 1997; 76(8):1017–1020.

151. Perez-Stable CM, Schwartz GG, Farinas A, Finegold M, Binderup L, Howard GA, et al. The G gamma/T-15 transgenic mouse model of androgen-independent prostate cancer: target cells of carcinogenesis and the effect of the vitamin D analogue EB 1089. *Cancer Epidemiol Biomarkers Prev* 2002; 11(6):555–563.

152. El Abdaimi K, Papavasiliou V, Rabbani SA, Rhim JS, Goltzman D, Kremer R. Reversal of hypercalcemia with the vitamin D analogue EB1089 in a human model of squamous cancer. *Cancer Res* 1999; 59:3325–3328.

153. Schwartz GG, Hill CC, Oeler TA, Becich MJ, Bahnson RR. 1,25-Dihydroxy-16-ene-23-yne-vitamin D_3 and prostate cancer cell proliferation in vivo. *Urology* 1995; 46(3):365–369.

154. Shternfeld IS, Lasudry JG, Chappell RJ, Darjatmoko SR, Albert DM. Antineoplastic effect of 1,25-dihydroxy-16-ene-23-yne-vitamin D_3 analogue in transgenic mice with retinoblastoma. *Arch Ophthalmol* 1996; 114(11):1396–1401.

155. Light BW, Yu WD, McElwain MC, Russell DM, Trump DL, Johnson CS. Potentiation of cisplatin antitumor activity using a vitamin D analogue in a murine squamous cell carcinoma model system. *Cancer Res* 1997; 57(17):3759–3764.

156. Zhou JY, Norman AW, Chen DL, Sun GW, Uskokovic M, Koeffler HP. 1,25-Dihydroxy-16-ene-23-yne-vitamin D_3 prolongs survival time of leukemic mice. *Proc Natl Acad Sci USA* 1990; 87(10):3929–3932.

157. Evans SR, Schwartz AM, Shchepotin EI, Uskokovic M, Shchepotin IB. Growth inhibitory effects of 1,25-dihydroxyvitamin D_3 and its synthetic analogue, 1alpha,25-dihydroxy-16-ene-23yne-26,27-hexafluoro-19-nor-cholecalcifero l (Ro 25-6760), on a human colon cancer xenograft. *Clin Cancer Res* 1998; 4(11):2869–2876.

158. Anzano MA, Smith JM, Uskokovic MR, Peer CW, Mullen LT, Letterio JJ, et al. 1 alpha,25-Dihydroxy-16-ene-23-yne-26,27-hexafluorocholecalciferol (Ro24-5531), a new deltanoid (vitamin D analogue) for prevention of breast cancer in the rat. *Cancer Res* 1994; 54(7):1653–1656.

159. Wali RK, Bissonnette M, Khare S, Hart J, Sitrin MD, Brasitus TA. 1 alpha,25-Dihydroxy-16-ene-23-yne-26,27,hexafluorocholecalciferol, a noncalcemic analogue of 1 alpha,25-dihydroxyvitamin D_3, inhibits azowymethane-induced colonic tumorigenesis. *Cancer Res* 1995; 55(14):3050–3054.

160. Lucia MS, Anzano MA, Slayter MV, Anver MR, Green DM, Shrader MW, et al. Chemopreventive activity of tamoxifen, N-(4-hydroxyphenyl)retinamide, and the vitamin D analogue Ro24-5531 for androgen-promoted carcinomas of the rat seminal vesicle and prostate. *Cancer Res* 1995; 55(23):5621–5627.

161. Otoshi T, Iwata H, Kitano M, Nishizawa Y, Morii H, Yano Y, et al. Inhibition of intestinal tumor development in rat multi-organ carcinogenesis and aberrant crypt foci in rat colon carcinogenesis by 22-oxa-calcitriol, a synthetic analogue of 1 alpha, 25-dihydroxyvitamin D_3. *Carcinogenesis* 1995; 16(9):2091–2097.

162. Barreto AM, Schwartz GG, Woodruff R, Cramer SD. 25-Hydroxyvitamin D_3, the prohormone of 1,25-dihydroxyvitamin D_3, inhibits the proliferation of primary prostatic epithelial cells. *Cancer Epidemiol Biomarkers Prev* 2000; 9(3):265–270.

163. Hsu JY, Feldman D, McNeal JE, Peehl DM. Reduced 1alpha-hydroxylase activity in human prostate cancer cells correlates with decreased susceptibility to 25-hydroxyvitamin D_3-induced growth inhibition. *Cancer Res* 2001; 61(7):2852–2856.

164. Minghetti P, Norman AW. 1,25(OH)2-vitamin D3 receptors: gene regulation and genetic circuitry [review]. *FASEB J* 1988; 2(15):3043–3053.

165. Binderup L, Binderup E, Godtfredsen WO. Development of new vitamin D analongs. In: Feldman D, Glorieux FH, Pike JW, eds. *Vitamin D*. San Diego, CA: Academic, 1997:1027–1043.

166. Colston KW, Berger U, Coombs RC. Possible role for witamin D incontrolling breast cancer cell proliferation. *Lancet* 1989; 28:188–191.

167. Krishnan AV, Feldman D. Regulation of vitamin D receptor abundance. In: Feldman D, Glorieux FH, Pike JW, eds. *Vitamin D*. San Diego, CA: Academic, 1997:179–200.

168. van den Bemd GC, Pols HA, Birkenhager JC, van Leeuwen JP. Conformational change and enhanced stabilization of the vitamin D receptor by the 1,25-dihydroxyvitamin D3 analog KH1060. *Proc Natl Acad Sci USA* 1996; 93(20):10,685–10,690.

169. Haussler MR, Jurutka PW, Hsieh JC, Nuclear vitamin D receptor: structure, function, phosphorylation and control of gene transcription. In: Feldman D, Glorieux FH, Pike JW, eds. *Vitamin D*. San Diego, CA: Academic, 1997:149–177.

170. Crofts LA, Hancock MS, Morrison NA, Eisman JA. Multiple promoters direct the tissue-specific expression of novel N-terminal variant human vitamin D receptor gene transcripts. *Proc Natl Acad Sci USA* 1998; 95(18):10,529–10,534.

171. Zou A, Elgort MG, Allegretto EA. Retinoid X receptor (RXR) ligands activate the human 25-hydroxyvitamin D3-24-hydroxylase promoter via RXR heterodimer binding to two vitamin D-responsive elements and elicit additive effects with 1,25-dihydroxyvitamin D3. *J Biol Chem* 1997; 272(30):19,027–19,034.

172. MacDonald PN, Dowd DR, Nakajima S, Galligan MA, Reeder MC, Haussler CA, et al. Retinoid X receptors stimulate and 9-cis retinoic acid inhibits 1,25-dihydroxyvitamin D3-activated expression of the rat osteocalcin gene. *Mol Cell Biol* 1993; 13:5907–5917.

173. Li M, Indra AK, Warot X, Brocard J, Messaddeq N, Kato S, et al. Skin abnormalities generated by temporally controlled RXRalpha mutations in mouse epidermis. *Nature* 2000; 407(6804):633–636.

174. Yagishita N, Yamamoto Y, Yoshizawa T, Sekine K, Uematsu Y, Murayama H, et al. Aberrant growth plate development in VDR/RXR gamma double null mutant mice. *Endocrinology* 2001; 142(12):5332–5341.

175. Haussler MR, Haussler CA, Jurutka PW, Thompson PD, Hsieh J-C, Remus LS, et al. The vitamin D hormone and its nuclear receptor: molecular actions and disease states. *J Endocrinol* 1997; 154:S57–S73.

176. Haussler MR, Whitfield GK, Haussler CA, Hsieh JC, Thompson PD, Selznick SH, et al. The nuclear vitamin D receptor: biological and molecular regulatory properties revealed. *J Bone Miner Res* 1998; 13:325–349.

177. Jurutka PW, Whitfield GK, Hsieh JC, Thompson PD, Haussler CA, Haussler MR. Molecular nature of the vitamin D receptor and its role in regulation of gene expression [review]. *Rev Endocr Metab Disord* 2001; 2(2):203–216.

178. Quack M. Selective recognition of vitamin D receptor conformations mediates promoter selectivity of vitamin D analogs. *Mol Pharmacol* 1999; 55(6):1077–1087.

179. Nayer S, Danielsson C, Kahlen JP, Schrader M, Mathiasen IS, Binderup L, et al. The anti-proliferative effect of vitamin D3 analogues is not mediated by inhibition of the AP-1 pathway, but may be related to promoter selectivity. *Oncogene* 1995; 11(9):1853–1858.

180. Denielsson C, Mathiasen IS, James SY, Nayeri S, Bretting C, Hansen CM, et al. Sensitive induction of apoptosis in breast cancer cells by a novel 1,25-dihydroxyvitamin D3 analogue shows relation to promoter selectivity. *J Cell Biochem* 1997; 66(4):552–562.

181. Kremer R, Karaplis AC, Henderson J, Gulliver W, Banville D, Hendy GN, et al. Regulation of parathyroid hormone-like peptide in cultured normal human keratinocytes: Effect of growth factors and 1,25 dihydroxyvitamin D_3 on gene expression and secretion. *J Clin Invest* 1991; 87:884–893.

182. Nishishita T, Okazaki T, Ishikawa T, Igarashi T, Hata K, Ogata E, et al. A negative vitamin D response DNA element in the human parathyroid hormone-related peptide gene binds to vitamin D receptor along with Ku antigen to mediate negative gene regulation by vitamin D. *J Biol Chem* 1998; 273 (18):10,901–10,907.

183. Mackey SL, Heymont JL, Kronenberg, HM, Demay MB. Vitamin D receptor binding to the negative human parathyroid hormone vitamin D response element does not require the retinoid X receptor. *Mol Endocrinol* 1996; 10:298–305.

184. Zhou GE, Hashimoto Y, Kwak I, Tsai SY, Tsai MJ. Role of the steroid receptor coactivator SRC-3 in cell growth. *Mol Cell Biol* 2003; 23(21):7742–7755.

185. Zhao C, Yasui K, Lee CJ, Kurioka H, Hosokawa Y, Oka T, et al. Elevated expression levels of NCOA3, TOP1, and TFAP2C in breast tumors as predictors of poor prognosis. *Cancer* 2003; 98(1): 18–23.

186. Bouras T, Southey MC, Venter DJ. Overexpression of the steroid receptor coactivator AIB1 in breast cancer correlates with the absence of estrogen and progesterone receptors and positivity for p53 and HER2/neu. *Cancer Res* 2001; 61(3):903–907.

187. Bai J, Uehara Y, Montell DJ. Regulation of invasive cell behavior by taiman, a Drosophila protein related to AIB1, a steroid receptor coactivator amplified in breast cancer. *Cell* 2000; 103(7):1047–1058.

188. Anzick SL, Kononen J, Walker RL, Azorsa DO, Tanner MM, Guan XY, et al. AIB1, a steroid receptor coactivator amplified in breast and ovarian cancer. *Science* 1997; 277(5328):965–968.

189. Nemere I, Schwartz Z, Pedrozo H, Sylvia VL, Dean DD, Boyan BD. Identification of a membrane receptor for 1,25-dihydroxyvitamin D3 which mediates rapid activation of protein kinase C. *J Bone Miner Res* 1998; 13(9):1353–1359.

190. Barsony J, Renyi I, McKoy W. Subcellular distribution of normal and mutant vitamin receptors in living cells. Studies with a novel fluorescent ligand. *J Biol Chem* 1997; 272:5774–5782.

191. Norman AW. Receptors for 1alpha,25(OH)2D3: past, present, and future. *J Bone Miner Res* 1998; 13(9):1360–1369.

192. Caelles C, Gonzalez-Sancho JM, Munoz A. Nuclear hormone receptor antagonism with AP-1 by inhibition of the JNK pathway. *Genes Dev* 1997; 11:3352–3364

193. Henderson J, Sebag M, Rhim J, Goltzman D, Kremer R. Dysregulation of parathyroid hormone-like peptide expression and secretion in a keratinocyte model of tumor progression. *Cancer Res* 1991; 51:6521–6528.

194. Solomon C, White JH, Kremer R. Mitogen-activated protein kinase inhibits 1,25-dihydroxyvitamin D_3-dependent signal transduction by phosphorylating human retinoid X receptor α. *J Clin Invest* 1999; 103:1729–1735.

195. Solomon C, Kremer R, White JH, Rhim JS. Vitamin D resistance in RAS-transformed keratinocytes: mechanism and reversal strategies. *Radiat Res* 2001; 155(1 Pt 2):156–162.

196. Macoritto M, Kremer R. Phosphorylation of the human retinoid X receptor α inhibits the signal transduction by heterodimeric partners. Meeting of the American Society for Bone and Mineral Research, San Antonio TX, 2002.

197. Lohnes D, Jones G. Side chain metabolism of vitamin D_3 in osteosarcoma cell line UMR-106. Characterization of products. *J Biol Chem* 1987; 262(30):14,394–14,401.

198. Reinhardt TA, Horst RL. Ketoconazole inhibits self-induced metabolism of 1,25-dihydroxyvitamin D_3 and amplifies 1,25-dihydroxyvitamin D_3 receptor up-regulation in rat osteosarcoma cells. *Arch Biochem Biophys* 1989; 272(2):459–465.

199. Ly LH, Zhao XY, Holloway L, Feldman D. Liarozole acts synergistically with 1alpha,25-dihydroxyvitamin D_3 to inhibit growth of DU 145 human prostate cancer cells by blocking 24-hydroxylase activity. *Endocrinology* 1999; 140(5):2071–2076.

200. Schuster I, Egger H, Astecker N, Herzig G, Schussler M, Vorisek G. Selective inhibitors of CYP24: mechanistic tools to explore vitamin D metabolism in human keratinocytes. *Steroids* 2001; 66(3–5): 451–462.

201. Stewart AF, Horst R, Deftos LJ, Cadman EC, Lang R, Broadus AE. Biochemical evaluation of patients with cancer-associated hypercalcemia: evidence for humoral and nonhumoral groups. *N Engl J Med* 1980; 303(24):1377–1383.

202. Burton PB, Moniz C, Quirke P, Malik A, Bui TD, Juppner H, et al. Parathyroid hormone-related peptide: expression in fetal and neonatal development. *J Pathol* 1992; 187:291–296;

203. Benitez-Verguizas J, Esbrit P. Proliferative effect of parathyroid hormone-related protein on the hypercalcemic Walker 256 carcinoma cell line. *Biochem Biophys Res Commun* 1994; 198(3):1281–1289.

204. Rabbani SA, Gladu J, Liu B, Goltzman D. Regulation in vivo of the growth of Leydig cell tumors by antisense ribonucleic acid for parathyroid hormone-related peptide. *Endocrinology* 1995; 136(12): 5416–5422.

205. Huang DC, Kremer R. Inhibition of metastasis in melanoma following targeted disruption of the PTHrP gene: Enhanced visualization of the invasion process with green fluorescent protein. 24th Annual Meeting of the American Society of Bone Miner Research, San Antonio, TX, 2002:20–24.

206. Bouizar Z, Spyratos F, Deytieux S, de Vernejoul MC, Jullienn A. Polymerase chain reaction analysis of parathyroid hormone-related protein gene expression in breast cancer patients and occurrence of bone metastases. *Cancer Res* 1993; 53:5076–5078.

207. Truong NU, deB Edwardes MD, Papavasiliou V, Goltzman D, Kremer R. Parathyroid hormone-related peptide and survival of patients with cancer and hypercalcemia. *Am J Med* 2003; 115(2):115–121.

208. Abe M, Akeno N, Ohida S, Horiuchi N. Inhibitory effects of 1,25-dihydroxyvitamin D_3 and 9-cis-retinoic acid on parathyroid hormone-related protein expression by oral cancer cells (HSC-3). *J Endocrinol* 1998; 156(2):349–357.

209. Inoue D, Matsumoto R, Ogata E, I keda K. 22-Oxacalcitriol, a noncalcemic analogue of calcitriol, suppresses both cell proliferation and parathyroid hormone-related peptide gene expression in human T lymphotrophic virus, type I-infected T cells. *J Biol Chem* 1993; 268:16,730–16,736.

210. Falzon M, Zong J. The noncalcemic vitamin D analogs EB1089 and 22-oxacalcitriol suppress serum-induced parathyroid hormone-related peptide gene expression in a lung cancer cell line. *Endocrinology* 1998; 139(3):1046–1053.

211. Gurney H, Grill V, Martin TJ. Parathyroid hormone-related protein and response to pamidronate in tumour-induced hypercalcaemia. *Lancet* 1993; 341(8861):1611–1613.

212. Powell GJ, Southby J, Danks JA, Stillwell RG, Hayman JA, Henderson MA, et al. Localization of parathyroid hormone-related protein in breast cancer metastases: increased incidence in bone compared with other sites. *Cancer Res* 1991; 51(11):3059–3061.

213. Southby J, Kissin MW, Danks JA, Hayman JA, Moseley JM, Henderson MA, et al. Immunohistochemical localization of parathyroid hormone-related protein in human breast cancer. *Cancer Res* 1990; 50(23):7710–7716.

214. Guise TA, Yin JJ, Taylor SD, Kumagai Y, Dallas M, Boyce BH, et al. Evidence for a causal role of parathyroid hormone-related protein in the pathogenesis of human breast cancer-mediated osteolysis. *J Clin Invest* 1996; 98:1544.

215. Achbarou A, Kaiser S, Tremblay G, Ste-Marie LG, Brodt P, Goltzman D, et al. Urokinase overproduction results in increased skeletal metastasis by prostate cancer cells in vivo. *Cancer Res* 1994; 54:2372–2377.

216. Arguello F, Baggs RB, Frantz CN. A murine model of experimental metastasis to bone and bone marrow. *Cancer Res* 1988; 48:6876–6881.

4 Role of TGF-β and IGF in Tumor Progression and Bone Metastases

Erin Giles, BSc and Gurmit Singh, PhD

1. INTRODUCTION

Metastatic disease contributes to a large proportion of cancer-related deaths, and bone is among the most common sites for metastases for tumors originating in the breast and prostate. The propensity for these cancers to form bone metastases is not completely understood; however, it undoubtedly involves a number of unique characteristics of both the tumor cells and the bone microenvironment. Such an explanation was proposed more than a decade ago with Paget's "seed and soil" hypothesis, which suggested that metastatic cells are dispersed throughout the body, yet they will only survive and grow upon reaching tissues that are optimal for their growth (reviewed in ref. *1*).

The bone is a unique microenvironment as it serves as a reservoir for many cytokines and growth factors, including transforming growth factor (TGF)-β and insulin-like growth factor (IGF)-I and IGF-II. Small amounts of these proteins are present in the local environment during normal bone remodeling, however, local concentrations of TGF-β and IGF-I and IGF-II become significantly increased in the presence of osteolytic bone metastases because of the high rates of bone degradation. There is substantial evidence to suggest that TGF-β, IGFs, and their associated family members are highly involved in this complex metastatic process. These growth factors have multiple roles acting both on the tumor cells and surrounding stroma, all of which promote cancer progression. Our current knowledge regarding these key roles will be the focus of this chapter.

From: *Cancer Drug Discovery and Development*
Bone Metastasis: Experimental and Clinical Therapeutics
Edited by: G. Singh and S. A. Rabbani © Humana Press Inc., Totowa, NJ

2. TRANSFORMING GROWTH FACTOR-β

The TGF-β family of extracellular peptides regulates a number of diverse physiological processes, including proliferation, extracellular matrix (ECM) synthesis, angiogenesis, immune responses, apoptosis, and differentiation. The effect of TGF-β on these actions is, to a large extent, cell- and tissue-specific, as it exhibits both stimulatory and inhibitory properties depending on the cell type. The TGF-β signaling pathways activated under normal physiologic conditions are reasonably well understood and have been reviewed extensively *(2–6)*. Briefly, TGF-β generates signals through two types of receptor serine/threonine kinases termed type I and type II TGF-β receptors (TβRI and TβRII). Signal transduction is initiated upon binding of the TGF-β ligand to the type II receptor. The type I receptor is then recruited to this complex, where it is phosphorylated by a constitutively active TβRII kinase, resulting in kinase activation and subsequent phosphorylation of the Smad cytoplasmic signaling molecules. Activated Smads are then translocated to the nucleus where they partner with transcription factors, resulting in the modulation of target gene transcription.

2.1. Alterations in TGF-β Signaling in Cancer Cells

In the early stages of tumor development, TGF-β acts as a tumor suppressor through its ability to inhibit cell growth; however, there is evidence to suggest that TGF-β signaling becomes deregulated in a number of cancers, thereby stimulating invasion and metastases of late-stage, more aggressive tumors (reviewed in refs. *7–9*). This biphasic role for TGF-β can be attributed to selective alterations in TβRs, Smads, and/or target genes that disrupt normal functions of TGF-β that are undesirable to tumor formation, while enhancing TGF-β-mediated effects that favor tumor growth and invasion. Furthermore, TGF-β can also affect many cell types in the local environment of the tumor, creating conditions that support tumor growth, invasion, and metastasis. Thus, in addition to disrupting the growth-inhibitory and apoptosis inducing actions of TGF-β, this growth factor can also enhance angiogenesis, immunosuppression, and matrix metalloproteinase (MMP) secretion.

2.1.1. MUTATIONS IN THE TGF-βRs

Mutations in TβRII have been identified in recurrent, but not primary breast tumors *(10)*, and loss of TβRII expression has been correlated with high tumor grade in both *in situ* and invasive breast cancers *(11)*. A mutation in the TβRI gene has also been linked to metastatic breast cancer *(12)*. Despite these findings, TβR mutations are not frequently found in breast cancers *(13)*. On the other hand, truncated and inactivated forms of the TβRII are often present in colon and gastric tumors, as well as gliomas (reviewed in ref. *14*). Similarly, mutations affecting TβRI have been identified in additional forms of cancers, including tumors of the ovary and pancreas and T-cell lymphomas *(15–18)*.

2.1.2. ALTERED SMAD FUNCTION

Alterations in Smad function are generally associated with deletion or mutation of Smad4. Smad4 was first identified as a tumor suppressor that is lost in approximately half of pancreatic cancers *(19)*, and mutations in this gene also occur in colorectal cancer, with an increased incidence of mutation in those with metastatic disease. Mouse models also support this association: Animals with mutations and deletions of Smad4 have been shown to develop gastrointestinal polyps (similar to those found in humans) that subsequently, progress to invasive adenocarcinomas. Although alterations in other Smads occur less frequently, mutations in Smad2 have been reported in human colorectal and lung cancers (20,21). A number of Smad-deficient mice have been created. Smad2- and Smad4-deficient mice are embryonically lethal, but Smad3-null mice remain viable, and although these animals appear more prone to infections as a result of immunodeficiency (22,23), one group has shown 100% penetrance of metastatic colon cancer in these animals (24). Alterations in Smad signaling have also been associated with a poor outcome in breast cancer patients: Xie and colleagues found that lack of phosphorylated Smad2 was associated with shorter overall survival in a cohort of stage II breast cancer patients (25), and decreased nuclear abundance of Smad3 was significantly correlated to tumor grade and size in a study of breast cancer tissue specimens (26).

2.1.3. Resistance to TGF-β-Mediated Cytostasis and Apoptosis

Although loss of receptor or Smad function might result in changes that promote tumor formation, it is more likely that loss of TGF-β-mediated growth arrest results from changes occurring further downstream in the TGF-β signaling pathway, through the specific loss of cytostatic gene transcription. TGF-β commonly exerts its growth-inhibitory effects by regulating components of the cell cycle machinery, thereby preventing transcription of genes required for the G1–S-phase transition. Common targets include (1) the cyclin-dependent kinases (Cdks), which are associated with early G1-phase progression, (2) Cdk inhibitors (CdkI), which halt the cell cycle prior to the G1 restriction point, and (3) retinoblastoma protein (Rb) that when present in the hypophosphorylated form, acts to repress genes that are crucial for progression of the cell cycle to the S-phase. Alteration in many of these cell-cycle-related genes have been identified with cancers, including deletion of Rb and the CdkIs p15 and p27, as well as overexpression of the cyclin-dependent kinases Cdk4 and Cdc25a (reviewed in refs. 27 and 28). Mutations in these molecules allow for progression of the cell cycle and increased cell growth and proliferation.

Cells that have intact TGF-β signaling but have lost the growth inhibitory signals become increasingly invasive and metastatic, and many such tumors show increased production of TGF-β (29). Associated with this increased invasive and metastatic phenotype are a series of morphologic changes, commonly referred to as an epithelial to mesenchymal transition (EMT). The ability for TGF-β to induce these changes has been demonstrated in cell cultures of normal and transformed breast epithelial cells, squamous carcinoma, ovarian adenosarcoma, and melanoma. The interaction between TGF-β and Ras signaling pathways appears to be important for EMT, and current evidence suggests that these two pathways act synergistically to induce epithelial to mesenchymal transition (30). This finding might partially explain why the invasive growth of Ras-transformed cells often depends on intact TGF-β signaling (31,32). Increased activation of the Ras pathway in breast cancer cells not only blocks the antiproliferative effects of TGF-β, but also increases the ability of cells to metastasize to the bone in response to TGF-β, suggesting that oncogenic Ras "reprograms" the TGF-β response of these cells (33).

2.2. Effects of TGF-β on the Tumor Environment

In addition to modulating the growth properties of tumor cells, TGF-β has additional actions on surrounding cells and tissues that help create an environment that that promotes the growth and colonization of tumors. Most notably, high levels of TGF-β promote angiogenesis, induce expression of matrix-degrading enzymes, and assist tumors in evading the immune system. Furthermore, high levels of TGF-β appear to play a key role in the development of bone metastases by enhancing bone degradation, which promotes colonization and growth of secondary tumors in the bone.

2.2.1. TGF-β STIMULATES ANGIOGENESIS

Sufficient blood supply to a tumor is critical for growth and invasion. Not only do blood vessels deliver oxygen and nutrients to the tumor, but it is through intravastation into the blood system that cancerous cells metastasize to distant organs. For this reason, angiogenesis is critical for the survival and metastasis of tumors. TGF-β exerts a number of effects, both direct and indirect, that stimulate angiogenesis, and animal studies have shown many components of the TGF-β pathway are essential for vascular development. Inactivation of the genes encoding TGF-β or TβRII results in defective vasculogenesis and angiogenesis, generating nonviable embryos *(34,35)*. Similarly, in vivo models of tumorigenesis have shown that angiogenesis is increased in both prostate cells and Chinese hamster ovary cells transfected with TGF-β1, and this effect could be reduced with the local administration of TGF-β-neutralizing antibodies *(36,37)*. Clinical data also supports an association between TGF-β and angiogenesis. High levels of TGF-β were associated with tumor microvessel density and poor prognosis in a cohort of breast cancer patients *(37)*, and similar associations have been observed in renal, prostate, and hepatic tumors *(38–41)*. This effect is, in part, explained by the ability of TGF-β to stimulate production of vascular endothelial growth factor (VEGF), a direct stimulator of endothelial cell proliferation and migration. In addition, TGF-β might contribute to angiogenesis by serving as a chemoattractant for monocytes, which secrete proangiogenic cytokines.

2.2.2. ESCAPE FROM IMMUNOSURVEILENCE IS MEDIATED BY TGF-β

Transforming growth factor also plays a role in suppressing local immune responses by inhibiting the proliferation and differentiation of a number of cell types that are necessary for immune surveillance. This presents a survival advantage for tumors that either produce high levels of this cytokine or reside in an environment where local levels of TGF-β are high. These immunosuppressive effects of TGF-β include (1) suppression of T-lymphocyte activation, proliferation, and function, (2) arrest of B-cells and a corresponding decrease in immunoglobulin synthesis, and (3) reduction in the activity of natural killer (NK) cells, neutrophils, and macrophages (reviewed in ref. *42*).

2.2.3. TGF-β INDUCES MMP EXPRESSION AND ACTIVITY

Matrix metalloproteinases (MMPs) are a family of proteolytic enzymes involved in the degradation and remodeling of the extracellular matrix. The ability for MMPs to degrade basement membranes implies that they are essential for a number of steps in the metastatic process, including neovascularization, extravasation of tumor cells into the circulation, and invasion of tumor cells into distant sites. TGF-β-mediated induction of MMPs has been well documented. TGF-β1 induces activity of MMP-9 and MMP-2 in cultures of breast, prostate, and osteosarcoma cells, as well as surrounding endothelial cells *(43–45)*. Additional studies have shown that by secreting MMPs, metastatic cancer cells are able to degrade mineralized bone, promoting osteolysis and the subsequent development of bone metastases *(46,47)*. Thus, by enhancing the activity of MMPs, TGF-β promotes an environment that fosters the migration and invasion of tumor cells.

2.2.4. TGF-β Stimulates Bone Degradation Via PTHrP

Breast cancers commonly metastasize to the bone, and upon reaching this secondary site, the increased tumor production of parathyroid hormone-related protein (PTHrP) promotes the activation of osteoclasts, resulting in increased bone resorption. This promotes the release of activated growth factors from the bone, including IGF and TGF-β, which stimulate proliferation of the surrounding cells, as discussed previously.

Using sequential passages of MDA-MB-231 breast cancer cells isolated from bone metastases, Yoneda and colleagues *(48)* have generated a bone-seeking MDA-MB-231 clone that has distinct biological characteristics compared to the parental cell line, suggesting that cells metastasizing to the bone undergo phenotypic changes that promote their survival and proliferative capacity in the bone environment. In particular, these bone-seeking clones produced increased amounts of PTHrP in response to TGF-β, and in contrast to the parental line, growth of the bone-seeking cells was not inhibited by TGF-β *(48)*. In vivo studies support these findings. In a mouse model of bone metastases, expression of breast cancer cells nonresponsive to TGF-β (because of a mutation in TβRII) resulted in decreased bone destruction, fewer tumors, and prolonged survival compared to control animals. Furthermore, expression of cells with a constitutively active TβRI resulted in increased PTHrP production and corresponding increase in osteolytic bone metastases and decreased survival *(49)*. Thus, TGF-β plays a key role in promoting bone degradation and the subsequent development of bone metastases.

3. INSULIN-LIKE GROWTH FACTOR AND IGF-BINDING PROTEINS

3.1. The IGF System

Insulin-like growth factor-I and IGF-II are known stimulators of cell growth, proliferation and differentiation, and there is significant evidence to support the role of the IGF system in the development and progression of certain cancers. The IGF system consists of the IGF ligands (IGF-I and IGF-II), the insulin and type I and type II IGF cell surface receptors (IR, IGF-IR, and IGF-IIR), and a family of IGF-binding proteins (IGFBPs). IGF signaling and its role in cancer has been reviewed extensively *(50–52)*. Briefly, signal transduction is initiated with the binding of IGF-I or IGF-II to the extracellular subunit of the IGF-IR, which generates a conformational change and subsequent receptor tyrosine kinase activation. This initiates signaling through the mitogen-activating protein (MAP) kinase and phosphatidylinositol (PI)3 kinase pathways, which ultimately results in transcription of target genes within the nucleus. In contrast, IGF-IIR has no tyrosine kinase activity and can bind IGF-II, but not IGF-I. Binding of IGF-II to this receptor results in degradation of the ligand, decreasing its activity.

Activity of the IGFs is regulated by a family of at least six structurally related proteins, termed IGF-binding proteins (IGFBP-1–6) (reviewed in refs. *53–55*). IGFBPs have a high affinity for IGF-I and IGF-II, and they function in the circulation to transport and stabilize circulating IGF. Secretion of IGFBPs into the local extracellular environment further allows these proteins to regulate tissue/cellular localization of IGF and to modulate IGF ligand–receptor interactions. In this manner, IGFBPs are believed to be important regulators of IGF-dependent proliferation, either inhibiting or enhancing IGF action, depending on the cellular conditions. In addition, these proteins appear to have a more recently identified role in controlling cell growth that is unrelated to their role in binding IGF (reviewed in refs. *56* and *57*). These IGF-independent actions are not yet completely understood, but direct binding of IGFBPs to the cell surface has been reported, and both IGFBP-3 and IGFBP-5 can be translocated to the nucleus, where they have the potential to influence target gene activation.

3.2. Role of IGFs in Cancer

The evidence demonstrating both direct and indirect roles for IGFs in cancer is substantial, and the role of the IGF system in cancer has been the focus of several reviews *(58–61)*. IGFs are overexpressed in many cancers, and both IGF-I and IGF-II are mitogenic for a number of cancer cell lines, including sarcoma, leukemia, and cancers of the prostate, breast, lung, colon, stomach, esophagus, liver, pancreas, kidney, thyroid, brain, ovary, and uterus *(62)*. In addition to stimulating proliferation, prolonged stimulation with IGFs can promote cellular transformation. Recent population-based studies indicate that high serum IGF-I is a risk factor for the development of breast, prostate, colorectal, and lung cancers; however, the strength of association varies greatly given the race, gender, and menopausal status (for breast cancer) of the population being studied.

Increased tumor expression of IGF-IR has been identified as an important factor in the maintenance of the transformed phenotype *(63)*, and its expression is strongly correlated with metastatic ability *(64)*. In addition, IGFs have additional indirect effects that both block the antiproliferative effects of tumor suppressor genes and synergize with mitogenic growth factors and steroids (particularly estrogens and epidermal growth factors [EGF]) to further promote cancer cell growth.

3.3. Role of IGFBPs in Cancer

The role of IGFBPs in cancer progression and metastasis was identified only recently, and the association between IGFBP-3 and breast cancer has been the most extensively studied. Evidence surrounding this association has been inconsistent. Not only are the responses to this protein cell-specific but they are also influenced by complex interplay between local concentrations of growth factors and proteases, and the signaling pathways activated.

3.3.1. ANTITUMOR EFFECTS OF IGFBPS

Given the positive association between the levels of circulating IGF-I and breast cancer risk, it seems logical that by binding IGF in the circulation, high levels of IGFBP-3 would inhibit cancer cell growth. Indeed, the growth-inhibitory effects of IGFBP-3 have been demonstrated in many malignant and nonmalignant cell lines, including a variety of breast cancer cell lines *(65,66)*. This inhibitory action is generally explained by the ability for IGFBP-3 to tightly bind the IGF ligand, thereby competing for binding with the IGF-IR and blocking downstream stimulation of cell growth and survival that result from receptor activation. In addition, cell growth can be inhibited by analogs of IGF that activate the IGF-IR, but cannot bind IGFBP-3. Thus, mechanisms independent of IGF must also be involved.

Apoptosis is fundamental in preventing the development of malignant disease, and there is evidence to suggest that in addition to inhibiting cell growth, IGFBP-3 also has direct and indirect apoptosis-inducing effects *(67)*. IGFBP-3 has been shown to increase cellular production of the pro-apoptotic proteins Bax and Bad and to sensitize cancer cells to the apoptosis-inducing effects of both ionizing radiation and ceramide. It has been suggested that this involves a positive feedback loop in which p53 stimulates IGFBP-3, and IGFBP-3 further enhances p53-mediated apoptosis. Furthermore, IGFBP-3 was reported to directly induce apoptosis through a p53- and IGF-independent mechanism; however, details of this mechanism have not been fully elucidated *(68)*.

3.3.2. IGFBPs May Promote Tumorigenesis: Developed Resistance?

Although IGFBP-3 inhibits the growth of many breast cancer cells in vitro, there are also studies demonstrating that IGFBP-3 has the ability to stimulate cell growth. Furthermore, increased expression of IGFBP-3 in breast tumors has been correlated with poor prognosis in some studies *(69–71)*, thereby suggesting that this protein exerts growth-stimulatory effects in some breast tumors.

The conflicting views on the role of IGFBP-3 in mediating cellular proliferation cannot be explained by variations in the cell lines being studied, as opposing actions have also been reported within one cell type. The most convincing explanation for this dual action is one of developed resistance. It has been postulated that, at the early stages of tumor development, IGFBP-3 might act to inhibit cell growth; however, as tumors become more advanced they become resistant to these growth-inhibitory effects, and in some cases IGFBP-3 actually generates a stimulatory signal. Resistance to the antiproliferative effects could represent a survival advantage to cancer cells, and evidence supporting this hypothesis is accumulating. The development of an aggressive breast cancer phenotype, including the progression from estrogen dependence to independence, has been associated with an increased production of IGFBP-3 *(72)*. Cellular resistance is also supported by studies in which IGFBP-3 was transfected into cells that do not normally express this gene. Initially the cells responded to increased IGFBP-3 in an expected manner, with inhibition of cell growth at the G1–S transition; yet at late-passage numbers, these cells became resistant to the inhibitory effects of IGFBP-3 and cell proliferation was enhanced *(73)*.

Currently, only one mechanism to explain this developed resistance has been described, and this work comes from a series of studies by Baxter and colleagues, who have demonstrated that the MAP kinase pathway is involved in this process. Their studies have shown that IGFBP-3 inhibits DNA synthesis in MCF-10A breast epithelial cells, but following expression of oncogenic Ras, these now malignant cells respond to IGFBP-3 with increased cell proliferation *(74)*. These transformed cells displayed increased EGF receptor phosphorylation and activation of the p44/42– and p38–MAP kinase pathways, indicating that enhanced EGF signaling was responsible for these stimulatory effects *(75)*. Additional processes are also likely involved in the development of a resistant phenotype; identification of these mechanisms will be critical for developing successful anticancer therapies targeting IGFBP-3.

3.4. Mechanisms of IGFBP Action

3.4.1. IGF-Dependent Activity

As mentioned previously, the ability for IGFBPs to bind IGFs is one of the primary means by which IGFBPs influence IGF activity. Because IGFBPs bind to IGF with greater affinity than to the IGF-IR, the presence of IGFBPs will inhibit IGF–IGF-IR interaction, thereby blocking IGF signaling. However, in the presence of IGFBP-specific proteases, IGFBPs are degraded, liberating free IGF, which can then bind to the IGF-IR and initiate signal transduction. A number of ligand-specific proteases have been identified. Many of these are upregulated in tumors, including prostate-specific antigen (PSA), MMPs, γ-nerve growth factor, cathepsin D, plasmin, and thrombin, which provides a further link between IGFBPs and cancer. For example, PSA, whose production spikes with prostate cancer, specifically cleaves IGFBP-3 and IGFBP-5. IGFBP-2, IGFBP-3, IGFBP-4, and IGFBP-5 can be degraded by various members of the MMP family; MMPs have been highly implicated in the metastatic process, and their role in IGFBP degradation further substantiates their prometastatic activity *(76–78)*.

3.4.2. IGF-INDEPENDENT EFFECTS OF IGFBP-3

In addition to modulating the activity of IGF, a number of early studies implicated activity of IGFBP-3 that was independent of IGF; however, Cohen et al. *(79)* were the first to present direct evidence for these IGF-independent effects. In their study, transfection of the IGFBP-3 gene into mouse fibroblasts lacking the IGF-I receptor resulted in decreased cell growth, demonstrating that IGFBP-3 action can occur independently of IGF signaling *(79)*. Subsequent studies have confirmed such IGF-independent effects in a number of systems, including breast *(80)* and prostate *(81)* cancer cells. Although the exact mechanisms are not fully understood, both signaling via cell surface receptors and nuclear localization of IGFBP-3 appear to be involved.

3.4.2.1. Signaling via IGFBP-3-Specific Cell Surface Receptors. Insulin-like growth factor binding protein-3 binds to the surface of many cell types. The positively charged C-terminal domain of IGFBP-3 (^{228}KGRKR) appears to be necessary for cell surface binding, as this interaction is inhibited in a recombinant IGFBP-3 protein with mutations in this region *(82)*, whereas synthetic peptides containing the ^{228}KGRKR sequence compete with IGFBP-3 for cell surface binding *(83)*. In contrast, in a screen of recombinant IGFBP-3 fragments, Yamanaka et al. found that a fragment containing IGFBP-3 amino acids 88–183 (the midregion of IGFBP-3) exhibited binding with the same affinity as the whole-length protein *(84)*. Therefore, there remains a discrepancy as to the region(s) of the protein required for cell surface binding.

Similarly, the identity of the receptor (or receptors) to which IGFBP-3 binds is also not yet known. In breast cancer cells, this binding has been shown to specifically occur with cell membrane proteins ranging from 20 to 50 kDa in size *(85)*. A series of studies in mink lung epithelial cells supported the type V TGF-β receptor (TβRV) as the putative IGFBP-3 receptor *(86,87)*, and in this model, this receptor appears necessary for cellular responses to both IGFBP-3 and TGF-β. The TβRV, however, has not yet been identified in breast tissue, and the majority of tumor-derived epithelial cell lines tested do not express this receptor. If this is, in fact, the IGFBP-3 receptor, then its variable expression could contribute to the contrasting stimulatory and inhibitory effects of IGFBP-3 described earlier. At this time, a specific cell-signaling role for TβRV has not been defined, and further studies will be required to substantiate its role as a putative IGFBP-3 receptor.

Additional roles for TGF-β receptors in IGFBP-3 signaling are slowly being identified. Fanayan and colleagues *(88)* have demonstrated that IGFBP-3 activates the promoter of a TGF-β responsive gene, *PAI-1*, by inducing phosphorylation of the TβRI cell surface receptor. This gene activation did not require nuclear translocation of IGFBP-3, indicating IGFBP-3 was likely signaling from the cell surface. Although it was demonstrated that TβR-II was necessary for this effect, the means by which IGFBP-3 initiates this signal has not yet been defined *(88)*.

3.4.2.2. Nuclear Localization. A feature unique to the IGFBP-3 and IGFBP-5 proteins is the presence of a positively charged region in the C terminal domain that functions as a nuclear localization signal (NLS) *(89)*. In human breast cancer cells, recombinant IGFBP-3 and IGFBP-5 are actively transported to the nucleus by a common pathway, mediated by the importin-β nuclear transport factor. Once in the nucleus, IGFBP-3 binds to insoluble nuclear components, thereby actively accumulating in this compartment. Mutations in the NLS sequence have been shown to diminish IGFBP-3 binding to importin-β in vitro and decrease nuclear import and/or accumulation, indicating that nuclear translocation is a NLS-dependent process *(90)*.

Many small proteins with a functional NLS have been identified as nuclear cotransporters for larger proteins that lack a NLS. This appears to be the case for IGFPB-3. Using a breast cancer cell line that does not normally express IGFBP-3, Schedlich and colleagues *(91)* found that fluorescently labeled IGF-I was translocated to the nucleus in cells expressing recombinant human IGFBP-3, but not in those expressing IGFBP-3 with mutations in the NLS sequence. Similarly, IGF-I analogs with decreased IGFBP-3 binding affinity were not translocated to the nucleus. Together, these findings suggest that in breast cancer cells, IGFBP-3 also acts as a carrier for IGF-I nuclear transport. It is also possible that IGFBP-3 serves as a nuclear transporter for other large proteins; however, to date, additional proteins exploiting this transport function have not been identified.

Nuclear uptake of IGFBP-3 has been associated with diving cells in a number of studies *(91–93)*, but the exact role of IGFBP-3 in the nucleus is still not fully understood. Interaction of IGFBP-3 with nuclear transcription factors were hypothesized based on the high homology between the C-terminal domain of this protein and the DNA-binding domain of many transcription factors. Using a yeast two-hybrid system, Liu et al. *(94)* demonstrated the interaction between nuclear IGFBP-3 and the retinoid X receptor (RXR). In this study, RXR and IGFBP-3 colocalized in both the cytoplasm and nucleus of prostate cancer cells and the incubation with a RXR specific ligand stimulated transport of the complex to the nucleus. More recently, Schedlich and colleagues *(95)* have extended these findings to breast cancer cells and have further demonstrated the interaction between IGFBP-3 and the retinoic acid receptor (RAR)-α. Retinoic acid (RA) is a nonsteroidal hormone that is a potent inhibitor of cell growth and a proapoptotic factor for both normal and malignant cells, but all-*trans*-RA resistance is common in aggressive breast cancers. RA signaling requires the formation of a RXR:RAR heterodimers, and the subsequent ligand-mediated activation of transcription factor complexes. Thus, upon translocation to the nucleus, IGFBP-3 prevents the formation of these heterodimers and, as a result, blocks the cellular response to RA. Retinoid has been shown to be an effective therapeutic agent in the treatment of some cancers, but has been unsuccessful in treating advanced breast cancer. Furthermore, increased secretion of IGFBP-3 has been reported following stimulation with RA *(96)*. If resistance to retinoid signaling in these patients is the result of upregulation and nuclear localization of IGFBP-3, then combining inhibitors of IGFBP-3 with retinoid receptor agonists might represent an effective means of treating such resistant tumors.

4. EFFECTS OF TGF-β ARE MEDIATED BY IGFBP-3

Secretion of IGFBP-3 has been demonstrated in response to a number of growth factors, including TGF-β, RA, TNF-α, antiestrogens, and vitamin D (reviewed in ref. *96*), suggesting that IGFBP-3 might be a common mediator of these effects. Interestingly, many of these factors have dual action in tumor cells, promoting cell survival in some cells while inhibiting survival in others. Of particular interest in regard to breast cancer development and progression is the increased production of IGFBP-3 in response to TGF-β.

As described previously, TGF-β inhibits proliferation and induces apoptosis in both normal breast epithelia and in early-stage tumors. As the tumor develops a more aggressive phenotype, TGF-β generates a mitogenic response. This switch from an inhibitory to stimulatory response mirrors that of IGFBP-3 in early-stage vs late-stage breast cancer, further implicating a common pathway for these factors in tumor development. TGF-β treatment results in a dose- and time-dependent increase in IGFBP-3 production, at both the mRNA and protein levels (97,98), and both the growth inhibitory and proliferative response to TGF-β are at least partially mediated by IGFBP-3 (99–103).

In a study of Hs578T breast cancer cells, Oh and colleagues observed that the growth-inhibitory effects of TGF-β were preceded by an increase in IGFBP-3 (104), and blocking the expression of IGFBP-3 was sufficient to prevent the TGF-β-mediated inhibition of cell growth. The authors proposed that IGFBP-3 likely exerts its effects by binding IGF, thereby inhibiting the access of IGF to the type I receptor, eliminating the downstream signaling cascade. Although this mechanism of action is quite possible, more recent evidence indicates that the role of IGFBP-3 in regulating cell growth is far more complex.

In the MDA-MB-231 breast cancer cell model, our lab has also demonstrated that the effect of TGF-β on proliferation is mediated in part by IGFBP-3. However, in this system, the response to TGF-β was concentration dependent. At very low concentrations (0.001–0.05 ng/mL), TGF-β was shown to stimulate cell proliferation, and this was directly linked to an increase in IGFBP-3. As concentrations were increased beyond 1 ng/mL, TGF-β exerted an inhibitory effect that was accompanied by a decrease in IGFBP-3. Furthermore, these cells did not respond to exogenous IGF, suggesting that the mitogenic effects of IGFBP-3 were independent of IGFBP-3:IGF-binding interactions (103).

It is clear that the interactions among TGF-β, IGFBP-3, and cell growth and survival are extremely complex. McCaig et al. (105) have further demonstrated that not only is the intrinsic ability for IGFBP-3 to either enhance or inhibit the growth and survival of breast epithelial cells dependent on concentration of the cytokines and the cell lines being tested, but simultaneous exposure to other cytokines might also be a determinant of the cellular response. They have found that the effect of IGFBPs on mediating cell death varies depending on the extracellular matrix components present in the environment (105). IGFBP-3 is undoubtedly involved in mediating the effects of TGF-β; however, our understanding of the nature of this interaction is far from being complete.

5. CONCLUSION

The development of bone metastases is a common outcome in advanced breast cancer, and this process appears to be driven, at least in part, by both TGF-β and the IGF family of growth factors. The key effects of these two growth factors in promoting the development of osteolytic bone metastases are summarized in Fig. 1. This includes activity on both tumor cells and the surrounding stroma. Because these growth factors are stored in the bone, they become highly concentrated at the site of metastases (where bone degradation is upregulated) in patients with osteolytic bone lesions. These growth factors

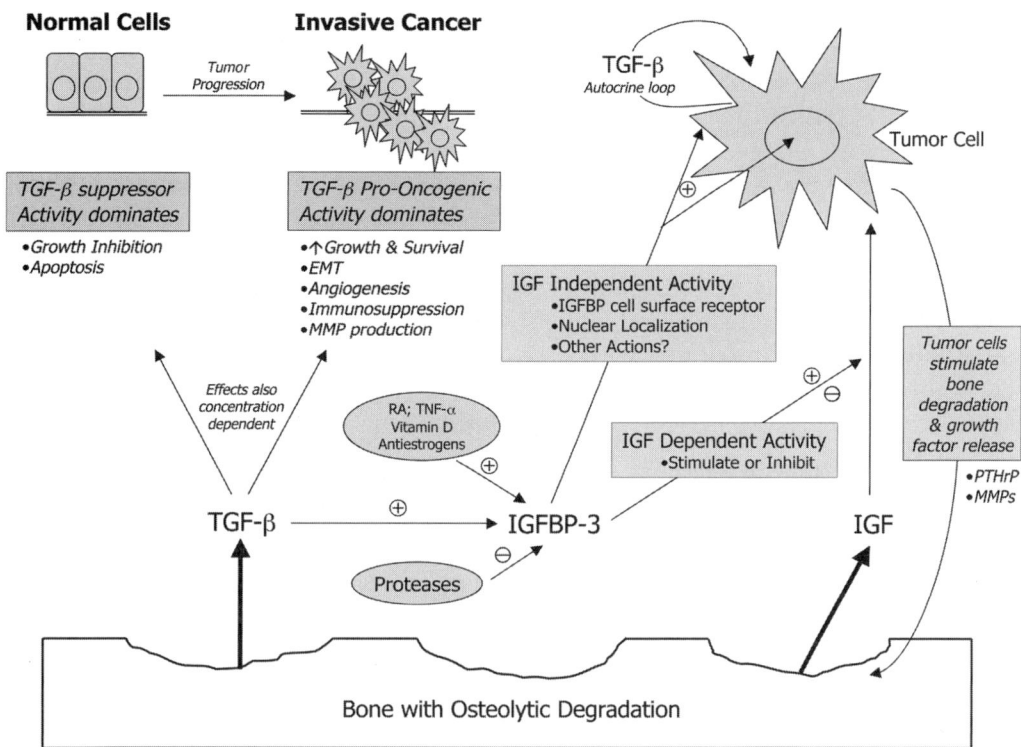

Fig. 1. Effects of IGFs and TGF-β on cancerous cells and surrounding stroma that promote the development of osteolytic bone metastases. Tumor cells stimulate bone degradation, thereby promoting release of growth factors into the local environment. TGF-β exerts both stimulatory and inhibitory effects on tumor cells, and these effects are both cell- and concentration-specific. IGFs have direct tumor-promoting effects that are modulated by the IGFBPs. Levels of IGFBP-3 are upregulated by a number of growth factors, including TGF-β, yet the activity of IGFBP-specific proteases can also degrade these proteins. IGFBP-3 acts through both IGF-dependent and IGF-independent mechanisms. The activity of these growth factors enhance proliferation and survival of advanced metastatic tumors, which further promotes bone breakdown, thereby creating a self-perpetuating cycle that facilitates the development of osteolytic bone metastases.

enhance proliferation and survival of advanced metastatic tumors, which further promotes bone breakdown, thereby creating a self-perpetuating cycle that facilitates the development of osteolytic bone metastases.

Although TGF-β inhibits the growth of many cells, we have presented evidence to suggest that in the late stages of tumourigenesis, TGF-β signaling becomes deregulated with specific loss of activity that is undesirable to tumor formation, including apoptosis and cytostasis. At the same time, TGF-β-mediated effects that enhance tumour growth are enhanced. This results in cancerous cells that are resistant to the apoptosis and growth inhibitory activity of TGF-β in an environment with increased blood supply because of enhanced angiogenesis, increased MMP production, and suppressed activity of immune cells.

Transforming growth facor-β also influences the IGF system, by directly stimulating production of IGFBP-3 in many cancer cells. Like TGF-β, IGFBP-3 has antitumor activity in both normal and some malignant cell lines, yet resistance to these effects is evident in advanced malignancy. In addition to regulating cell growth by modulating the interaction between IGF and the IGF receptors, IGFBP-3 has bioactivity independent of its binding to IGF. IGFBP-3 binds to the cell surface, suggesting the presence of IGFBP-3-specific receptors, which could activate intracellular signaling. In addition, IGFBP-3 can be translocated to the nucleus, where this protein could interact directly with other molecules to regulate target gene transcription. On the other hand, the ability for IGFBP-3 to be translocated to the nucleus might provide a means of shuttling larger proteins to the nucleus, and in this way, IGFPB-3 might serve as a nuclear transporter. These possibilities are not mutually exclusive, and future studies will be required to determine the exact role of IGFBP-3 in many of these processes.

REFERENCES

1. Orr FW, Lee J, Duivenvoorden WC, Singh G. Pathophysiologic interactions in skeletal metastasis. *Cancer* 2000; 88:2912–2918.
2. Shi Y, Massague J. Mechanisms of TGF-beta signaling from cell membrane to the nucleus. *Cell* 2003; 113:685–700.
3. Derynck R, Feng XH. TGF-beta receptor signaling. *Biochim Biophys Acta* 1997; 1333:F105–F150.
4. Itoh S, Itoh F, Goumans MJ, ten Dijke P. Signaling of transforming growth factor-beta family members through Smad proteins. *Eur J Biochem* 2000; 267:6954–6967.
5. Zimmerman CM, Padgett RW. Transforming growth factor beta signaling mediators and modulators. *Gene* 2000; 249:17–30.
6. Massague J, Chen YG. Controlling TGF-beta signaling. *Genes Dev* 2000; 14:627–644.
7. Derynck R, Akhurst RJ, Balmain A. TGF-beta signaling in tumor suppression and cancer progression. *Nat Genet* 2001; 29:117–129.
8. Massague J, Blain SW, Lo RS. TGFbeta signaling in growth control, cancer, and heritable disorders. *Cell* 2000; 103:295–309.
9. Rich J, Borton A, Wang X. Transforming growth factor-beta signaling in cancer. *Microsc Res Tech* 2001; 52:363–373.
10. Lucke CD, Philpott A, Metcalfe JC, et al. Inhibiting mutations in the transforming growth factor beta type 2 receptor in recurrent human breast cancer. *Cancer Res* 2001; 61:482–485.
11. Gobbi H, Arteaga CL, Jensen RA, et al. Loss of expression of transforming growth factor beta type II receptor correlates with high tumour grade in human breast in-situ and invasive carcinomas. *Histopathology* 2000; 36:168–177.
12. Chen T, Carter D, Garrigue-Antar L, Reiss M. Transforming growth factor beta type I receptor kinase mutant associated with metastatic breast cancer. *Cancer Res* 1998; 58:4805–4810.
13. Anbazhagan R, Bornman DM, Johnston JC, Westra WH, Gabrielson E. The S387Y mutations of the transforming growth factor-beta receptor type I gene is uncommon in metastases of breast cancer and other common types of adenocarcinoma. *Cancer Res* 1999; 59:3363,3364.
14. Siegel PM, Massague J. Cytostatic and apoptotic actions of TGF-beta in homeostasis and cancer. *Nat Rev Cancer* 2003; 3:807–821.
15. Wang D, Kanuma T, Mizunuma H, et al. Analysis of specific gene mutations in the transforming growth factor-beta signal transduction pathway in human ovarian cancer. *Cancer Res* 2000; 60:4507–4512.
16. Schiemann WP, Pfeifer WM, Levi E, Kadin ME, Lodish HF. A deletion in the gene for transforming growth factor beta type I receptor abolishes growth regulation by transforming growth factor beta in a cutaneous T-cell lymphoma. *Blood* 1999; 94:2854–2861.
17. Siegel PM, Massague J. Cytostatic and apoptotic actions of TGF-beta in homeostasis and cancer. *Nat Rev Cancer* 2003; 3:807–821.
18. Chen T, Triplett J, Dehner B, et al. Transforming growth factor-beta receptor type I gene is frequently mutated in ovarian carcinomas. *Cancer Res* 2001; 61:4679–4682.
19. Hahn SA, Schutte M, Hoque AT, et al. DPC4, a candidate tumor suppressor gene at human chromosome 18q21.1. *Science* 1996; 271:350–353.

20. Uchida K, Nagatake M, Osada H, et al. Somatic in vivo alterations of the JV18-1 gene at 18q21 in human lung cancers. *Cancer Res* 1996; 56:5583–5585.

21. Eppert K, Scherer SW, Ozcelik H, et al. MADR2 maps to 18q21 and encodes a TGFbeta-regulated MAD-related protein that is functionally mutated in colorectal carcinoma. *Cell* 1996; 86:543–552.

22. Datto MB, Frederick JP, Pan L, Borton AJ, Zhuang Y, Wang XF. Targeted disruption of Smad3 reveals an essential role in transforming growth factor beta-mediated signal transduction. *Mol Cell Biol* 1999; 19:2495–2504.

23. Yang X, Letterio J., Lechleider RJ, et al. Targeted disruption of SMAD3 results in impaired mucosal immunity and diminished T cell responsiveness to TGF-beta. *EMBO J* 1999; 18:1280–1291.

24. Eppert K, Scherer SW, Ozcelik H, et al. MADR2 maps to 18q21 and encodes a TGFbeta-regulated MAD-related protein that is functionally mutated in colorectal carcinoma. *Cell* 1996; 86:543–552.

25. Xie W, Mertens JC, Reiss DJ, et al. Alterations of Smad signaling in human breast carcinoma are associated with poor outcome: a tissue microarray study. *Cancer Res* 2002; 62:497–505.

26. Jeruss JS, Sturgis CD, Rademaker AW, Woodruff TK. Down-regulation of activin, activin receptors, and Smads in high-grade breast cancer. *Cancer Res* 2003; 63:3783–3790.

27. Vermeulen K, Van Bockstaele DR, Berneman ZN. The cell cycle: a review of regulation, deregulation and therapeutic targets in cancer. *Cell Prolif* 2003; 36:131–149.

28. Park MT, Lee SJ. Cell cycle and cancer. *J Biochem Mol Biol* 2003; 36:60–65.

29. Oft M, Heider KH, Beug H. TGFbeta signaling is necessary for carcinoma cell invasiveness and metastasis. *Curr Biol* 1998; 8:1243–1252.

30. Oft M, Peli J, Rudaz C, Schwarz H, Beug H, Reichmann E. TGF-beta1 and Ha-Ras collaborate in modulating the phenotypic plasticity and invasiveness of epithelial tumor cells. *Genes Dev* 1996; 10: 2462–2477.

31. Lehmann K, Janda E, Pierreux CE, et al. Raf induces TGFbeta production while blocking its apoptotic but not invasive responses: a mechanism leading to increased malignancy in epithelial cells. *Genes Dev* 2000; 14:2610–2622.

32. Oft M, Heider KH, Beug H. TGFbeta signaling is necessary for carcinoma cell invasiveness and metastasis. *Curr Biol* 1998; 8:1243–1252.

33. Yin JJ, Selander K, Chirgwin JM, et al. TGF-beta signaling blockade inhibits PTHrP secretion by breast cancer cells and bone metastases development. *J Clin Invest* 1999; 103:197–206.

34. Dickson RB, Kasid A, Huff KK, et al. Activation of growth factor secretion in tumorigenic states of breast cancer induced by 17 beta-estradiol or v-Ha-ras oncogene. *Proc Natl Acad Sci USA* 1987; 84: 837–841.

35. Oshima M, Oshima H, Taketo MM. TGF-beta receptor type II deficiency results in defects of yolk sac hematopoiesis and vasculogenesis. *Dev Biol* 1996; 179:297–302.

36. Ueki N, Nakazato M, Ohkawa T, et al. Excessive production of transforming growth-factor beta 1 can play an important role in the development of tumorigenesis by its action for angiogenesis: validity of neutralizing antibodies to block tumor growth. *Biochim Biophys Acta* 1992; 1137:189–196.

37. de Jong JS, van Diest PJ. van der Valk P, Baak JP. Expression of growth factors, growth-inhibiting factors, and their receptors in invasive breast cancer. II: Correlations with proliferation and angiogenesis. *J Pathol* 1998; 184:53–57.

38. Ito N, Kawata S, Tamura S, et al. Positive correlation of plasma transforming growth factor-beta 1 levels with tumor vascularity in hepatocellular carcinoma. *Cancer Lett* 1995; 89:45–48.

39. Ivanovic V, Melman A, Davis-Joseph B, Valcic M, Geliebter J. Elevated plasma levels of TGF-beta 1 in patients with invasive prostate cancer. *Nat Med* 1995; 1:282–284.

40. Wikstrom P, Stattin P, Franck-Lissbrant I, Damber JE, Bergh A. Transforming growth factor beta1 is associated with angiogenesis, metastasis, and poor clinical outcome in prostate cancer. *Prostate* 1998; 37:19–29.

41. Stiles JD, Ostrow PT, Balos LL, et al. Correlation of endothelin-1 and transforming growth factor beta 1 with malignancy and vascularity in human gliomas. *J Neuropathol Exp Neurol* 1997; 56:435–439.

42. Beck C, Schreiber H, Rowley D. Role of TGF-beta in immune-evasion of cancer. *Microsc Res Tech* 2001; 52:387–395.

43. Duivenvoorden WC, Hirte HW, Singh G. Transforming growth factor beta1 acts as an inducer of matrix metalloproteinase expression and activity in human bone-metastasizing cancer cells. *Clin Exp Metastasis* 1999; 17:27–34.

44. Edwards DR, Murphy G, Reynolds JJ, et al. Transforming growth factor beta modulates the expression of collagenase and metalloproteinase inhibitor. *EMBO J* 1987; 6:1899–1904.

45. Wilson MJ, Sellers RG, Wiehr C, Melamud O, Pei D, Peehl DM. Expression of matrix metalloproteinase-2 and -9 and their inhibitors, tissue inhibitor of metalloproteinase-1 and -2, in primary cultures of human prostatic stromal and epithelial cells. *J Cell Physiol* 2002; 191:208–216.

46. Sanchez-Sweatman OH, Lee J, Orr FW, Singh G. Direct osteolysis induced by metastatic murine melanoma cells: role of matrix metalloproteinases. *Eur J Cancer* 1997; 33:918–925.

47. Sanchez-Sweatman OH, Orr FW, Singh G. Human metastatic prostate PC3 cell lines degrade bone using matrix metalloproteinases. *Invasion Metastasis* 1998; 18:297–305.

48. Yoneda T, Williams PJ, Hiraga T, Niewolna M, Nishimura R. A bone-seeking clone exhibits different biological properties from the MDA-MB-231 parental human breast cancer cells and a brain-seeking clone in vivo and in vitro. *J Bone Miner Res* 2001; 16:1486–1495.

49. Yin JJ, Selander K, Chirgwin JM, et al. TGF-beta signaling blockade inhibits PTHrP secretion by breast cancer cells and bone metastases development. *J Clin Invest* 1999; 103:197–206.

50. LeRoith D, Roberts CT, Jr. The insulin-like growth factor system and cancer. *Cancer Lett* 2003; 195: 127–137.

51. Baxter RC. Changes in the IGF-IGFBP axis in critical illness. *Best Pract Res Clin Endocrinol Metab* 2001; 15:421–434.

52. Yu H, Rohan T. Role of the insulin-like growth factor family in cancer development and progression. *J Natl Cancer Inst* 2000; 92:1472–1489.

53. Collett-Solberg PF, Cohen P. The role of the insulin-like growth factor binding proteins and the IGFBP proteases in modulating IGF action. *Endocrinol Metab Clin N Am* 1996; 25:591–614.

54. Kelley KM, Oh Y, Gargosky SE, et al. Insulin-like growth factor-binding proteins (IGFBPs) and their regulatory dynamics. *Int J Biochem Cell Biol* 1996; 28:619–637.

55. Rosenzweig SA. What's new in the PGF-binding proteins? *Growth Horm IGF Res* 2004; 14:329–336.

56. Mohan S, Baylink DJ. IGF-binding proteins are multifunctional and act via IGF-dependent and -independent mechanisms. *J Endocrinol* 2002; 175:19–31.

57. Lee KW, Cohen P. Nuclear effects: unexpected intracellular actions of insulin-like growth factor binding protein-3. *J Endocrinol* 2002; 175:33–40.

58. Yu H, Rohan T. Role of the insulin-like growth factor family in cancer development and progression. *J Natl Cancer Inst* 2000; 92:1472–1489.

59. LeRoith D, Roberts CT, Jr. The insulin-like growth factor system and cancer. *Cancer Lett* 2003; 195: 127–137.

60. O'Connor R. Regulation of IGF-I receptor signaling in tumor cells. *Horm Metab Res* 2003; 35: 771–777.

61. Baxter RC. Changes in the IGF-IGFBP axis in critical illness. *Best Pract Res Clin Endocrinol Metab* 2001; 15:421–434.

62. Yu H, Rohan T. Role of the insulin-like growth factor family in cancer development and progression. *J Natl Cancer Inst* 2000; 92:1472–1489.

63. Baserga R, Peruzzi F, Reiss K. The IGF-1 receptor in cancer biology. *Int J Cancer* 2003; 107: 873–877.

64. LeRoith D, Roberts CT, Jr. The insulin-like growth factor system and cancer. *Cancer Lett* 2003; 195: 127–137.

65. Oh Y, Muller HL, Pham H, Rosenfeld RG. Demonstration of receptors for insulin-like growth factor binding protein-3 on Hs578T human breast cancer cells. *J Biol Chem* 1993; 268:26,045–26,048.

66. Baxter RC. Signalling pathways involved in antiproliferative effects of IGFBP-3: a review. *Mol Pathol* 2001; 54:145–148.

67. Rajah R, Valentinis B, Cohen P. Insulin-like growth factor (IGF)-binding protein-3 induces apoptosis and mediates the effects of transforming growth factor-beta1 on programmed cell death through a p53- and IGF-independent mechanism. *J Biol Chem* 1997; 272:12,181–12,188.

68. Hollowood AD, Lai T, Perks CM, Newcomb PV, Alderson D, Holly JM. IGFBP-3 prolongs the p53 response and enhances apoptosis following UV irradiation. *Int J Cancer* 2000; 88:336–341.

69. Goodwin PJ, Ennis M, Pritchard KI, et al. Insulin-like growth factor binding proteins 1 and 3 and breast cancer outcomes. *Breast Cancer Res Treat* 2002; 74:65–76.

70. Rocha RL, Hilsenbeck SG, Jackson JG, Lee AV, Figueroa JA, et al. Correlation of insulin-like growth factor-binding protein-3 messenger RNA with protein expression in primary breast cancer tissues: detection of higher levels in tumors with poor prognostic features. *J Natl Cancer Inst* 1996; 88:601–606.

71. Yu H, Levesque MA, Khosravi MJ, Papanastasiou-Diamandi A, Clark GM, Diamandis EP. Insulin-like growth factor-binding protein-3 and breast cancer survival. *Int J Cancer* 1998; 79:624–628.

72. Figueroa JA, Jackson JG, McGuire WL, Krywicki RF, Yee D. Expression of insulin-like growth factor binding proteins in human breast cancer correlates with estrogen receptor status. *J Cell Biochem* 1993; 52:196–205.

73. Firth SM, Fanayan S, Benn D, Baxter RC. Development of resistance to insulin-like growth factor binding protein-3 in transfected T47D breast cancer cells. *Biochem Biophys Res Commun* 1998; 246: 325–329.

74. Martin JL, Baxter RC. Oncogenic ras causes resistance to the growth inhibitor insulin-like growth factor binding protein-3 (IGFBP-3) in breast cancer cells. *J Biol Chem* 1999; 274:16,407–16,411.

75. Martin JL, Weenink SM, Baxter RC. Insulin-like growth factor-binding protein-3 potentiates epidermal growth factor action in MCF-10A mammary epithelial cells. Involvement of p44/42 and p38 mitogen-activated protein kinases. *J Biol Chem* 2003; 278:2969–2976.

76. Chambers AF, Matrisian LM. Changing views of the role of matrix metalloproteinases in metastasis. *J Natl Cancer Inst* 1997; 89:1260–1270.

77. DeClerck YA, Perez N, Shimada H, Boone TC, Langley KE, Taylor SM. Inhibition of invasion and metastasis in cells transfected with an inhibitor of metalloproteinases. *Cancer Res* 1992; 52:701–708.

78. Orr FW, Lee J, Duivenvoorden WC, Singh G. Pathophysiologic interactions in skeletal metastasis. *Cancer* 2000; 88:2912–2918.

79. Cohen P, Lamson G, Okajima T, Rosenfeld RG. Transfection of the human insulin-like growth factor binding protein-3 gene into Balb/c fibroblasts inhibits cellular growth. *Mol Endocrinol* 1993; 7:380–386.

80. Gill ZP, Perks CM, Newcomb PV, Holly JM. Insulin-like growth factor-binding protein (IGFBP-3) predisposes breast cancer cells to programmed cell death in a non-IGF-dependent manner. *J Biol Chem* 1997; 272:25,602–25,607.

81. Rajah R, Valentinis B, Cohen P. Insulin-like growth factor (IGF)-binding protein-3 induces apoptosis and mediates the effects of transforming growth factor-beta1 on programmed cell death through a p53- and IGF-independent mechanism. *J Biol Chem* 1997; 272:12,181–12,188.

82. Firth SM, Ganeshprasad U, Baxter RC. Structural determinants of ligand and cell surface binding of insulin-like growth factor-binding protein-3. *J Biol Chem* 1998; 273:2631–2638.

83. Booth BA, Boes M, Andress DL, et al. IGFBP-3 and IGFBP-5 association with endothelial cells: role of C-terminal heparin binding domain. *Growth Reg* 1995; 5:1–17.

84. Yamanaka Y, Fowlkes JL, Wilson EM, Rosenfeld RG, Oh Y. Characterization of insulin-like growth factor binding protein-3 (IGFBP-3) binding to human breast cancer cells: kinetics of IGFBP-3 binding and identification of receptor binding domain on the IGFBP-3 molecule. *Endocrinology* 1999; 140: 1319–1328.

85. Oh Y, Muller HL, Lamson G, Rosenfeld RG. Insulin-like growth factor (IGF)-independent action of IGF-binding protein-3 in Hs578T human breast cancer cells. Cell surface binding and growth inhibition. *J Biol Chem* 1993; 268:14,964–14,971.

86. Leal SM, Liu Q, Huang SS, Huang JS. The type V transforming growth factor beta receptor is the putative insulin-like growth factor-binding protein 3 receptor. *J Biol Chem* 1997; 272:20,572–20,576.

87. Leal SM, Huang SS, Huang JS. Interactions of high affinity insulin-like growth factor-binding proteins with the type V transforming growth factor-beta receptor in mink lung epithelial cells. *J Biol Chem* 1999; 274:6711–6717.

88. Fanayan S, Firth SM, Baxter RC. Signaling through the Smad pathway by insulin-like growth factor-binding protein-3 in breast cancer cells. Relationship to transforming growth factor-beta 1 signaling. *J Biol Chem* 2002; 277:7255–7261.

89. Radulescu RT. Nuclear localization signal in insulin-like growth factor-binding protein type 3. *Trends Biochem Sci* 1994; 19:278.

90. Schedlich LJ, Le Page SL, Firth SM, Briggs LJ, Jans DA, Baxter RC. Nuclear import of insulin-like growth factor-binding protein-3 and -5 is mediated by the importin beta subunit. *J Biol Chem* 2000; 275:23,462–23,470.

91. Schedlich LJ, Young TF, Firth SM, Baxter RC. Insulin-like growth factor-binding protein (IGFBP)-3 and IGFBP-5 share a common nuclear transport pathway in T47D human breast carcinoma cells. *J Biol Chem* 1998; 273:18,347–18,352.

92. Li W, Fawcett J, Widmer HR, Fielder PJ, Rabkin R, Keller GA. Nuclear transport of insulin-like growth factor-I and insulin-like growth factor binding protein-3 in opossum kidney cells. *Endocrinology* 1997; 138:1763–1766.

93. Wraight CJ, Liepe IJ, White PJ, Hibbs AR, Werther GA. Intranuclear localization of insulin-like growth factor binding protein-3 (IGFBP-3) during cell division in human keratinocytes. *J Invest Dermatol* 1998; 111:239–242.

94. Liu B, Lee HY, Weinzimer SA, et al. Direct functional interactions between insulin-like growth factor-binding protein-3 and retinoid X receptor-alpha regulate transcriptional signaling and apoptosis. *J Biol Chem* 2000; 275:33,607–33,613.

95. Schedlich LJ, O'Han MK, Leong GM, Baxter RC. Insulin-like growth factor binding protein-3 prevents retinoid receptor heterodimerization: implications for retinoic acid-sensitivity in human breast cancer cells. *Biochem Biophys Res Commun* 2004; 314:83–88.

96. Schedlich LJ, Graham LD. Role of insulin-like growth factor binding protein-3 in breast cancer cell growth. *Microsc Res Tech* 2002; 59:12–22.

97. Kveiborg M, Flyvbjerg A, Eriksen EF, Kassem M. Transforming growth factor-beta1 stimulates the production of insulin-like growth factor-I and insulin-like growth factor-binding protein-3 in human bone marrow stromal osteoblast progenitors. *J Endocrinol* 2001; 169:549–561.

98. Martin JL, Baxter RC. Transforming growth factor-beta stimulates production of insulin-like growth factor-binding protein-3 by human skin fibroblasts. *Endocrinology* 1991; 128:1425–1433.

99. Oh Y, Muller HL, Ng L, Rosenfeld RG. Transforming growth factor-beta-induced cell growth inhibition in human breast cancer cells is mediated through insulin-like growth factor-binding protein-3 action. *J Biol Chem* 1995; 270:13,589–13,592.

100. Cohen P, Rajah R, Rosenbloom J, Herrick DJ. IGFBP-3 mediates TGF-beta1-induced cell growth in human airway smooth muscle cells. *Am J Physiol Lung Cell Mol Physiol* 2000; 278:L545–L551.

101. Kansra S, Ewton DZ, Wang J, Friedman E. IGFBP-3 mediates TGF beta 1 proliferative response in colon cancer cells. *Int J Cancer* 2000; 87:373–378.

102. McCaig C, Fowler CA, Laurence NJ, et al. Differential interactions between IGFBP-3 and transforming growth factor-beta (TGF-beta) in normal vs cancerous breast epithelial cells. *Br J Cancer* 2002; 86:1963–1969.

103. Giles ED, Singh G. Role of insulin-like growth factor binding proteins (IGFBPs) in breast cancer proliferation and metastasis. *Clin Exp Metastasis* 2003; 20:481–487.

104. Oh Y, Muller HL, Ng L, Rosenfeld RG. Transforming growth factor-beta-induced cell growth inhibition in human breast cancer cells is mediated through insulin-like growth factor-binding protein-3 action. *J Biol Chem* 1995; 270:13,589–13,592.

105. McCaig C, Perks CM, Holly JM. Intrinsic actions of IGFBP-3 and IGFBP-5 on Hs578T breast cancer epithelial cells: inhibition or accentuation of attachment and survival is dependent upon the presence of fibronectin. *J Cell Sci* 2002; 115:4293–4303.

5

Biologic and Therapeutic Implications of Osteomimicry and Epithelial–Mesenchymal Transition in Prostate Cancer

Wen-Chin Huang, PhD, Valerie Odero-Marah, PhD, and Leland W. K. Chung PhD

CONTENTS

INTRODUCTION
OSTEOMIMICRY
EPITHELIAL–MESENCHYMAL TRANSITION
THERAPEUTIC TARGETING
REFERENCES

1. INTRODUCTION

Death from prostate cancer is usually attributable to the development of bone and visceral organ metastases. The spine, pelvic bones, and ribs are among the most frequent sites of prostate cancer bone metastases. The peripheral skeleton and skull are less frequent sites (1,2). There are two hypotheses for the preferential homing of prostate cancer cells to bone. The first is that the mechanical hemodynamics of blood flow from prostate to bone favor the spread of prostate cancer cells to specific anatomical sites (3). A second theory holds that prostate cancer cells have a specific affinity to bone, which attracts and colonizes prostate cancer cells in a relationship like the "seed" (cancer cell) and "soil" (bone microenvironment) hypothesis originally proposed by Paget (4). Understanding the molecular mechanism underlying prostate cancer tropism to bone and the evolutionary process leading to androgen independence and invasiveness will allow us to develop better therapies for the management of prostate cancer bone metastasis.

Cancer cells reside in an organotypic host microenvironment, the importance of which has long been underemphasized because it is perceived only as a silent bystander (5,6). Past understandings of the organ-specific profile of cancer and metastasis have led to the idea that pre-existing subpopulations of cancer cells must have successfully completed a rather inefficient metastatic process (7,8). Strong experimental evidence supported the

From: *Cancer Drug Discovery and Development*
Bone Metastasis: Experimental and Clinical Therapeutics
Edited by: G. Singh and S. A. Rabbani © Humana Press Inc., Totowa, NJ

concept that primary tumors are heterogeneous, and upon subsequent metastasis, a non-random, sequential, multistep selective process occurred among pre-existing cell subtypes *(7,9,10)*. Kauffman et al. *(11)* reviewed the roles of metastatic suppressor genes whose loss might prompt the selective growth and survival of cancer cells at certain secondary sites. Chambers et al. *(12)* suggested that the molecular interaction between cancer cells and their metastatic organ site determines the success of cancer colonization.

These selective processes are generally believed to occur rarely and in the late stages of tumor progression *(8,11)*. Conceptually, this conflicts with the idea that molecular signatures in the primary cancer prior to metastasis can reliably predict clinical outcome *(13,14)*. A compromise idea was proposed by Kang et al. *(15)*, who suggested that the expression of certain genes in primary breast cancer might indeed, be prognostic, but organ-specific tropism can be achieved only after the cancer cells have expressed a concrete set of overt bone-metastasis genes. In this understanding, the tumor microenvironment is the "missing link" that not only provides fertile "soil" for cancer growth but also exerts dominant inductive influences on the evolution and subsequent selection of critical cancer cell clones at both primary and metastatic sites.

In this context, we focus our review on two important contemporary biologic questions concerning prostate cancer bone metastasis that could be considered as attractive therapeutic targets. These two biologic processes are osteomimicry, the ability of prostate cancer cells to mimic "bone-like" properties, and the epithelial–mesenchymal transition (EMT), which coincides with the ability of prostate cancer cells to gain migratory, invasive, and metastatic potential (see following sections). Understanding the fundamental molecular links between the processes of osteomimicry and EMT and clinical prostate cancer metastases could reveal novel future molecular targets for the treatment of prostate cancer bone metastasis.

2. OSTEOMIMICRY

Koeneman and colleagues *(16)* proposed that osseous metastatic prostate cancer cells must be osteomimetic (bone-cell-like) in order to migrate, grow, and survive in the bone microenvironment. Immunohistochemical staining and Western blot analyses have shown that the osteoblast-restricted proteins osteocalcin (OC), bone sialoprotein (BSP), and osteopontin (OPN) are highly expressed in malignant skeletal metastatic prostate specimens and bone metastatic prostate cancer cell lines *(17–21)*. These bone proteins regulate the differentiation, development, and mineralization of the skeleton. OC (5–6 kDa) is a member of the Gla family of proteins containing γ-carboxyglutamic acid residues. It is also one of the major noncollagenous bone matrix proteins. The functions of OC are regulation of the maturation and mineralization of bone at the late stage and bone remodeling *(22,23)*. BSP (70–80 kDa) is a highly sulfated, phosphorylated, and glycosylated protein that mediates cell attachment to the matrix through the RGD (Arg-Gly-Asp) motif *(24)*. BSP has been hypothesized to play a role in bone mineralization, where its high degree of negative charge could function in calcium sequestration or in hydroxyapatite crystal nucleation *(25)*. OPN (approx 60 kDa) is a secreted glycoprotein in both phosphorylated and nonphosphorylated forms. OPN also contains an integrin-binding RGD *(26–28)*. OPN receptors include two families of proteins, integrins ($\alpha v \beta 3$, $\alpha v \beta 1$, $\alpha v \beta 5$ *[29]*, $\alpha 9 \beta 1$ *[18]*, and $\alpha 4 \beta 1$ *[30]*) and CD44 *(31)*, which are ubiquitous, multistructural, and multifunctional transmembrane glycoproteins that mediate cell–cell and cell–matrix interactions *(32)*. OPN is involved in regulating bone formation and the remodeling of mineralized tissues and mediating cell migration *(33)*.

Many articles have reported that these bone-specific proteins are involved in cancer skeletal metastasis. For example, OC expressed in prostate cancer could serve as a chemoattractant for recruiting osteoblasts and stimulating bone remodeling *(34)*. Overexpression of BSP protein in normal or cancer cells could enhance their attachment to osteoblasts and osteoclasts and stimulate osteoblast differentiation *(35–37)*. OPN stimulates anchorage-independent growth of human prostate cancer cell lines *(21)*. The amounts of BSP and OPN in serum were elevated in colon, breast, prostate, and lung cancers *(38)*. Plasma OPN levels were associated with tumor burden and survival in patients with metastatic prostate cancer *(39)*. Fedarko and co-workers *(40)* suggested that BSP and OPN interact with Factor H on the surface of cancer cells, leading to the evasion of complement-mediated attack. These data collectively suggest that the increased expression of the bone-specific proteins OC, BSP, and OPN in prostate tumor cells promotes acquisition of bone-like or osteomimetic properties and escape from immune system surveillance when migrating and invading the skeletal microenvironment, thus enabling cancer cells to grow and survive under highly restrictive circumstances.

How is the bone-related gene expression turned on in cancer cells? The expression of OC, BSP, and OPN is regulated by various factors, including soluble protein factors (transforming growth factor [TGF]-β, basic fibroblast growth factor [bFGF], insulin-like growth factor [IGF]-I, IGF-II, tumor necrosis factor [TNF]-α, and BMPs) *(41–45)*, 1, 25-dihydroxyvitamin D3 *(46,47)*, glucocorticoids *(48,49)*, parathyroid hormone (PTH) and parathyroid hormone-related peptide (PTHrP) *(50–54)*, prostaglandin E2 *(55)*, and cyclic AMP (cAMP) *(53,56–58)*. These regulators stimulate osteoblast-specific genes through cAMP-dependent protein kinase A (PKA) *(50,53,55,57)*, the protein kinase C (PKC) pathway *(43,52)*, and mitogen-activating protein kinase (MAPK) signaling pathways *(42,52,59)*.

Many nuclear transcription factors that bind to their cognate cis-acting elements on OC, BSP, and OPN promoter regions have also been identified. These nuclear proteins are Runx2 *(47,60,61)*, MSX2 *(61,62)*, SP1 *(47)*, AP1 *(47,63)*, Dlx-5 *(64)*, and CREB *(55)*. Runx2 (Cbfa1/AML3) is an osteoblast-related transcription factor with an important role in bone development and differentiation *(60,65,66)*. This transcription factor binds a cis-acting element, OSE2, in the target genes of OC, BSP, OPN, and type I collagen *(47,60,61,67–69)*. In addition to Runx2 overexpression in bone metastatic prostate cancer cells *(47)*, high levels of the bone-specific OC, BSP, and OPN proteins were also observed in aggressive cancer cells. Hence, the actions of these nuclear transcription factors on the initiation of osteoblast-specific gene expressions might be the molecular basis for switching the phenotype of prostate epithelial cells to become bone-like and undertake skeletal metastasis.

The expression of the bone-specific proteins OC, BSP, and OPN is upregulated in aggressive skeletal metastatic prostate specimens and bone metastatic prostate cancer cell lines, which is one of the critical steps to cause prostate tumor cells to acquire bone-like properties. Figure 1 depicts the important regulatory steps that control prostate cancer cell osteomimicry. Increased insight into the molecular basis of prostate cancer's osteomimetic properties could lead to future treatments for bone metastasis. Novel preventive and therapeutic strategies can be designed to target these soluble factors, signaling pathways, and nuclear transcription factors as a cancer therapy.

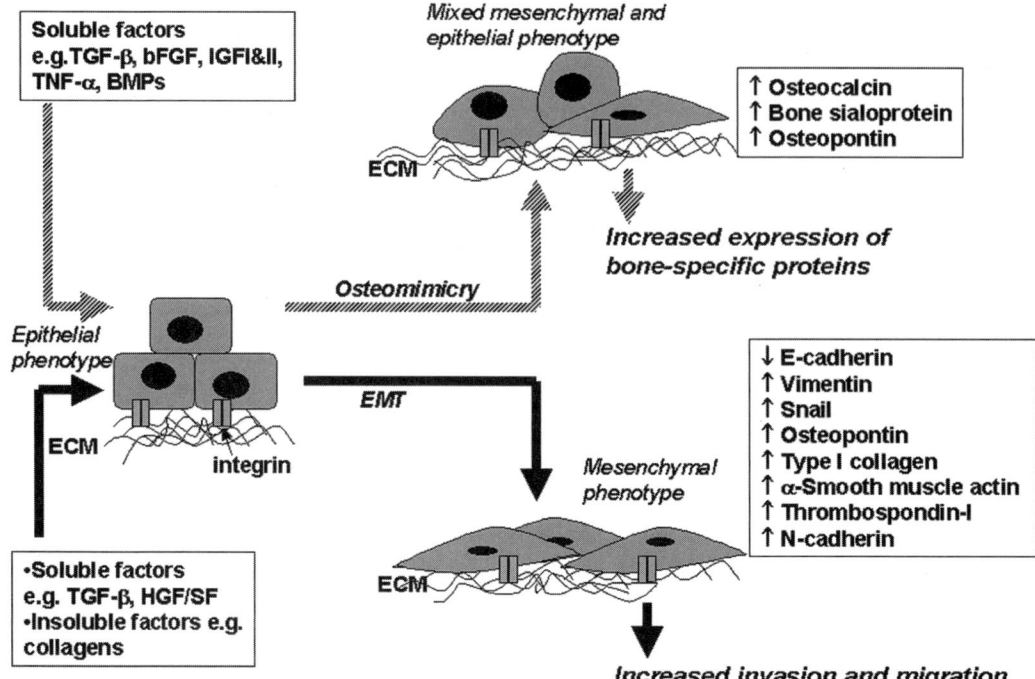

Fig. 1. Osteomimicry and epithelial–mesenchymal transition (EMT) in prostate cancer correlates with progression of tumor cells toward an invasive and metastatic phenotype with propensity toward colonization of bone. Osteomimicry is triggered by soluble growth factors from the stroma that act on normal epithelial cells leading to upregulation of the bone-specific proteins osteocalcin, bone sialoprotein, and osteopontin. This allows the cancer cells to escape immune surveillance and successfully colonize the bone microenvironment. Soluble growth factors as well as insoluble matrix proteins such as collagen can also induce EMT in normal epithelial cells, leading to downregulation of cell adhesion-associated proteins, such as E-cadherin, and upregulation of mesenchymal proteins, such as vimentin, Snail, osteopontin, and N-cadherin among others, resulting in increased invasion and migration. EMT has also been associated with a change in morphology from an epithelioid to a more elongated fibroblasticlike shape.

3. EPITHELIAL–MESENCHYMAL TRANSITION

Epithelial–mesenchymal transition (EMT) was first described by developmental biologists in terms of the morphological changes epithelial cells undergo at specific sites during embryonic development, resulting in more migratory cells (70). In mammals, EMT occurs during gastrulation, limb formation, and organogenesis of the lungs, kidneys, gut, and heart. EMT is involved in the formation of parietal endoderm, mesoderm, and definitive endoderm at the primitive streak during gastrulation (71,72). In addition, EMT leads to the transition of dorsal neural epithelium into neural crest cells and subsequent migration and differentiation into various cell types such as neurons and glia of the peripheral nervous system, pigment cells, and connective tissue in the heart, face, and neck (73,74).

In vivo studies have shown that during EMT, polarized epithelial cells expressing keratin intermediate filaments, desmosomes, and adherens junctions switch off genes encoding cell adhesion proteins and modify the type of intermediate filaments expressed, as they acquire mesenchymal characteristics such as vimentin expression, synthesis of extracellular matrix molecules such as fibronectin and certain types of collagen, and a flattened phenotype. These cells subsequently become more migratory, express gelatinase and invasive activity, and traverse underlying basement membrane. Following EMT, cells can differentiate into other cell types or revert back to an epithelial cell *(70,75,76)*.

It is important to note that not all EMTs undergo all the changes listed, but EMT is always associated with cell migration. It has been widely reported that epithelial tumor cells also undergo an EMT phase reminiscent of embryonic development. This involves loss of epithelial characteristics and acquisition of mesenchymal markers as the cells become more invasive and metastatic *(76–78)*. During neoplastic growth and development, tumor survival can be related to an EMT process by which tumor epithelial cells switch their phenotype toward the development of functional vascular endothelium ("vasculogenic mimicry") under hypoxic conditions, possibly through the activation of HIF-1α transcription factor *(79,80)*.

What initiates EMT? Signals originating from outside the epithelial cell can induce EMT. This includes extracellular matrix molecules such as collagen, soluble factors such as epidermal growth factor (EGF), scatter factor/hepatocyte growth factor (SF/HGF), and members of the TGF-β and FGF family *(81)*. These molecules can lead to a signaling cascade whereby signals are transduced from the cell surface to the nucleus, resulting in transcriptional regulation of specific genes. Because complex interactions between stromal and epithelial/tumor cells exist, the question arises as to whether EMT represents a coordinated response to instructive cues derived from stroma or whether EMT is a response to the intrinsic factors produced by a reactive epithelium.

Cancer studies have yielded some interesting clues. TGF-β can play dual roles in cancer; it acts as a tumor suppressor in primary tumors by inhibiting cell proliferation, but stimulates growth and invasion as the tumor progresses. Indeed, many epithelial tumors overexpress TGF-β and it has been found to act in both an autocrine manner on the tumor cells as well as a paracrine manner to modulate the stroma (82). The reactive stroma can be formed in response to TGF-β secreted by both tumor epithelium and host stroma and it could lead to increased local inflammatory reaction such as lymphocyte infiltration and angiogenesis. The stroma reaction promotes subsequent tumor cell growth, invasion, motility and survival and increased angiogenesis that triggers the metastatic cascade *(78,83,84)*. Using a colon carcinoma spheroid model, Bates et al. found that activated macrophages produced TNF-α and could trigger autocrine TNF-α production by the tumor cells themselves, and, subsequently, accelerated TGF-β-mediated EMT *(85)*. It seems that EMT is the result of a complex interplay between epithelial and stromal cells, mediated by soluble factors that could be produced under a positive feedback loop that fuels cancer progression (Fig. 1).

Crucial questions with relevance for therapeutic intervention are whether TGF-β-induced EMT occurs in most or all metastatic carcinomas and whether reversing EMT by promoting the mesenchymal-to-epithelial transition (MET) can reverse the malignant phenotype of cancer cells. Several genetic mouse models seem to support this idea, although residual metastases still occur after antagonizing TGF-β-receptor signaling; it remains to be clarified whether this is the result of TGF-β-receptor independent pathways or is a consequence of participating host immune surveillance *(86)*.

The canonical Ras pathway has been shown to be important for EMT both in vitro and in vivo. The Ras effect is mediated by several distinct pathways. For example, activation of the MAPK pathway is required for EMT in EpH4 mammary epithelial cells in vitro and in nude mice. In addition, activated MEK, an activator of MAPK, and Rac, a member of the Rho GTPase family, can induce EMT in a bladder carcinoma cell line *(87)*. Certain master genes have been described that can regulate the entire EMT process. These include Fos transcription factor, which can induce EMT via a Wnt-like pathway, and Snail transcription factor, which can downregulate E-cadherin *(76)*. Loss of E-cadherin expression can also result in EMT. In fact, the majority of epithelial cancers are characterized by the loss of E-cadherin expression either by silencing mutations in the gene or transcriptional repression *(76)*.

How does the EMT signal result in cell motility? This is probably the result of growth-factor-induced changes in the actin/myosin motility machinery *(76)*. Growth factor signaling might affect the Rho GTPase family, leading to cytoskeletal reorganization and altered cell motility. Alternatively, integrin engagement by extracellular signals might regulate various effector molecules such as paxillin, which can result in modulation of the actin cytoskeleton *(76)*. An important distinction needs to be made to differentiate scattering from EMT. Scattering refers to cell cultures on plastic treated with growth factors, inhibitors, or inducible oncogenes that lead to a fibroblastoid shape, redistribution/decreased expression of E-cadherin, and a migratory pheonotype but no increase of the mesenchymal genes within 48 h *(87)*. This effect is dependent on cell type and involves MAPK, phosphoinositide 3 kinase (PI3K), and the Rac and Rho GTPase signaling pathways. For complete EMT to occur, at least 4–6 d of exposure to several signals is necessary. It might occur more efficiently in certain cell types, and in some cases three-dimentional (3D) culture conditions might be required *(87)*.

Epithelial–mesenchymal transition in prostate cancer is a relatively unexplored area. Prostate cancer cells have been shown to overexpress TGF-β1, which stimulates angiogenesis and metastasis and inhibits immune responses directed against tumor cells, thus promoting cancer growth *(88)*. Untergasser et al. have shown that treatment of human prostate epithelial cells with TGF-β1, TGF-β2, and TGF-β3 led to increased expression of the mesenchymal marker vimentin after 24 h, suggesting that EMT had occurred *(88)*. Zhau et al. *(89)* observed increased invasion and growth of human prostate PC-3 cells following transfection with c-erbB2/neu, which corresponded with their ability to overexpress vimentin. A different study by Putz et al. revealed that disseminated tumor cells recovered from the bone marrow of patients with cancer of the prostate, breast, lung, and colon coexpressed cytokeratin and vimentin, indicative of EMT *(90)*. However, unlike established EMT models in breast cancer *(91)*, up to now there are no good EMT models that can be used to evaluate the prostate cancer metastatic cascade.

Although EMT has been studied widely in vitro and in vivo, some discrepancy remains as to how exactly to describe it, because the requirements to induce EMT in vitro or in vivo can differ, and it is often difficult to recapitulate in vitro experiments in vivo. Thus, it is not surprising to find studies that vary in their stringency for defining EMT. Overall, EMT occurs as a tumor progresses and involves loss of epithelial markers such as E-cadherin, gain of mesenchymal markers such as vimentin, and cytoskeletal rearrangements that result in increased cell motility as a cancer becomes more invasive and metastatic. Changes in genes involved in EMT could potentially be used to predict metastatic outcome. The genes involved in EMT could also be regarded as a new class of targets for therapy.

4. THERAPEUTIC TARGETING

The host microenvironment could participate actively in the rather inefficient but nonrandom metastatic process by which cancer cell variants evolve increased growth and survival advantages via tumor–stroma interaction at primary or secondary sites of tumor growth. The molecular processes associated with this interaction have been reviewed in the context of a reciprocal cancer cell–microenvironment interaction that facilitates the development of osteomimicry and EMT, both of which are likely to participate in the metastatic cascade of prostate cancer cells.

Men with advanced prostate cancer often develop debilitating metastatic disease for which there is no effective therapy, but an increased understanding at the molecular level of osteomimicry and EMT might be the key to novel therapeutic developments. Figure 2 shows possible points of interference that could trigger the reversal of these biochemical and behavioral changes in cancer cells and their microenvironment, restoring the phenotype (but not the genotype) of cancer cells. These strategies include the following:

1. *Targeting intracellular transcription factors.* Based on the requirement of Runx2 (Cbfa1/AML3) for osteomimicry and HIF-1α for vasculogenic mimicry, these two transcription factors could be excellent therapeutic targets.

2. *Targeting growth factors and their receptor signaling.* TGF-β and IGF-I/bFGF have been associated with EMT and osteomimicry and are potentially attractive therapeutic targets. Additional novel mediators in the tumor–stroma communication that determines osteomimicry are being evaluated by our laboratory and others and could yield interesting therapeutic effects.

3. *Targeting the extracellular matrix (ECMs) at the interphase between tumor and stroma.* The promotion of osteomimicry and EMT by collagen I, mediated by integrin α2β1, and the development of new blood vessels through the expression of αvβ3 reveal new targeting opportunities using designed antibodies or peptides *(92,93)*.

4. *Targeting bone turnover.* Once prostate cancer cells acquire bone-like properties, they can participate actively in osteoclastogenesis and new bone formation *(94–96)*. Thus, new therapeutic drugs that interfere with bone turnover, including bisphosphonates, OPG, and endothelin receptor antagonists such as Astrasenten, could interfere with the growth of prostate cancer in bone, although they are not likely to be effective in targeting local tumor growth and soft tissue metastasis because of the different mediators involved in tumor–stroma interaction (95).

5. *Targeting matrix metalloproteinases (MMPs).* The interrelationship between stroma and epithelium involves critical participation by MMPs that activate invasion and colonization of cancer cells in bone *(97)*. Studies using prostate and other cancer models reveal the role of MMPs in cancer progression driven by cancer-associated stroma *(97,98)* and inflammatory macrophages *(99)* and are often associated with EMT and osteomimicry.

Although the above molecular targeting strategies might be revealed by the study of osteomimicry and EMT, they closely parallel current therapeutic developments intended to block tumor angiogenesis (RGD peptide and thalidomide), selective bone targeting (Astrasenten, bisphosphonate, and OPG), and cancer invasion (MMPs). Further novel therapeutic strategies can present themselves for development after further dissection of the molecular steps involved in osteomimicry and EMT in prostate cancer.

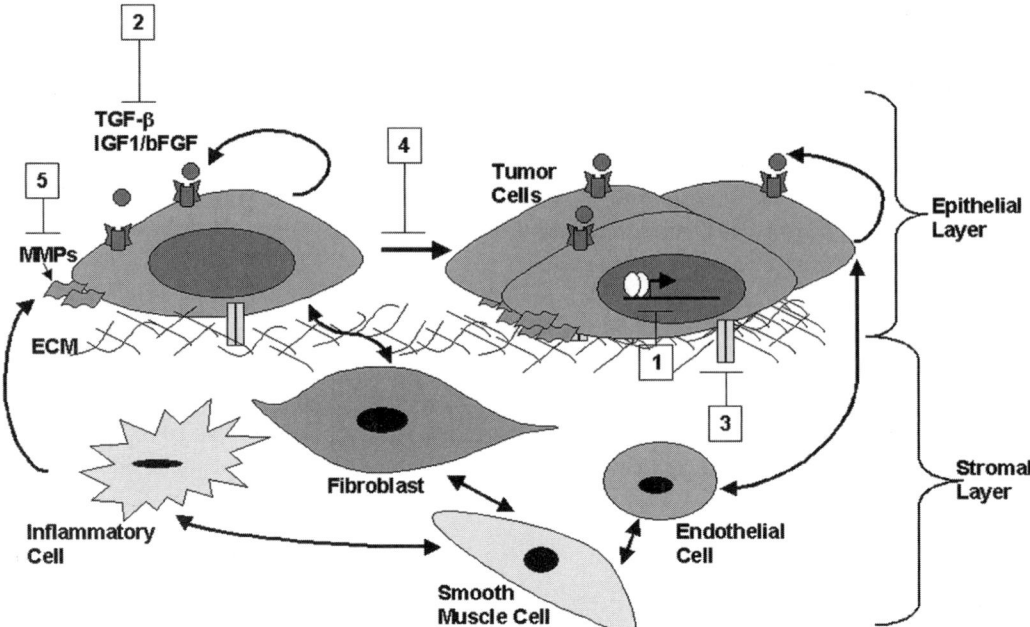

Fig. 2. Possible therapeutic targets that might be used to reverse the biochemical and behavioral changes in cancer cells and their microenvironment include (1) various transcription factors that contribute to cancer progression, including Runx2, which promotes osteomimicry, and HIF-1α, which has been implicated in vasculogenic mimicry, (2) growth factors such as TGF-β and IGF-I/bFGF that have been associated with EMT and osteomimicry, (3) integrins such as α2β1, which promotes attachment to collagen I during osteomimicry and EMT, and αvβ3, which mediates development of new blood vessels, (4) bone-like proteins and endothelin receptor on prostate cancer cells that have metastasized to bone and on osteoblasts, which could be targeted by bisphosphonates, OPG, and endothelin receptor antagonists such as Astrasenten, and (5) MMPs that are important for invasion through the extracellular matrix (ECM) and subsequent colonization of bone.

REFERENCES

1. Bubendorf L, Schopfer A, Wagner U, et al. Metastatic patterns of prostate cancer: an autopsy study of 1,589 patients. *Hum Pathol* 2000; 31:578.
2. Cher ML. Mechanisms governing bone metastasis in prostate cancer. *Curr Opin Urol* 2001; 11:483.
3. Batson OV. The function of the vertebral veins and their role in the spread of metastases. 1940. *Ann Surg* 1940; 112:138.
4. Paget S. The distribution of secondary growths in cancer of the breast. *Lancet* 1889; 1:571.
5. Hanahan D, Weinberg RA. The hallmarks of cancer. *Cell* 2000; 100:57.
6. Muller WJ, Sinn E, Pattengale PK, et al. Single-step induction of mammary adenocarcinoma in transgenic mice bearing the activated c-neu oncogene. *Cell* 1998; 54:105.
7. Kerbel RS, Waghorne C, Korczak B, et al. Clonal dominance of primary tumours by metastatic cells: genetic analysis and biological implications. *Cancer Surv* 1988; 7:597.
8. Poste G, Fidler IJ. The pathogenesis of cancer metastasis. *Nature* 1980; 283:139.
9. Herlyn D, Iliopoulos D, Jensen PJ, et al. In vitro properties of human melanoma cells metastatic in nude mice. *Cancer Res* 1990; 50:2296.
10. Semenza GL. Hypoxia, clonal selection, and the role of HIF-1 in tumor progression. *Crit Rev Biochem Mol Biol* 2000; 35:71.

11. Kauffman EC, Robinson VL, Stadler WM, et al. Metastasis suppression: the evolving role of metastasis suppressor genes for regulating cancer cell growth at the secondary site. *J Urol* 2003; 169:1122.

12. Chambers AF, Groom AC, MacDonald IC. Dissemination and growth of cancer cells in metastatic sites. *Nat Rev Cancer* 2002; 2:563.

13. van 't Veer LJ, Dai H, van de Vijver MJ, et al. Gene expression profiling predicts clinical outcome of breast cancer. *Nature* 2002; 415:530.

14. Ramaswamy S, Ross KN, Lander ES, et al. A molecular signature of metastasis in primary solid tumors. *Nat Genet* 2003; 33:49.

15. Kang Y, Siegel PM, Shu W, et al. A multigenic program mediating breast cancer metastasis to bone. *Cancer Cell* 2003; 3:537.

16. Koeneman KS, Yeung F, Chung LW. Osteomimetic properties of prostate cancer cells: a hypothesis supporting the predilection of prostate cancer metastasis and growth in the bone environment. *Prostate* 1999; 39:246.

17. Matsubara S, Wada Y, Gardner TA, et al. A conditional replication-competent adenoviral vector, Ad-OC-E1a, to cotarget prostate cancer and bone stroma in an experimental model of androgen-independent prostate cancer bone metastasis. *Cancer Res* 2001; 61:6012.

18. Curatolo C, Ludovico GM, Correale M, et al. Advanced prostate cancer follow-up with prostate-specific antigen, prostatic acid phosphatase, osteocalcin and bone isoenzyme of alkaline phosphatase. *Eur Urol* 1992; 21(Suppl 1):105.

19. Waltregny D, Bellahcene A, Van Riet I, et al. Prognostic value of bone sialoprotein expression in clinically localized human prostate cancer. *J Natl Cancer Inst* 1998; 90:1000.

20. Brown LF, Papadopoulos-Sergiou A, Berse B, et al. Osteopontin expression and distribution in human carcinomas. *Am J Pathol* 1994; 145:610.

21. Thalmann GN, Sikes RA, Devoll RE, et al. Osteopontin: possible role in prostate cancer progression. *Clin Cancer Res* 1999; 5:2271.

22. Roach HI. Why does bone matrix contain non-collagenous proteins? The possible roles of osteocalcin, osteonectin, osteopontin and bone sialoprotein in bone mineralisation and resorption. *Cell Biol Int* 1994; 18:617.

23. Stein GS, Lian JB, Owen TA. Relationship of cell growth to the regulation of tissue-specific gene expression during osteoblast differentiation. *FASEB J* 1990; 4:3111.

24. Ganss B, Kim RH, Sodek J. Bone sialoprotein. *Crit Rev Oral Biol Med* 1999; 10:79.

25. Hunter GK, Goldberg HA. Nucleation of hydroxyapatite by bone sialoprotein. *Proc Natl Acad Sci USA* 1993; 90:8562.

26. Oldberg A, Franzen A, Heinegard D. Cloning and sequence analysis of rat bone sialoprotein (osteopontin) cDNA reveals an Arg-Gly-Asp cell-binding sequence. *Proc Natl Acad Sci USA* 1986; 83:8819.

27. Fisher LW, Hawkins GR, Tuross N, et al. Purification and partial characterization of small proteoglycans I and II, bone sialoproteins I and II, and osteonectin from the mineral compartment of developing human bone. *J Biol Chem* 1987; 262:9702.

28. Senger DR, Perruzzi CA, Papadopoulos A. Elevated expression of secreted phosphoprotein I (osteopontin, 2ar) as a consequence of neoplastic transformation. *Anticancer Res* 1989; 9:1291.

29. Ruoslahti E, Pierschbacher MD. New perspectives in cell adhesion: RGD and integrins. *Science* 1987; 238:491.

30. Bayless KJ, Meininger GA, Scholtz JM, et al. Osteopontin is a ligand for the alpha4beta1 integrin. *J Cell Sci* 1998; 111(Pt 9):1165.

31. Weber GF, Ashkar S, Glimcher MJ, et al. Receptor-ligand interaction between CD44 and osteopontin (Eta-1). *Science* 1996; 271:509.

32. Xie Y, Sakatsume M, Nishi S, et al. Expression, roles, receptors, and regulation of osteopontin in the kidney. *Kidney Int* 2001; 60:1645.

33. Butler WT. The nature and significance of osteopontin. *Connect Tissue Res* 1989; 23:123.

34. Glowacki J, Lian JB. Impaired recruitment and differentiation of osteoclast progenitors by osteocalcin-deplete bone implants. *Cell Differ* 1987; 21:247.

35. Bianco P, Fisher LW, Young MF, et al. Expression of bone sialoprotein (BSP) in developing human tissues. *Calcif Tissue Int* 1991; 49:421.

36. Cooper LF, Yliheikkila PK, Felton DA, et al. Spatiotemporal assessment of fetal bovine osteoblast culture differentiation indicates a role for BSP in promoting differentiation. *J Bone Miner Res* 1998; 13:620.

37. Zhang JH, Tang J, Wang J, et al. Over-expression of bone sialoprotein enhances bone metastasis of human breast cancer cells in a mouse model. *Int J Oncol* 2003; 23:1043.

38. Fedarko NS, Jain A, Karadag A, et al. Elevated serum bone sialoprotein and osteopontin in colon, breast, prostate, and lung cancer. *Clin Cancer Res* 2001; 7:4060.

39. Hotte SJ, Winquist EW, Stitt L, et al. Plasma osteopontin: associations with survival and metastasis to bone in men with hormone-refractory prostate carcinoma. *Cancer* 2002; 95:506.

40. Fedarko NS, Fohr B, Robey PG, et al. Factor H binding to bone sialoprotein and osteopontin enables tumor cell evasion of complement-mediated attack. *J Biol Chem* 2000; 275:16666.

41. Alliston T, Choy L, Ducy P, et al. TGF-beta-induced repression of CBFA1 by Smad3 decreases cbfa1 and osteocalcin expression and inhibits osteoblast differentiation. *EMBO J* 2001; 20:2254.

42. Xiao G, Jiang D, Gopalakrishnan R, et al. Fibroblast growth factor 2 induction of the osteocalcin gene requires MAPK activity and phosphorylation of the osteoblast transcription factor, Cbfa1/Runx2. *J Biol Chem* 2002; 277:36181.

43. Kim HJ, Kim JH, Bae SC, et al. The protein kinase C pathway plays a central role in the fibroblast growth factor-stimulated expression and transactivation activity of Runx2. *J Biol Chem* 2003; 278:319.

44. Gilbert L, He X, Farmer P, et al. Expression of the osteoblast differentiation factor RUNX2 (Cbfa1/AML3/Pebp2alpha A) is inhibited by tumor necrosis factor-alpha. *J Biol Chem* 2002; 277:2695.

45. Samoto H, Shimizu E, Matsuda-Honjo Y, et al. TNF-alpha suppresses bone sialoprotein (BSP) expression in ROS17/2.8 cells. *J Cell Biochem* 2002; 87:313.

46. Morrison NA, Shine J, Fragonas JC, et al. 1,25-dihydroxyvitamin D-responsive element and glucocorticoid repression in the osteocalcin gene. *Science* 1989; 246:1158.

47. Yeung F, Law WK, Yeh CH, et al. Regulation of human osteocalcin promoter in hormone-independent human prostate cancer cells. *J Biol Chem* 2002; 277:2468.

48. Morrison N, Eisman J. Role of the negative glucocorticoid regulatory element in glucocorticoid repression of the human osteocalcin promoter. *J Bone Miner Res* 1993; 8:969.

49. Lian JB, Shalhoub V, Aslam F, et al. Species-specific glucocorticoid and 1,25-dihydroxyvitamin D responsiveness in mouse MC3T3-E1 osteoblasts: dexamethasone inhibits osteoblast differentiation and vitamin D down-regulates osteocalcin gene expression. *Endocrinology* 1997; 138:2117.

50. Yang R, Gerstenfeld LC. Signal transduction pathways mediating parathyroid hormone stimulation of bone sialoprotein gene expression in osteoblasts. *J Biol Chem* 1996; 271:29839.

51. Ouyang H, Franceschi RT, McCauley LK, et al. Parathyroid hormone-related protein down-regulates bone sialoprotein gene expression in cementoblasts: role of the protein kinase A pathway. *Endocrinology* 2000; 141:4671.

52. Miao D, Tong XK, Chan GK, et al. Parathyroid hormone-related peptide stimulates osteogenic cell proliferation through protein kinase C activation of the Ras/mitogen-activated protein kinase signaling pathway. *J Biol Chem* 2001; 276:32204.

53. Boguslawski G, Hale LV, Yu XP, et al. Activation of osteocalcin transcription involves interaction of protein kinase A- and protein kinase C-dependent pathways. *J Biol Chem* 2000; 275:999.

54. Jiang D, Franceschi RT, Boules H, et al. PTH induction of the osteocalcin gene: Requirement for an OSE1 sequence in the promoter and involvement of multiple signaling pathways. *J Biol Chem* 2004; 279:5329.

55. Samoto H, Shimizu E, Matsuda-Honjyo Y, et al. Prostaglandin E2 stimulates bone sialoprotein (BSP) expression through cAMP and fibroblast growth factor 2 response elements in the proximal promoter of the rat BSP gene. *J Biol Chem* 2003; 278:28659.

56. Stein GS, Lian JB, Stein JL, et al. Transcriptional control of osteoblast growth and differentiation. *Physiol Rev* 1996; 76:593.

57. Boudreaux JM, Towler DA. Synergistic induction of osteocalcin gene expression: identification of a bipartite element conferring fibroblast growth factor 2 and cyclic AMP responsiveness in the rat osteocalcin promoter. *J Biol Chem* 1996; 271:7508.

58. Yu XP. Chandrasekhar S. Parathyroid hormone (PTH 1-34) regulation of rat osteocalcin gene transcription. *Endocrinology* 1997; 138:3085.

59. Xiao G, Gopalakrishnan R, Jiang D, et al. Bone morphogenetic proteins, extracellular matrix, and mitogen-activated protein kinase signaling pathways are required for osteoblast-specific gene expression and differentiation in MC3T3-E1 cells. *J Bone Miner Res* 2002; 17:101.

60. Ducy P, Zhang R, Geoffroy V, et al. Osf2/Cbfa1: a transcriptional activator of osteoblast differentiation. *Cell* 1997; 89:747.

61. Barnes GL, Javed A, Waller SM, et al. Osteoblast-related transcription factors Runx2 (Cbfa1/AML3) and MSX2 mediate the expression of bone sialoprotein in human metastatic breast cancer cells. *Cancer Res* 2003; 63:2631.

62. Newberry EP, Boudreaux JM, Towler DA. Stimulus-selective inhibition of rat osteocalcin promoter induction and protein-DNA interactions by the homeodomain repressor Msx2. *J Biol Chem* 1997; 272:29607.

63. Aslam F, McCabe L, Frenkel B, et al. AP-1 and vitamin D receptor (VDR) signaling pathways converge at the rat osteocalcin VDR element: requirement for the internal activating protein-1 site for vitamin D-mediated trans-activation. *Endocrinology* 1999; 140:63.

64. Ryoo HM, Hoffmann HM, Beumer T, et al. Stage-specific expression of Dlx-5 during osteoblast differentiation: involvement in regulation of osteocalcin gene expression. *Mol Endocrinol* 1997; 11:1681.

65. Komori T, Yagi H, Nomura S, et al. Targeted disruption of Cbfa1 results in a complete lack of bone formation owing to maturational arrest of osteoblasts. *Cell* 1997; 89:755.

66. Otto F, Thornell AP, Crompton T, et al. Cbfa1, a candidate gene for cleidocranial dysplasia syndrome, is essential for osteoblast differentiation and bone development. *Cell* 1997; 89:765.

67. Banerjee C, McCabe LR, Choi JY, et al. Runt homology domain proteins in osteoblast differentiation: AML3/CBFA1 is a major component of a bone-specific complex. *J Cell Biochem* 1997; 66:1.

68. Steitz SA, Speer MY, Curinga G, et al. Smooth muscle cell phenotypic transition associated with calcification: upregulation of Cbfa1 and downregulation of smooth muscle lineage markers. *Circ Res* 2001; 89:1147.

69. Kern B, Shen J, Starbuck M, et al. Cbfa1 contributes to the osteoblast-specific expression of type I collagen genes. *J Biol Chem* 2001; 276:7101.

70. Hay ED. An overview of epithelio-mesenchymal transformation. *Acta Anat (Basel)* 1995; 154:8.

71. Veltmaat JM, Orelio CC, Ward-Van Oostwaard D, et al. Snail is an immediate early target gene of parathyroid hormone related peptide signaling in parietal endoderm formation. *Int J Dev Biol* 2000; 44:297.

72. Ciruna B, Rossant J. FGF signaling regulates mesoderm cell fate specification and morphogenetic movement at the primitive streak. *Dev Cell* 2001; 1:37.

73. Nieto MA. The early steps of neural crest development. *Mech Dev* 2001; 105:27.

74. Tucker RP. Neural crest cells: a model for invasive behavior. *Int J Biochem Cell Biol* 2004; 36:173.

75. Savagner P, Valles AM, Jouanneau J, et al. Alternative splicing in fibroblast growth factor receptor 2 is associated with induced epithelial-mesenchymal transition in rat bladder carcinoma cells. *Mol Biol Cell* 1994; 5:851.

76. Boyer B, Valles AM, Edme N. Induction and regulation of epithelial-mesenchymal transitions. *Biochem Pharmacol* 2000; 60:1091.

77. Thiery JP. Epithelial-mesenchymal transitions in tumour progression. *Nat Rev Cancer* 2002; 2:442.

78. Petersen OW, Nielsen HL, Gudjonsson T, et al. Epithelial to mesenchymal transition in human breast cancer can provide a nonmalignant stroma. *Am J Pathol* 2003; 162:391.

79. Pugh CW, Ratcliffe PJ. Regulation of angiogenesis by hypoxia: role of the HIF system. *Nat Med* 2003; 9:677.

80. Hendrix MJ, Seftor EA, Hess AR, et al. Vasculogenic mimicry and tumour-cell plasticity: lessons from melanoma. *Nat Rev Cancer* 2003; 3:411.

81. Savagner P. Leaving the neighborhood: molecular mechanisms involved during epithelial-mesenchymal transition. *Bioessays* 2001; 23:912.

82. Gold LI. The role for transforming growth factor-beta (TGF-beta) in human cancer. *Crit Rev Oncog* 1999; 10:303.

83. Thomasset N, Lochter A, Sympson CJ, et al. Expression of autoactivated stromelysin-1 in mammary glands of transgenic mice leads to a reactive stroma during early development. *Am J Pathol* 1998; 153:457.

84. Rowley DR. What might a stromal response mean to prostate cancer progression? *Cancer Metastasis Rev* 1998; 17:411.

85. Bates RC, Mercurio AM. Tumor necrosis factor-alpha stimulates the epithelial-to-mesenchymal transition of human colonic organoids. *Mol Biol Cel* 2003; 14:1790.

86. Thiery JP. Epithelial-mesenchymal transitions in development and pathologies. *Curr Opin Cell Biol* 2003; 15:740.

87. Grunert S, Jechlinger M, Beug H. Diverse cellular and molecular mechanisms contribute to epithelial plasticity and metastasis. *Nat Rev Mol Cell Biol* 2003; 4:657.

88. Untergasser G, Gander R, Rumpold H, et al. TGF-beta cytokines increase senescence-associated beta-galactosidase activity in human prostate basal cells by supporting differentiation processes, but not cellular senescence. *Exp Gerontol* 2003; 38:1179.

89. Zhau HY, Zhou J, Symmans WF, et al. Transfected neu oncogene induces human prostate cancer metastasis. *Prostate* 1996; 28:73.
90. Putz E, Witter K, Offner S, et al. Phenotypic characteristics of cell lines derived from disseminated cancer cells in bone marrow of patients with solid epithelial tumors: establishment of working models for human micrometastases. *Cancer Res* 1999; 59:241.
91. Gotzmann J, Mikula M, Eger A, et al. Molecular aspects of epithelial cell plasticity: implications for local tumor invasion and metastasis. *Mutat Res* 2004; 566:9.
92. Arap W, Pasqualini R, Ruoslahti E. Cancer treatment by targeted drug delivery to tumor vasculature in a mouse model. *Science* 1998; 279:377.
93. Tucker GC. Alpha v integrin inhibitors and cancer therapy. *Curr Opin Investig Drugs* 2003; 4:722.
94. Leder BZ, Smith MR, Fallon MA, et al.: Effects of gonadal steroid suppression on skeletal sensitivity to parathyroid hormone in men. *J Clin Endocrinol Metab* 2001; 86:511.
95. Lin DL, Tarnowski CP, Zhang J, et al. Bone metastatic LNCaP-derivative C4-2B prostate cancer cell line mineralizes in vitro. *Prostate* 2001; 47:212.
96. Carducci MA, Nelson JB, Bowling MK, et al. Atrasentan, an endothelin-receptor antagonist for refractory adenocarcinomas: safety and pharmacokinetics. *J Clin Oncol* 2002; 20:2171.
97. Nemeth JA, Yousif R, Herzog M, et al. Matrix metalloproteinase activity, bone matrix turnover, and tumor cell proliferation in prostate cancer bone metastasis. *J Natl Cancer Inst* 2002; 94:17.
98. Singer CF, Kronsteiner N, Marton E, et al. MMP-2 and MMP-9 expression in breast cancer-derived human fibroblasts is differentially regulated by stromal-epithelial interactions. *Breast Cancer Res Treat* 2002; 72:69.
99. Migita T, Sato E, Saito K, et al. Differing expression of MMPs-1 and -9 and urokinase receptor between diffuse- and intestinal-type gastric carcinoma. *Int J Cancer* 1999; 84:74.

6 Roles of Immune-Cell-Derived Matrix Metalloproteinases in Tumor Growth and Metastasis

Kristina A. Szabo, MSc and Gurmit Singh, PhD

1. INTRODUCTION

A considerable amount of clinical and experimental data has shown that proteolytic enzymes affecting the composition and function of the extracellular matrix (ECM) and cell surface molecules appear to be essential for the metastatic process. Certain structural changes of the ECM accompany cell migration during physiological tissue remodeling and tumor cell invasion. The ECM forms basement membranes that modulate cell adhesion, cell motility, and the selective exchange of molecules between cells and interstitial fluids. In mediating immune surveillance, inflammatory cells routinely cross this barrier. Matrix metalloproteinases (MMPs) are a family of zinc-containing endopeptidases that share structural domains and have the capacity to degrade ECM components as well as to alter biological functions of ECM macromolecules [1]. The specific proteolytic targets of MMPs include many other proteinases, proteinase inhibitors, clotting factors, chemotactic molecules, latent growth factors, growth-factor-binding proteins, cell surface receptors, as well as cell–cell and cell–matrix adhesion molecules [2–10]. ECM fragments of laminin, collagen, and fibrin also have biological roles in modulating inflammatory cell infiltration and cell proliferation. Such activities further underscore the importance of immune-cell-derived matrix-degrading enzymes, such as MMPs, during tumor growth and metastasis.

From: *Cancer Drug Discovery and Development*
Bone Metastasis: Experimental and Clinical Therapeutics
Edited by: G. Singh and S. A. Rabbani © Humana Press Inc., Totowa, NJ

Immune cells are important sources of MMPs and utilize these enzymes to mediate extravasation into tissues during inflammation *(11)*. The net effect of a mixture of active MMPs is determined by their substrate specificity, cellular sources, area of distribution, and the type and level of their regulatory proteins *(11)*. Under normal physiological conditions, MMP transcripts are generally expressed at low levels, but these levels rise rapidly when tissues are locally induced to undergo remodeling *(12,13)*, at which time, MMPs likely serve specialized roles to sustain homeostasis. Cancer cells can orchestrate the activity of various proteases, receptors, and polypeptide inhibitors, channeling all of them in the invasion process. In addition, recent studies emphasize not only soluble factors but also cell–matrix and cell–cell interactions as key factors in the regulation of MMPs. This chapter details the structures, functions, and regulatory mechanisms of MMPs and presents an overview of the biological activities of immune-cell-derived MMPs in tumor progression.

2. CLASSIFICATION OF THE MATRIX METALLOPROTEINASE FAMILY

Matrix metalloproteinases have a descriptive name and an MMP number. The nomenclature does not accurately reflect the actual number of enzymes because MMP-4, MMP-5, and MMP-6 have been eliminated owing to duplication *(14)*. The MMPs are organized into three major functional groups, in part based on substrate specificity: the interstitial collagenases (MMP-1, MMP-8, and MMP-13), which act on collagen types I, II, and III, the stromelysins (MMP-3, MMP-10, and MMP-11) with specificity for laminin, fibronectin and proteoglycans, and the gelatinases (MMP-2 and MMP-9), which most effectively cleave type IV and V collagen *(15,16)*. This classification is somewhat arbitrary because the physiological substrates are still a matter of debate. The substrate specificity of distinct MMPs has been determined by their ability to degrade various components of the ECM in vitro. It is now recognized that there is some functional overlap between members of the MMP family, although direct evidence for the proteolytic activity of MMPs in vivo is still limited *(17)*. Because an overlap of substrate specificity might exist among the different proteolytic pathways, several enzymes may be operational simultaneously in a tumor and act in a cascade-like manner. Therefore, taken together, the MMPs can degrade most ECM components, whether by a redundant action on similar substrates, or by a cooperative effect of several MMPs on distinct components.

Matrix metalloproteinases share a common domain structure, although not all domains are represented in all family members *(18)*. Domains located on either side of the catalytic core define the substrate affinities, which are used to categorize the MMPs into their subfamilies. In general, MMPs share a pre-domain, which is a signal peptide for secretion, a pro-domain to maintain latency, a catalytic domain containing a highly conserved zinc-binding site, a hinge region, and a C-terminal domain also known as a hemopexinlike domain *(19)*. Two family members, MMP-2 and MMP-9, have a gelatin-binding domain containing three fibronectin type II repeats inserted into the catalytic domain. Five members, known as membrane-type matrix metalloproteinases (MT-MMPs), have a carboxyl-terminal transmembrane domain after the hemopexin domain. They reside on the cell surface, in contrast to the other family members, which are secreted as proenzymes into the extracellular milieu *(20)*. MMPs are functional at neutral pH and are produced by a variety of cells including fibroblasts, neutrophils, eosinophils, macrophages, T-cells, chondrocytes, and osteoblasts.

3. REGULATION OF MATRIX METALLOPROTEINASE ACTIVITY

The modeling, disassembly, and remodeling of connective tissue matrices by one or more MMPs involves secretion and proteolytic activation of the precursor MMPs. Transcription of MMP genes can take place on demand in response to growth factors (such as epidermal growth factor [EGF], fibroblast growth factor [FGF], and platelet-derived growth factor [PDGF]) (21,22), cytokines, hormones, chemical agents (phorbol esters, actin stress fiber-disrupting drugs), physical stress, cellular transformation, and components of infectious pathogens, among others (23). Enhanced MMP gene expression can be downregulated by suppressive factors, which include transforming growth factor-β (TGF-β), retinoic acids, and glucocorticoids (24–28). TGF and insulin-like growth factor (IGF) are components of the ECM, where they are both linked to corresponding binding proteins. Proteolytic remodeling of the ECM might favor the release of TGF and IGF from their receptors, influencing cell functions and MMP production (29,30).

There are two known in vivo mechanisms of MMP inhibition. The first is α_2-macroglobulin, a large protein (approx 750 kDa) produced by the liver (1). The second, more specific, mechanism of inhibition is a family of proteins known as tissue inhibitors of metalloproteinases (TIMPs) that comprises four members (TIMP-1, TMP-2, TMP-3, and TMP-4). TIMPs are specific endogenous inhibitors of MMPs that form noncovalent-binding complexes in a 1:1 stoichiometry with pro-forms and activated forms of MMPs and inhibit enzymatic activity. Although TIMPs bind tightly to most MMPs and are highly similar in their quaternary structure, their tissue distribution, regulation, and function are diverse, suggesting that each TIMP can have a specific physiological role. Similar to MMPs, TIMPs are also regulated by a network of different signaling molecules. TIMPs can also inhibit the MT-MMPs, however, unlike soluble MMPs, MT-MMPs exhibit significant differences in affinities for the various TIMPs (20).

Matrix metalloproteinases are synthesized and secreted as inactive zymogens; they share an N-terminal inhibitory pro-peptide sequence with a cysteine (Cys) that chelates the zinc (Zn^{2+}) ion and keeps the enzyme in a latent pro-form (12). Various factors can activate MMPs via a conformational change that disrupts the Cys-Zn^{2+} binding (cysteine switch) and leads to intermediate activation followed by autocatalytic cleavage of the pro-peptide from the core protein that renders the enzyme fully active (31,32). In vivo, most pro-MMPs are likely to be activated by tissue or plasma proteinases. Using transgenic mice deficient in urokinase-type plasminogen activator (uPA), Carmeliet and colleagues have suggested that the uPA–plasmin system is a pathophysiologically significant activator of pro-MMPs (33). Furthermore, MMPs and plasma proteases can regulate one anothers activity by degrading their respective inhibitors. MMP-12, MMP-7, and the stromelysins are able to degrade the serine protease inhibitor (serpin) α1PI (34–36). Conversely, plasmin has proteolytic activity against MMP inhibitors such as TIMP-2 (37).

Although not all MT-MMPs are fully characterized, there is evidence that one of their functions is to localize and activate secreted MMPs. The activation of pro-MMP-2 is thought to take place primarily on the cell surface. Recent studies propose that this activation process requires both active MT1-MMP and the TIMP-2-bound MT1-MMP. The C-terminus of pro-MMP-2 forms a noncovalent complex with TIMP-2, whereas the free part of MT1-MMP can remove the pro-domain portion of the molecule (38,39). Full activation of pro-MMP-2 is achieved by a second cleavage event in which the intermediate MMP-2 species is autocatalytically processed to the fully active enzyme (40). The

MT1-MMP/TIMP-2/pro-MMP-2 complex *(41–43)*, referred to as the ternary complex, only occurs at low TIMP-2 concentrations relative to MT1-MMP to permit availability of enough inhibitor-free MT1-MMP to initiate pro-MMP-2 activation *(44)*. This dual function of TIMP-2 is both a controversial and intriguing issue. In all, the action of MMPs can be regulated at the level of gene transcription, translation, and secretion of latent enzyme, pro-enzyme activation, and inactivation by endogenous inhibitors. Under physiological conditions, the activity of MMPs is tightly regulated to prevent excessive proteolytic activity and tissue destruction.

4. IMMUNE CELLS AND MATRIX METALLOPROTEINASE EXPRESSION

Components of the inflammatory environment include monocytes, macrophages, B- and T-lymphocytes, neutrophils, eosinophils, and mast cells. Each of these cells has distinct functions in inflammation and in the restoration of homeostasis *(45,46)*. Although specialized in their multiple effector functions, these cells may interact with each other in order to modify such activities as the expression of surface receptors, the production of inflammatory cytokines, or the level of activation. The production, secretion, and activation of MMPs by immune cells follows cell-specific patterns of representation. MMPs prepare vascular and immune tissues for macrophage and T-cell adhesion, facilitate the secretion of membrane-bound cytokines, and enable extravascular tissue access. Which MMPs the macrophage will produce depends upon its level of differentiation and on tight regulation by many physiologic, pathologic, and pharmacologic stimuli *(47–51)*. Macrophages have been shown to secrete MMP-1, MMP-2, MMP-3, MMP-7, and MMP-9, as well as a unique elastase designated MMP-12 *(48,50–58)*. Neutrophil-derived MMPs, such as MMP-8 and MMP-9, play a key role in the degradation of ECM constituents during inflammatory diseases *(59–62)*. Neutrophils have been found to release a soluble factor that can activate endothelial cell MMP-2 independent of cell–cell contact *(63)*. MMP-9 in neutrophils can be prepackaged in granules prior to activation; thus, it can be present without detectable *de novo* synthesis during inflammatory responses involving neutrophils *(62)*. Furthermore, MMP-12 has been shown to cleave α_1-antitrypsin, releasing a 4-kDa fragment that is chemotactic for neutrophils *(64)*. T-Cells predominantly secrete the gelatinases MMP-2 and MMP-9, after β1-integrin- or vascular cell adhesion molecule (VCAM)-1-dependent stimulation by cytokines and inflammatory mediators *(65–69)*. Leukocyte extravasation requires the secretion of MMPs, which allows leukocytes to penetrate through the basement membrane and into the tissue stroma *(70,71)*. It is likely that gelatinase expression facilitates T-lymphocyte traffic across subendothelial basal lamina, because MMP inhibitors have been observed to inhibit the migration of resting T-cells across a basal lamina equivalent in vitro *(67)*. Furthermore, stimulation of T-cells with interleukin (IL)-2 and IL-4 increases both cell migration as well as MMP-2 and MMP-9 production *(68,69,72,73)* and enhances their migration across reconstituted basement membranes. Invasive leukocytes have been shown to constitutively produce substantial quantities of MMPs, and recent studies suggest that MMP-9 inactivates the primary physiologic inhibitor of leukocyte elastase, α_1-proteinase inhibitor (α_1PI [α_1-antitrypsin]); this step is central to leukocyte migration *(74)*. Taken together, these studies suggest a role for MMPs in the process of immune cell recruitment to the site of inflammation.

Unlike other MMPs, which are expressed or released in response to injury, disease, or inflammation, MMP-7 is expressed by noninjured, noninflamed exocrine and mucosal epithelium. Thus, this enzyme likely serves a common homeostatic function among epithelia and several observations implicate a role for MMP-7 in innate immunity *(75,76)*. All tissues in which MMP-7 is constitutively expressed are more available to the external environment and, hence, are vulnerable to bacterial exposure. Bacterial exposure is a potent and relevant process that controls MMP-7 expression and activation in human and murine epithelial tissues, suggesting a novel role for micro-organisms in the regulation of this MMP *(75–78)*. An important common role of mucosal epithelium is to function as an active barrier against the external environment, and the secretion of antibiotic peptides (defensins) by epithelial cells appears to be an important component of innate immunity. MMP-7 was found to regulate the activity of defensins in internal mucosal defense *(78)*, thus aiding mucosal immune cells by regulating the level of active antimicrobial peptides. Stromal–epithelial interactions are complex and can involve paracrine factors, ECM interactions, and cell–cell contact.

4.1. Cytokines and Chemokines

In the context of immunity, MMPs function not only as effectors of tissue remodeling but also interact with the cytokine and chemokine networks. Chemokines are produced primarily by leukocytes and have been implicated directly and indirectly in the generation of immunity as well as specific antimicrobial/fungal activity during inflammation and disease. The role of chemokines in the recruitment of neutrophils, monocytes, and lymphocytes into inflammatory sites has been described by a number of laboratories *(79)*. The cleavage of various chemokines by MMPs can modify their functional properties and limit their bioavailability and activity to target foci of inflammation. This can then ensure the localization of the responding immune cells to restricted sites and allow a migratory immune cell to actively orchestrate its own fate, as it traverses into extravascular spaces, by tailoring ECM composition to facilitate its passage and its response to a given inflammatory stimulus *(80,81)*. The biological activities of chemoattractants might augment inflammatory processes in concert with the ECM environment, thereby fine-tuning the duration and intensity of the immune response as needed.

In addition to this regulatory effect of MMPs on cytokines and chemokines, the latter are often involved in MMP regulation. Inflammatory mediators such as TNF-α/β and IL-1α/β modulate the expression and regulation of MMPs via different pathways *(68,70,82–86)*. For example, they have been shown to induce the expression of MMPs in human macrophage cells *(87)*. Many of these agents, such as TNF-α and several interleukins, are themselves upregulated in epithelial cells in response to bacterial infection *(88)*. They have been shown to stimulate lymphocyte motility and are secreted by a number of different cell types in response to acute inflammatory stimuli. Macrophage colony-stimulating factor (M-CSF) is one of the several factors known to regulate the survival *(89)*, proliferation *(90)*, differentiation, and accumulation of mononuclear phagocytic lineage cells *(91,92)*. MMP gene expression in macrophages can be controlled by the relative levels of M-CSF and granulocyte–macrophage colony-stimulating factor (GM-CSF) *(93)*, because GM-CSF was found to stimulate expression of MMP-12, whereas M-CSF repressed MMP-12 in murine macrophages *(51)*. Zhang and colleagues reported that whereas TNF-α, GM-CSF or IL-1β when added individually stimulated only MMP-9 and TIMP-1, the combination of GM-CSF with TNF-α or IL-1β, or all three cytokines, induced the synthesis of MMP-1 and caused a further increased production of MMP-9 and TIMP-1 *(94)*.

The susceptibility of the pro-inflammatory cytokine IL-1β to degradation by MMPs introduces a new important aspect in understanding the progression of inflammation and tissue damage, because IL-1α is also an inducer of MMP gene transcription *(95)*. While normal tissues contain little MMP activity, the production of pro-MMP-1, pro-MMP-3, pro-MMP-7, and pro-MMP-9 is enhanced by IL-1β secreted from activated macrophages and many other cell types. These MMPs are synthesized and secreted from cells as inactive precursors, but once activated, they can control the activity of IL-1β but not IL-1α. It is notable that the major type of IL-1 found in rheumatoid synovium is IL-1β *(96)*.

In contrast, inflammatory mediators can act as inhibitors of MMP production, as demonstrated by the ability of interferon-γ (IFN-γ), IL-4, and IL-10, progesterone, and corticosteroids to suppress MMP synthesis *(49,68,97–102)*. It has been well established that macrophage chemotactic protein-1 (MCP-1) is chemotactic for monocytes, but TNF-α could regulate such movement by rapidly downregulating the expression of CCR2, the chemokine receptor for MCP-1 *(103,104)*. The relative amounts of intact and cleaved MCP-3 that are present after pathophysiological cleavage regulates chemotaxis and the extent of inflammation. Identification of the importance of MMP-2 in the pathophysiological processing of MCP-3 *(8)* reveals the intersection of two distinct pathways that regulate the extracellular environment and the inactivation of a cytokine in vivo by MMP activity. Growing evidence also suggests that the same cytokines that influence MMP expression not only associate with the ECM components but are also subject to enzymatic processing by these enzymes *(95,105,106)*. Collectively, these findings suggest that cytokines such as TNF-α could serve not only in activating circulating immune cells but also in modulating their behavior when cells are in the context of an inflamed ECM microenvironment *(84)*. Therefore, it is clear that the interaction of MMPs with cytokines and chemokines provides a self-attenuating network to dissipate pro-inflammatory activities and determine the extent of connective tissue degradation.

4.2. Cell–Cell and Cell–Matrix Interactions

Recent studies emphasize not only soluble factors but also cell–matrix and cell–cell interactions as initiators in the expression of MMPs. MMPs are also known to solubilize cell-surface and matrix-bound factors that can then act in an autocrine or paracrine manner to influence cellular properties such as growth, death, and migration. Studies have indicated a role for direct cell–cell contact in potentiating MMP expression, notably MMP-1 and MMP–9 in monocytes *(107,108)* and T-lymphoma cells *(109,110)*, as well as mast cell-T–cell contact *(111)*. Mast cells were found to degranulate in response to direct contact with activated T-cells as well as to produce tumor necrosis factor-α (TNF-α) *(112)*. Furthermore, T-cells are capable of directly inducing MMP-9 expression in fibroblasts *(113)*, neutrophils *(114)*, and monocytes *(107,115)*, through cell–cell contact. As mentioned previously, MMPs are responsible for the matrix degradation required for leukocyte extravasation during inflammation *(72)*. They have also been shown to mediate the release of Fas ligand (FasL) *(116)* and process the inflammatory cytokine TNF-α, releasing the biologically active form from the surface of cells *(105,117,118)*. The bidirectional signaling that occurs upon adhesion of T-lymphoma cells to endothelial cells is a determinant in the production of MMP-9 and TIMP-1 in both cell types *(109)*.

Extracellular proteases modulate cellular behavior by altering cell surface–ECM interactions and regulating the processing of growth factors. A possible mechanism might be the release of growth factors from the ECM, thus favoring tumor growth in a paracrine manner. The spectrum of MMPs is broad, including proteins involved in homeostasis such as fibrinogen *(2,5)*, Factor XII *(7)*, plasminogen *(3)*, and plasmin *(4)*. MMP activity has been implicated in the cleavage of E-cadherin *(119)*, the shedding of L-selectin *(120,121)*, and the hyaluronan proteoglycan receptor CD44 *(122,123)* from various cells. There is evidence that inhibition of E-cadherin function can be mediated through the shedding of its ectodomain as a result of cleavage by MMP-7 and MMP-3 *(9,119)*. Activated human T-cells localized in atherosclerotic plaques have been demonstrated to mediate contact-dependent expression of MMP-1, MMP-2, MMP-3, and MMP–9 in vascular smooth muscle cells through T-lymphocyte surface molecule CD40 ligand signaling *(124)*. In addition, although insulin-like growth factor-binding proteins (IGFBPs) can confer latency on IGF-I and IGF-II, their degradation not only can restore the activity of these growth factors but also influence the IGF-independent effect of IGFBP on cell growth. IGFBP-1 has been identified as a potential physiological substrate for MMP-11 *(125)*. Collectively, the actions of MMPs demonstrate their significance in governing inflammatory responses not only by creating a trail for immune cells to migrate into inflamed tissues but also by modifying the contextual molecules that affect cell behavior and enzyme secretion itself *(84)*. Thus, MMP activity on nontraditional substrates could exert a biological impact on inflammatory processes that is as profound as the effects caused by ECM degradation *(80)*.

Interleukin-1β and TNF-α have a number of overlapping biological effects, including the increased expression of intercellular adhesion molecule-1 (ICAM-1) and VCAM-1 by endothelial cells (ECs), which promotes increased adhesion to capillary ECs and extravasation. ICAM-1 is implicated in a broad range of transient cellular interactions that regulate leukocyte homing, activation, and effector functions. Thus, the interaction between ICAM-1 and its physiological ligand LFA-1 is implicated in leukocyte arrest on endothelial cells, stabilization of cognate interactions between antigen-presenting cells and T-lymphocytes and adhesion of cytotoxic T-cells and natural killer (NK) cells to target organs *(126,127)*. More directly, the shedding of ICAM-1 has been observed to inhibit cell-mediated cytotoxicity and provide primary tumor cells, as well as tumor cell lines, with a mechanism of defense against cytolytic T-cells and NK cells *(128–132)*. Recently, the release of ICAM-1 from the cell surface has been attributed to MMP activity *(133)*. Stimulation of ICAM-1 by LFA-1 has been observed to induce expression of MMP-9 *(109)*. Similarly, adhesion of leukocytes to vascular ECs via VCAM-1 induces expression of MMP-2 *(134)*, and cell–matrix interaction via β1-integrins control MMP-dependent migration through basement membranes *(135)*. These observations provide evidence that MMPs might also contribute to tumor evasion of immune surveillance. Thus, MMPs can inactivate or shed proteins from cell surfaces and transform membrane-bound cytokines, cytokine receptors, and adhesion molecules to their soluble forms, leading to potential mediation of inflammatory reactions *(12)*. Protease activation and substrate cleavage can occur more rapidly than downregulation of cell surface receptor expression, providing a potentially tighter control over specific adhesion events *(136)*. Shedding of cell surface receptors, as a result of proteolytic cleavage of a portion of their extracellular domain, could provide a regulatory mechanism that helps terminate cell–cell and cell–ECM interactions *(137,138)*.

5. IMMUNE CELLS AND MATRIX METALLOPROTEINASES IN TUMORS

In order for tumor cell invasion to successfully occur, a balance between proteases and inhibitors is necessary. An optimal invasion phenotype requires that tumor cells have the ability to form attachments with each other and with matrix proteins. Uninhibited matrix degradation leading to complete dissolution of matrix proteins would not be conducive to metastatic spread. MMPs are believed to play an important role in the sequential, interrelated steps necessary for tumor growth and metastasis. They have the potential to create an environment that supports the growth of primary tumors, to enhance tumor angiogenesis and neovascularization, and to enable the disruption of local tissue architecture and penetration of connective tissue barriers which allows for the dissemination of cancer cells *(139)*.

It is well established that solid tumors comprise a heterogeneous population of cells. The malignant cells are usually surrounded and infiltrated by a stromal compartment consisting of fibroblasts, myofibroblasts, vascular endothelial cells, pericytes, macrophages, lymphocytes, and neutrophils *(140–144)*. Stromal reactions occurring in cancer tissues do not efficiently suppress tumour growth because of the presumptive immunosuppressive effects of carcinoma cells. Although, initially, it was assumed that tumor cells were the origin of MMPs found in this environment, *in situ* hybridization techniques have shown that whereas some MMPs are expressed by tumor cells, MMPs are predominantly produced by adjacent host stromal and inflammatory cells in response to factors released by tumors *(see* Fig. 1) *(16,19)*.

Among the stromal cells, the presence of macrophages is frequently noted in aggressive malignant tumors, indicating a relation to the degree of tumor cell differentiation *(145–153)*. These tumor-associated macrophages (TAMs), which likely represent a unique subset of macrophage cells, can enhance angiogenesis by producing growth factors *(154)*, favoring fibrin deposition, and by releasing MMPs *(50,155–160)*. Invading blood vessels provide nutrition and oxygen for the malignant cell population as well as a route for metastasizing tumor cells into the systemic circulation *(140)*. TAMs are now thought to play an important role in regulating the development of new blood vessels by producing factors that promote angiogenesis *(140,158)*. For example, implanted syngeneic fibrosarcomas were observed to be markedly less vascularized when their murine hosts were depleted of monocytes *(158)*. Furthermore, Leibovich and colleagues *(161)* showed that TAMs and their conditioned medium could induce neovascularization in various in vivo assays, In addition, the vascularization of tumors formed by several human tumor cell lines in vivo has been correlated with the degree of macrophage infiltration *(158)*. Also, TAMs are the major cell type in breast carcinoma containing immunoreactive TNF-α and TNF-β receptors (p55 and p75) are upregulated in endothelial cells as well as leukocytes in these tumors *(162,163)*. Interestingly, the systemic administration of relatively specific macrophage toxins, such as silica, carrageenen, and trypan blue, reduces the size of primary murine tumors but enhances growth of metastases *(156,164–166)*.

Whereas MMPs, secreted largely by stromal cells, commonly facilitate tumor progression, their proteolytic cleavage products might inhibit angiogenesis and, thus, limit metastatic growth by the generation of antiangiogenic agents *(167)*. This was first apparent with the isolation of angiostatin from the urine of mice with Lewis lung cell (LLC)

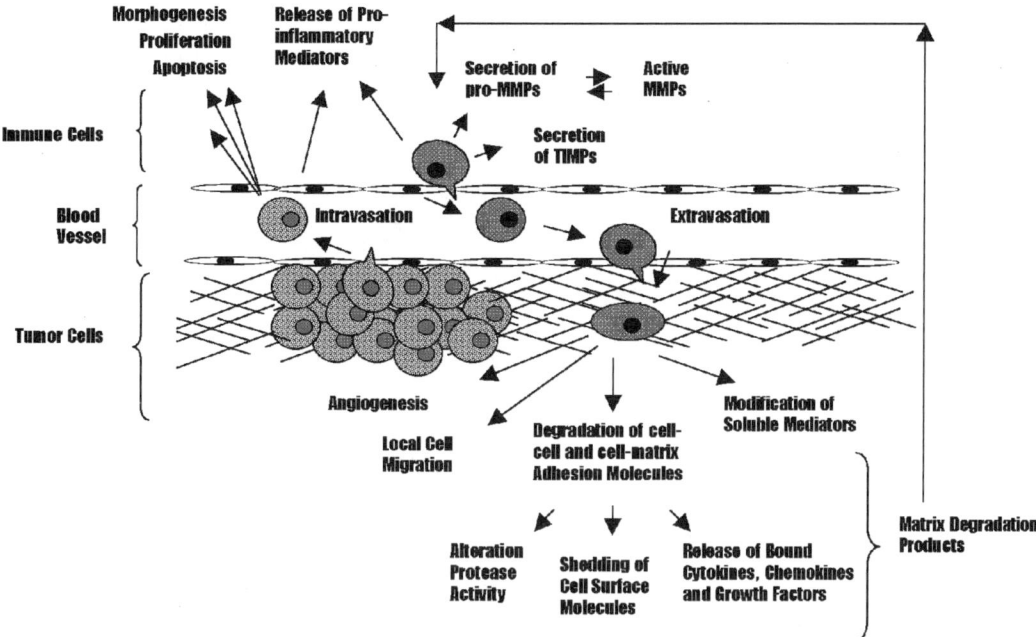

Fig. 1. Schematic representation of the various roles of MMPs. During the development of primary tumors, metastatic spread, and growth of tumors at secondary sites, MMPs have significant functional overlap and, therefore, the actions that take place at one stage of tumor growth or development might play a role in the other stages. Furthermore, fragments of matrix proteins released by MMP proteolysis can further act as chemoattractants for distant immune cells and, thus, participate in a feedback loop to modulate protease production and leukocyte recruitment.

carcinoma *(169)*. Angiostatin, a plasminogen cleavage product, inhibits EC proliferation and thereby angiogenesis *(3)* and is believed to be responsible for maintaining LLC metastases in a dormant state. Dong and colleagues demonstrated that the generation of angiostatin in the LLC model was not caused by tumor cell proteinases but, rather, was associated with the presence of macrophages in the primary tumor, presumably the result of the production of MMP-12 by the macrophage cells *(169)*. It has recently been shown that MMP-3, MMP-7, MMP-9, and MMP-12 can generate angiostatin from plasminogen, indicating that their expression in peritumoral areas could, in fact, serve to limit angiogenesis and, therefore, inhibit tumor growth and invasion *(3,168–170)*. In addition the ability of MMPs to degrade and inactivate IL-1β *(95)* and cleave the precursor of TNF-α, leaving a biologically active form *(105,171)* indicates that MMPs and TIMPs might regulate the availability and activity of inflammatory cytokines at the site of tumor invasion. Whalen *(172)* has suggested that tumor-derived signals might be misconstrued by immune cells, as those signals normally present at sites of inflammation, and in their efforts to heal the perceived wound, these cells might inadvertently aid tumor growth. Thus, the contribution of macrophage cells to angiogenesis must depend on the fine regulation and balance of proangiogenic and antiangiogenic factors *(173,174)*.

The expression of MMPs in tumors is regulated in a paracrine manner by growth factors and cytokines secreted by tumor-infiltrating inflammatory cells as well as by tumor or stromal cells. Recent studies have suggested that continuous crosstalk takes place between tumor cells, stromal cells, and inflammatory cells during the invasion process *(175–178)*. For example, tumor-derived MMPs, such as MMP-9, are able to induce the proteolytic cleavage of IL-2R (the receptor essential for the proliferation of T-cells), thereby suppressing signaling and the proliferative capability of cancer-encountered T-cells (i.e., tumor-specific cytotoxic lymphocytes) *(179)*. MMPs, in this case also MMP-9, activate TGF-β *(180)*, an inhibitor of the T-lymphocyte response against tumors *(181)*, thereby promoting tumor invasion. An example of the manner in which the action of MMPs may promote tumor progression via evasion of mechanisms of immunosurveillance is seen from the effect of their degradation of tumor-derived α_1-PI *(182)*. Here, the cleavage of α_1-PI, principally by MMP-11, results in the generation of the carboxyl-terminal fragment α_1PI-C. α_1PI-C has been shown to enhance the growth and invasiveness of tumor cells in nude mice. It has been hypothesized that this molecule can modulate the activity of tumor–host immune reactions, principally the activity of NK cells *(182)*.

Studies using transgenic models demonstrate that TIMP-1 expression in vivo can either increase or decrease tumor invasion in a tumor-cell-specific manner *(183,184)*. It is possible that TIMP overexpression is the host response to tumor invasion in an attempt to control MMP activity and retain ECM integrity. However, there are indications that TIMPs can have growth stimulatory activity on certain cell types, including lymphoma cells and tumors of various origins *(185,186)*. Consistently, gelatinases have been found to be upregulated at the advancing edge of invasive malignancies, where they are coexpressed with MT1-MMP and TIMP-2 and with some ECM proteins, suggesting their interaction in cancer cell invasion and metastasis *(187–189)*. In this regard, it is noteworthy that certain invasive tumors express high levels of stromal TIMP-2, which were found to be associated with malignant parameters *(190)*. In particular, studies using *in situ* hybridization provided evidence for a predominantly stromal-cell-associated production of MMP-2 mRNA *(191–196)*. Once the protein is secreted, it becomes bound to the invasive front of the tumor cells, where it is localized to the surface of the tumor cells themselves *(191,194,197–201)*. It is also possible that host-derived MMP-2 binds membrane-bound molecules such as MT-MMP *(202)* or integrin $\alpha_v\beta_3$ *(203)* at the surface of tumor cells and, thus, localizes MMPs at sites proximal to important ECM ligands that would facilitate cellular invasion. An explanation as to why the peritumoral stromal cells express MT1-MMP, MMP-2, and MMP-9 might be that both the tumor cells and the stromal cells contribute to a different part of the metastatic cascade. The tumor cell MMPs could contribute to the invasive growth of the tumor, whereas the stromal elements contribute to the remodeling process and the desmoplastic reaction that occurs in the tissue adjacent to the tumor *(204)*. In general, the induction of MMPs in the stroma within tumors and in adjacent normal tissue represents a direct or indirect host response to the presence of tumor cells.

6. CONCLUSION

With the extensive new information provided in the field of MMP research over the past several years, researchers have begun to acquire a better appreciation of the significance of the proteolytic and destructive potential of the MMP family in biology and pathology. The interactions of tumor cells with their microenvironment determine many of the essential factors that will impact the fate of the tumor cells. MMPs contribute to the malignant process by their ability to promote the degradation of a variety of biologically relevant molecules that are not limited to ECM compounds. Instead, these molecules include a growing family of MMP substrates, among them cytokines, growth factor receptors, and cell–cell and cell–matrix adhesion molecules. It is likely that the activity of MMPs on nonmatrix substrates yields the critical response required for tumor progression. Although the expression of MMPs in malignancies has been widely studied and debated, the specific role of distinct immune-cell-derived MMPs in the progression of cancer might be more complex than previously assumed. Various studies are currently investigating the selective roles of protease families in specific tumors. Also, relevant are the interesting aspects of the cooperation between classes of proteases and proteolytic cascades, as well as the hierarchical relationship between individual MMPs and cells, cytokines, and chemokines of the immune system. Consequently, further studies could reveal many new pathophysiological implications of MMPs in their regulation of immune cells, cytokine and chemokine networks, and matrix proteolysis during the metastatic process.

ACKNOWLEDGMENTS

This work was supported by Canadian Institute of Health Research and Canadian Breast Cancer Research Alliance.

REFERENCES

1. Nagase H, Woessner JF Jr. Matrix Metalloproteinases. *J Biol Chem* 1999; 274:21,491–21,494.
2. Bini A, Itoh Y, Kudryk BJ, Nagase H. Degradation of cross-linked fibrin by matrix metalloproteinase 3 (stromelysin 1): hydrolysis of the gamma Gly 404-Ala 405 peptide bond. *Biochemistry* 1996; 35: 13,056–13,063.
3. Patterson BC, Sang QA. Angiostatin-converting enzyme activities of human matrilysin (MMP-7) and gelatinase B/Type IV collagenase (MMP-9). *J Biol Chem* 1997; 272:28,823–28,825.
4. Cornelius LA, Nehring LC, Harding E, Bolanowski M, Welgus HG, Kobayashi DK, et al. Matrix metalloproteinases generate angiostatin: effects on neovascularization. *J Immunol* 1998; 161:6845–6852.
5. Bini A, Wu D, Schnuer J, Kudryk BJ. Characterization of stromelysin 1 (MMP-3), matrilysin (MMP-7, and membrane type 1 matrix metalloproteinase (MT1-MMP) derived fibrin(ogen) fragments D-dimer and D-like monomer: NH_2-terminal sequences of late-stage digest fragments. *Biochemistry* 1999; 38:13,928–13,936.
6. Bergers G, Coussens LM. Extrinsic regulators of epithelial tumour progression: metalloproteinases. *Curr Opin Genet Dev* 2000; 10:120–127.
7. Hiller O, Lichte A, Oberpichler A, Kocourek A, Tschesche H. Matrix metalloproteinases collagenase-2, macrophage elastase, collagenase-3, and membrane type-1 matrix metalloproteinase impair clotting by degradation of fibrinogen and factor XII. *J Biol Chem* 2000; 275:33,008–33,013.
8. McQuibban GA, Gong JH, Tam EM, McCulloch CA, Clark-Lewis I, Overall CM. Inflammation dampened by gelatinase A cleavage of monocyte chemoattractant protein-3. *Science* 2000; 289:1202–1206.
9. Noë V, Fingleton B, Jacobs K, Crawford HC, Vermeulen S, Steelant W, Bruyneel E, Matrisian LM, Mareel M. Release of an invasion promotor E-cadherin fragment by matrilysin and stromelysin-1. *J Cell Sci* 2001; 114:111–118.
10. McCawley LJ, Matrisian LM. Matrix metalloproteinases: they're not just for matrix anymore! *Curr Opin Cell Biol* 2001; 13:534–540.
11. Goetzl E, Banda MJ, Leppert D. Matrix metalloproteinases in immunity. *J Immunol* 1996; 156:1–4.
12. Leppert D, Lindberg RL, Kappos L, Leib SL. Matrix metalloproteinases: multifunctional effectors of inflammation in multiple sclerosis and bacterial meningitis. *Brain Res Rev* 2001; 36:249–257.

13. Coussens LM, Fingleton B, Matrisian LM. Matrix metalloproteinase inhibitors and cancer: trials and tribulations. *Science* 2002; 295:2387–2392.

14. Woessner JF Jr. MMPs and TIMPs - an historical perspective. *Mol Biotechnol* 2002; 22:33–49.

15. Borkakoti N. Structural studies of matrix metalloproteinases. *J Mol Med* 2000; 78:261–268.

16. Nelson AR, Fingleton B, Rothenberg ML, Matrisian LM. Matrix metalloproteinases: biologic activity and clinical implications. *J Clin Oncol* 2000; 18:1135–1149.

17. Westermarck J, Kähäri V. Regulation of matrix metalloproteinase expression in tumor invasion. *FASEB J* 1999; 13:781–792.

18. Stetler-Stevenson WG, Yu AE. Proteases in invasion: matrix metalloproteinases. *Semin Cancer Biol* 2001; 11:143–152.

19. Hoekstra R, Eskens FA, Verweij E. Matrix metalloproteinase inhibitors: current developments and future perspectives. *Oncologist* 2001; 6:415–427.

20. Hernandez-Barrantes S, Bernardo M, Toth M, Fridman R. Regulation of membrane type-matrix metalloproteinases. *Semin Cancer Biol* 2002; 12:131–138.

21. Mauviel A. Cytokine regulation of metalloproteinase gene expression. *J Cell Biochem* 1993; 53: 288–295.

22. Madlener M, Mauch C, Conca W, Brauchle M, Parks WC, Werner S. Regulation of the expression of stromelysin-2 by growth factors in keritanocytes: implications for normal and impaired wound healing. *Biochem J* 1996; 320:659–664.

23. Fini ME, Cook JR, Mohan R. Regulation of MMP gene expression. In: Parks WC and Mecham RP, eds. Matrix metalloproteinases. San Diego, CA: Academic, 1998:299–356.

24. Frisch SM, Ruley HE. Transcription from the stromelysin promotor is induced by interleukin-1 and repressed by dexamethasone. *J Biol Chem* 1987; 262:16,300–16,304.

25. Kerr LD, Miller DB, Martrisian LM. TGF-beta 1 inhibition of transin/stromelysin gene expression is mediated through a Fos binding sequence. *Cell* 1990; 61:267–278.

26. Lafyatis R, Kim SJ, Angel P, Roberts AB, Sporn MB, Karin M, Wilder RL. Interleukin-1 stimulates and all-trans-retinoic acid inhibits collagenase gene expression through its 5' activator protein-1-binding site. *Mol Endocrinol* 1990; 4:973–980.

27. Nicholson RC, Mader S, Nagpal S, Leid M, Rochette-Egly C, Chambon P. Negative regulation of the rat stromelysin gene promotor by retinoic acid is mediated by an AP1 binding site. *EMBO J* 1990; 9:4443–4454.

28. Delany AM, Brinckerhoff CE. Post-transcriptional regulation of collagenase and stromelysin gene expression by epidermal growth factor and dexamethasone in cultured human fibroblasts. *J Cell Biochem* 1992; 50:400–410.

29. Parker A, Gockerman A, Busby WH, Clemmons DR. Properties of an insulin-like growth factor-binding protein-4 protease that is secreted by smooth muscle cells. *Endocrinology* 1995; 136:2470–2476.

30. Imai Y, Busby WH Jr, Smith CE, Clarke JB, Garmong AJ, Horwitz GD, Rees C, Clemmons DR. Protease-resistant form of insulin-like growth factor-binding protein 5 is an inhibitor of insulin-like growth factor-I actions on porcine smooth muscle cells in culture. *J Clin Invest* 1997; 100:2596–2605.

31. Springman EB, Angleton EL, Birkedal-Hansen H, Van Wart HE. Multiple modes of activation of latent human fibroblast collagenase: evidence for the role of a Cys73 active-site zinc complex in latency and a "cysteine switch" mechanism for activation. *Proc Natl Acad Sci USA* 1990; 87:364–368.

32. Morgunova E, Tuuttila A, Bergmann U, Isupov M, Lindqvist Y, Schneider G, Tryggvason K. Structure of human pro-matrix metalloproteinase-2: activation mechanism revealed. *Science* 1999; 284:1667–1670.

33. Carmeliet P, Moons L, Lijnen R, Baes M, Lemaitre V, Tipping P, et al. Urokinase-generated plasmin activates matrix metalloproteinases during aneurysm formation. *Nat Genet* 1997; 17:439–444.

34. Zhang Z, Winyard PG, Chidwick K, Murphy G, Wardell M, Carrell RW, Blake DR. Proteolysis of human native and oxidised alpha 1-proteinase inhibitor by matrilysin and stromelysin. *Biochim Biophys Acta* 1994; 1199:224–228.

35. Sires UI, Murphy G, Baragi VM, Fliszar CJ, Welgus HG, Senior RM. Matrilysin is much more efficient than other matrix metalloproteinases in the proteolytic inactivation of alpha 1-antitrypsin. *Biochem Biophys Res Commun* 1994; 204:613–620.

36. Noel A, Santavicca M, Stoll I, L'Hoir C, Staub A, Murphy G, et al. Identification of structural determinants controlling human and mouse stromelysin-3 proteolytic activities. *J Biol Chem* 1995; 270:22,866–22,872.

37. Noel A, Gilles C, Bajou K, Devy L, Kebers F, Lewalle JM, et al. Emerging roles for proteinases in cancer. *Invasion Metastasis* 1997; 17:221–239.

38. Itoh Y, Binner S, Nagase H. Steps involved in activation of the complex of pro-matrix metalloproteinase 2 (progelatinase A) and tissue inhibitor of metalloproteinases (TIMP)-2 by 4-aminophenylmercuric acetate. *Biochem J* 1995; 308:645–651.

39. Kinoshita T, Sato H, Okada A, Ohuchi E, Imai K, Okada Y, Seiki M. TIMP-2 promotes activation of progelatinase A by membrane-type 1 matrix metalloproteinase immobilized on agarose beads. *J Biol Chem* 1998; 273:16,098–16,103.

40. Atkinson SJ, Crabbe T, Cowell S, Ward RV, Butler MJ, Sato H, et al. Intermolecular autolytic cleavage can contribute to the activation of progelatinase A by cell membranes. *J Biol Chem* 1995; 270:30,479–30,485.

41. Zucker S, Drews M, Conner C, Foda HD, DeClerck YA, Langley KE, et al. Tissue inhibitor of metalloproteinase-2 (TIMP-2) binds to the catalytic domain of the cell surface receptor, membrane type 1-matrix metalloproteinase 1 (MT1-MMP). *J Biol Chem* 1998; 273:1216–1222.

42. Butler GS, Butler MJ, Atkinson SJ, Will H, Tamura T, van Westrum SS, et al. The TIMP2 membrane type 1 metalloproteinase "receptor" regulates the concentration and efficient activation of progelatinase A. A kinetic study. *J Biol Chem* 1998; 273:871–880.

43. Strongin AY, Collier I, Bannikov G, Marmer BL, Grant GA, Goldberg GI. Mechanism of cell surface activation of 72-kDa type IV collagenase. Isolation of the activated form of the membrane metalloprotease. *J Biol Chem* 1995; 270:5331–5338.

44. Jo Y, Yeon J, Kim HJ, Lee ST. Analysis of tissue inhibitor of metalloproteinases-2 effect on pro-matrix metalloproteinase-2 activation by membrane-type 1 matrix metalloproteinase using baculovirus/insect-cell expression system. *Biochem J* 2000; 345 Pt3:511–519.

45. Kerr LD, Olashaw NE, Matrisian LM. Transforming growth factor beta 1 and cAMP inhibit transcription of epidermal growth factor and oncogene-induced transin RNA. *J Biol Chem* 1988; 263:16,999–17,005.

46. Overall CM, Wrana JL, Sodek J. Transcriptional and post-transcriptional regulation of a 72-kDa gelatinase/type IV collagenase by transforming growth factor-beta 1 in human fibroblasts: Comparisons with collagenase and tissue inhibitor of matrix metalloproteinase gene expression. *J Biol Chem* 1991; 266:14,064–14,071.

47. Welgus HG, Campbell EJ, Bar-Shavit Z, Senior RM, Teitelbaum SL. Human alveolar macrophages produce a fibroblast-like collagenase and collagenase inhibitor. *J Clin Invest* 1985; 76:219–224.

48. Busiek DF, Ross FP, McDonnell S, Murphy G, Matrisian LM, Welgus HG. The matrix metalloproteinase matrilysin (PUMP) is expressed in developing human mononuclear phagocytes. *J Biol Chem* 1992; 267:9087–9092.

49. Lacraz S, Nicod L, Galve-de Rochemonteix B, Baumberger C, Dayer JM, Welgus HG. Suppression of metalloproteinase biosynthesis in human alveolar macrophages by interleukin-4. *J Clin Invest* 1992; 90:382–388.

50. Xie B, Dong Z, Fidler IJ. Regulatory mechanisms for the expression of type IV collagenases/gelatinases in murine macrophages. *J Immunol* 1994; 152:3637–3644.

51. Kumar R, Dong Z, Fidler IJ. Differential regulation of metalloelastase activity in murine peritoneal macrophages by granulocyte-macrophage colony-stimulating factor and macrophage colony-stimulating factor. *J Immunol* 1996; 157:5104–5111.

52. Cury JD, Campbell EJ, Lazarus CJ, Albin RJ, Welgus HG. Selective up-regulation of human alveolar macrophage collagenase production by lipopolysaccharide and comparison to collagenase production by fibroblasts. *J Immunol* 1988; 141:4306–4312.

53. Welgus HG, Campbell EJ, Cury JD, Eisen AZ, Senior RM, Wilhelm SM, Goldberg GI. Neutral metalloproteinases produced by human alveolar mononuclear phagocytes. Enzyme profile, regulation, and expression during cellular development. *J Clin Invest* 1990; 86:1496–1502.

54. Campbell EJ, Cury JD, Shapiro SD, Goldberg GI, Welgus HG. Neutral proteinases of human mononuclear phagocytes. Cellular differentiation markedly alters cell phenotype for serine proteinases, metalloproteinases, and tissue inhibitor of metalloproteinases. *J Immunol* 1991; 146:1286–1293.

55. Shapiro SD, Kobayashi DK, Ley TJ. Cloning and characterization of a unique elastolytic metalloproteinase produced by human alveolar macrophages. *J Biol Chem* 1993; 268:23,824–23,829.

56. Shapiro SD. Elastolytic metalloproteinases produced by human mononuclear phagocytes. Potential roles in destructive lung disease. *Am J Respir Crit Care Med* 1994; 150:S160–S164.

57. Belaaouaj A, Shipley JM, Kobayashi DK, Zimonjic DB, Popescu N, Silverman GA, Shapiro SD. Human macrophage metalloelastase. Genomic organization, chromosomal location, gene linkage, and tissue-specific expression. *J Biol Chem* 1995; 270:14,568–14,575.

58. Chizzolini C, Rezzonico R, De Luca C, Burger D, Dayer JM. Th2 cell membrane factors in association with IL-4 enhance matrix metalloproteinase-1 (MMP-1) while decreasing MMP-9 production by granulocyte-macrophage colony-stimulating factor-differentiated human monocytes. *J Immunol* 2000; 164:5952–5960.

59. Weiss SJ. Tissue destruction by neutrophils. *N Engl J Med* 1989; 320:365–376.

60. Tschesche H, Groeger C, Wenzel HR. Enzymatic fragment substitution as a tool in protein design. *Biomed Biochim Acta* 1991; 50:S175–180.

61. Sorsa T, Ding Y, Salo T, Lauhio A, Teronen O, Ingman T, et al. Effects of tetracyclines on neutrophil, gingival, and salivary collagenases. A functional and western-blot assessment with special reference to their cellular sources in periodontal diseases. *Ann NY Acad Sci* 1994; 732:112–131.

62. Opdenakker G, Van den Steen PE, Dubois B, Nelissen I, Van Coillie E, Masure S, et al. Gelatinase B functions as regulator and effector in leukocyte biology. *J Leukoc Biol* 2001; 69:851–859.

63. Schwartz JD, Monea S, Marcus SG, Patel S, Eng K, Galloway AC, Mignatti P, Shamamian P. Soluble factor(s) released from neutrophils activates endothelial cell matrix metalloproteinase-2. *J Surg Res* 1998; 76:79–85.

64. Banda MJ, Rice AG, Griffin GL, Senior RM. Alpha 1-proteinase inhibitor is a neutrophil chemoattractant after proteolytic inactivation by macrophage elastase. *J Biol Chem* 1988; 263:4481–4484.

65. Montgomery AM, Sabzevari H, Reisfeld RA. Production and regulation of gelatinase B by human T-cells. *Biochim Biophys Acta* 1993; 1176:265–268.

66. Zhou H, Bernhard EJ, Fox FE, Billings PC. Induction of metalloproteinase activity in human T-lymphocytes. *Biochim Biophys Acta* 1993; 1177:174–178.

67. Leppert D, Waubant E, Galardy R, Bunnett NW, Hauser SL. T cell gelatinases mediate basement membrane transmigration in vitro. *J Immunol* 1995; 154:4379–4389.

68. Johnatty RN, Taub DD, Reeder SP, Turcovski-Corrales SM, Cottam DW, Stephenson TJ, Rees RC. Cytokine and chemokine regulation of proMMP-9 and TIMP-1 production by human peripheral blood lymphocytes. *J Immunol* 1997; 158:2327–2333.

69. Xia M, Leppert D, Hauser SL, Sneedharan SP, Nelson PJ, Krensky AM, Goetzl EJ. Stimulus specificity of matrix metalloproteinase dependence of human T cell migration through a model basement membrane. *J Immunol* 1996; 156:160–167.

70. Leber TM, Balkwill FR. Regulation of monocyte MMP-9 production by TNF-alpha and a tumour-derived soluble factor (MMPSF). *Br J Cancer* 1998; 78:724–732.

71. Ismair MG, Ries C, Lottspeich F, Zang C, Kolb HJ, Petrides PE. Autocrine regulation of matrix metalloproteinase-9 gene expression and secretion by tumor necrosis factor-alpha (TNF-alpha) in NB4 leukemic cells: specific involvement of TNF receptor type 1. *Leukemia* 1998; 12:1136–1143.

72. Leppert D, Hauser SL, Kishiyama JL, An S, Zeng L, Goetzl EJ. Stimulation of matrix metalloproteinase-dependent migration of T cells by eicosanoids. *FASEB J* 1995; 9:1473–1481.

73. Leppert D, Waubant E, Burk MR, Oksenberg JR, Hauser SL. Interferon beta-1b inhibits gelatinase secretion and in vitro migration of human T cells: a possible mechanism for treatment efficacy in multiple sclerosis. *Ann Neurol* 1996; 40:846–852.

74. Liu Z, Shipley JM, Vu TH, Zhou X, Diaz LA, Werb Z, Senior RM. Gelatinase B-deficient mice are resistant to experimental bullous pemphigoid. *J Exp Med* 1998; 188:475–482.

75. López-Boado YS, Wilson CL, Hooper LV, Gordon JI, Hultgren SJ, Parks WC. Bacterial exposure induces and activates matrilysin in mucosal epithelial cells. *J Cell Biol* 2000; 148:1305–1315.

76. Parks WC, Lopez-Boado YS, Wilson CL. Matrilysin in epithelial repair and defense. *Chest* 2001; 120:36S–41S.

77. Dunsmore SE, Saarialho-Kere UK, Roby JD, Wilson CL, Matrisian LM, Welgus HG, Parks WC. Matrilysin expression and function in airway epithelium. *J Clin Invest* 1998; 102:1321–1331.

78. Wilson CL, Ouellette AJ, Satchell DP, Ayabe T, López-Boada YS, Stratman JL, et al. Regulation of intestinal alpha-defensin activation by the metalloproteinase matrilysin in innate host defense. *Science* 1999; 286:113–117.

79. Taub DD, Oppenheim JJ. Chemokines, inflammation and the immune system. *Ther Immunol* 1994; 1:229–246.

80. McQuibban GA, Gong JH, Wong JP, Wallace JL, Clark-Lewis I, Overall CM. Matrix metalloproteinase processing of monocyte chemoattractant proteins generates CC chemokine receptor antagonists with anti-inflammatory properties in vivo. *Blood* 2002; 100:1160–1167.

81. Vaday GG, Lider O. Extracellular matrix moieties, cytokines, and enzymes: dynamic effects on immune cell behavior and inflammation. *J Leukocyte Biol* 2000; 67:149–159.

82. Unemori EN, Hibbs MS, Amento EP. Constitutive expression of a 92-kD gelatinase (type V collagenase) by rheumatoid synovial fibroblasts and its induction in normal human fibroblasts by inflammatory cytokines. *J Clin Invest* 1991; 88:1656.

83. Hanemaaijer R, Sorsa T, Konttinen YT, Ding Y, Sutinen M, Visser H, et al. Matrix metalloproteinase-8 is expressed in rheumatoid synovial fibroblasts and endothelial cells. *J Biol Chem* 1997; 272:31,504–31,509.

84. Vaday GG, Hershkoviz R, Rahat MA, Lahat N, Cahalon L, Lider O. Fibronectin-bound TNF-alpha stimulates monocyte matrix metalloproteinase-9 expression and regulates chemotaxis. *J Leukocyte Biol* 2000; 68:737–747.

85. Vaday GG, Schor H, Rahat MA, Lahat N, Lider O. Transforming growth factor-beta suppresses tumor necrosis factor alpha-induced matrix metalloproteinase-9 expression in monocytes. *J Leukocyte Biol* 2001; 69:613–621.

86. Robinson SC, Scott KA, Balkwill FR. Chemokine stimulation of monocyte matrix metalloproteinase-9 requires endogenous TNF-alpha. *Eur J Immunol* 2002; 32:404–412.

87. Sarén P, Welgus HG, Kovanen PT. TNF-alpha and IL-1 beta selectively induce expression of 92-kDa gelatinase by human macrophages. *J Immunol* 1996; 157:4159–4165.

88. Jung HC, Eckmann L, Yang SK, Panja A, Fierer J, Morzycka-Wroblewska E, Kagnoff MF. A distinct array of proinflammatory cytokines is expressed in human colon epithelial cells in response to bacterial invasion. *J Clin Invest* 1995; 95:55–65.

89. Marsh CB, Pomerantz RP, Parker JM, Winnard AV, Mazzaferri EL, Moldovan N, et al. Regulation of monocyte survival in vitro by deposited IgG: role of macrophage colony-stimulating factor. *J Immunol* 1999; 162:6217–6225.

90. Akagawa KS, Kamoshita K, Tokunaga T. Effects of granulocyte-macrophage colony-stimulating factor and colony-stimulating factor-1 on the proliferation and differentiation of murine alveolar macrophages. *J Immunol* 1988; 141:3383–3390.

91. Held TK, Mielke ME, Unger M, Trautmann M, Cross AS. Kinetics and dose dependence of macrophage colony-stimulating factor-induced proliferation and activation of murine mononuclear phagocytes in situ: differences between lungs, liver and spleen. *J Interferon Cytokine Res* 1996; 16:159–168.

92. Stanley ER, Berg KL, Einstein DB, Lee PS, Pixley FJ, Wang Y, Yeung YG. Biology and activation of colony-stimulating factor-1. *Mol Reprod Dev* 1997; 46:4–10.

93. Hashimoto S, Suzuki T, Dong HY, Yamazaki N, Matsushima K. Serial analysis of gene expression in human monocytes and macrophages. *Blood* 1999; 94:837–844.

94. Zhang Y, McCluskey K, Fujii K, Wahl LM. Differential regulation of monocyte matrix metalloproteinase and TIMP-1 production by TNF-alpha, granulocyte-macrophage CSF, and IL-1 beta through prostaglandin-dependent and independent mechanisms. *J Immunol* 1998; 161:3071–3076.

95. Ito A, Mukaiyama A, Itoh Y, Nagase H, Thogersen IB, Enghild JJ, Sasaguri Y, Mori Y. Degradation of interleukin 1 beta by matix metalloproteinases. *J Biol Chem* 1996; 271:14,657–14,660.

96. Arend WP, Dayer JM. Cytokines and cytokine inhibitors or antagonists in rheumatoid arthritis. *Arthritis Rheum* 1990; 33:305–315.

97. Shapiro SD, Campbell EJ, Kobayashi DK, Welgus HG. Immune modulation of metalloproteinase production in human macrophages. Selective pretranslational suppression of interstitial collagenase and stromelysin biosynthesis by interferon-gamma. *J Clin Invest* 1990; 86:1204–1210.

98. Wahl LM, Corcoran ME, Mergenhagen SE, Finbloom DS. Inhibition of phospholipase activity in human monocytes by IFN-gamma blocks endogenous prostaglandin E2-dependent collagenase production. *J Immunol* 1990; 144:3518–3522.

99. Woessner JF Jr. Matrix metalloproteinases and their inhibitors in connective tissue remodeling. *FASEB J* 1991; 5:2145–2154.

100. Corcoran ML, Stetler-Stevenson WG, Brown PD, Wahl LM. Interleukin 4 inhibition of prostaglandin E2 synthesis blocks interstitial collagenase and 92-kDa type IV collagenase/gelatinase production by human monocytes. *J Biol Chem* 1992; 267:515–519.

101. Mertz PM, DeWitt DL, Stetler-Stevenson WG, Wahl LM. Interleukin 10 suppression of monocyte prostaglandin H synthase-2. Mechanism of inhibition of prostaglandin-dependent matrix metalloproteinase production. *J Biol Chem* 1994; 269:21,322–21,329.

102. Lacraz S, Nicod L, Chicheportiche R, Welgus HG, Dayer JM. IL-10 inhibits metalloproteinase and stimulates TIMP-1 production in human mononuclear phagocytes. *J Clin Invest* 1995; 96:2304–2310.

103. Sica A, Saccani A, Borsatti A, Power CA, Wells TN, Luini W, et al. Bacterial lipopolysaccharide rapidly inhibits expression of C-C chemokine receptors in human monocytes. J Exp Med 1997; 185: 969–974.

104. Weber C, Draude G, Weber KS, Wubert J, Lorenz RL, Weber PC. Downregulation by tumor necrosis factor-alpha of monocyte CCR2 expression and monocyte chemotactic protein-1-induced transendothelial migration is antagonized by oxidized low-density lipoprotein: a potential mechanism of monocyte retention in atherosclerotic lesions. *Atherosclerosis* 1999; 145:115–123.

105. Gearing AJ, Beckett P, Christodoulou M, Churchill M, Clements J, Davidson AH, et al. Processing of tumour necrosis factor-alpha precursor by metalloproteinases. *Nature* 1994; 370:555–557.

106. McGeehan GM, Becherer JD, Bast RC, Boyer CM, Champion B, Connolly KM, Conway JG, Furdon P, Karp S, Kidao S, et al. Regulation of tumour necrosis factor-alpha processing by a metalloproteinase inhibitor. *Nature* 1994; 370:558–561.

107. Lacraz S, Isler P, Vey E, Welgus HG, Dayer JM. Direct contact beween T lymphocytes and monocytes is a major pathway for induction of metalloproteinase expression. *J Biol Chem* 1994; 269:22,027–22,033.

108. Miltenburg AM, Lacraz S, Welgus HG, Dayer JM. Immobilized anti-CD3 antibody activates T cell clones to induce the production of interstitial collagenase, but not tissue inhibitor of metalloproteinases, in monocytic THP-1 cells and dermal fibroblasts. *J Immunol* 1995; 154:2655–2667.

109. Aoudjit F, Potworowski EF, St-Pierre Y. Bi-directional induction of matrix metalloproteinase-9 and tissue inhibitor of matrix metalloproteinase-1 during T lymphoma/endothelial cell contact: implication of ICAM-1. *J Immunol* 1998; 160:2967–2973.

110. Aoudjit F, Esteve PO, Desrosiers M, Potworowski EF, St-Pierre Y. Gelatinase B (MMP-9) production and expression by stromal cells in the normal and adult thymus and experimental thymic lymphoma. *Int J Cancer* 1997; 71:71–78.

111. Baram D, Vaday GG, Salamon P, Drucker I, Hershkoviz R, Mekori YA. Human mast cells release metalloproteinase-9 on contact with activated T cells: juxtacrine regulation by TNF-alpha. *J Immunol* 2001; 167:4008–4016.

112. Bhattacharyya SP, Drucker I, Reshef T, Kirshenbaum AS, Metcalfe DD, Mekori YA. Activated T lymphocytes induce degranulation and cytokine production by human mast cells following cell-to-cell contact. *J Leukocyte Biol* 1998; 63:337–341.

113. Burger D, Rezzonico R, Li JM, Modoux C, Pierce RA, Welgus HG, Dayer JM. Imbalance between interstitial collagenase and tissue inhibitor of metalloproteinases 1 in synoviocytes and fibroblasts upon direct contact with stimulated T lymphocytes: involvement of membrane-associated cytokines. *Arthritis Rheum* 1998; 41:1748–1759.

114. Zhang JH, Ferrante A, Arrigo AP, Dayer JM. Neutrophil stimulation and priming by direct contact with activated human T lymphocytes. *J Immunol* 1992; 148:177–181.

115. Malik N, Greenfield BW, Wahl AF, Kiener PA. Activation of human monocytes through CD40 induces matrix metalloproteinases. *J Immunol* 1996; 156:3952–3960.

116. Kayagaki N, Kawasaki A, Ebata T, Ohmoto H, Ikeda S, Inoue S, Yoshino K, Okumura K, Yagita H. Metalloproteinase-mediated release of human Fas ligand. *J Exp Med* 1995; 182:1777–1783.

117. Chandler S, Cossins J, Lury J, Wells G. Macrophage metalloelastase degrades matrix and myelin proteins and processes a tumour necrosis factor-alpha fusion protein. *Biochem Biophys Res Commun* 1996; 228:421–429.

118. Amour A, Slocombe PM, Webster A, Butler M, Knight CG, Smith BJ, Stephens PE, Shelley C, Hutton M, Knauper V, Docherty AJ, Murphy G. TNF-alpha converting enzyme (TACE) is inhibited by TIMP-3. *FEBS Lett* 1998; 435:39–44.

119. Perl A.K, Wilgenbus P, Dahl U, Semb H, Christofori G. A casual role for E-cadherin in the translation from adenocarcinoma to carcinoma. *Nature* 1998; 392:190–193.

120. Gu B, Bendall LJ, Wiley JS. Adenosine triphosphate-induced shedding of CD23 and L-selectin (CD62L) from lymphocytes is mediated by the same receptor but different metalloproteinases. *Blood* 1998; 92:946–951.

121. Zhao L, Shey M, Farnsworth M, Dailey MO. Regulation of membrane metalloproteolytic cleavage of L-selectin (CD62l) by the epidermal growth factor domain. *J Biol Chem* 2001; 276:30,631–30,640.

122. Okamoto I, Kawano Y, Tsuiki H, Sasaki J, Nakao M, Matsumoto M, Suga M, Ando M, Nakajima M, Saya H. CD44 cleavage induced by a membrane-associated metalloproteinase plays a critical role in tumor cell migration. *Oncogene* 1999; 18:1435–1446.

123. Kajita M, Itoh Y, Chiba T, Mori H, Okada A, Kinoh H, Seiki M. Membrane-type 1 matrix metalloproteinase cleaves CD44 and promotes cell migration. *J Cell Biol* 2001; 153:893–904.

124. Schönbeck U, Mach F, Sukhova GK, Murphy C, Bonnefoy JY, Fabunmi RP, Libby P. Regulation of matrix metalloproteinase expression in human vascular smooth muscle cells by T lymphocytes: a role for CD40 signaling in plaque rupture? *Circ Res* 1997; 81:448–454.

125. Manes S, Mira E, Barbacid MM, Cipres A, Fernandez-Resa P, Buesa JM, et al. Identification of insulin-like growth factor-binding protein-1 as a potential physiological substrate for human stromelysin-3. *J Biol Chem* 1997; 272:25,706–25,712.

126. Springer TA. The sensation and regulation of interactions with the extracellular environment: the cell biology of lymphocyte adhesion receptors. *Annu Rev Cell Biol* 1990; 6:359–402.

127. Springer TA. Traffic signals for lymphocyte recirculation and leukocyte emigration: the multistep paradigm. *Cell* 1994; 76:301–314.

128. Altomonte M, Gloghini A, Bertola G, Gasparollo A, Carbone A, Ferrone S, Maio M. Differential expression of cell adhesion molecules CD54/CD11a and CD58/CD2 by human melanoma cells and functional role in their interaction with cytotoxic cells. *Cancer Res* 1993; 53:3343–3348.

129. Becker JC, Brocker EB. Lymphocyte-melanoma interaction: role of surface molecules. *Recent Results Cancer Res* 1995; 139:205–214.

130. Becker JC, Dummer R, Hartmann AA, Burg G, Schmidt RE. Shedding of ICAM-1 from human melanoma cell lines induced by IFN-gamma and tumor necrosis factor-alpha. Functional consequences on cell-mediated cytotoxicity. *J Immunol* 1991; 147:4398–4401.

131. Fonsatti E, Altomonte M, Coral S, Cattarossi I, Nicotra MR, Gasparollo A, et al. Tumour-derived interleukin 1alpha (IL-1alpha) up-regulates the release of soluble intercellular adhesion molecule-1 (sICAM-1) by endothelial cells. *Br J Cancer* 1997; 76:1255–1261.

132. Sanchez-Rovira P, Jimenez E, Carracedo J, Barneto IC, Ramirez R, Aranda E. Serum levels of intercellular adhesion molecule 1 (ICAM-1) in patients with colorectal cancer: inhibitory effect on cytotoxicity. *Eur J Cancer* 1998; 34:394–398.

133. Lyons PD, Benveniste EN. Cleavage of membrane-associated ICAM-1 from astrocytes: involvement of a metalloprotease. *Glia* 1998; 22:103–112.

134. Romanic AM, Madri JA. The induction of 72-kD gelatinase in T cells upon adhesion to endothelial cells is VCAM-1 dependent. *J Cell Biol* 1994; 125:1165–1178.

135. Xia M, Sreedharan SP, Dazin P, Damsky CH, Goetzl EJ. Integrin-dependent role of human T cell matrix metalloproteinase activity in chemotaxis through a model basement membrane. *J Cell Biochem* 1996; 61:452–458.

136. Fiore E, Fusco C, Romero P, Stamenkovic I. Matrix metalloproteinase 9 (MMP-9/gelatinase B) proteolytically cleaves ICAM-1 and participates in tumor cell resistance to natural killer cell-mediated cytotoxicity. *Oncogene* 2002; 21:5213–5223.

137. Peschon JJ, Slack JL, Reddy P, Stocking KL, Sunnarborg SW, Lee DC, Russell WE, Castner BJ, Johnson RS, Fitzner JN, Boyce RW, Nelson N, Kozlosky CJ, Wolfson MF, Rauch CT, Cerretti DP, Paxton RJ, March CJ, Black RA. An essential role for ectodomain shedding in mammalian development. *Science* 1998; 282:1281–1284.

138. Hafezi-Moghadam A, Thomas KL, Prorock AJ, Huo Y, Ley K. L-selectin shedding regulates leukocyte recruitment. *J Exp Med* 2001; 193:863–872.

139. Ohtani H. Stromal reaction in cancer tissue: pathophysiologic significance of the expression of matrix-degrading enzymes in relation to matrix turnover and immune/inflammatory reactions. *Pathol Int* 1998; 48:1–9.

140. Leek RD, Harris AL, Lewis CE. Cytokine networks in solid human tumors: regulation of angiogenesis. *J Leukocyte Biol* 1994; 56:423–435.

141. Neville MC, Medina D, Monks J, Hovey RC. The mammary fat pad. *J Mammary Gland Biol Neoplasia* 1998; 3:109–116.

142. Alexander CM, Selvarajan S, Mudgett J, Werb Z. Stromelysin-1 regulates adipogenesis during mammary gland involution. *J Cell Biol* 2001; 152:693–703.

143. Giannelli G, Fransvea E, Marinosci F, Bergamini C, Daniele A, Colucci S, et al. Gelatinase levels in male and female breast cancer. *Biochem Biophys Res Commun* 2002; 292:161–166.

144. Atula S, Grenman R, Syrjanen S. Fibroblasts can modulate the phenotype of malignant epithelial cells in vitro. *Exp Cell Res* 1997; 235:180–187.

145. Göttlinger HG, Rieber P, Gokel JM, Lohe KJ, Riethmuller G. Infiltrating mononuclear cells in human breast carcinoma: predominance of T4+ monocytic cells in the tumor stroma. *Int J Cancer* 1985; 35: 199–205.

146. Kelly PM, Davison RS, Bliss E, McGee JO. Macrophages in human breast disease: a quantitative immunohistochemical study. *Br J Cancer* 1988; 57:174–177.

147. Leek RD, Lewis CE, Whitehouse R, Greenall M, Clarke J, Harris AL. Association of macrophage infiltration with angiogenesis and prognosis in invasive breast carcinoma. *Cancer Res* 1996; 56:4625–4629.

148. O'Sullivan C, Lewis CE. Tumour-associated leukocytes: friends or foes in breast carcinoma. *J Pathol* 1994; 172:229–235.

149. Normann SJ. Macrophage infiltration and tumor progression. *Cancer Metastasis Rev* 1985; 4:277–291.

150. Ring P, Johansson K, Hoyhtya M, Rubin K, Lindmark G. Expression of tissue inhibitor of metalloproteinases TIMP-2 in human colorectal cancer - a predictor of tumour stage. *Br J Cancer* 1997; 76:805–811.

151. Jaalinoja J, Herva R, Korpela M, Hoyhtya M, Turpeenniemi-Hujanen T. Matrix metalloproteinase 2 (MMP-2) immunoreactive protein is associated with poor grade and survival in brain neoplasms. *J Neurooncol* 2000; 46:81–90.

152. Zuk JA, Walker RA. Immunohistochemical analysis of HLA antigens and mononuclear infiltrates of benign and malignant breast. *J Pathol* 1987; 152:275–285.

153. Van Netten JP, Ashmead BJ, Parker RL, Thornton IG, Fletcher C, Cavers D, et al. Macrophage-tumor cell associations: a factor in metastasis of breast cancer? *J Leukocyte Biol* 1993; 54:360–362.

154. Nathan CF. Secretory products of macrophages. *J Clin Invest* 1987; 79:319–326.

155. Turnock K, Bulmer JN, Gray C. Phenotypic characterization of macrophage subpopulations and localization of factor XIII in the stromal cells of carcinomas. *Histochem J* 1990; 22:661–666.

156. Mantovani A, Bottazzi B, Colotta F, Sozzani S, Ruco L. The origin and function of tumor-associated macrophages. *Immunol Today* 1992; 13:265–270.

157. Van Netten JP, George EJ, Ashmead BJ, Fletcher C, Thornton IG, Coy P. Macrophage-tumor cell associations in breast cancer. *Lancet* 1993; 342:872,873.

158. Graves DT, Valent AJ. Monocyte chemotactic proteins from human tumor cells. *Biochem Pharmacol* 1991; 41:333–337.

159. Fu YX, Cai JP, Chin YH, Watson GA, Lopez DM. Regulation of leukocyte binding protein to endothelial tissues by tumor-derived granulocyte macrophage colony-stimulating factor (GM-CSF). *Int J Cancer* 1992; 50:585–588.

160. Stewart T, Tsai SC, Grayson H, Henderson R, Opelz G. Incidence of de-novo breast cancer in women chronically immunosuppressed after organ transplantation. *Lancet* 1995; 346:796–798.

161. Leibovich SJ, Polverini PJ, Fong TW, Harlow LA, Koch AE. Production of angiogenic activity by human monocytes requires an L-arginine/nitric oxide-synthase-dependent effector mechanism. *Proc Natl Acad Sci USA* 1994; 91:4190–4194.

162. Miles DW, Happerfield LC, Naylor MS, Bobrow LG, Rubens RD, Balkwill FR. Expression of tumour necrosis factor (TNF alpha) and its receptors in benign and malignant breast tissue. *Int J Cancer* 1994; 56:777–782.

163. Pusztai L, Clover LM, Cooper K, Starkey PM, Lewis CE, McGee JO. Expression of tumour necrosis factor alpha and its receptors in carcinoma of the breast. *Br J Cancer* 1994; 70:289–292.

164. Jones PD, Castro JE. Immunological mechanisms in metastatic spread and the antimetastatic effects of C. parvum. *Br J Cancer* 1977; 35:519–527.

165. Mantovani A, Giavazzi R, Polentarutti N, Spreafico F, Garattini S. Divergent effects of macrophage toxins on growth of primary tumors and lung metastases in mice. *Int J Cancer* 1980; 25:617–620.

166. Keller R. Mononuclear phagocytes in the control of primary and secondary tumor growth. *Adv Exp Med Biol* 1982; 155:289–302.

167. O'Reilly MS, Holmgren L, Shing Y, Chen C, Rosenthal RA, Moses M, et al. Angiostatin: a novel angiogenesis inhibitor that mediates the suppression of metastases by a Lewis lung carcinoma. *Cell* 1994; 79:315–328.

168. O'Reilly MS, Boehm T, Shing Y, Fukai N, Vasios G, Lane WS, et al. Endostatin: an endogenous inhibitor of angiogenesis and tumor growth. *Cell* 1997; 88:277–285.

169. Dong, Z, Kumar R, Yang X, Fidler IJ. Macrophage-derived metalloproteinase is responsible for the generation of angiostatin in Lewis lung carcinoma. *Cell* 1997; 88:801–810.

170. Lijnen HR, Ugwu F, Bini A, Collen D. Generation of an angiostatin-like fragment from plasminogen by stromelysin-1 (MMP-3). *Biochemistry* 1998; 37:4699–4702.

171. Moss ML, Jin SL, Milla ME, Bickett DM, Burkhart W, Carter HL, et al. Cloning of a disintegrin metalloproteinase that processes precursor tumour-necrosis factor-alpha. *Nature* 1997; 385:733–736.

172. Whalen GF. Solid tumours and wounds: transformed cells misunderstood as injured tissue? *Lancet* 1990; 336:1489–1492.

173. Polverini PJ, Leibovich SJ. Induction of neovascularization in vivo and endothelial proliferation in vitro by tumor-associated macrophages. *Lab Invest* 1984; 51:635–642.

174. Sunderkotter C, Steinbrink K, Goebeler M, Bhardwaj R, Sorg C. Macrophages and angiogenesis. *J Leukocyte Biol* 1994; 55:410–422.

175. Basset P, Okada A, Chenard MP, Kannan R, Stoll I, Anglard P, et al. Matrix metalloproteinases as stromal effectors of human carcinoma progression: therapeutic implications. *Matrix Biol* 1997; 15:535–541.

176. Uria JA, Stahle-Backdahl M, Seiki M, Fueyo A, Lopez-Otin C. Regulation of collagenase-3 expression in human breast carcinomas is mediated by stromal-epithelial cell interactions. *Cancer Res* 1997; 57: 4882–4888.

177. Johnsen M, Lund LR, Romer J, Almholt K, Dano K. Cancer invasion and tissue remodeling: common themes in proteolytic matrix degradation. *Curr Opin Cell Biol* 1998; 10:667–671.

178. Johansson N, Vaalamo M, Grenman S, Hietanen S, Klemi P, Saarialho-Kere U, Kahari VM. Collagenase-3 (MMP-13) is expressed by tumor cells in invasive vulvar squamous cell carcinomas. *Am J Pathol* 1999; 154:469–480.

179. Sheu B-C, Hsu S-M, Ho H-N, Lien H-C, Huang S-C, Lin R-H. A novel role of metalloproteinase in cancer-mediated immunosuppression. *Cancer Res* 2001; 61:237–242.

180. Yu Q, Stamenkovic I. Cell surface-localized matrix metalloproteinase-9 proteolytically activates TGF-b and promotes tumor invasion and angiogenesis. *Genes Dev* 2000; 14:163–176.

181. Gorelik L, Flavell RA. Immune-mediated eradication of tumors through the blockade of transforming growth factor-β signaling in T cells. *Nature Med* 2001; 7:1118–1122.

182. Kataoka H, Uchino H, Iwamura T, Sseiki M, Nabeshima K, Koono M. Enhanced tumor growth and invasiveness in vivo by a carboxyl-terminal framgent of α1-Proteinase inhibitor generated by m atrix metalloproteinases. *Am J Pathol* 1999; 154:457–468.

183. Martin DC, Ruther U, Sanchez-Sweatman OH, Orr FW, Khokha R. Inhibition of SV40 T antigen-induced hepatocellular carcinoma in TIMP-1 transgenic mice. *Oncogene* 1996; 13:569–576.

184. Soloway PD, Alexander CM, Werb Z, Jaenisch R. Targeted mutagenesis of Timp-1 reveals that lung tumor invasion is influenced by Timp-1 genotype of the tumor but not by that of the host. *Oncogene* 1996; 13:2307–2314.

185. Hayakawa T, Yamashita K, Tanzawa K, Uchijima E, Iwata K. Growth-promoting activity of tissue inhibitor of metalloproteinases-1 (TIMP-1) for a wide range of cells. A possible new growth factor in serum. *FEBS Lett* 1992; 298:29–32.

186. Nemeth JA, Rafe A, Steiner M, Goolsby CL. TIMP-2 growth-stimulatory activity: a concentration- and cell type-specific response in the presence of insulin. *Exp Cell Res* 1996; 224:110–115.

187. Chen WT. Membrane proteases: roles in tissue remodeling and tumour invasion. *Curr Opin Cell Biol* 1992; 4:802–809.

188. Birkedal-Hansen H. Proteolytic remodeling of extracellular matrix. *Curr Opin Cell Biol* 1995; 7: 728–735.

189. Kohn EC, Liotta LA. Molecular insights into cancer invasion: strategies for prevention and intervention. *Cancer Res* 1995; 55:1856–1862.

190. Visscher DW, Hoyhtya M, Ottosen SK, Liang CM, Sarkar FH, Crissman JD, Fridman R. Enhanced expression of tissue inhibitor of metalloproteinase-2 (TIMP-2) in the stroma of breast carcinomas correlates with tumor recurrence. *Int J Cancer* 1994; 59:339–344.

191. Polette M, Gilbert N, Stas I, Nawrocki B, Noel A, Remacle A, et al. Gelatinase A expression and localization in human breast cancers. An in situ hybridization study and immunohistochemical detection using confocal microscopy. *Virchows Arch* 1994; 424:641–645.

192. MacDougall JR, Matrisian LM. Contributions of tumor and stromal matrix metalloproteinases to tumor progression, invasion and metastasis. *Cancer Metastasis Rev* 1995; 14:351–362.

193. Heppner KJ, Matrisian LM, Jensen RA, Rodgers WH. Expression of most matrix metalloproteinase family members in breast cancer represents a tumor-induced host response. *Am J Pathol* 1996; 149:273–282.
194. Soini Y, Hurskainen T, Hoyhtya M, Oikarinen A, Autio-Harmainen H. 72 KD and 92 KD type IV collagenase, type IV collagen, and laminin mRNAs in breast cancer: a study by in situ hybridization. *J Histochem Cytochem* 1994; 42:945–951.
195. Stetler-Stevenson WG, Aznavoorian S, Liotta LA. Tumor cell interactions with the extracellular matrix during invasion and metastasis. *Annu Rev Cell Biol* 1993; 9:541–573.
196. Coussens LM, Werb Z. Matrix metalloproteinases and the development of cancer. *Chem Biol* 1996; 3:895–904.
197. Hoyhtya M, Fridman R, Komarek D, Porter-Jordan K, Stetler-Stevenson WG, Liotta LA, Liang CM. Immunohistochemical localization of matrix metalloproteinase 2 and its specific inhibitor TIMP-2 in neoplastic tissues with monoclonal antibodies. *Int J Cancer* 1994; 56:500–505.
198. Davies B, Miles DW, Happerfield LC, Naylor MS, Bobrow LG, Rubens RD, Balkwill FR. Activity of type IV collagenases in benign and malignant breast disease. *Br J Cancer* 1993; 67:1126–1131.
199. Monsky WL, Kelly T, Lin CY, Yeh Y, Stetler-Stevenson WG, Mueller SC, Chen WT. Binding and localization of M(r) 72,000 matrix metalloproteinase at cell surface invadopodia. *Cancer Res* 1993; 53:3159–3164.
200. Monteagudo C, Merino MJ, San-Juan J, Liotta LA, Stetler-Stevenson WG. Immunohistochemical distribution of type IV collagenase in normal, benign, and malignant breast tissue. *Am J Pathol* 1990; 136:585–592.
201. Clavel C, Polette M, Doco M, Binninger I, Birembaut P. Immunolocalization of matrix metalloproteinases and their tissue inhibitor in human mammary pathology. *Bull Cancer* 1992; 79:261–270.
202. Sato H, Takino T, Okada Y, Cao J, Shinagawa A, Yamamoto E, Seiki M. A matrix metalloproteinase expressed on the surface of invasive tumour cells. *Nature* 1994; 370:61–65.
203. Brooks PC, Stromblad S, Sanders LC, von Schalscha TL, Aimes RT, Stetler-Stevenson WG, Quigley JP, Cheresh DA. Localization of matrix metalloproteinase MMP-2 to the surface of invasive cells by interaction with integrin alpha v beta 3. *Cell* 1996; 85:683–693.
204. John A, Tuszynski G. The role of matrix metalloproteinases in tumor angiogenesis and tumor metastasis. *Pathol Oncol Res* 2001; 7:14–23.

7

Contribution of Osteopontin to the Development of Bone Metastasis

Alison L. Allan, PhD, *Alan B. Tuck,* MD, PhD,
Vivien H. C. Bramwell, PhD, MBBS,
Theodore A. Vandenberg, MD,
Eric W. Winquist, MSc, MD, *and Ann F. Chambers,* PhD

CONTENTS

1. INTRODUCTION

Metastasis is the spread of cancer cells from a primary site, resulting in the establishment of secondary tumors in distant locations *(1–3)*. Certain types of cancer have organ-specific preferences for metastatic growth, and breast and prostate cancers often preferentially metastasize to bone *(2,3)*. In fact, it has been estimated that the majority of breast and prostate cancer patients who succumb to their disease will have bone metastases at the time of death *(4,5)*. Bone metastasis has significant clinical and quality-of-life implications for cancer patients, including severe bone pain, increased susceptibility to fractures, bone deformability, neurological impingement, hypercalcemia, and compromise of bone marrow function (reviewed in refs. *6–8*).

In order for cancer cells to metastasize to bone, they must successfully complete a series of sequential steps. These steps include dissemination of tumor cells from the primary tumor into the bloodstream (a process called intravasation), survival and migration in the circulation, arrival in the bone marrow sinus, extravasation into the bone marrow cavity, and colonization and growth in the bone via interactions with bone cells

From: *Cancer Drug Discovery and Development*
Bone Metastasis: Experimental and Clinical Therapeutics
Edited by: G. Singh and S. A. Rabbani © Humana Press Inc., Totowa, NJ

(1,2,7,9–11). Cells can also disseminate from the primary tumor through the lymphatic system, although the lack of direct flow from the lymphatic system to the bone marrow means that cancer cells escaping via this route must still enter the arterial system in order to be distributed to the skeleton *(3,12)*. The movement of tumor cells within and between secondary sites is not random; rather, it depends to a large extent on the location of the primary tumor relative to the body's natural pattern of blood flow. For example, tumor cells that enter the circulation from most parts of the body (e.g., liver, breast, prostate, bone) are carried by the systemic venous system directly to the heart and then circulated to all organs of the body via the systemic arterial system *(3,10)*. However, meta-analysis of a series of autopsy studies by Weiss *(13)* documented that for breast and prostate cancer, there were greater numbers of bone metastases present than would be expected based solely on blood-flow patterns. A number of theories have been proposed to explain the propensity of certain types of cancer cells to preferentially metastasize to specific secondary sites such as bone. The most central of these theories is the "seed and soil" theory of metastasis, first proposed in 1889 by Paget *(3,14,15)*. Paget predicted that a cancer cell (the "seed") can survive and proliferate only in secondary sites (the "soil") that produce growth factors appropriate to that type of cell. The bone microenvironment is richly vascularized and contains cells that can produce and/or regulate many of the molecular factors utilized by breast and prostate tumor cells for survival, adhesion, migration, invasion, and growth. This suggests that the bone might provide a fertile "soil" for the establishment of metastases *(16)*. The contribution of one of these molecular factors, the phosphoprotein osteopontin (OPN), is the topic of this chapter.

Osteopontin is one of the most abundant noncollagenous proteins in bone, and it plays an important role in bone development, bone remodeling, and regulation of bone homeo-stasis *(17)*. OPN is also involved in a number of other normal and pathologic conditions, such as mammary gland development, lactation, vascular remodeling, immune reactiv-ity/inflammation, renal disease, and cancer (reviewed in refs. *18* and *19*). OPN can be produced by many types of cells, including bone cells (osteoblasts, osteocytes, osteo-clasts), fibroblasts, inflammatory cells, endothelial cells, and tumor cells *(17,20)*. Clini-cal studies have demonstrated that OPN is overexpressed by many human cancers, and in some cases, this is associated with cancer progression *(19–23)*. In particular, it has been shown that there is a strong correlation between elevated OPN levels in patients with breast or prostate cancer and increased tumor aggressiveness, increased tumor burden, and poor prognosis/survival rates *(24–27)*.

The OPN protein contains several highly conserved structural elements including heparin- and calcium-binding domains, a thrombin-cleavage site, a CD44-binding site, and an RGD (Arg-Gly-Asp) integrin-binding amino acid sequence *(18)*. Based on the presence of these domains, it is not surprising that experimental studies have shown that the importance of OPN lies in its ability to interact with a diverse range of factors, including cell surface receptors (integrins, CD44), secreted proteases (matrix metalloproteinases, urokinase plasminogen activator), and growth factor–receptor path-ways (transforming growth factor-α/epithelial growth factor receptor [TGF-α/EGFR], hepatocyte growth factor [HGF]/Met, vascular endothelial growth factor [VEGF]). These complex signaling interactions can result in changes in gene expression, which ultimately lead to alterations in cell properties involved in malignancy such as adhesion, migration, invasion, enhanced tumor cell survival, tumor angiogenesis, and metastasis *(28–38)*.

Downregulation of OPN by antisense strategies results in decreased tumorigenicity of transformed fibroblasts *(39,40)*, whereas OPN-deficient mice injected with melanoma cells show reduced experimental metastasis to bone and soft tissues compared to wild-type controls *(41)*. Taken together with the clinical observations, these experimental studies indicate that OPN is not merely associated with cancer, but that it actually plays a multifaceted functional role in malignancy.

2. OSTEOPONTIN AND PROSTATE CANCER METASTASIS TO BONE

Prostate cancer is the most common male cancer and the second leading cause of cancer-related deaths in North American men *(42,43)*, and patients with metastatic prostate cancer usually have lymph node and bone involvement. Prostate cancer metastasis to bone typically results in osteoblastic (sclerotic) lesions involving bones of the vertebrae, the sternum, the pelvis, and other bones in the axial skeleton. The occurrence of bone metastasis in prostate cancer patients can be identified by the presence of symptoms such as bone pain, bone scintigraphy, and measurement of serum alkaline phosphatase, a marker of increased osteoblast activity *(44,45)*. However, despite the high frequency of skeletal involvement in prostate cancer causing morbidity and mortality, the molecular mechanisms responsible for prostatic bone metastasis remain largely unexplained.

Clinical studies in this and other laboratories have shown that OPN is overexpressed in the blood *(21,27)* and tumor tissue *(46,47)* of prostate cancer patients. Thalmann et al. *(46)* showed that increased OPN mRNA and protein expression in tumor specimens correlated with cancer stage and the occurrence of lymph node and bone metastases. Multivariable analysis by Hotte et al. *(27)* demonstrated that OPN levels in the blood of prostate cancer patients positively correlated with the occurrence of bone metastasis and negatively and independently correlated with survival. Blood OPN levels were also positively correlated with surrogate measures of bone tumor burden, such as increased serum alkaline phosphatase levels and the need for palliative treatment. Experimentally, it has been shown that treatment of cultured prostate cancer cells with OPN can influence Ca^{2+} signaling *(48)*, proliferation *(49)*, and anchorage-independent growth *(46)*. These clinical and experimental studies provide strong evidence that there is an association between increased levels of OPN and prostate cancer progression, and they suggest that OPN might play a functional role in prostate cancer metastasis to bone.

3. OSTEOPONTIN AND BREAST CANCER METASTASIS TO BONE

Breast cancer is a leading cause of morbidity and mortality in women *(42,43)*, mainly because of the propensity of primary breast tumors to metastasize to distant sites such as lymph nodes, lungs, liver, brain, and bone *(2,3,5)*. Breast cancer metastasis to bone is predominantly osteolytic but may be osteosclerotic or mixed, and is accompanied by severe bone pain, osteoporosis, fractures of the long bones, spinal cord compression, and hypercalcemia. The severe impact on patient quality of life and the long clinical course of the disease (the median survival of patients diagnosed with solely bone metastases is significantly longer than the average survival with metastases at multiple sites) *(5)* highlights the need for a better understanding of the causative mechanisms of breast cancer metastasis to bone.

We and others have found that OPN levels are elevated in the blood *(21,24,25)* and primary tumors *(20,25,26,47,50,51)* of patients with breast cancer, and in some cases, this has been correlated with poor prognosis and survival *(24–26)*. Singhal et al. *(24)* observed that metastasis to bone and other sites was associated with increased levels of circulating OPN in patients' blood, and a number of other studies have demonstrated that OPN mRNA and protein is expressed in tissue specimens of clinical bone metastases from the breast *(25,47,50,51)*. In experimental models of breast cancer, enhanced expression of OPN has been associated with increased malignancy and metastasis *(31,32,34,37,38,52–54)*. Mouse models utilizing intracardiac injection of human breast cancer cells to target the bone demonstrate that the resultant bone metastases express high levels of OPN *(53,54)*. In functional studies, we have shown that transfection of breast cancer cells with endogenous OPN or treatment with exogenous OPN can result in increased malignant cell behavior, including enhanced adhesion, migration, invasion, and metastasis. This OPN-mediated malignancy is largely dependent on its interaction with other factors such as integrins, proteases, and growth factor–receptor pathways *(29,31,32,34,37,38)*. Additionally, we have found that breast carcinoma cells of higher in vivo malignancy not only tend to express more OPN but might also be more responsive to OPN *(31)*.

The above-described studies provide strong circumstantial evidence that OPN is involved in bone metastasis during breast and prostate cancer progression. However, the molecular mechanisms by which OPN might functionally contribute to this process remain largely hypothetical. Before discussing these potential mechanisms, it might be helpful to first review what is known about the cellular and molecular aspects of normal bone homeostasis and the disruptions that occur during bone metastasis.

4. MOLECULAR MECHANISMS OF BONE METASTASIS DEVELOPMENT

The performance of normal bone function (i.e., support of hematopoiesis, maintenance of blood calcium levels, and support and protection of soft tissues) requires continuous tissue renewal, called bone remodeling, to occur throughout the skeleton. A delicate and tightly regulated balance between bone destruction ("resorption") and bone formation is, therefore, required for maintenance of bone homeostasis and function. The cells that are responsible for bone resorption are hematopoietically derived and are called osteoclasts. Bone-forming cells, called osteoblasts, are derived from the mesenchyme and are responsible for rebuilding the resorbed bone via development of new mineralized bone matrix. Bone resorption and bone formation are "coupled" by feedback mechanisms that are regulated by a number of different molecular factors (reviewed in ref. *55*). The occurrence of bone metastasis results in dysregulation of this coupling, which ultimately favors either bone formation (osteoblastic metastasis) or bone resorption (osteolytic metastasis). However, the concept that there are basically two separate types of bone metastasis is probably too simplistic because there is evidence that both osteoblastic and osteoclastic components are activated in most bone metastases *(8,56–58)*. The mechanisms that disrupt normal bone resorption and formation during bone metastasis are largely unknown, although differences in the growth factor milieu within the bone microenvironment can influence different metabolic changes that lead to the final shift in homeostasis favoring the development of clinically detectable lytic or sclerotic lesions *(47,58)*.

Before tumor cells can begin to mediate these alterations in the bone, they must leave the primary site via the bloodstream, survive in the circulation, invade into, migrate through, and survive in the bone microenvironment and initiate adhesive interactions

with bone cells *(1,2,7,9,16)*. Tumor cell secretion of proteases such as urokinase plasminogen activator (uPA) and matrix metalloproteinases (MMPs) allows invasion through
the basement membrane and access to the metastatic site, as well as facilitating growth
factor release from the extracellular matrix *(59,60)*. Expression of integrins (in particular,
$\alpha v \beta 3$) by either tumor cells or bone cells is believed to be important in facilitating
migration and adhesion *(61,62)*. A number of studies have examined specific molecular
factors thought to be involved in the development of osteoblastic bone metastasis during
prostate cancer progression. It is believed that the production of growth factors such as
epidermal growth factor (EGF), insulin-like growth factor (IGF), platelet-derived growth
factor (PDGF), TGF-β, and bone morphogenic proteins (BMPs, members of the TGF-β
family) by prostate cancer cells in the bone microenvironment can stimulate osteoblast
activity and induce new bone formation as well as promote tumor cell growth (reviewed
in refs. *8* and *63*). In addition, proteases such as uPA and PSA (prostatic-specific antigen)
can activate latent growth factors and inactivate parathyroid hormone-related peptide
(PTHrP), a key mediator of bone resorption *(8,64,65)*. The production of growth factors
by prostate cancer cells can, thus, act in both an autocrine and a paracrine manner to
stimulate tumor cell proliferation and new bone formation, ultimately resulting in the
development of osteoblastic bone metastases.

The major pathway thought to be involved in osteolytic bone metastases is the receptor
activator of nuclear factor-κB ligand (RANKL) system (8,61). PTHrP and other factors,
including PTH and the cytokines interleukin (IL)-11, IL-6, and IL-1, can be produced by
breast cancer cells to stimulate the production of RANKL by osteoblasts and bone stromal cells. RANKL then binds to its receptor, RANK, on osteoclast progenitor cells and
stimulates osteoclast differentiation and bone resorption. PTHrP also downregulates the
expression of osteoprotegrin (OPG), a decoy receptor that blocks RANKL from binding
to RANK. The production of osteoclast-stimulating factors such as PTHrP by breast
cancer cells in the bone microenvironment results in osteolysis and a subsequent release
of sequestered growth factors from the bone matrix, which, in turn, can stimulate tumor
cell proliferation (reviewed in refs. *8* and *61*). TGF-β is one of the growth factors released
during bone resorption, and TGF-β has been shown to increase PTHrP production by
tumor cells, thus stimulating more bone resorption *(61,66,67)*. This cyclical and mutually
beneficial relationship between breast cancer cells and osteoclasts results in a net effect
of disruption in bone homeostasis favoring bone degradation and growth of the tumor
cells into osteolytic bone metastases. Clinical studies have shown that PTHrP expression
in primary breast tumors can be correlated with the development of bone metastases,
although not with standard prognostic factors, recurrence, or survival *(68)*. Interestingly,
breast cancer cells seem to express higher levels of PTHrP when they are present in the
bone, as opposed to visceral metastatic sites such as lung *(69,70)*. This observation
underlines the importance of tumor–bone interactions in the development of osteolytic
bone metastasis.

It has long been recognized that the ability of tumor cells to develop and maintain a
metastatic phenotype is reliant on factors intrinsic to each tumor cell, factors intrinsic to
the host environment, and the complex interactions between the two. This concept of a
tumor–host microenvironment seems to be particularly relevant to bone metastasis
(7,16,71). It is likely that both tumor-cell-derived OPN and host-cell-derived OPN (i.e.,
from the bone matrix, bone cells, immune cells, and vascular endothelial cells) are
important to the process of bone metastasis, although the relative importance and contri-

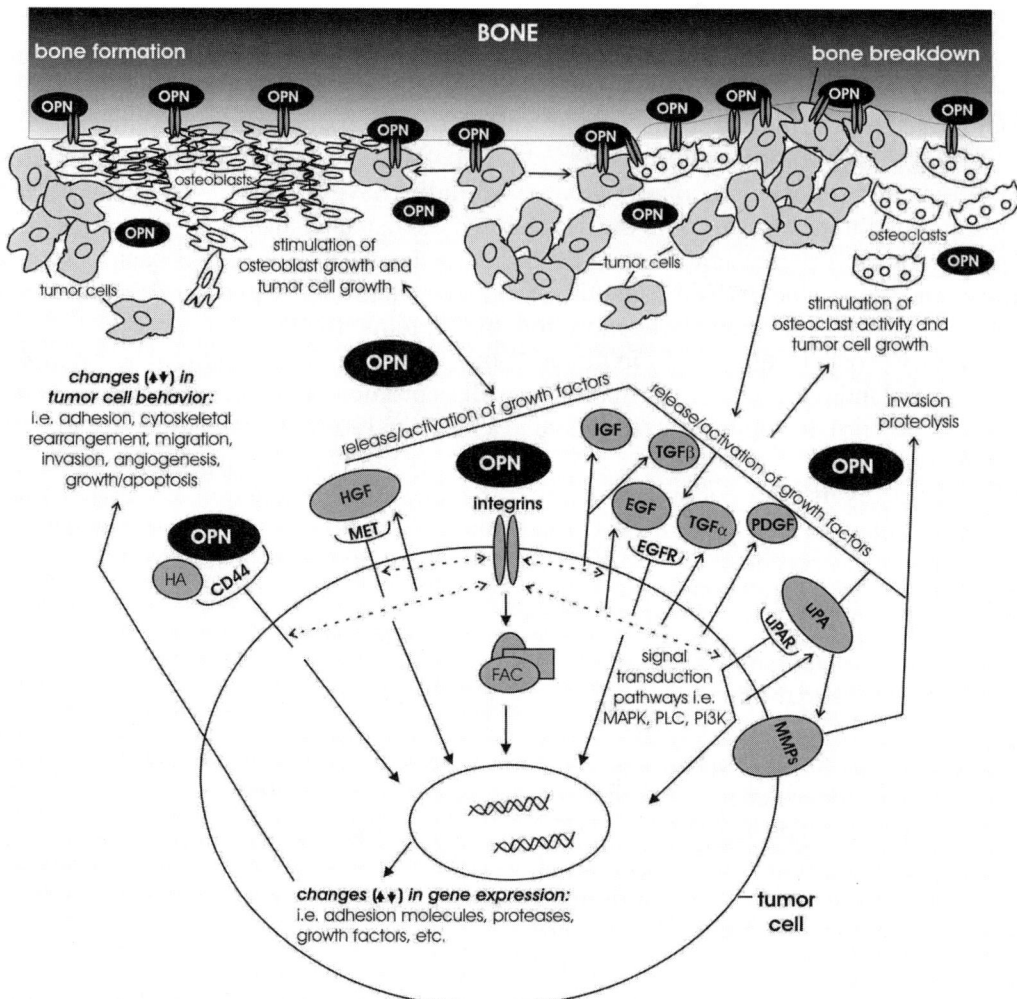

Fig. 1. Contribution of OPN to the development of bone metastasis. This schematic is a hypothetical representation of how OPN might help tumor cells to both respond to and influence the bone microenvironment. Sources of OPN might include the bone matrix, osteoblasts, osteoclasts, and the tumor cells themselves, as well as other host cells such endothelial cells and immune cells. As discussed in the text, OPN-mediated molecular crosstalk between itself and other tumor-derived and host-derived factors such as integrins, proteases, and growth factor–receptor pathways has the potential to influence tumor and bone cell behavior through multiple different signaling pathways.

bution of each remains poorly understood. However, a growing number of studies have supplied evidence of possible mechanisms by which OPN can contribute to the establishment of bone metastasis during breast and prostate cancer progression. These mechanisms, discussed next and represented schematically in Fig. 1, might be active at a number of steps during the metastatic process, including survival, invasion, migration, adhesion, angiogenesis, and growth.

5. PROPOSED MOLECULAR MECHANISMS
OF OPN DURING BONE METASTASIS

5.1. Influence of OPN on Tumor Cell Survival

After dissemination from the primary tumor, one of the first requirements of a successful metastatic tumor cell is survival in the circulation. This survival requires that the cell can overcome two types of challenges: physical challenges from hemodynamic shear stresses in the circulation and biological challenges from host antitumor immune responses *(3,10)*. One of the primary defenses that the host employs is the production of reactive oxygen species (i.e., nitric oxide, OH, and O_2^-) by activated monocytes, macrophages, or endothelial cells upon contact with the tumor cell, a process called oxidative burst. This can result in the death of both the tumor cell and the host cell as a result of the inactivation of critical metabolic pathways. One of these reactive oxygen species, nitric oxide (NO), is a nitrogen radical that is the product of nitric oxide synthase (NOS). Inducible nitric oxide synthase (iNOS) is the enzyme responsible for producing NO in response to extracellular stimuli (reviewed in ref. *72*). Studies have shown that OPN can inhibit induction of iNOS, suggesting that OPN may play a role in tumor defenses against the immune system *(28,73,74)*. It is possible that tumor cell secretion of OPN might promote metastasis by protecting the tumor cell against NO produced by vascular cells or immune cells in the circulation and/or the bone microenvironment.

Another possible contribution of OPN to tumor cell survival has been suggested by Koeneman et al. *(75)*, who hypothesized that in order for tumor cells to survive in the bone microenvironment, they must become "osteomimetic." That is to say, a switch of tumor cell gene expression toward a bone-like phenotype (i.e., expression of OPN and other bone proteins) must occur in order to facilitate survival and reciprocal cellular interactions between tumor cells and bone cells, ultimately allowing tumor cells to successfully establish themselves as metastases in the bone.

Finally, OPN has been shown to regulate cell-death-suppression signaling in breast cancer cells via interactions with the $\alpha v \beta 3$ integrin *(76)*. This suggests that autocrine effects of OPN–$\alpha v \beta 3$ interactions could protect tumor cells in the circulation and/or that adhesive interactions between tumor cells expressing $\alpha v \beta 3$ and bone cells expressing OPN might provide a survival advantage to tumor cells in the bone. The importance of these integrin-mediated interactions is discussed in further detail next.

5.2. Interaction of OPN With Cell Surface Receptors

Integrins are a family of dimeric transmembrane receptors comprised of α- and β-subunits. At least 24 different heterodimers can be formed by noncovalent associations between 18 α- and 8 β-subunits, and each heterodimer can bind a variety of class-specific ligands, including extracellular matrix proteins (i.e., laminin, vitronectin), E-cadherin, and OPN. Integrin–ligand interactions can induce activation and clustering of the focal adhesion complex (FAC), which serves to assemble structural and regulatory proteins such that they can mediate cytoskeletal shape and migration and create a framework for the association of signaling molecules. Integrins can coordinate with proteases and growth factor pathways to activate a number of intracellular signaling cascades, consequently altering gene expression and influencing a dynamic range of cellular processes, including migration, proliferation, differentiation, survival, and angiogenesis (reviewed in refs. *77* and *78*). During normal bone remodeling, there is evidence that osteoblast differentiation and bone mineralization can be negatively modulated by the αvβ3 integrin *(79)* and that OPN might be involved in osteoclast-mediated bone resorption via binding to αvβ3 *(80)*.

Various integrins have been shown to have prognostic value for a number of human cancers, and depending on the stage of tumor progression, some integrins could be upregulated or downregulated *(81)*. In particular, increased expression of the αvβ3 integrin has been observed in a variety of metastatic cancers, including those of the breast and prostate *(62,81,82)*. The expression of αvβ3 has been observed to be increased in more aggressive primary breast tumors, invasive breast cancer cell lines, and breast cancer bone metastases *(82–84)* and has been shown to be important in experimental models of breast and prostate cancer metastasis *(85–87)*. Recently, an elegant study by Bakewell et al. *(88)* demonstrated that knockout mice deficient in the β3 integrin subunit are resistant to bone metastasis after intracardiac injection of tumor cells. The αvβ3 integrin, via binding to bone matrix proteins such as vitronectin, bone sialoprotein (BSP), and OPN, has been observed to mediate breast cancer cell adhesion and migration to bone *(89)*. A study by Zheng et al. *(90)* showed that αvβ3 is expressed by the invasive prostate cancer cell line PC-3 and by primary prostate adenocarcinoma cells, although not by noninvasive LNCaP prostate cancer cells or by normal primary prostate epithelial cells. The authors of this study also observed that the expression of αvβ3 promotes a migratory phenotype in prostate cancer cells through activation of the FAK signaling pathway. Other studies have shown that exogenous OPN can stimulate integrin-mediated growth of prostate epithelial cells with high proliferative potential *(49)* and induce αvβ3-dependent Ca^{2+} signaling in cultured PC-3 prostate cancer cells *(48)*. It is believed that Ca^{2+} signaling in tumor cells is important for the regulation of proliferation, invasion, and metastatic potential *(91)*.

We have observed that OPN-induced breast cancer cell adhesion, migration, invasion, and metastasis occur via integrin-dependent mechanisms *(29,34,38)*. Interestingly, breast epithelial cells of differing degrees of malignancy utilize different cell surface integrins in this process. We found that nonmetastatic 21NT breast epithelial cells migrate toward OPN in an αvβ5- and αvβ1-dependent fashion and, in fact, do not express αvβ3. In contrast, highly metastatic breast cancer cells such as MDA-MB-435 cells do express αvβ3 and migrate toward OPN in an αvβ3-dependent fashion *(34,38)*. These findings suggested that differential integrin utilization might be an important component of OPN-mediated metastatic ability in breast cancer cells. Stable transfection and overexpression of β3 in the nonmetastatic 21NT cells conferred upon these cells a more aggressive phenotype via an enhanced ability to respond to OPN both in vitro and in vivo *(38)*. Although we or others have not investigated the importance of OPN–integrin interactions in specific models of bone metastasis, our studies provide evidence that increased αvβ3 integrin expression could contribute to breast cancer metastasis in general, by making the tumor cells more responsive to the malignancy-enhancing effects of OPN.

One of the most fascinating aspects of the OPN/αvβ3 story is the fact that both OPN and αvβ3 can be produced either by tumor cells or by bone cells, suggesting several possible scenarios of OPN involvement in the promotion of bone metastasis. For example, expression of αvβ3 by the tumor cells would allow them to interact with OPN produced within the bone matrix, hence mediating tumor–bone interactions. However, along the same lines of reasoning, tumor-cell-derived OPN could also interact closely with αvβ3 expressed on the surface of osteoclasts in order to mediate osteolytic bone resorption. The fact that highly metastatic tumor cells express OPN suggests that tumor-derived OPN is important to the metastatic process, likely via its ability to upregulate proteolytic enzymes, growth factors, and its own cell surface receptors, as well as by its ability to influence the behavior of other cells in the bone microenvironment (*31–37*, discussed further in the subsequent subsections). This potential for OPN to influence bone metastasis in a variety of different ways is particularly important, considering the inherent heterogeneity found both within and between tumor types. It remains to be elucidated whether the specific functional consequences of OPN–integrin interactions on tumor cell malignancy differ depending on the cellular source of OPN and whether these consequences are different in osteolytic vs osteoblastic bone metastasis. However, it is clear that OPN and integrins produced by various cell types in the bone could influence cell behavior using both autocrine and paracrine mechanisms.

In addition to mediating cell behavior through binding to cell surface integrins, OPN can also bind to other cell surface receptors such as CD44. The CD44 family is made up of multiple protein isoforms generated by alternative splicing of a single-gene product. Although there is some indication that expression of specific CD44 variants (in particular, CD44v5 and CD44v6) might be associated with the propensity for breast carcinoma to metastasize *(92)*, this issue remains controversial, and there is evidence that such "high-risk" CD44 variant isoforms are rare in bony metastases *(93)*. This notwithstanding, it has been shown that bone cells (osteoblasts, osteocytes, and osteoclasts) can express CD44 *(94)* and that the interaction between OPN and CD44 in the normal bone microenvironment is important for osteoclast motility (via integrin-mediated mechanisms) and bone remodeling *(95,96)*. It has also been demonstrated that OPN can induce CD44v6 protein expression and promote cell adhesion of tumor cells in an integrin-dependent manner *(97)*. Interestingly, CD44v6 has been shown to be required for HGF activation of its receptor Met in rat and human prostate carcinoma cells *(98)*, and we have observed that activation of Met by OPN in breast carcinoma cells is integrin-dependent *(34*, discussed in the following subsections). Therefore, although further studies are clearly required to determine if or how the interaction of OPN and CD44 can influence bone metastasis, the observation that both tumor cells and bone cells can express these molecules suggests that binding of OPN to CD44 could mediate tumor–bone interactions in ways similar to those discussed for integrins.

5.3. Interaction of OPN With Proteases

Increased expression of proteolytic enzymes such as uPA and members of the MMP family has been observed in many human cancers and has been positively correlated with tumor progression *(99,100)*. These proteases provide cells with the ability to generate localized proteolytic activity at the tumor–host interface in order to mediate cell invasion and migration through the extracellular matrix (ECM). Additionally, association between these proteases and cell surface integrins (and the resulting induction of intracellular signaling cascades) has been linked to increased malignant cell behavior, including tumor cell adhesion, migration, invasion, and proliferation (reviewed in refs. *59* and *60*). During bone metastasis development, it is believed that proteases such as uPA and MMPs utilize both direct proteolytic mechanisms (i.e., breakdown of the bone matrix) and indirect nonproteolytic mechanisms (i.e., signaling through integrins and/ or the release of sequestered growth factors from the bone matrix, which promote tumor growth) in order to potentiate invasive cellular events that allow tumor cells to establish themselves and grow in the bone *(8,61,101)*.

Clinical studies have shown that the expression of uPA in tumor tissue can be positively correlated with the occurrence of bone metastasis in prostate cancer patients *(102)* and that expression of uPA in disseminated tumor cells recovered from the bone marrow of breast cancer patients can be associated with poor prognosis *(103)*. In cultured breast cancer cells, we have shown that OPN (either transfected or added exogenously) can upregulate the expression and enzymatic activity of uPA and that OPN-mediated breast carcinoma cell migration and invasion is uPA dependent *(31,32)*. A study by Fisher et al. *(50)* reported increased levels of tumor-derived uPA and its receptor uPAR in clinical tissue specimens of primary human breast carcinoma and its bone metastases. This study also showed increased levels of OPN in primary malignant tumors and bone metastases specimens, suggesting a possible interaction between OPN and the uPA system during bone metastasis development. Interestingly, it was observed that the majority of OPN expression in the bone metastases was localized to the stromal cells rather than the tumor cells, although some OPN was expressed by the tumor cells themselves. It has been postulated that crosstalk between tumor cells and bone cells in the bone microenvironment could cause an increase in bone cell OPN (18). Combined with our experimental findings, the observations by Fisher and colleagues suggests the possibility that both host-cell-derived OPN and tumor-cell-derived OPN might be influential in upregulating uPA production by tumor cells in order to mediate invasion into the bone matrix and the release of growth factors into the bone microenvironment.

The expression of MMP-2 has been associated with clinical disease progression to bone metastasis in prostate cancer patients *(104)*, and MMPs have been shown to be important for bone turnover and tumor cell growth in an experimental model of prostatic bone metastasis *(105)*. Other experimental studies have shown that inhibitors of MMPs are effective in reducing bone metastasis burden in prostate and breast cancer models *(106,107)*. Although the relationship between MMPs and OPN and their joint involvement in bone metastasis development requires further investigation, a number of studies suggest that OPN-mediated changes in malignant behavior (i.e., alterations in cellular adhesion, migration, and invasion) might involve MMPs. We have not seen consistent upregulation of MMPs in breast cancer cells in response to either exogenous or endogenous OPN. However, the possibility that MMPs might be linked to OPN-mediated cell invasion is supported by the observation that OPN can induce MMP-2 activation in some cell types *(35,108)*. In addition, MMP-3 and MMP-7 have been shown to be capable of cleaving OPN, and the resulting OPN cleavage product has increased bioactivity in terms of promoting cell migration and integrin-dependent cell adhesion *(109)*. Finally, the finding that both MMPs *(110)* and uPA *(111)* can be localized to the cell surface by interactions with integrins that could also bind OPN suggests that molecular crosstalk between OPN, integrins, and proteases might be one mechanism by which OPN promotes metastasis to the bone and elsewhere.

5.4. Interaction of OPN With Growth Factor–Receptor Pathways

The availability of active growth factors in the bone microenvironment is essential for bone metastasis development, although the mechanisms by which these factors act might be different in osteoblastic vs osteolytic metastasis. For example, during osteoblastic bone metastasis, the growth factor requirements for prostate tumor cells and osteoblasts are remarkably similar. Growth factors such as EGF, TGF-α, HGF, IGF, and PDGF have all been shown to be critical for both prostate cancer cell growth in the bone and the formation

of new bone matrix by osteoblasts. During osteolytic bone metastasis, the release of sequestered growth factors from the bone matrix might influence tumor cells by increasing proliferation and other malignant cell behaviors via interaction with cell surface receptors and
initiation of intracellular signaling cascades (reviewed in refs. *8, 16, 75,* and *112*).

The expression of OPN can be upregulated by a number of these growth factors,
including EGF, HGF, PDGF, TGF-β, and BMPs *(18,19,113)*. In addition, there is evidence that growth factors such as HGF can activate integrin receptors (in particular,
αvβ3) and enhance OPN-mediated migration of bone cells *(114)*. In experimental models
of breast cancer, we have found that OPN can interact specifically with the HGF/Met *(34)*
and EGF/TGF-α/EGFR *(37)* growth factor–receptor pathways. Studies from our laboratory have shown that integrin-dependant OPN-induced cell migration of breast cancer
cells involves activation and increased expression of the HGF receptor Met *(34)*. OPN-
mediated cell migration also increases the expression of EGF, TGF-α, and EGFR *(37)*,
indicating that the influence of OPN on tumor cell behavior involves a cascade of events,
including at least two growth factor–receptor pathways and multiple downstream signal
transduction pathways. Although it has not yet been shown whether these signaling
interactions hold true in prostate cancer cells and/or in experimental models of bone
metastasis, our results suggest some intriguing possibilities in terms of the importance of
OPN–growth factor interactions during bone metastasis. For example, OPN in the bone
microenvironment (be it tumor derived or bone derived) could serve to upregulate growth
factor receptors on the surface of tumor cells and/or the expression of their cognate
ligands, making them more responsive to circulating growth factors. OPN-mediated
upregulation of growth factor receptors on the cell surface of osteoblasts might similarly
be important to osteoblastic proliferation and the formation of new bone. Additionally,
the upregulation of OPN by growth factors released from the bone matrix during osteolysis or by the tumor cells themselves could create a synergistic feedback mechanism
within and between tumor cells and bone cells that could conceivably contribute to both
osteolytic and osteoblastic processes.

Although the importance and participation of OPN–growth factor interactions during bone metastasis development remains largely speculative, it is likely that the function of OPN in the bone microenvironment involves multiple interactions with the
growth factors discussed earlier as well as other interactions that have not yet been
uncovered. This idea is supported by the findings of a recent study by Kang et al. *(54)*,
who showed concomitant expression and cooperative functionality of OPN, connective
tissue growth factor (CTGF), and the cytokine IL-11 in breast cancer cells during
experimental bone metastasis. Interestingly, combined transfection and overexpression
of OPN, CTGF, and IL-11 in cells caused a significant increase in the occurrence of
osteolytic bone metastasis relative to cells that expressed only one or two of these
factors, suggesting that a multigenic program is involved in mediating breast cancer
metastasis to bone.

6. CONCLUSION

Considerable advances have been made in the last decade toward identifying molecular factors that are important to bone metastasis development. However, further elucidation of the specific mechanistic details by which these factors functionally contribute
to the metastatic process is required in order to develop effective therapeutic strategies
to combat bone metastasis. In particular, the growing evidence that tumor–host interac-

tions are absolute requirements for bone metastasis development and the observation that both tumor cells and host cells can produce metastasis-associated factors continues to validate Paget's classical theory of "seed and soil" at both the cellular and molecular levels. The inappropriate response of tumor cells to normal host signaling and/or the inability of the host to appropriately regulate tumor cell behavior creates a vicious cycle resulting in the development of metastasis in the bone and elsewhere.

The importance of the tumor–host interface during bone metastasis development suggests that disruption of tumor–bone interactions might be a useful therapeutic strategy. The ability of OPN to utilize multiple different signaling pathways to facilitate interactions between tumor cells and bone cells, combined with the observation that it can be produced by both tumor cells and host cells in the bone microenvironment (Fig. 1) suggests that OPN might be a candidate therapeutic target for the treatment and/or prevention of bone metastasis. One potential strategy would be to target OPN directly using antisense molecules or antibodies to block OPN expression and function. Alternatively, indirect targeting via inhibition of OPN-induced molecular pathways (individually or in combination) that are involved in bone metastasis might also be an effective approach. For example, small-molecule antagonists that interfere with critical ligand interactions of cell signaling receptors such as EGFR *(115)* and the $\alpha v \beta 3$ integrin *(116–118)* might help to block OPN-mediated interactions between tumor and bone. Other strategies, such as inhibition of protease activity or tyrosine kinase activity, might also be effective. Further elucidation of the molecular details by which OPN contributes to bone metastasis is required in order to assess (1) the prognostic value of OPN in determining disease progression and/or monitoring of bone metastasis and (2) whether specifically tailored therapy regimens aimed at blocking pathways activated by OPN are useful for clinical management or prevention of bone metastasis. These studies will complement the current knowledge about mechanisms of bone metastasis development and hopefully provide an opportunity to improve patient quality of life.

ACKNOWLEDGMENTS

We thank members of our laboratory and our collaborators for their research work and helpful discussions. Studies from our laboratory are supported by grants 12078 and 15323 from the Canadian Breast Cancer Research Alliance (to A.B.T., V.H.B., T.A.V., and A.F.C.), a grant from the Prostate Cancer Research Foundation of Canada (to E.W.W. and A.F.C.), and grant 42511 from the Canadian Institutes of Health Research (to A.F.C.) A.F.C. is the recipient of a Canada Research Chair in Oncology and an award from the Lloyd Carr-Harris Foundation. A.L.A. is supported by the H.L. Holmes Postdoctoral Award from the National Research Council of Canada.

Wherever possible, we have cited review articles and we refer the reader to these for citations of primary works. We apologize to the authors whose work we could not cite directly because of space restrictions.

REFERENCES

1. Fidler IJ. The biology of human cancer metastasis. *Acta Oncol* 1991; 30:668–675.
2. Chambers AF. The metastatic process: basic research and clinical implications. *Oncol Res* 1999; 11:161–168.
3. Chambers AF, Groom AC, MacDonald IC. Dissemination and growth of cancer cells in metastatic sites. *Nat Rev Cancer* 2002; 2:563–572.

 4. Arnheim FK. Carcinoma of the prostate: a study of post-mortem findings on one hundred and seventy-six cases. *J Urol* 1948; 60:599–603.
 5. Coleman RE, Rubens RD. The clinical course of bone metastases from breast cancer. *Br J Cancer* 1987; 55:61–66.
 6. Coleman RE. Skeletal complications of malignancy. *Cancer* 1997; 80:1588–1594.
 7. Mundy GR. Mechanisms of bone metastasis. *Cancer* 1997; 80:1546–1556.
 8. Mundy GR. Metastasis to bone: causes, consequences and therapeutic opportunities. *Nat Rev Cancer* 2002; 2:584–593.
 9. Chambers AF, Naumov GN, Varghese HJ, Nadkarni KV, MacDonald IC, Groom AC. Critical steps in hematogenous metastasis: an overview. *Surg Oncol Clin North Am* 2001; 10:243–255, vii.
10. MacDonald IC, Groom AC, Chambers AF. Cancer spread and micrometastasis development: quantitative approaches for in vivo models. *BioEssays* 2002; 24:885–893.
11. Woodhouse EC, Chuaqui RF, Liotta LA. General mechanisms of metastasis. *Cancer* 1997; 80:1529–1537.
12. Swartz MA, Skobe M. Lymphatic function, lymphangiogenesis, and cancer metastasis. *Microsc Res Tech* 2001; 55:92–99.
13. Weiss L. Comments on hematogenous metastatic patterns in humans as revealed by autopsy. *Clin Exp Metastasis* 1992; 10:191–199.
14. Paget S. The distribution of secondary growths in cancer of the breast. *Lancet* 1889; 1:99–101.
15. Paget S. The distribution of secondary growths in cancer of the breast. 1889. *Cancer Metastasis Rev* 1989; 8:98–101.
16. Mastro AM, Gay CV, Welch DR. The skeleton as a unique environment for breast cancer cells. *Clin Exp Metastasis* 2003; 20:275–284.
17. Heinegard D, Andersson G, Reinholt FP. Roles of osteopontin in bone remodeling. *Ann NY Acad Sci* 1995; 760:213–222.
18. Sodek J, Ganss B, McKee MD. Osteopontin. *Crit Rev Oral Biol Med* 2000; 11:279–303.
19. Furger KA, Menon RK, Tuck AB, Bramwell VH, Chambers AF. The functional and clinical roles of osteopontin in cancer and metastasis. *Curr Mol Med* 2001; 1:621–632.
20. Brown LF, Papadopoulos-Sergiou A, Berse B, Manseau EJ, Tognazzi K, Perruzzi CA, et al. Osteopontin expression and distribution in human carcinomas. *Am J Pathol* 1994; 145:610–623.
21. Fedarko NS, Jain A, Karadag A, Van Eman MR, Fisher LW. Elevated serum bone sialoprotein and osteopontin in colon, breast, prostate, and lung cancer. *Clin Cancer Res* 2001; 7:4060–4066.
22. Agrawal D, Chen T, Irby R, Quackenbush J, Chambers AF, Szabo M, et al. Osteopontin identified as lead marker of colon cancer progression, using pooled sample expression profiling. *J Natl Cancer Inst* 2002; 94:513–521.
23. Ye QH, Qin LX, Forgues M, He P, Kim JW, Peng AC, et al. Predicting hepatitis B virus-positive metastatic hepatocellular carcinomas using gene expression profiling and supervised machine learning. *Nat Med* 2003; 9:416–423.
24. Singhal H, Bautista DS, Tonkin KS, O'Malley FP, Tuck AB, Chambers AF, et al. Elevated plasma osteopontin in metastatic breast cancer associated with increased tumor burden and decreased survival. *Clin Cancer Res* 1997; 3:605–611.
25. Tuck AB, O'Malley FP, Singhal H, Tonkin KS, Harris JF, Bautista D, et al. Osteopontin and p53 expression are associated with tumor progression in a case of synchronous, bilateral, invasive mammary carcinomas. *Arch Pathol Lab Med* 1997; 121:578–584.
26. Tuck AB, O'Malley FP, Singhal H, Harris JF, Tonkin KS, Kerkvliet N, et al. Osteopontin expression in a group of lymph node negative breast cancer patients. *Int J Cancer* 1998; 79:502–508.
27. Hotte SJ, Winquist EW, Stitt L, Wilson SM, Chambers AF. Plasma osteopontin: associations with survival and metastasis to bone in men with hormone-refractory prostate carcinoma. *Cancer* 2002; 95:506–512.
28. Denhardt DT, Chambers AF. Overcoming obstacles to metastasis—defenses against host defenses: osteopontin (OPN) as a shield against attack by cytotoxic host cells. *J Cell Biochem* 1994; 56:48–51.
29. Xuan JW, Hota C, Shigeyama Y, D'Errico JA, Somerman MJ, Chambers AF. Site-directed mutagenesis of the arginine-glycine-aspartic acid sequence in osteopontin destroys cell adhesion and migration functions. *J Cell Biochem* 1995; 57:680–690.
30. Weber GF, Ashkar S, Cantor H. Interaction between CD44 and osteopontin as a potential basis for metastasis formation. *Proc Assoc Am Physicians* 1997; 109:1–9.

31. Tuck AB, Arsenault DM, O'Malley FP, Hota C, Ling MC, Wilson SM, et al. Osteopontin induces increased invasiveness and plasminogen activator expression of human mammary epithelial cells. *Oncogene* 1999; 18:4237–4246.

32. Tuck AB, Hota C, Chambers AF. Osteopontin(OPN)-induced increase in human mammary epithelial cell invasiveness is urokinase (uPA)-dependent. *Breast Cancer Res Treat* 2001; 70:197–204.

33. Shijubo N, Uede T, Kon S, Nagata M, Abe S. Vascular endothelial growth factor and osteopontin in tumor biology. *Crit Rev Oncog* 2000; 11:135–146.

34. Tuck AB, Elliott BE, Hota C, Tremblay E, Chambers AF. Osteopontin-induced, integrin-dependent migration of human mammary epithelial cells involves activation of the hepatocyte growth factor receptor (Met). *J Cell Biochem* 2000; 78:465–475.

35. Philip S, Bulbule A, Kundu GC. Osteopontin stimulates tumor growth and activation of promatrix metalloproteinase-2 through nuclear factor-kappa B-mediated induction of membrane type 1 matrix metalloproteinase in murine melanoma cells. *J Biol Chem* 2001; 276:44,926–44,935.

36. Geissinger E, Weisser C, Fischer P, Schartl M, Wellbrock C. Autocrine stimulation by osteopontin contributes to antiapoptotic signalling of melanocytes in dermal collagen. *Cancer Res* 2002; 62:4820–4828.

37. Tuck AB, Hota C, Wilson SM, Chambers AF. Osteopontin-induced migration of human mammary epithelial cells involves activation of EGF receptor and multiple signal transduction pathways. *Oncogene* 2003; 22:1198–1205.

38. Furger KA, Allan AL, Wilson SM, Hota C, Vantyghem SA, Postenka CO, et al. β3 integrin expression increases breast carcinoma cell responsiveness to the malignancy-enhancing effects of osteopontin. *Mol Cancer Res* 2003; 1:810–819.

39. Behrend EI, Craig AM, Wilson SM, Denhardt DT, Chambers AF. Reduced malignancy of ras-transformed NIH 3T3 cells expressing antisense osteopontin RNA. *Cancer Res* 1994; 54:832–837.

40. Gardner HA, Berse B, Senger DR. Specific reduction in osteopontin synthesis by antisense RNA inhibits the tumorigenicity of transformed Rat1 fibroblasts. *Oncogene* 1994; 9:2321–2326.

41. Nemoto H, Rittling SR, Yoshitake H, Furuya K, Amagasa T, Tsuji K, et al. Osteopontin deficiency reduces experimental tumor cell metastasis to bone and soft tissues. *J Bone Miner Res* 2001; 16: 652–659.

42. National Cancer Institute of Canada: Canadian cancer statistics, 2003. Toronto: National Cancer Institute of Canada, 2003.

43. Jemal A, Murray T, Samuels A, Ghafoor A, Ward E, Thun MJ. Cancer statistics, 2003. CA: *Cancer J Clin* 2003; 53:5–26.

44. Oh WK, Kantoff PW. Management of hormone refractory prostate cancer: current standards and future prospects. *J Urol* 1998; 160:1220–1229.

45. McMurtry CT, McMurtry JM. Metastatic prostate cancer: complications and treatment. *J Am Geriatr Soc* 2003; 51:1136–1142.

46. Thalmann GN, Sikes RA, Devoll RE, Kiefer JA, Markwalder R, Klima I, et al. Osteopontin: possible role in prostate cancer progression. *Clin Cancer Res* 1999; 5:2271–2277.

47. Carlinfante G, Vassilioul D, Svensson O, Wendel M, Heinegard D, Andersson G. Differential expression of osteopontin and bone sialoprotein in bone metastasis of breast and prostate carcinoma. *Clin Exp Metastasis* 2003; 20:437–444.

48. Lecrone V, Li W, Devoll RE, Logothetis C, Farach-Carson MC. Calcium signals in prostate cancer cells: specific activation by bone-matrix proteins. *Cell Calcium* 2000; 27:35–42.

49. Elgavish A, Prince C, Chang PL, Lloyd K, Lindsey R, Reed R. Osteopontin stimulates a subpopulation of quiescent human prostate epithelial cells with high proliferative potential to divide in vitro. *Prostate* 1998; 35:83–94.

50. Fisher JL, Field CL, Zhou H, Harris TL, Henderson MA, Choong PF. Urokinase plasminogen activator system gene expression is increased in human breast carcinoma and its bone metastases—a comparison of normal breast tissue, non-invasive and invasive carcinoma and osseous metastases. *Breast Cancer Res Treat* 2000; 61:1–12.

51. Reinholz MM, Iturria SJ, Ingle JN, Roche PC. Differential gene expression of TGF-beta family members and osteopontin in breast tumor tissue: analysis by real-time quantitative PCR. *Breast Cancer Res Treat* 2002; 74:255–269.

52. Oates AJ, Barraclough R, Rudland PS. The identification of osteopontin as a metastasis-related gene product in a rodent mammary tumour model. *Oncogene* 1996; 13:97–104.

53. Sung V, Gilles C, Murray A, Clarke R, Aaron AD, Azumi N, et al. The LCC15-MB human breast cancer cell line expresses osteopontin and exhibits an invasive and metastatic phenotype. *Exp Cell Res* 1998; 241:273–284.

54. Kang Y, Siegel PM, Shu W, Drobnjak M, Kakonen SM, Cordon-Cardo C, et al. A multigenic program mediating breast cancer metastasis to bone. *Cancer Cell* 2003; 3:537–549.

55. Harada S, Rodan GA. Control of osteoblast function and regulation of bone mass. *Nature* 2003; 423:349–355.

56. Percival RC, Urwin GH, Harris S, Yates AJ, Williams JL, Beneton M, et al. Biochemical and histological evidence that carcinoma of the prostate is associated with increased bone resorption. *Eur J Surg Oncol* 1987; 13:41–49.

57. Vinholes JJ, Purohit OP, Abbey ME, Eastell R, Coleman RE. Relationships between biochemical and symptomatic response in a double-blind randomised trial of pamidronate for metastatic bone disease. *Ann Oncol* 1997; 8:1243–1250.

58. Yi B, Williams PJ, Niewolna M, Wang Y, Yoneda T. Tumor-derived platelet-derived growth factor-BB plays a critical role in osteosclerotic bone metastasis in an animal model of human breast cancer. *Cancer Res* 2002; 62:917–923.

59. Chambers AF, Matrisian LM. Changing views of the role of matrix metalloproteinases in metastasis. *J Natl Cancer Inst* 1997; 89:1260–1270.

60. Blasi F, Carmeliet P. uPAR: a versatile signalling orchestrator. *Nature Rev Mol Cell Biol* 2002; 3: 932–943.

61. Yoneda T. Cellular and molecular basis of preferential metastasis of breast cancer to bone. *J Orthop Sci* 2000; 5:75–81.

62. Cooper CR, Chay CH, Pienta KJ. The role of alpha(v)beta(3) in prostate cancer progression. *Neoplasia* 2002; 4:191–194.

63. Ware JL. Growth factors and their receptors as determinants in the proliferation and metastasis of human prostate cancer. *Cancer Metastasis Rev* 1993; 12:287–301.

64. Achbarou A, Kaiser S, Tremblay G, Ste-Marie LG, Brodt P, Goltzman D, et al. Urokinase overproduction results in increased skeletal metastasis by prostate cancer cells in vivo. *Cancer Res* 1994; 54: 2372–2377.

65. Iwamura M, Hellman J, Cockett AT, Lilja H, Gershagen S. Alteration of the hormonal bioactivity of parathyroid hormone-related protein (PTHrP) as a result of limited proteolysis by prostate-specific antigen. *Urology* 1996; 48:317–325.

66. Pfeilschifter J, Mundy GR. Modulation of type beta transforming growth factor activity in bone cultures by osteotropic hormones. *Proc Natl Acad Sci USA* 1987; 84:2024–2028.

67. Yin JJ, Selander K, Chirgwin JM, Dallas M, Grubbs BG, Wieser R, et al. TGF-beta signaling blockade inhibits PTHrP secretion by breast cancer cells and bone metastases development. *J Clin Invest* 1999; 103:197–206.

68. Bundred NJ, Walker RA, Ratcliffe WA, Warwick J, Morrison JM, Ratcliffe JG. Parathyroid hormone related protein and skeletal morbidity in breast cancer. *Eur J Cancer* 1992; 28:690–692.

69. Kohno N, Kitazawa S, Fukase M, Sakoda Y, Kanbara Y, Furuya Y, et al. The expression of parathyroid hormone-related protein in human breast cancer with skeletal metastases. *Surg Today* 1994; 24:215–220.

70. Powell GJ, Southby J, Danks JA, Stillwell RG, Hayman JA, Henderson MA, et al. Localization of parathyroid hormone-related protein in breast cancer metastases: increased incidence in bone compared with other sites. *Cancer Res* 1991; 51:3059–3061.

71. Liotta LA, Kohn EC. The microenvironment of the tumour-host interface. *Nature* 2001; 411:375–379.

72. Bogdan C. Nitric oxide and the immune response. *Nature Immunol* 2001; 2:907–916.

73. Feng B, Rollo EE, Denhardt DT. Osteopontin (OPN) may facilitate metastasis by protecting cells from macrophage NO-mediated cytotoxicity: evidence from cell lines down-regulated for OPN expression by a targeted ribozyme. *Clin Exp Metastasis* 1995; 13:453–462.

74. Rollo EE, Laskin DL, Denhardt DT. Osteopontin inhibits nitric oxide production and cytotoxicity by activated RAW264.7 macrophages. *J Leukocyte Biol* 1996; 60:397–404.

75. Koeneman KS, Yeung F, Chung LW. Osteomimetic properties of prostate cancer cells: a hypothesis supporting the predilection of prostate cancer metastasis and growth in the bone environment. *Prostate* 1999; 39:246–261.

76. Noti JD. Adherence to osteopontin via alphavbeta3 suppresses phorbol ester-mediated apoptosis in MCF-7 breast cancer cells that overexpress protein kinase C-alpha. *Int J Oncol* 2000; 17:1237–1243.

77. Newham P, Humphries MJ. Integrin adhesion receptors: structure, function and implications for biomedicine. *Mol Med Today* 1996; 2:304–313.
78. Giancotti FG, Ruoslahti E. Integrin signaling. *Science* 1999; 285:1028–1032.
79. Cheng SL, Lai CF, Blystone SD, Avioli LV. Bone mineralization and osteoblast differentiation are negatively modulated by integrin alpha(v)beta3. *J Bone Miner Res* 2001; 16:277–288.
80. Ohshima S, Kobayashi H, Yamaguchi N, Nishioka K, Umeshita-Sasai M, Mima T, Nomura S, et al. Expression of osteopontin at sites of bone erosion in a murine experimental arthritis model of collagen-induced arthritis: possible involvement of osteopontin in bone destruction in arthritis. *Arthritis Rheum* 2002; 46:1094–1101.
81. Varner JA, Cheresh DA. Integrins and cancer. *Curr Opin Cell Biol* 1996; 8:724–730.
82. Liapis H, Flath A, Kitazawa S. Integrin alpha V beta 3 expression by bone-residing breast cancer metastases. *Diagn Mol Pathol* 1996; 5:127–135.
83. Kitazawa S, Maeda S. Development of skeletal metastases. *Clin Orthop* 1995; 312:45–50.
84. Wong NC, Mueller BM, Barbas CF, Ruminski P, Quaranta V, Lin EC, et al. Alphav integrins mediate adhesion and migration of breast carcinoma cell lines. *Clin Exp Metastasis* 1998; 16:50–61.
85. Felding-Habermann B, O'Toole TE, Smith JW, Fransvea E, Ruggeri ZM, Ginsberg MH, et al. Integrin activation controls metastasis in human breast cancer. *Proc Natl Acad Sci USA* 2001; 98:1853–1858.
86. De S, Chen J, Narizhneva NV, Heston W, Brainard J, Sage EH, et al. Molecular pathway for cancer metastasis to bone. *J Biol Chem* 2003; 278:39,044–39,050.
87. Nemeth JA, Cher ML, Zhou Z, Mullins C, Bhagat S, Trikha M. Inhibition of alpha(v)beta3 integrin reduces angiogenesis, bone turnover, and tumor cell proliferation in experimental prostate cancer bone metastases. *Clin Exp Metastasis* 2003; 20:413–420.
88. Bakewell SJ, Nestor P, Prasad S, Tomasson MH, Dowland N, Mehrotra M, et al. Platelet and osteoclast β3 integrins are critical for bone metastasis. *Proc Natl Acad Sci USA* 2003; 100:14,205–14,210.
89. van der Pluijm, Vloedgraven H, Papapoulos S, Lowick C, Grzesik W, Kerr J, et al. Attachment characteristics and involvement of integrins in adhesion of breast cancer cell lines to extracellular bone matrix components. *Lab Invest* 1997; 77:665–675.
90. Zheng DQ, Woodard AS, Fornaro M, Tallini G, Languino LR. Prostatic carcinoma cell migration via alpha(v)beta3 integrin is modulated by a focal adhesion kinase pathway. *Cancer Res* 1999; 59:1655–1664.
91. Cole K, Kohn E. Calcium-mediated signal transduction: biology, biochemistry, and therapy. *Cancer Metastasis Rev* 1994; 13:31–44.
92. Lackner C, Moser R, Bauernhofer T, Wilders-Truschnig M, Samonigg H, Berghold A, et al. Soluble CD44 v5 and v6 in serum of patients with breast cancer. Correlation with expression of CD44 v5 and v6 variants in primary tumors and location of distant metastasis. *Breast Cancer Res Treat* 1998; 47:29–40.
93. Putz E, Witter K, Offner S, Stosiek P, Zippelius A, Johnson J, et al. Phenotypic characteristics of cell lines derived from disseminated cancer cells in bone marrow of patients with solid epithelial tumors: establishment of working models for human micrometastases. *Cancer Res* 1999; 59:241–248.
94. Nakamura H, Kenmotsu S, Sakai H, Ozawa H. Localization of CD44, the hyaluronate receptor, on the plasma membrane of osteocytes and osteoclasts in rat tibiae. *Cell Tissue Res* 1995; 280:225–233.
95. Chellaiah MA, Hruska KA. The integrin alpha(v)beta(3) and CD44 regulate the actions of osteopontin on osteoclast motility. *Calcif Tissue Int* 2003; 72:197–205.
96. Yamazaki M, Nakajima F, Ogasawara A, Moriya H, Majeska RJ, Einhorn TA. Spatial and temporal distribution of CD44 and osteopontin in fracture callus. *J Bone Joint Surg Br* 1999; 81:508–515.
97. Gao C, Guo H, Downey L, Marroquin C, Wei J, Kuo PC. Osteopontin-dependent CD44v6 expression and cell adhesion in HepG2 cells. *Carcinogenesis* 2003 [Epub ahead of print].
98. Orian-Rousseau V, Chen L, Sleeman JP, Herrlich P, Ponta H. CD44 is required for two consecutive steps in HGF/c-Met signaling. *Genes Dev* 2002; 16:3074–3086.
99. Stetler-Stevenson WG, Hewitt R, Corcoran M. Matrix metalloproteinases and tumor invasion: from correlation and causality to the clinic. *Semin Cancer Biol* 1996; 7:147–154.
100. Brunner N, Nielsen HJ, Hamers M, Christensen IJ, Thorlacius-Ussing O, Stephens RW. The urokinase plasminogen activator receptor in blood from healthy individuals and patients with cancer. *APMIS* 1999; 107:160–167.
101. Sloan EK, Anderson RL. Genes involved in breast cancer metastasis to bone. *Cell Mol Life Sci* 2002; 59:1491–1502.

102. Ohta S, Fuse H, Fujiuchi Y, Nagakawa O, Furuya Y. Clinical significance of expression of urokinase-type plasminogen activator in patients with prostate cancer. *Anticancer Res* 2003; 23:2945–2950.

103. Solomayer EF, Diel IJ, Wallwiener D, Bode S, Meyberg G, Sillem M, et al. Prognostic relevance of urokinase plasminogen activator detection in micrometastatic cells in the bone marrow of patients with primary breast cancer. *Br J Cancer* 1997; 76:812–818.

104. Kanoh Y, Akahoshi T, Ohara T, Ohtani N, Mashiko T, Ohtani S, et al. Expression of matrix metalloproteinase-2 and prostate-specific antigen in localized and metastatic prostate cancer. *Anticancer Res* 2002; 22:1813–1817.

105. Nemeth JA, Yousif R, Herzog M, Che M, Upadhyay J, Shekarriz B, et al. Matrix metalloproteinase activity, bone matrix turnover, and tumor cell proliferation in prostate cancer bone metastasis. *J Natl Cancer Inst* 2002; 94:17–25.

106. Winding B, NicAmhlaoibh R, Misander H, Hoegh-Andersen P, Andersen TL, Holst-Hansen C, et al. Synthetic matrix metalloproteinase inhibitors inhibit growth of established breast cancer osteolytic lesions and prolong survival in mice. *Clin Cancer Res* 2002; 8:1932–1939.

107. Corey E, Brown LG, Quinn JE, Poot M, Roudier MP, Higano CS, et al. Zoledronic acid exhibits inhibitory effects on osteoblastic and osteolytic metastases of prostate cancer. *Clin Cancer Res* 2003; 9:295–306.

108. Teti A, Farina AR, Villanova I, Tiberio A, Tacconelli A, Sciortino G, et al. Activation of MMP-2 by human GCT23 giant cell tumour cells induced by osteopontin, bone sialoprotein and GRGDSP peptides is RGD and cell shape change dependent. *Int J Cancer* 1998; 77:82–93.

109. Agnihotri R, Crawford HC, Haro H, Matrisian LM, Havrda MC, Liaw L. Osteopontin, a novel substrate for matrix metalloproteinase-3 (stromelysin-1) and matrix metalloproteinase-7 (matrilysin). *J Biol Chem* 2001; 276:28,261–28,267.

110. Brooks PC, Stromblad S, Sanders LC, von Schalscha TL, Aimes RT, Stetler-Stevenson WG, et al. Localization of matrix metalloproteinase MMP-2 to the surface of invasive cells by interaction with integrin alpha v beta 3. *Cell* 1996; 85:683–693.

111. Yebra M, Parry GC, Stromblad S, Mackman N, Rosenberg S, Mueller BM, Cheresh DA. Requirement of receptor-bound urokinase-type plasminogen activator for integrin alphavbeta5-directed cell migration. *J Biol Chem* 1996; 271:29393–29399.

112. Roodman GD. Role of stromal-derived cytokines and growth factors in bone metastasis. *Cancer* 2003; 97:733–738.

113. Ariztia EV, Subbarao V, Solt DB, Rademaker AW, Iyer AP, Oltvai ZN. Osteopontin contributes to hepatocyte growth factor-induced tumor growth and metastasis formation. *Exp Cell Res* 2003; 288: 257–267.

114. Faccio R, Grano M, Colucci S, Villa A, Giannelli G, Quaranta V, et al. Localization and possible role of two different alpha v beta 3 integrin conformations in resting and resorbing osteoclasts. *J Cell Sci* 2002; 115:2919–2929.

115. Ciardiello F, Tortora G. A novel approach in the treatment of cancer: targeting the epidermal growth factor receptor. *Clin Cancer Res* 2001; 7:2958–2970.

116. Tucker GC. Inhibitors of integrins. *Curr Opin Pharmacol* 2002; 2:394–402.

117. Teti A, Migliaccio S, Baron R. The role of the alphaVbeta3 integrin in the development of osteolytic bone metastases: a pharmacological target for alternative therapy? *Calcif Tissue Int* 2002; 71:293–299.

118. Harms JF, Welcch DR, Samant RS, Shevde LA, Miele ME, Babu GR, et al. A small molecule antagonist of the $\alpha(v)\beta3$ integrin suppresses MDA-MB-435 skeletal metastasis. *Clin Exp Metastasis* 2004; 21:119–128.

8

Role of Interleukin-11 in Osteolytic Bone Metastasis

Ryan R. Simon, MSc, *Martin K. Butcher,* HONBSc, *and Stephen G. Shaughnessy,* PhD

1. INTRODUCTION

Interleukin (IL)-11 is a pleiotropic cytokine that belongs to the IL-6 family of cytokines *(1)*. Other cytokines belonging to this family include oncostatin M (OSM), leukemia inhibitory factor (LIF), cardiotrophin (CT)-1, and ciliary neurotrophic factor (CNTF). All members of this cytokine family have their own unique α-chain receptors, which, when occupied, initiate signal transduction via the recruitment and subsequent homodimerization or heterodimerization of membrane-associated glycoprotein (gp) 130 *(2)*. Members of this cytokine family, therefore, often share overlapping biological activities and have multiple effects on both hematopoietic and nonhematopoietic cell populations *(2)*. For example, IL-11 has been shown to synergize with a number of growth factors to enhance megakaryocytopoiesis *(3–5)* and erythropoiesis in vivo *(6–8)* and to enhance both platelet and neutrophil recovery following sublethal irradiation *(9)*. In addition, IL-11 has been shown to stimulate the production of acute-phase reactants and to act as an effective inhibitor of adipogenesis *(10–14)*. Finally, IL-11 is secreted by both bone marrow stromal cells and mature osteoblasts, and is known to function as a potent stimulator of both osteoclast formation and activity *(15–17)*. As a result, IL-11 is thought to play a role in such diverse pathologies as heparin-induced osteoporosis *(18)*, postmenopausal bone loss *(19)*, and, as reviewed in this chapter, osteolytic bone metastasis.

From: *Cancer Drug Discovery and Development*
Bone Metastasis: Experimental and Clinical Therapeutics
Edited by: G. Singh and S. A. Rabbani © Humana Press Inc., Totowa, NJ

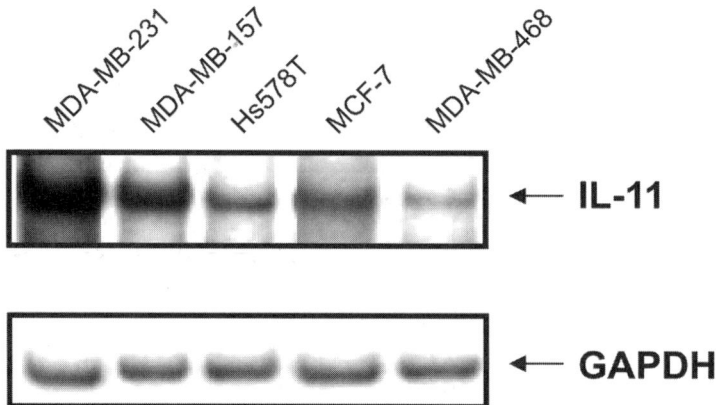

Fig. 1. Interleukin-11 expression by human breast cancer cell lines. Total RNA from various human breast cancer cell lines was harvested and subjected to semiquantitative reverse–transcription–polymerase chain reaction (RT-PCR) using IL-11 specific primers. Glyceraldehyde-3-phosphate dehydrogenase (GAPDH) was used as a control for equal loading.

2. IL-11 PRODUCTION BY CANCER CELLS

Several groups have detected IL-11 expression by human breast cancers. Thus, Selander et al. detected IL-11 transcripts in 14 of 17 tissue biopsies that they obtained from patients with primary breast cancer *(20)*. In addition, we have detected IL-11 expression in several commonly available breast cancer cell lines, including MDA-MB-231, MDA-MB-157, Hs578T, MCF-7, and MDA-MB-468 cells (Fig. 1). Subsequent experiments using IL-11-specific enzyme-linked immunosorbent assays (ELISAs) confirmed these later findings and demonstrated that these cell lines not only express but also secrete IL-11. Thus, by using IL-11-specific ELISAs, we detected in IL-11 the culture medium of these cancer cell lines at concentrations that reached as high as 10 ng/million cells/d. Similar findings were reported by Suarez-Cuervo et al. when they quantified the release of IL-11 into the culture medium of MDA-MB-231 cells *(21)*. These findings suggest that primary human breast cancer cells not only express but also secrete significant quantities of IL-11.

In addition to constitutively expressing IL-11, there is now ample evidence to suggest that human breast cancer cells might upregulate IL-11 production when exposed to various cytokines and/or growth factors that are normally found within the bone microenvironment *(22–24)*. In accordance with this concept, we and others have shown that human breast cancer cells increase their expression of IL-11 when treated with transforming growth factor-β (TGF-β). Thus, we found that IL-11 expression was increased in a dose-dependent manner when MDA-MB-231 cells were cultured in the presence of increasing concentrations of TGF-β (Fig. 2). These findings are in agreement with those of Chen et al., who used oligonucleotide array expression analysis to demonstrate an 18-fold enhancement of IL-11 message when MDA-MB-231 cells were treated with TGF-β *(23)*. Similar findings have also been reported by Lacroix et al. *(24)*. Whether other bone regulatory factors such as tumor necrosis factor-α (TNF-α), IL-1, or parathyroid hormone (PTH) also stimulate cancer cells to produce large amounts of IL-11 is not known.

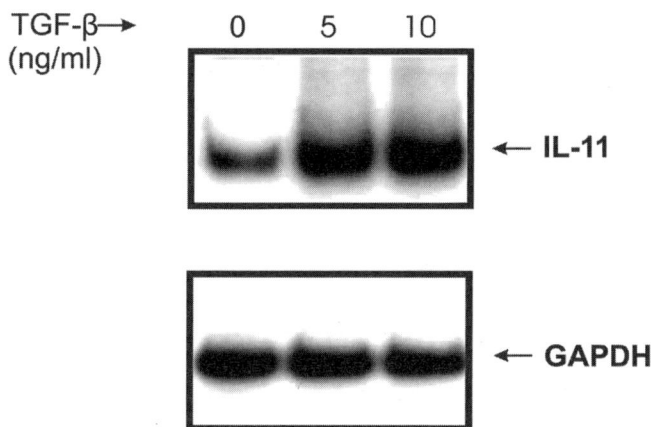

Fig. 2. The effect of TGF-β on MDA-MB-231 expression of IL-11. MDA-MB-231 cells were either left untreated or treated with TGF-β for 24 h before harvesting their total RNA and subjecting it to semiquantitative RT-PCR using IL-11 specific primers. GAPDH was used as a control for equal loading.

However, such factors have been shown to increase IL-11 expression in both human and murine osteoblast-like cells *(15–17)*.

3. EVIDENCE THAT CANCER CELLS STIMULATE OSTEOBLASTS TO PRODUCE IL-11

Several groups, including our own, have shown that the conditioned media from human breast cancer cell lines can stimulate IL-11 expression in both murine and human osteoblast cell cultures (Fig. 3) *(25)*. Thus, we have shown that the conditioned medium of MDA-MB-231 cells can stimulate IL-11 expression in primary cultures of murine calvaria cells by fivefold. Similarly, Morinaga et al. demonstrated that the conditioned media from MDA-MB-231 cells could stimulate IL-11 expression in the human osteoblastlike cell line SaOS-2 and that this effect was at least partially mediated by TGF-β *(25)*. Whether or not other factors secreted by cancer cells can induce the expression of IL-11 in either murine or human osteoblasts is unknown. However, studies using human osteosarcoma cell lines and primary mouse osteoblasts have shown that a number of factors are capable of directly inducing osteoblast expression of IL-11 *(15–17)*. For example, Elias et al. demonstrated that factors such as IL-1, TGF-β, PTH, parathyroid hormone-related protein (PTHrP), and prostaglandin E_2 (PGE$_2$) are all capable of inducing IL-11 expression in SaOS-2 cells *(17)*. Similarly, Romas et al. demonstrated that the addition of IL-1, TNF-α, PGE$_2$, PTH, and 1,25-dihydroxyvitamin D_3 (1α,25[OH]$_2$D$_3$) to primary murine osteoblast cultures could also induce the expression of IL-11, both at the protein and mRNA levels *(15)*. However, to what extent these factors can mediate the ability of cancer cells to induce osteoblast expression of IL-11 is not known.

4. POTENTIAL ROLES FOR IL-11 IN OSTEOLYTIC BONE METASTASIS

Several steps are thought to be critical to the metastatic spread of cancer to bone. These include a cancer cell's ability to: (1) respond to bone-specific growth factors

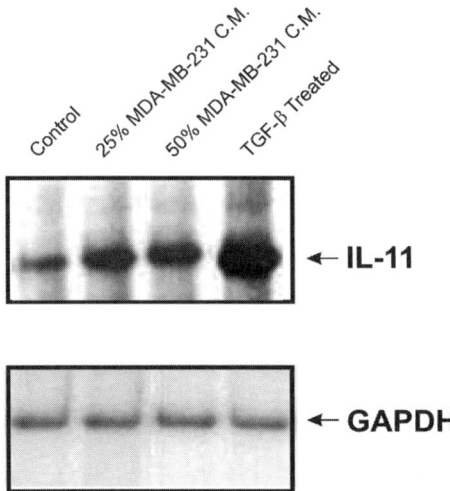

Fig. 3. The effect of cancer cell conditioned media and TGF-β treatment on IL-11 expression by primary murine calvaria cells. Primary murine calvaria cells (osteoblasts) were isolated and treated with either MDA-MB-231 cell conditioned media or TGF-β. Twenty-four hours later, total RNA from the calvaria cells was harvested and subjected to semiquantitative RT-PCR using IL-11 specific primers. GAPDH was used as a control for equal loading.

(26–30), (2) respond to chemotactic factors produced within the bone microenvironment *(31–35)*, (3) adhere to bone microvasculature/stromal cells and/or matrix *(36–41)*, and, (4) induce the osteolysis of the bone matrix *(42–45)*. Whether IL-11 is playing a role in any of these processes has not been established. However, when Selander et al. transfected human IL-11 into MDA-MB-231 cells and then inoculated nude mice with both high- and low-expressing clones, they found that tumor burden was significantly greater in those mice that had been inoculated with the high-IL-11-producing clones *(20)*. Although the mechanism for this effect is unknown, one possible explanation is that IL-11 is providing a growth advantage to those cancer cells that are expressing high levels of the cytokine.

To date, few studies have attempted to define a role for IL-11 in osteolytic bone metastasis. As such, there have been no studies to address the issue of whether IL-11 might promote the homing of cancer cells to bone by inducing cancer cell adhesion to either bone-derived endothelial cells or bone marrow stromal cells. In addition, few studies have addressed whether IL-11 can act as either a growth factor and/or a chemotactic factor for cancer cells when they metastasize to bone. Lacroix et al. investigated whether IL-11 could stimulate DNA synthesis in five different human breast cancer cell lines (MCF-7, T-47D, MDA-MB-231, Hs578T, and BT-20) *(24)*. However, they found that IL-11 could not stimulate cell proliferation in any of the cell lines tested. In contrast, when Arihiro et al. investigated IL-11's ability to facilitate the chemotactic motility of three human breast carcinoma cell lines (MDA-MB-231, T-47D, and MCF-7), they found that IL-11 appeared to elicit a chemotactic response in MDA-MB-231 cells when used at supraphysiological concentrations (i.e., greater than 100 ng/mL) *(46)*. Therefore, although very high concentrations of IL-11 were required in order to elicit a response, these results do support the possibility that IL-11 might elicit a chemotactic response in some cancers.

Perhaps one of the most important mechanisms by which IL-11 could be involved in the metastatic spread of cancer to bone is through its potential to stimulate both osteoclast formation and activity *(15–17)*. However, to our knowledge, no one has demonstrated that cancer cells by secreting IL-11 can induce osteoclast formation either in vitro or in vivo. Indeed, in experiments by Tumber et al., anti-IL-11 antibodies failed to suppress the effect that MDA-MB-231 conditioned media had on osteoclastogenesis in murine metatarsal explants *(47)*. Why neutralization of IL-11 activity in this assay failed to have any effect on osteoclastogenesis remains unexplained. It might be that the constitutive expression of IL-11 by MDA-MB-231 cells is too low to have any effect on osteoclast formation and that a significantly different outcome might occur if the MDA-MB-231 cells were first exposed to TGF-β. However, a slightly more complicated explanation is suggested by the experiments of Kang et al. *(22)*. Kang et al. selected for a highly metastatic subpopulation of human breast cancer cells by inoculating nude mice with MDA-MB-231 cells and then recovering only those cells that had successfully metastasized to bone. By repeating this process several times and then characterizing the various subpopulations that they obtained, Kang et al. discovered that those cells that had a high propensity to metastasize to bone had five genes that were highly overexpressed. These genes were, matrix metalloproteinase-1 (MMP-1), chemokine (C-X-C motif) receptor 4 (CXCR4), connective tissue growth factor (CTGF), osteopontin (OPN), and, not surprisingly, IL-11. The authors then demonstrated that the overexpression of IL-11 alone was not sufficient to induce an aggressive osteolytic phenotype. However, when IL-11 was overexpressed with OPN in the parental cell line, a highly metastatic phenotype was generated. Most importantly, this phenotype was also associated with a significant increase in the number of TRAP+ multinucleated cells (osteoclasts) that were found in the bone lesions. Because overexpression of OPN alone, like IL-11, was insufficient to induce an aggressive metastatic phenotype, it remains unclear how IL-11 and OPN expression together might cooperate to achieve such a change. It is possible that OPN augments IL-11's ability to induce osteoclast formation and activity, and that by doing so, TGF-β is released into the bone microenvironment. The newly released TGF-β could then stimulate the surrounding cancer cells or osteoblasts to secrete even more IL-11. This, in turn, might result in additional tumor cell growth and osteolysis, thus perpetuating the cycle. This scenario typifies a classic "vicious cycle" of tumor-cell-induced osteoclastogenesis (Fig. 4).

5. CLINICAL RELEVANCE

Given the poor prognosis that patients face following colonization of their bones by cancer, much interest has been expressed in developing prognostic indicators that would predict if a patient is likely to develop bone metastasis. Although the expression in primary cancers of PTHrP was initially believed to be predictive of patients developing osteolytic bone metastasis *(43,48)*, a recent clinical study by Henderson et al. challenges this belief *(49)*. In addition, a study by Guise et al. demonstrated that the overexpression of PTHrP in mammary tumors inoculated into the arterial circulation of nude mice resulted in hypercalcemia, but not bone metastasis *(50)*. Given these findings, Sotiriou et al.

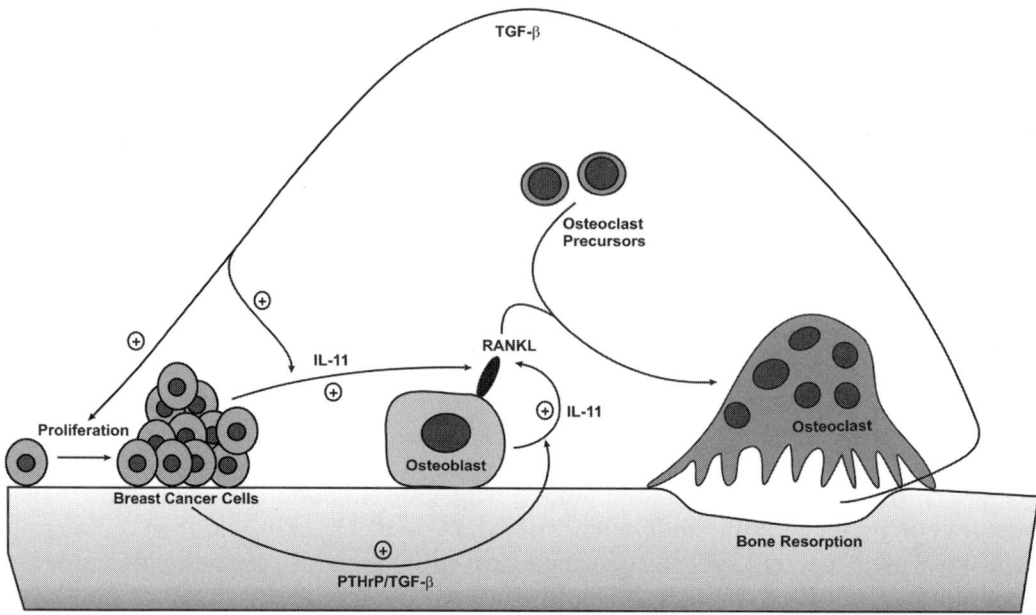

Fig. 4. Postulated mechanism by which IL-11 might be involved in osteolytic bone metastasis. We propose that increased osteoclast formation is responsible for the osteolysis and hypercalcemia associated with some bone metastases and that cancer cells induce osteoclast formation by either directly or indirectly promoting the synthesis and release of IL-11. This, in turn, might further stimulate the metastatic process by releasing chemotactic factors, and/or growth factors, such as TGF-β, back into the bone microenvironment.

explored the possibility that IL-11 might be a better prognostic indicator than PTHrP in determining whether a cancer might metastasize to bone *(51)*. Using immunohistochemistry and *in situ* hybridization techniques to study IL-11 and IL-6 expression in 99 invasive primary breast biopsies, Sotiriou et al., found that a significantly higher incidence ($p = 0.002$) of bone metastasis occurred in those patients whose tumors expressed IL-11. Interestingly, none of the 10 normal breast tissues sampled were positive for IL-11 expression. These findings support the possibility of using IL-11 expression as a prognostic indicator for the development of bone metastasis.

REFERENCES

1. Paul SR, Bennett F, Calvetti JA, Kelleher K, Wood CR, O'Hare RM, et al. Molecular cloning of a cDNA encoding interleukin-11, a stromal cell derived lymphopoietic cytokine. *Proc Natl Acad Sci USA* 1990; 87:7512–7516.
2. Du X, Williams DA. Interleukin-11: review of molecular, cell biology, and clinical use. *Blood* 1997; 89:3897–3908.
3. Bruno E, Briddell RA, Cooper RJ, Hoffman R. Effects of recombinant interleukin 11 on human megakaryocyte progenitor cells. *Exp Hematol* 1991; 19:378–381
4. Neben TY, Loebelenz J, Hayes L, McCarthy K, Stoudemire J, Schaub R, et al. Recombinant human interleukin-11 stimulates megakaryocytopoiesis and increases peripheral platelets in normal and splenectomized mice. *Blood* 1993; 81:901–908.

5. Weich NS, Wang A, Fitzgerald M, Neben TY, Donaldson D, Giannotti J, et al. Recombinant human interleukin-11 directly promotes megakaryocytopoiesis in vitro. *Blood* 1997; 90:3893–3902.
6. Quesniaux VF, Clark SC, Turner K, Fagg B. Interleukin-11 stimulates multiple phases of erythropoiesis in vitro. *Blood* 1992; 80:1218–1223.
7. Rodriguez MH, Arnaud S, Blanchet JP. IL-11 directly stimulates murine and human erythroid burst formation in semisolid cultures. *Exp Hematol* 1995; 23:545–550.
8. de Haan G, Dontje B, Engel C, Loeffler M, Nijhof W. In vivo effects of interleukin-11 and stem cell factor in combination with erythropoietin in the regulation of erythropoiesis. *Br J Haematol* 1995; 90: 783–790.
9. Galmiche MC, Vogel CA, Delaloye AB, Schmidt PM, Healy F, Mach JP, Buchegger F. Combined effects of interleukin-3 and interleukin-11 on hematopoiesis in irradiated mice. *Exp Hematol* 1996; 24: 1298–1306.
10. Baumann H, Schendel P. Interleukin-11 regulates the hepatic expression of the same plasma protein genes as interleukin-6. *J Biol Chem* 1991; 266:20,424–20,427.
11. Fukuda Y, Sassa S. Effect of interleukin-11 on the levels of mRNAs encoding heme oxygenase and haptoglobin in human HepG2 hepatoma cells. *Biochem Biophys Res Commun* 1993; 193:297–302.
12. Gordon MS, McCaskill-Stevens WJ, Battiato LA, Loewy J, Loesch D, Breeden E, et al. A phase I trial of recombinant human interleukin-11 (neumega rhIL-11 growth factor) in women with breast cancer receiving chemotherapy. *Blood* 1996; 87:3615–3624.
13. Ohsumi J, Miyadai K, Kawashima I, Ishikawa-Ohsumi H, Sakakibara S, Mita-Honjo K, et al. Adipogenesis inhibitory factor. A novel inhibitory regulator of adipose conversion in bone marrow. *FEBS Lett* 1991; 288:13–16.
14. Keller DC, Du XX, Srour EF, Hoffman R, Williams DA. Interleukin-11 inhibits adipogenesis and stimulates myelopoiesis in human long-term marrow cultures. *Blood* 1993; 82:1428–1435.
15. Romas E, Udagawa N, Zhou H, Tamura T, Saito M, Taga T, et al. The role of gp130-mediated signals in osteoclast development: regulation of interleukin 11 production by osteoblasts and distribution of its receptor in bone marrow cultures. *J Exp Med* 1996; 183:2581–2591.
16. Girasole G, Passeri G, Jilka RL, Manolagas SC. Interleukin II: a new cytokine critical for osteoclast development. *J Clin Invest* 1994; 93:1516–1524.
17. Elias JA, Tang W, Horowitz MC. Cytokine and hormonal stimulation of human osteosarcoma interleukin-11 production. *Endocrinology* 1995; 136(2):489–498.
18. Walton KJ, Duncan JM, Deschamps P, Shaughnessy SG. Heparin acts synergistically with interleukin-11 to induce STAT3 activation and in vitro osteoclast formation. *Blood* 2002; 100:2530–2536.
19. Shaughnessy SG, Walton KJ, Deschamps P, Butcher M, Beaudin SM. Neutralization of interleukin-11 activity decreases osteoclast formation and increases cancellous bone volume in ovariectomized mice. *Cytokine* 2002; 20:78–85.
20. Selander KS, Reddi S, Harris KW, Valve E, Harjonen P, Dean P, et al. Increased interleuken-11 expression by breast cancer cells results in increased bone metastasis in mice. *Calcif Tissue Int* 2000; S68.
21. Suarez-Cuervo C, Harris KW, Kallman L, Vaananen HK, Selander KS. Tumor necrosis factor-alpha induces interleukin-6 production via extracellular-regulated kinase 1 activation in breast cancer cells. *Breast Cancer Res Treat* 2003; 80:71–78.
22. Kang Y, Siegel PM, Shu W, Drobnjak M, Kakonen SM, Cordon-Cardo C, et al. A multigenic program mediating breast cancer metastasis to bone. *Cancer Cell* 2003; 3:537–549.
23. Chen CR, Kang Y, Massague J. Defective repression of c-myc in breast cancer cells: A loss at the core of the transforming growth factor beta growth arrest program. *Proc Natl Acad Sci USA* 2001; 98(3): 992–999.
24. Lacroix M, Siwek B, Marie PJ, Body JJ. Production and regulation of interleukin-11 by breast cancer cells. *Cancer Lett* 1998; 127:29–35.
25. Moringa Y, Fujita N, Ohishi K, Tsuruo T. Stimulation of interleukin-II production from osteoblast-like cells by transforming growth factor-β and tumor cell factors. *Int J Cancer* 1997; 71:422–428.
26. Yin JJ, Selander K, Chirgwin JM, Dallas M, Grubbs BG, Wieser R, et al. TGF-beta signaling blockade inhibits PTHrP secretion by breast cancer cells and bone metastases development. *J Clin Invest* 1999; 103(2):197–206.
27. Lahm H, Suardet L, Laurent PJ, et al. Growth regulation and co-stimulation of human colorectal cancer cell lines by insulin-like growth factors I, II and transforming growth factor β. *Br J Cancer* 1992; 65:341–346.

28. Chackal-Roy M, Niemeyer C, Moore M, Zetter BR. Stimulation of human prostatic carcinoma cell growth by factors present in human bone marrow. *J Clin Invest* 1989; 84:43–50.
29. Gleave M, Hsieh JT, Gao C, von Eschenbach AC, Chung LWK. Acceleration of human prostate cancer growth in vivo by factors produced by prostate and bone fibroblasts. *Cancer Res* 1991; 51:3753–5761.
30. Millar-Book W, Orr FW, Singh G: In vitro effects of bone and platelet-derived transforming growth factor-β on the growth of walker 256 carcinosarcoma cells. *Clin Expl Metastasis* 1990; 8:503–510.
31. Muller A, Homey B, Soto H, Ge N, Catron D, Buchanan ME, et al. Involvement of chemokine receptors in breast cancer metastasis. *Nature* 2001; 410:50–56.
32. Orr FW, Millar-Book W, Singh G. Chemotactic activity of bone and platelet-derived TGF-beta for bone metastasizing rat walker 256 carcinosarcoma cells. *Invasion Metastasis* 1990; 10:241–252.
33. Orr W, Varani J, Gondek MD, Ward PA, Mundy GR. Chemotactic responses of tumor cells to products of resorbing bone. *Science* 1979; 203:176–179.
34. Magro C, Orr FW, Manishen WJ, Sivananthan K, Mokashi S. Adhesion, chemotaxis, and aggregation of Walker carcinosarcoma cells in response to products of resorbing bone. *J Natl Cancer Inst* 1985; 74: 829–838.
35. Mundy GR, Poser JW. Chemotactic activity of the gamma-carboxyglutamic acid containing protein in bone. *Calcif Tissue Int* 1983; 35:164–168.
36. Sung V, Stubbs JT 3rd, Fisher L, Aaron AD, Thompson EW. Bone sialoprotein supports breast cancer cell adhesion proliferation and migration through differential usage of the alpha(v)beta3 and alpha(v)beta5 integrins. *J Cell Physiol* 1998; 176(3):482–494.
37. Haq M, Goltzman D, Tremblay G, Brodt P. Rat prostate adenocarcinoma cells disseminate to bone and adhere preferentially to bone marrow-derived endothelial cells. *Cancer Res* 1992; 52:4613–4619
38. Nakai M, Mundy GR, Williams PJ, Boyce B, Yoneda T. A synthetic antagonist to laminin inhibits the formation of osteolytic metastases by human melanoma cells in nude mice. *Cancer Res* 1992; 52:5395–5399.
39. Caligaris-Cappio F, Bergui L, Gregretti MG. Role of bone marrow stromal cells in the growth of human multiple myeloma. *Blood* 1991; 77:2688–2693.
40. Uchiyama H, Barut BA, Mohrbacher AF, Chauhan D, Anderson KC. Adhesion of human myeloma-derived cell lines to bone marrow stromal cells stimulates interleukin-6 secretion. *Blood* 1993; 82: 3712–3720.
41. Kostenuik PJ, Singh G, Orr FW. Preferential adhesion of PC-3 prostate cancer cells to osteoblast-like matrix. *Proc Am Assoc Cancer Res* 1994; 25:56 (Abstract).
42. Honore P, Luger NM, Sabino MA, Schwei MJ, Rogers SD, Mach DB, et al. Osteoprotegerin blocks bone cancer-induced skeletal destruction, skeletal pain and pain-related neurochemical reorganization of the spinal cord. *Nature Med* 2000; 6(5):521–528.
43. Guise TA, Yin JJ, Taylor SD, Kumagai Y, Dallas M, Boyce BF, et al. Evidence for a causal role of parathyroid hormone-related protein in the pathogenesis of human breast cancer-mediated osteolysis. *J Clin Invest* 1996; 98(7):1544–1549.
44. Elion G, Mundy GR. Direct resorption of bone by human breast cancer cells in vitro. *Nature* 1978; 276:726–728.
45. Garrett IR. Bone destruction in cancer. *Semin Oncol* 1993, 20:4–9.
46. Arihiro K, Oda H, Kaneko M, Inai K. Cytokines facilitate chemotactic motility of breast carcinoma cells. *Breast Cancer* 2000; 7(3):221–230.
47. Tumber A, Morgan HM, Meikle MC, Hill PA. Human breast-cancer cells stimulate the fusion, migration, and resorptive activity of osteoclasts in bone explants. *Int J Cancer* 2001; 91:665–672.
48. Gallwitz WE, Guise TA, Mundy GR. Guanosine nucleotides inhibit different syndromes of PTHrP excess caused by human cancers in vivo. *J Clin Invest* 2002; 110:1559–1572.
49. Henderson M, Danks J, Moseley J, Slavin J, Harris T, McKinlay M, et al. Parathyroid hormone-related protein production by breast cancers, improved survival, and reduced bone metastases. *J Natl Cancer Inst* 2000; 93:234–237.
50. Wysolmerski JJ, Dann PR, Zelazny E, Dunbar ME, Insogna KL, Guise TA, et al. Overexpression of parathyroid hormone-related protein causes hypercalcemia but not bone metastases in a murine model of mammary tumorigenesis. *J Bone Miner Res* 2002; 17:1164–1170.
51. Sotiriou C, Lacroix M, Lespagnard L, Larsimont D, Paesmans M, Body JJ. Interleukins-6 and -11 expression in primary breast cancer and subsequent development of bone metastases. *Cancer Lett* 2001; 169:87–95.

9 Cell Adhesion Molecules in Tumor Metastasis

Sujata Persad, PhD, and Gurmit Singh, PhD

CONTENTS

INTRODUCTION
ADHESION MOLECULES
INTEGRIN ADHESION RECEPTORS IN TUMOR METASTASIS
E-CADHERIN CELL ADHESION SYSTEM IN TUMOR METASTASIS
REFERENCES

1. INTRODUCTION

When tumors progress to greater malignancy, cells within the tumor develop an increasing ability to detach from neighboring cells and invade through surrounding tissues and tissue boundaries to form new growths (metastasis) at sites distinct from that of the primary tumor. The molecular mechanisms involved in the metastatic process are diverse and not completely understood; however, the processes of cell–cell and cell–extracellular matrix (ECM) adhesion and degradation of the extracellular matrix are accepted as critical. In this chapter, we will focus on the current knowledge of the roles of cell–cell and cell–ECM adhesions in the initiation and maintenance of metastasis at new sites.

Tumor progression and metastasis are thought to involve a complex array of genetic and epigenetic changes in the tumor cells that result in heterogeneity in the characteristics of cells that are specific for different tumors and for different sites of metastasis from the same primary tumor. These phenotypic differences can modify and be modified by the manner in which the cell interacts with its environment, with respect to both interaction with other cells and interaction with the ECM *(1)*. Tumor cell detachment from the primary tumor, cell chemotaxis, adhesion, and selective tumor growth at preferred sites are important steps required for site-specific metastasis *(2)*. This process is best described by the "decathalon champion" model introduced by Fiddler et al. *(3)*. This model describes that the invasive/metastatic cell must escape from the primary tumor, intravasate into the blood vascular or lymphatic system, survive in the circulation, avoid host defense mechanisms, arrest and extravasate into a new site, and successfully grow at the new site (*see* Fig. 1).

From: *Cancer Drug Discovery and Development*
Bone Metastasis: Experimental and Clinical Therapeutics
Edited by: G. Singh and S. A. Rabbani © Humana Press Inc., Totowa, NJ

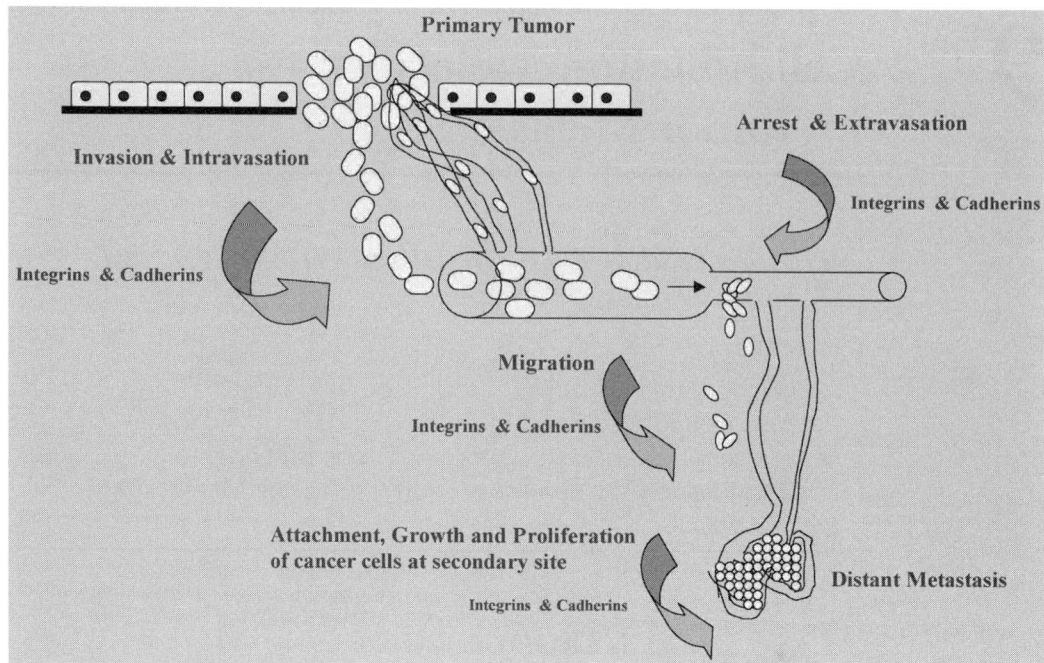

Fig. 1. The sequential steps of the metastatic cascade highlighting the adhesion molecules involved in each stage. Adhesion molecules that are involved in promoting the metastatic process exert their effect at multiple points of the cascade, effectively regulating the final outcome of the process.

Abnormality of cell adhesion is the basis for human cancer morphogenesis and affects the biological characteristics of human cancers. Therefore, it is not unexpected that the clinico-pathological parameters of various cancers are quite frequently and significantly associated with molecular events inactivating cell adhesion systems. Further understanding of genetic and epigenetic events in cell adhesion systems will cast further light on the mechanism of multistage human carcinogenesis. Moreover, it is expected that molecules participating in such genetic epigenetic changes will emerge as the targets of new strategies for prevention and therapy of multistage human carcinogenesis.

2. ADHESION MOLECULES

Over the last decade, the perception that cell adhesion molecules anchor cells to the ECM and to each other has undergone a major transition as it has become apparent that these molecules play a major role in cellular signal transduction, both outside-in and inside-out signaling. By this token, they control cellular responses to various external stimuli and, thus, play an important role in how a cell senses and interacts with its local environment. This is true for both cells at the primary tumor site as well as at the site of new metastasis *(4)*. The different classes of adhesion molecule include integrins, cadherins, selectins, members of the immunoglobulin superfamily, and hyaluronate-binding proteins. Members from each of these families of adhesion molecules have been implicated in carcinogenesis and/or progression.

3. INTEGRIN ADHESION RECEPTORS IN TUMOR METASTASIS

Integrins contribute to tumor growth and metastasis in a variety of ways. These adhesion receptors mediate tumor cell attachment, migration, and invasion and support arrest of metastatic cells within the vasculature of target organs, processes that are all necessary for successful metastasis of cancer. Cancer progression is associated with a multitude of changes in integrin expression and functionality, which collectively mediate transition of cancer cells from a sessile stationary cell phenotype to a disseminating migratory/invasive cell phenotype. In this transition, tumor cells acquire specific abilities that allow them to interact in a very dynamic manner with the ECM and with host cells within the lymphatic system, the blood vascular system, and target organ tissue. To fully support these processes, tumor cell integrins often cooperate with growth factor receptors, a variety of proteases including the matrix metalloproteinases, the cytoskeleton, and intracellular signaling molecules. Tumor cell integrin functions are regulated by endogenous and exogenous mechanisms that control integrin activation by mechanisms that are not fully understood. The activation state of the integrins directly affects the metastatic activity of tumor cells.

3.1. The Integrin Receptors

Integrins are transmembrane glycoproteins composed of noncovalantly linked α- and β-subunits. Combinations of 18α- and 9β-chains allow formation of an array of (at least 24) integrin heterodimers, each of which supports interaction with a unique set of extracellular matrix proteins and sometimes-soluble ligand proteins in a cell-type-specific manner. Each integrin subunit spans the plasma membrane and typically possesses a short cytoplasmic domain. Receptor diversity and versatility in ligand binding is determined by the extracellular domains of specifically paired α- and β-subunits. The intracellular tail of the β-subunit can interact with focal adhesion plaques in the cell, which are sites of interaction with the actin cytoskeleton and contain and interact with a number of protein kinases such as focal adhesion kinase (FAK), integrin-linked kinase (ILK), Src, and protein kinase C (PKC). Further, integrin-mediated adhesion, specifically integrin clustering in focal adhesions at sites of cell–matrix contact, involves cytoskeletal reorganization and leads to changes in cell shape. Integrin signaling has profound consequences that impact not only on cell adhesive, migratory, and tumor cell functions but also on tumor cell survival and proliferation. Intracellular signaling from integrin receptors occurs in response to integrin binding to ECM proteins (outside-in signaling). In turn, integrin signaling is controlled by intracellular mechanisms, which modulate the ligand-binding properties of the receptors (inside-out signaling) (5–7).

When clustered in focal adhesions, integrins interact with cytoplasmic and plasma-membrane-bound partner molecules, some of which enhance metastasis and some that suppress metastasis. One such group of integrin-associated proteins is the tetraspanins, a family of glycoproteins with four transmembrane domains (8). Tetraspanins have the ability to assemble into tightly packed microdomains, which are thought to stabilize and control the signaling activity and special orientation of integrins within a tetraspanin complex (9,10). These are generally categorized as metastasis suppressor genes/proteins. Loss of the expression of members of the tetraspanin family of proteins has been associated with metastasis and progression in a variety of human malignancies including prostate, breast, and colon cancer (11). In contrast, association of integrins with osteopontin, a protein that is consistently upregulated in relation to tumor progression *(12)*, has been shown to enhance metastasis *(13)*. Osteopontin appears to function as a secreted integrin-binding protein that can also affect cell motility and proteinase activity in an integrin-independent manner *(14)*.

A characteristic of malignant tumor cells is that they can upregulate their integrin functionality not only through intrinsic mechanisms but also through aberrant response to growth factors and, perhaps, other still unidentified stimuli. Crosstalk between integrins and growth factor receptors adds an interesting twist to the control of integrin functionality and signaling during tumor progression. For example, breast cancer cells respond to binding of heregulin-β to the endothelial growth factor (EGF) family member receptor erbB3 with dimerization of erbB3 and erbB2. This leads to rapid and robust upregulation of β1 integrin function and results in increased cell adhesion and migration *(15)*. Similarly, association of integrin α6β4 and erbB2 promotes phosphatidylinositol 3 (PI3)-kinase-dependent tumor cell invasion *(16)*. The interaction between the cytoplasmic tails of integrin subunits and growth factor receptors involves paxillin, a focal adhesion adaptor protein that coordinates changes in the actin cytoskeleton that are associated with cell motility and cell adhesion *(17,18)*. These findings might explain the functional link between overexpression of growth factor receptors, such as the c-erbBs, and altered integrin-mediated adhesive, migratory, and invasive tumor cell behaviors. Alterations in integrin-supported invasive functions can be the result of ligation of growth factor receptors that likely act in concert with altered production and activity of degrading enzymes such as the metalloproteinases *(19)*.

3.2. Integrin Receptor Activation

Integrins can exist in distinct states of activation, and these determine ligand affinity, can alter ligand specificity, and modulate intracellular signals resulting from integrin ligation. Integrin activation has profound consequences on cell adhesion, migration, and invasion. Activated integrins can endow tumor cells in many ways with crucial functions that permit or facilitate a disseminating phenotype. In general, integrin activation controls cell adhesion. Such control is particularly important in the vasculature, where dynamic flow physically opposes tumor cell attachment *(20,21)*. Constitutive activation of tumor cell integrins has been suggested to promote hematogenous dissemination and colonization of bone matrix as a target site for metastasis. In this regard, tumor cell interaction with bone matrix proteins osteopontin and sialoprotein has been reported to be enhanced when integrin αvβ3 is activated *(22,23)*. Evidence for this concept was established for several tumor cell types such as breast and prostate cancer cells that typically seed bone metastasis. Further, there seems to be a general tendency that integrin activation promotes a more dynamic interaction of adhesion receptors with their substrates. A prominent feature in this regard is tumor cell migration *(22,24,25)*. Integrin activation is thought to promote transition from a sessile, stationary to a migratory cell phenotype *(24)*.

Recently, the first integrin crystal structure was solved for the extracellular segment of αvβ3 *(26)*. Further studies has shown that the presence of a ligand bound to αvβ3 resulted in tertiary and quaternary conformational changes that caused an altered orientation of αv relative to β3 *(27)*. A recent molecular model for integrin αLβ2 with its ligand intercellular adhesion molecule (ICAM)-1 also supports conformational changes of the integrin from a low-affinity to a high-affinity state *(28)*. Thus, it appears that distinct functional activation states of the integrin receptors have distinct molecular conformations. Transition between these activation states and their stable expression are regulated by intracellular constraints involving cytoskeletal elements and their adaptor molecules (29–32), signal transduction molecules (33,34), and/or crosstalk between integrins and growth factor receptors (35–37). They can further involve modification of the extracellular integrin subunit domains by metalloproteinases (25,38).

Importantly, metastatic tumor cells seem to possess mechanisms that permanently upregulate the activation state of key integrin receptors or which allow them to switch to a highly activated state very quickly under specific conditions that the cell might encounter en route to a target site of metastasis. It has been suggested that certain clonal cell populations within the primary tumor already express such intrinsic regulatory mechanisms and that these cells are selected during tumor progression and metastatic dissemination. Another suggestion is that cell clones with constitutively activated integrins or those that posses mechanisms to respond to exogenous triggers of integrin activation evolve during tumor formation and prevail during tumor progression.

3.3. Integrins in Migration/Invasion

Migratory and invasive tumor cell functions are supported by a number of different integrins and depend on certain matrix proteins on which the cells migrate. Increased cell migration in metastatic tumor cells is regulated by changes in integrin expression or by their activation state and intracellular signal processing. *De novo* expression or upregulation of certain integrins, including $\alpha v\beta 3$ and $\alpha 3\beta 1$, is associated with a metastatic phenotype and increased motility in a variety of cancer cells, such as melanoma, breast, and prostate cancer (39–42). The migration supporting integrins acts in concert with signaling proteins, cytoskeletal adaptor proteins, growth factor receptors, and metalloproteinases for optimized motility and invasive activity. A key molecule that is central to these processes is the focal adhesion kinase (FAK), which transmits signals from integrin matrix contact points also referred to as focal adhesions. In migratory cells, FAK is generally phosphorylated and activated, although in some cell types, FAK tyrosine phosphorylation correlated with reduced migration (43). In most metastatic cancer cell types, enhanced migration, altered integrin expression profile, and/or integrin activation is associated with downstream FAK phosphorylation and activation of Src (40,42–44). In addition to participating in transduction of signals from integrin matrix interaction, FAK provides an important link between growth factor receptor and integrin signaling pathways, which affect tumor cell migration.

Control of cell migration also depends on cytoskeletal rearrangements and an ordered distribution of integrin molecules at the cell surface, as cells establish and detach matrix contacts while they move forward and constantly change their shape. This process requires the constant recycling of integrin molecules from the rear part of the cell to the leading edge, where lamellipodia are protruding. It has been suggested that directional motility involves, at least partially, integrin internalization at the retracting margin and their redistribution to the front of the cell (45). To support locomotion, integrins cluster at discrete sites of cell–matrix contact referred to as focal adhesions. At the focal adhesions, integrins connect with elements of the cytoskeleton via adaptor proteins. Key adaptor proteins are paxillin and the actin-binding proteins filamin and talin (18,46,47). Paxillin, in turn, binds to several other proteins such as vinculin and actopaxin that are involved in controlling the organization of the actin cytoskeleton. Several of the paxillin-binding proteins are known to have oncogenic equivalents, such as v-Src, v-Crk, and BCR-ABL. It is thought that these proteins use paxillin as a docking site to perturb and perhaps bypass normal integrin-dependent adhesion signaling pathways that are necessary for controlled cell proliferation *(48,49)*. The cytoplasmic tails of several integrin β-subunits bind to filamin, each with a unique binding strength. This has direct consequences for cell migration: Tight integrin β tail–filamin binding restricts cell migration by inhibiting transient membrane protrusion and cell polarization *(50)*. In contrast, strong binding of integrin β tail to paxillin promotes cell migration *(51)*. Thus, it has been suggested that increased migratory propensity in metastatic cells might be achieved by changes in the expression ratios of specific integrin heterodimers favoring α/β combinations that bind less tightly to talin and more strongly to paxillin.

Growth factors and proteases provide yet another level of control of integrin-mediated motility. For example, transforming growth factor-β1 (TGF-β1) has been shown to affect cancer cell migration and invasion by controlling the expression of a number of relevant genes. TGF-β1 has been shown to upregulate paxillin expression in malignant astrocytoma cells, promoting attachment and cell spreading *(52)*. Further, TGF-β1 was shown to promote migration in a variety of cancer cells by upregulating expression of certain integrins, such as integrin avβ3 in glioma cells *(53)* or α5β1 and α3β1 in hepatocellular carcinoma cells *(54,55)*. The contribution of proteases, specifically matrix metalloproteinases (MMPs), to tumor cell invasion has long been established *(56)*. Processing of ECM proteins by MMPs can profoundly alter the way the matrix is recognized by integrins. As a result, integrin-mediated interaction of tumor cells with the processed matrix can switch from support of firm adhesion to dynamic migration *(57)*. Conversely, MMPs can also directly modify integrin subunit proteins and thereby alter the functional activation state of integrins, which can lead to increased tumor cell migration *(38)*. All of these mechanisms seem to be intertwined because integrin expression and ligation to matrix, in turn, affects the production of MMPs and other matrix-degrading proteases *(25,38,58)*.

3.4. Integrins in Cell Survival

A very important link between integrin-mediated tumor cell migration/invasion and the ultimately successful metastasis is that signals that induce cell invasion also promote tumor cell survival. It has been demonstrated that tumor cells invading ECM coordinately regulate migration and survival mechanisms through activation of the extracellular regulated kinase (ERK) and molecular coupling of the adaptor proteins CAS (p130 Crk-associated substate) and Crk *(59)*. This association enables the transduction of external signals into changes in cell motility and modulation of the gene expression of members of the mitogen-activating protein (MAP) kinase cascade. Integrin-mediated cell attachment to certain substrates also prevents apoptosis of cells in growth-factor-deprived enviroment, as is often the case when a migrating tumor cell first extravasates into a new site. In many instances, integrin-mediated cell–matrix anchorage promotes cell survival. If cells are prevented from matrix attachment, a specific form of apoptosis called anoikis is often induced *(60)*. However, tumor cells might develop phenotypes that might lose the ability to undergo anoikis and this, too, promotes successful metastasis. To further improve the chance of survival under limiting growth conditions, tumor cells are able to recruit new blood vessels. This process is supported by tumor cell integrins. For example, expression of the integrin a6b4 enhances translation of vascular endothelial growth factor

VEGF. This mechanism involves the ability of a6b4 to activate the PI3-kinase–AKT signaling pathway *(61)*. The resultant secretion of VEGF by the tumor cells not only promotes angiogenesis to new tumor but also supports tumor cell growth in a paracrine manner. Interestingly, it has been observed that apoptosis of adherent cells is mediated by unligated integrins *(62)*. It is understood that the cytoplasmic domain of the b-subunit of unligated integrins recruits the apoptosis initiator caspase-8 to the plasma membrane, where it becomes activated in a death-receptor-independent manner. When integrin ligation occurs, the integrin–caspase-8-containing complex is disrupted, resulting in cell survival *(62)*.

3.5. Integrins in Angiogenesis

The formation of new blood vessels is essential for the successful growth of tumors and successful establishment of metastasis. Integrins have been shown to be positive mediators of this process referred to as angiogenesis, a process that is necessary for the hematogenous dissemination of tumor cells and to support the development of large lesions at the secondary site *(63)*. For example, migration of cultured endothelial cells on vitronectin and collagen has been shown to be mediated by $\alpha v\beta 3$ and $\alpha 2\beta 1$, respectively. The $\alpha v\beta 3$ integrin is reported to bind the metalloproenase MMP-2 to promote vascular invasion during angiogenesis *(64)* and its expression has been observed to be increased in newly formed blood vessels in human wound granulation tissue and in chick chorioallantoic membranes treated with the positive angiogenic factor basic fibroblast growth factor. In addition to promoting angiogenesis, the $\alpha v\beta 3$ integrin has also been reported to mediate motility and migration of cancer cells (murine melanoma) *(40,65)*, to assist in the arrest of melanoma and breast carcinoma cells under dynamic flow conditions *(20,21)*, to associate with the urokinase receptor and MMP2 in promoting an invasive phenotype in ovarian carcinoma cells *(66,67)*, and to enhance bone metastasis in a human mammary carcinoma cell line *(68)*. These observations suggest that integrins play a role at almost every stage of the metastatic process via different mechanisms at the different stages. Integrin expression and function in endothelial cells and tumor cells play an important role, directly and indirectly, in tumor development and establishment of new blood vessels that sustain and support further tumor growth and metastasis.

4. E-CADHERIN CELL ADHESION SYSTEM IN TUMOR METASTASIS

Cell–cell adhesion determines the polarity of cells and participates in maintaining societies of associated cells called tissues. Cell–cell adhesiveness is generally reduced in human cancers, which allows cancer cells to disobey the social order within tissues, resulting in destruction of histological structure. This is the morphological hallmark of the development of malignant tumors. Reduced intercellular adhesiveness is also indispensable for cancer invasion and metastasis. A tumor suppressor gene product, E-cadherin *(69)*, and its associated proteins, the catenins, which connect cadherins to the cytoskeletal actin filaments, are located at the lateral borders, concentrating on adherens junctions of epithelial cells and establish firm cell–cell contact.

The cell–cell adherens junction is a specialized region of the plasma membrane, connected to the actin cytoskeleton, where cadherins act as Ca^{2+}-dependent adhesion molecules *(70)*. Cadherins molecules are integral membrane glycoproteins with a single transmembrane domain. The extracellular domain of E-cadherin, the major type of cadherin in epithelial cells, is made up of five domains. Cadherins generally interact in a homophilic manner and, thus, E-cadherin binds selectively to E-cadherins and not other types of cadherin. The cytoplasmic undercoat proteins associated with the cadherins are the catenins. β-Catenin interacts with cadherins through its cytoplasmic domain, which exhibits the strongest degree of homology among members of the cadherin family. α-Catenin connects the β-catenin–E-cadherin complex to actin filaments. Interaction between cadherins and cytoskeletal proteins via the catenins confers stability on cell–cell adherens junctions.

The strategic position of E-cadherin at the major points of cell–cell interaction, adherens junction, suggest that suppression of E-cadherin expression or activity may trigger the release of cancer cells from the primary cancer tissue. Indeed, early in vitro experiments using cultured cells revealed that E-cadherin has invasion-suppressing properties (71,72). In fact, studies have shown that the E-cadherin gene satisfies the criteria for tumor suppressor genes (73). The major bulk of the evidence that cadherins are involved in the suppression of tumor invasion, and metastasis derives from analysis of cadherin expression in tumors at various stages of differentiation and from mutational analysis of cadherins in tumors. Reduced or absent E-cadherin expression has been reported in poorly differentiated, invasive, or high-grade tumors of squamous cell carcinoma of the head and neck, basal cell carcinoma, female genital tract tumors, and carcinomas of the stomach, bladder, breast, colon, and lung (70). Loss of E-cadherin is thought to initiate epithelial-to-mesenchymal transitions in epithelial cells, resulting in increased proportion of the inherently migratory mesenchymal cells in tumors. Generally, E-cadherin expression is strong in well-differentiated cancers, which maintain cell–cell adhesiveness and are less invasive, but are reduced, in undifferentiated cancers, which have lost their cell–cell adhesion and show strong invasive tendency (74,75). Significant correlation between abnormalities of E-cadherin expression and the clinical outcome of patients with cancers have been reported (76). The reduction of E-cadherin expression in tumors has been attributed to a variety of mechanisms, including mutations/deletions, transcriptional regulation as a result of hypermethylation or chromatin rearrangements (77). More recently, transcriptional repression of E-cadherin gene expression by the DNA-binding protein snail has been noted as a frequent cause for reduced expression of E-cadherin in invasive tumors (77). Silencing of the E-cadherin gene by DNA hypermethylation around the promoter region occurs frequently in many cancers, even in precancerous conditions (78,79). It is now widely recognized that many tumor suppressor genes are silenced by hypermethylation in various human cancers, and correction of DNA methylation status has gained recognition as a new anticancer strategy.

In diffuse infiltrating cancers, the most frequently observed condition are mutations in the genes for E-cadherin and α- and β-catenins (80,81). The tumor cells in diffuse-type cancers are dispersed throughout the tumor mass. Immuno-histochemical examination of these cancers normally shows a strong expression signal for E-cadherin. However, the E-cadherin molecules are not localized at the cell membrane but are distributed throughout the cytoplasm, suggesting that they lack cell–cell adhesive properties. These findings suggested that inactivation of the E-cadherin cell adhesion system might also be caused by genetic alterations. To this end, genetic alteration to α-catenin has been observed in lung cancer cell line (82,83). This cell line regained its cell–cell adhesiveness when transfected with wild-type α-catenin (84), providing evidence that this molecule is mandatory for E-cadherin adhesion system. However, mutational inactivation of the α-catenin gene is a rare event in vivo in human cancers. Mutations of the E-cadherin gene itself have been detected in human cancer cell lines and in vivo *(85–89)*. Reduced or completely undetectable expression of E-cadherin is frequently detected in poorly differentiated carcinomas. The gene mutations are most often in the introns that result in skipping of exon 9 of the gene *(87)*. Mutations of the β-catenin gene have also been reported to abolish cell–cell adhesiveness in carcinoma cells *(90)*. Further, at the invading front of many invasive cancer cells, the E-cadherin adhesion system has been shown to be inactivated by tyrosine phosphorylation of β-catenin *(91)*. Strong tyrosine phosphorylation of β-catenin has been observed in loosely adherent cancer cells that had no mutations and did not show reduced expression of E-cadherin or α- or β-catenins *(92)*. This aberrant tyrosine phosphorylation of β-catenin is catalyzed by an oncogene product, c-erbB-2 protein, which associates directly with β-catenin in cancer cells *(93,94)*. Tyrosine phosphorylation of β-catenin by c-erbB-2 is now known to be initiated by epidermal growth factor, which has been shown to induce scattering of cancer cell lines *(95)*. The E-cadherin cell adhesion system also crosstalks with the Wingless/Wnt signaling pathway through β-catenin and therefore expression of genes, which participate in cancer morphogenesis, may be regulated in conjunction with the Wingless/Wnt signaling pathway *(4)*.

In contrast to the tumor suppressor properties of E-cadherin, increased expression levels of another member of the cadherin family of proteins, N-cadherin, is correlated with cellular invasiveness *(96,97)*. N-Cadherin has been shown to link different N-cadherin-linked cell types *(98)* and is related to b1 integrin expression levels through intracellular signals *(99)*, which suggests an importance of this cadherin in metastatic invasion. It has been suggested that a switch from cellular expression of E-cadherin to N-cadherin in tumor cells might play an important role on tumor progression. Thus, cadherins, like integrins, might play diverse roles in the metastatic process from modulating cell motility and invasion to affecting the growth of cells at a new site.

Recently, a new cancer-associated cell membrane glycoprotein, dysadherin, has been identified which downregulates E-cadherin and promotes cancer metastasis *(100)*. Dysadherin transfected cells are able to form markedly higher number of metastatic nodules in mice than mock transfectants, suggesting the metastasis-promoting ability of dysadherin *(100)*. Colorectal carcinomas frequently show dysadherin immunoreactivity at the cell membrane, whereas there is no dysadherin expression in normal mucosa *(101)*. Furthermore, colorectal cancers exhibiting expression of dysadherin in conjunction with reduced expression of E-cadherin was significantly associated to lung metastsis and showed the worst prognosis *(101)*. Increased dysadherin expression by pancreatic ductal adenocarcinomas is also significantly correlated with an infitrative-type growth pattern and distant metastasis *(102)*. Thus, dysadherin expression might become a biological predictor of tumor aggressiveness and poor prognosis in human cancers.

REFERENCES

1. Roskelley CD Bissell MJ. The dominance of the microenvironment in breast and ovarian cancer. *Semin Cancer Biol* 2002; 12:97–104.
2. Yoneda T. Mechanism of preferential metastasis of breast cancer to bone. *Int J Oncol* 1996; 9:103–109.
3. Fidler IJ. Critical factors in the biology of human cancer metastasis:twenty-eighth G.H.A. Clowes memorial award lecture. *Cancer Res* 1990; 50:6130–6138.

4. Juliano RL. Signal transduction by cell adhesion receptors and the cytoskeleton:functions of integrins, cadherins, selectins, and immunoglobulin-superfamily members. *Annu Rev Pharmacol Toxicol* 2002; 42:283–323.

5. Schwartz MA, Assoian RK. Integrins and cell proliferation:regulation of cyclin-dependent kinases via cytoplasmic signaling pathways. *J Cell Sci* 2001; 114:2553–2560

6. Schwartz MA, Ginsberg MH. Networks and crosstalk:integrin signalling spreads. *Nat Cell Biol* 2002; 4:E65–E68.

7. Shattil SJ. Signaling through platelet integrin alpha IIb beta 3:inside-out, outside-in, and sideways. *Thromb Haemost* 1999; 82:318–325.

8. Maecker HT, Todd SC, Levy S. The tetraspanin superfamily:molecular facilitators. *FASEB J* 1997; 11: 428–442.

9. Bienstock RJ, Barrett JC. KAI1, a prostate metastasis suppressor:prediction of solvated structure and interactions with binding partners; integrins, cadherins, and cell-surface receptor proteins. *Mol Carcinog* 2001; 32:139–153.

10. Zhang XA, Bontrager AL, Hemler ME. Transmembrane-4 superfamily proteins associate with activated protein kinase C (PKC) and link PKC to specific beta(1) integrins. *J Biol Chem* 2001; 276: 25,005–25,013.

11. Yoshida BA, Sokoloff MM, Welch DR, Rinker-Schaeffer CW. Metastasis-suppressor genes:a review and perspective on an emerging field. *J Natl Cancer Inst* 2000; 92:1717–1730.

12. Agrawal D, Chen T, Irby R, Quackenbush J, Chambers AF, Szabo M, et al. Osteopontin identified as lead marker of colon cancer progression, using pooled sample expression profiling. *J Natl Cancer Inst* 2002; 94:513–521.

13. Chambers AF, Naumov GN, Vantyghem SA, Tuck AB. Molecular biology of breast cancer metastasis. Clinical implications of experimental studies on metastatic inefficiency. *Breast Cancer Res* 2000; 2:400–407.

14. Tuck AB, Hota C, Chambers AF. Osteopontin(OPN)-induced increase in human mammary epithelial cell invasiveness in urokinase (UPA)-dependent. *Breast Cancer Res Treast* 2001; 70:197–204.

15. Adelsman MA, McCarthy JB, Shimizu Y. Stimulation of beta1-integrin function by epidermal growth factor and heregulin-beta has distinct requirements for erbB2 but a similar dependence on phosphoinositide 3-OH kinase. *Mol Biol Cell* 1999; 10:2861–2878.

16. Gambaletta D, Marchetti A, Benedetti L, Mercurio AM, Sacchi A, et al. Cooperative signaling between alpha(6)beta(4) integrin and ErbB-2 receptor is required to promote phosphatidylinositol 3-kinase-dependent invasion. *J Biol Chem* 2000; 275:10,604–10,610.

17. Fernandez-Valle C, Tang Y, Ricard J, Rodenas-Ruano A, Taylor A, Hackler E, et al. Paxillin binds schwannomin and regulates its density-dependent localization and effect on cell morphology. *Nat Genet* 2002; 31:354–362.

18. Tumbarello DA, Brown MC, Turner CE. The paxillin LD motifs. *FEBS Lett* 2002; 513:114–118.

19. Eccles SA. The potential role of c-erb B oncogen signalling. *Cancer Res* 2002; 157:41–54.

20. Felding-Habermann B, O'Toole TE, Smith JW, Fransvea E, Ruggeri ZM, Ginsberg MH, et al. Integrin activation controls metastasis in human breast cancer. *Proc Natl Acad Sci USA* 2001; 98:1853–1858.

21. Pilch J, Habermann R, Felding-Habermann B. Unique ability of integrin alpha(v)beta 3 to support tumor cell arrest under dynamic flow conditions. *J Biol Chem* 2002; 277:21,930–21,938.

22. Byzova TV, Kim W, Midura RJ, Plow EF. Activation of integrin alpha(V)beta(3) regulates cell adhesion and migration to bone sialoprotein. *Exp Cell Res* 2000; 254:299–308.

23. Helluin O, Chan C, Vilaire G, Mousa S, DeGrado WF, Bennett JS. The activation state of alphavbeta 3 regulates platelet and lymphocyte adhesion to intact and thrombin-cleaved osteopontin. *J Biol Chem* 2000; 275:18,337–18,343.

24. Kiosses WB, Shattil SJ, Pampori N, Schwartz MA. Rac recruits high-affinity integrin alphavbeta3 to lamellipodia in endothelial cell migration. *Nat Cell Biol* 2001; 3:316–320.

25. Ratnikov BI, Rozanov DV, Postnova TIea. Alternative processing of integrin alpha subunit in tumour cells by membrane type-1 matrix metalloproteinase. *J Biol Chem* 2001; 277:7377–7385.

26. Xiong JP, Stehle T, Diefenbach B, Zhang R, Dunker R, Scott DL, et al. Crystal structure of the extracellular segment of integrin alpha Vbeta3. *Science* 2001; 294:339–345.

27. Xiong JP, Stehle T, Zhang R, Joachimiak A, Frech M, Goodman SL, et al. Crystal structure of the extracellular segment of integrin alpha Vbeta3 in complex with an Arg-Gly-Asp ligand. *Science* 2002; 296:151–155.

28. Legge GB, Morris GM, Sanner MF, Takada Y, Olson AJ, Grynszpan F. Model of the alphaLbeta2 integrin I-domain/ICAM-1 DI interface suggests that subtle changes in loop orientation determine ligand specificity. *Proteins* 2002; 48:151–160.

29. Jenkins AL, Nannizzi-Alaimo L, Silver D, Sellers JR, Ginsberg MH, Law DA, et al. Tyrosine phosphorylation of the beta3 cytoplasmic domain mediates integrin-cytoskeletal interactions. *J Biol Chem* 1998; 273:13,878–13,885.

30. Tzima E, del Pozo MA, Shattil SJ, Chien S, Schwartz MA. Activation of integrins in endothelial cells by fluid shear stress mediates Rho-dependent cytoskeletal alignment. *EMBO J* 2001; 20:4639–4647.

31. Zfou X, Li J, Kicik DF. The microtabule cytoskeleton participates in control of beta 2 integrin auidity. *J Biol Chem* 2001; 276:44,762–44,769.

32. Wang J, Chen H, Brown EJ. L-plastin peptide activation of alphabeta-mediated adhesion requires integrin conformational change and actin filament desassembly. *J Biol Chem* 2001; 276:14,474–14,481.

33. Calderwood DA, Yan B, de Pereda JM, Alvarez BG, Fujioka Y, Liddington RC, et al. The phosphotyrosine binding-like domain of talin activates integrins. *J Biol Chem* 2002; 277:21,749–21,758.

34. Jones SL. Protein kinase A regulates beta2 integrin avidity in neutrophils. *J Leukocyte Biol* 2002; 71: 1042–1048.

35. Baeckstrom D, Lu PJ, Taylor-Papadimitriou J. Activation of the alpha2beta1 integrin prevents c-erbB2-induced scattering and apoptosis of human mammary epithelial cells in collagen. *Oncogene* 2000; 19:4592–4603.

36. Byzova TV, Goldman CK, Pampori N, Thomas KA, Bett A, Shattil SJ, et al. A mechanism for modulation of cellular responses to VEGF:activation of the integrins. *Mol Cell* 2000; 6:851–860.

37. Faccio R, Grano M, Colucci S, Villa A, Giannelli G, Quaranta V, et al. Localization and possible role of two different alpha v beta 3 integrin conformations in resting and resorbing osteoclasts. *J Cell Sci* 2002; 115:2919–2929.

38. Ratnikov BI, Deryugina EI, Strongin AY. Gelatin zymography and substrate cleavage assays of matrix metalloproteinase-2 in breast carcinoma cells overexpressing membrane type-1 matrix metalloproteinase. *Lab Invest* 2002; 82:1583–1590.

39. Giannelli G, Fransvea E, Marinosci F, Bergamini C, Colucci S, Schiraldi O, et al. Transforming growth factor-beta1 triggers hepatocellular carcinoma invasiveness via alpha3beta1 integrin. *Am J Pathol* 2002; 161:183–193.

40. Li X, Regezi J, Ross FP, Blystone S, Ilic D, Leong SP, et al. Integrin alphavbeta3 mediates K1735 murine melanoma cell motility in vivo and in vitro. *J Cell Sci* 2001; 114:2665–2672.

41. Wong NC, Mueller BM, Barbas CF, Ruminski P, Quaranta V, Lin EC, et al. Alphav integrins mediate adhesion and migration of breast carcinoma cell lines. *Clin Exp Metast* 1998; 16:50–61.

42. Zheng DQ, Woodard AS, Fornaro M, Tallini G, Languino LR. Prostatic carcinoma cell migration via alpha(v)beta3 integrin is modulated by a focal adhesion kinase pathway. *Cancer Res* 1999; 59: 1655–1664.

43. Hauck CR, Hsia DA, Ilic D, Schlaepfer DD. v-Src SH3-enhanced interaction with focal adhesion kinase at beta 1 integrin-containing invadopodia promotes cell invasion. *J Biol Chem* 2002; 277: 12,487–12,490.

44. Sieg DJ, Hauck CR, Ilic D, Klingbeil CK, Schaefer E, Damsky CH, et al. FAK integrates growth-factor and integrin signals to promote cell migration. *Nat Cell Biol* 2000; 2:249–256.

45. Peirini LM, Lawson MA, Eddy RJea. Oriented endocytic recycling of alpha5 beta1 in mobile neutrophils. *Blood* 2000; 95:2471–2480.

46. Critchley DR. Focal adhesions—the cytoskeletal connection. *Curr Opin Cell Biol* 2000; 12:133–139.

47. Liu S, Calderwood DA, Ginsberg MH. Integrin cytoplasmic domain-binding proteins. *J Cell Sci* 2000; 113(Pt 20):3563–3571.

48. Sattler M, Pisick E, Morrison PT, Salgia R. Role of the cytoskeletal protein paxillin in oncogenesis. *Crit Rev Oncog* 2000; 11:63–76.

49. Turner CE. Paxillin interactions. *J Cell Sci* 2000; 113(Pt 23):4139,4140.

50. Calderwood DA, Huttenlocher A, Kiosses WBea. Increased filamin binding to beta-integrin cytoplasmic domains inhibits cell migration. *Nat Cell Biol* 2001; 3:1060–1068.

51. Liu S, Kiosses WB, Rose DM, Slepak M, Salgia R, Griffin JD, et al. A fragment of paxillin binds the alpha 4 integrin cytoplasmic domain (tail) and selectively inhibits alpha 4-mediated cell migration. *J Biol Chem* 2002; 277:20,887–20,894.

52. Han X, Stewart JE, Jr, Bellis SL, Benveniste EN, Ding Q, Tachibana K. et al. TGF-beta1 up-regulates paxillin protein expression in malignant astrocytoma cells: requirement for a fibronectin substrate. *Oncogene* 2001; 20:7976–7986.
53. Wick W, Platten M, Weller M. Glioma cell invasion:regulation of metalloproteinase activity by TGF-beta. *J Neurooncol* 2001; 53:177–185.
54. Cai T, Lei QY, Wang LY, Zha XL. TGF-beta 1 modulated the expression of alpha 5 beta 1 integrin and integrin-mediated signaling in human hepatocarcinoma cells. *Biochem Biophys Res Commun* 2000; 274:519–525.
55. Giannelli G, Astigiano S, Antonaci S, Morini M, Barbieri O, Noonan DM, et al. Role of the alpha3beta1 and alpha6beta4 integrins in tumor invasion. *Clin Exp Metast* 2002; 19:217–223.
56. Stetler-Stevenson WG, Yu AE. Proteases in invasion: matrix metalloproteinases. *Semin Cancer Biol* 2001; 11:143–152.
57. Giannelli G, Falk-Marzillier J, Schiraldi O, Stetler-Stevenson WG, Quaranta V. Induction of cell migration by matrix metalloprotease-2 cleavage of laminin-5. *Science* 1997; 277:225–228.
58. Ahmed N, Pansino F, Clyde R, Murthi P, Quinn MA, Rice GE, et al. Overexpression of alpha(v)beta6 integrin in serous epithelial ovarian cancer regulates extracellular matrix degradation via the plasminogen activation cascade. *Carcinogenesis* 2002; 23:237–244.
59. Shi C, Zhang X, Chen Z, Robinson MK, Simon DI. Leukocyte integrin Mac-1 recruits toll/interleukin-1 receptor superfamily signaling intermediates to modulate NF-kappaB activity. *Circ Res* 2001; 89:859–865.
60. Frisch SM, Screaton RA. Anoikis mechanisms. *Curr Opin Cell Biol* 2001; 13:555–562.
61. Chung J, Bachelder RE, Lipscomb EA, Shaw LM, Mercurio AM. Integrin (alpha 6 beta 4) regulation of eIF-4E activity and VEGF translation: a survival mechanism for carcinoma cells. *J Cell Biol* 2002; 158:165–174.
62. Stupack DG, Puente XS, Boutsaboualoy S, Storgard CM, Cheresh DA. Apoptosis of adherent cells by recruitment of caspase-8 to unligated integrins. *J Cell Biol* 2001; 155:459–470.
63. Jung YD, Ahmad SA, Liu W, Reinmuth N, Parikh A, Stoeltzing O, et al. The role of the microenvironment and intercellular cross-talk in tumor angiogenesis. *Semin Cancer Biol* 2002; 12:105–112.
64. Silletti S, Kessler T, Goldberg J, Boger DL, Cheresh DA. Disruption of matrix metalloproteinase 2 binding to integrin alpha vbeta 3 by an organic molecule inhibits angiogenesis and tumor growth in vivo. *Proc Natl Acad Sci USA* 2001; 98:119–124.
65. Voura EB, Ramjeesingh RA, Montgomery AM, Siu CH. Involvement of integrin alpha(v)beta(3) and cell adhesion molecule L1 in transendothelial migration of melanoma cells. *Mol Biol Cell* 2001; 12:2699–2710.
66. Hapke S, Kessler H, Arroyo dP, Benge A, Schmitt M, Lengyel E, et al. Integrin alpha(v)beta(3)/vitronectin interaction affects expression of the urokinase system in human ovarian cancer cells. *J Biol Chem* 2001; 276:26,340–26,348.
67. Chatterjee N, Chatterjee A. Role of Alpha V Beta3 integrin receptor in the invasive potential of human cervical cancer (sita) cells. *J Environ Pathol Toxicol Oncol* 2001; 20:211–221.
68. Pecheur I, Peyruchaud O, Serre CM, Guglielmi J, Voland C, Bourre F, et al. Integrin alpha(v)beta3 expression confers on tumor cells a greater propensity to metastasize to bone. *FASEB J* 2002; 16:1266–1268.
69. Takeichi M. Cadherin cell adhesion receptors as a morphogenetic regulator. *Science* 1991; 251:1451–1455.
70. Takeichi M. The cadherins:cell-cell adhesion molecules controlling animal morphogenesis. *Development* 1998; 102:639–655.
71. Behrens J, Mareel MM, Van Roy FM, Birchmeier W. Dissecting tumor cell invasion:epithelial cells acquire invasive properties after the loss of uvomorulin-mediated cell-cell adhesion. *J Cell Biol* 1989; 108:2435–2447.
72. Vleminckx K, Vakaet L, Jr, Mareel M, Fiers W, van Roy F. Genetic manipulation of E-cadherin expression by epithelial tumor cells reveals an invasion suppressor role. *Cell* 1991; 66:107–119.
73. Guilford P, Hopkins J, Harraway J, McLeod M, McLeod N, Harawira P, et al. E-cadherin germline mutations in familial gastric cancer. *Nature* 1998; 392:402–405.
74. Shimoyama Y, Hirohashi S, Hirano S, Noguchi M, Shimosato Y, Takeichi M, et al. Cadherin cell-adhesion molecules in human epithelial tissues and carcinomas. *Cancer Res* 1989; 49:2128–2133.
75. Shimoyama Y, Hirohashi S. Expression of E- and P-cadherin in gastric carcinomas. *Cancer Res* 1991; 51:2185–2192.

76. Bringuier PP, Umbas R, Schaafsma HE, Karthaus HF, Debruyne FM, Schalken JA. Decreased E-cadherin immunoreactivity correlates with poor survival in patients with bladder tumors. *Cancer Res* 1993; 53:3241–3245.

77. Cavallaro U, Schaffhauser B, Christofori G. Cadherins and the tumour progression: is it all in a switch? *Cancer Lett* 2002; 176:123–128.

78. Kanai Y, Ushijima S, Hui AM, Ochiai A, Tsuda H, Sakamoto M, Hirohashi S. The E-cadherin gene is silenced by CpG methylation in human hepatocellular carcinomas. *Int J Cancer* 1997; 71:355–359.

79. Yoshiura K, Kanai Y, Ochiai A, Shimoyama Y, Sugimura T, Hirohashi S. Silencing of the E-cadherin invasion-suppressor gene by CpG methylation in human carcinomas. *Proc Natl Acad Sci USA* 1995; 92:7416–7419.

80. Nakanishi Y, Ochiai A, Akimoto S, Kato H, Watanabe H, Tachimori Y, et al. Expression of E-cadherin, alpha-catenin, beta-catenin and plakoglobin in esophageal carcinomas and its prognostic significance: immunohistochemical analysis of 96 lesions. *Oncology* 1997; 54:158–165.

81. Ochiai A, Akimoto S, Shimoyama Y, Nagafuchi A, Tsukita S, Hirohashi S. Frequent loss of alpha catenin expression in scirrhous carcinomas with scattered cell growth. *Jpn J Cancer Res* 1994; 85:266–273.

82. Oda T, Kanai Y, Shimoyama Y, Nagafuchi A, Tsukita S, Hirohashi S. Cloning of the human alpha-catenin cDNA and its aberrant mRNA in a human cancer cell line. *Biochem Biophys Res Commun* 1993; 193:897–904.

83. Shimoyama Y, Nagafuchi A, Fujita S, Gotoh M, Takeichi M, Tsukita S, et al. Cadherin dysfunction in a human cancer cell line: possible involvement of loss of alpha-catenin expression in reduced cell-cell adhesiveness. *Cancer Res* 1992; 52:5770–5774.

84. Hirano S, Kimoto N, Shimoyama Y, Hirohashi S, Takeichi M. Identification of a neural alpha-catenin as a key regulator of cadherin function and multicellular organization. *Cell* 1992; 70:293–301.

85. Becker KF, Atkinson MJ, Reich U, Becker I, Nekarda H, Siewert JR, et al. E-cadherin gene mutations provide clues to diffuse type gastric carcinomas. *Cancer Res* 1994; 54:3845–3852.

86. Kanai Y, Oda T, Tsuda H, Ochiai A, Hirohashi S. Point mutation of the E-cadherin gene in invasive lobular carcinoma of the breast. *Jpn J Cancer Res* 1994; 85:1035–1039.

87. Muta H, Noguchi M, Kanai Y, Ochiai A, Nawata H, Hirohashi S. E-cadherin gene mutations in signet ring cell carcinoma of the stomach. *Jpn J Cancer Res* 1996; 87:843–848.

88. Oda T, Kanai Y, Oyama T, Yoshiura K, Shimoyama Y, Birchmeier W, et al. E-cadherin gene mutations in human gastric carcinoma cell lines. *Proc Natl Acad Sci USA* 1994; 91:1858–1862.

89. Saito A, Kanai Y, Maesawa C, Ochiai A, Torii A, Hirohashi S. Disruption of E-cadherin-mediated cell adhesion systems in gastric cancers in young patients. *Jpn J Cancer Res* 1999; 90:993–999.

90. Oyama T, Kanai Y, Ochiai A, Akimoto S, Oda T, Yanagihara K, et al. A truncated beta-catenin disrupts the interaction between E-cadherin and alpha-catenin: a cause of loss of intercellular adhesiveness in human cancer cell lines. *Cancer Res* 1994; 54:6282–6287.

91. Matsuyoshi N, Hamaguchi M, Taniguchi S, Nagafuchi A, Tsukita S, Takeichi M. Cadherin-mediated cell-cell adhesion is perturbed by v-src tyrosine phosphorylation in metastatic fibroblasts. *J Cell Biol* 1992; 118:703–714.

92. Shibata T, Gotoh M, Ochiai A, Hirohashi S. Association of plakoglobin with APC, a tumor suppressor gene product, and its regulation by tyrosine phosphorylation. *Biochem Biophys Res Commun* 1994; 203:519–522.

93. Kanai Y, Ochiai A, Shibata T, Oyama T, Ushijima S, Akimoto S, et al. c-erbB-2 gene product directly associates with beta-catenin and plakoglobin. *Biochem Biophys Res Commun* 1995; 208:1067–1072.

94. Ochiai A, Akimoto S, Kanai Y, Shibata T, Oyama T, Hirohashi S. c-erbB-2 gene product associates with catenins in human cancer cells. *Biochem Biophys Res Commun* 1994; 205:73–78.

95. Hoschuetzky H, Aberle H, Kemler R. Beta-catenin mediates the interaction of the cadherin-catenin complex with epidermal growth factor receptor. *J Cell Biol* 1994; 127:1375–1380.

96. Hazan RB, Phillips GR, Qiao RF, Norton L, Aaronson SA. Exogenous expression of N-cadherin in breast cancer cells induces cell migration, invasion, and metastasis. *J Cell Biol* 2000; 148:779–790.

97. Nieman MT, Prudoff RS, Johnson KR, Wheelock MJ. N-cadherin promotes motility in human breast cancer cells regardless of their E-cadherin expression. *J Cell Biol* 1999; 147:631–644.

98. Navarro P, Ruco L, Dejana E. Differential localization of VE- and N-cadherins in human endothelial cells: VE-cadherin competes with N-cadherin for junctional localization. *J Cell Biol* 1998; 140:1475–1484.

99. Arregui C, Pathre P, Lilien J, Balsamo J. The nonreceptor tyrosine kinase fer mediates cross-talk between N-cadherin and beta1-integrins. *J Cell Biol* 2000; 149:1263–1274.
100. Ino Y, Gotoh M, Sakamoto M, Tsukagoshi K, Hirohashi S. Dysadherin, a cancer-associated cell membrane glycoprotein, down-regulates E-cadherin and promotes metastasis. *Proc Natl Acad Sci USA* 2002; 99:365–370.
101. Aoki S, Shimamura T, Shibata T, Nakanishi Y, Moriya Y, Sato Y, et al. Prognostic significance of dysadherin expression in advanced colorectal carcinoma. *Br J Cancer* 2003; 88:726–732.
102. Shimamura T, Sakamoto M, Ino Y, Sato Y, Shimada K, Kosuge T, et al. Dysadherin overexpression in pancreatic ductal adenocarcinoma reflects tumor aggressiveness: relationship to e-cadherin expression. *J Clin Oncol* 2003; 21:659–667.

10 PTHrP and Cancer

Prostate and Lung

Leonard J. Deftos, MD, JD, *D. W. Burton,* BSc,
and Randolph H. Hastings, MD, PhD

1. INTRODUCTION

1.1. PTHrP

Originally discovered as a product of cancers that produce hypercalcemia, parathyroid hormone-related protein (PTHrP) has been demonstrated to be a product of many malignant tissues, including prostate and lung cancer, where it can regulate growth and proliferation in vivo and in vitro *(1–8)*. The amino-terminus of PTHrP reacts with the PTH/PTHrP receptor (PTHrPR) and produces most of the biological effects of native PTH, including hypercalcemia *(1,2)*. A second family of PTH-specific receptors has recently been identified *(1,9–11)*. However, there is accumulating and compelling evidence that non-amino-terminal forms of PTHrP, also generated through processing of the native isoforms, can exert biological effects *(1–4)*. The PTHrP gene expresses three forms of the polypeptide through alternate mRNA splicing: PTHrP1–141, a truncated 1–139 form, and a human-specific 1–173 residue *(11)*. Whereas PTHrP1–139 is quite similar to PTHrP1–141, PTHrP1–173 completely diverges from both at its own carboxy terminus *(1,2,11)*. The PTHrP gene sequence spans more than 15 kb and is composed of three primary regions: a complex promoter region, a coding region, and a multiple 3'-noncoding region *(3,11)*. The promoter region contains three different promoter elements, designated P1, P2, and P3. P1 and P3 are "TATA box"-like, and the P2 element is a GC-rich region *(1,11)*.

From: *Cancer Drug Discovery and Development*
Bone Metastasis: Experimental and Clinical Therapeutics
Edited by: G. Singh and S. A. Rabbani © Humana Press Inc., Totowa, NJ

1.2. PTHrP Processing

In addition to mRNA splicing, processing of PTHrP into peptides is an important regulatory mechanism *(1,3,11)*. Distinct biological properties have been attributed to the different PTHrP peptides, and specific receptors and effects have been postulated *(2,11)*. For example, PTHrP1–34/36 usually mediates the growth-regulating and hypercalcemic effects of the molecule, PTHrP38–94 promotes mineral transport, and peptides included in PTHrP107–141 inhibit osteoclast function in vitro *(1–3,11)*, and we have recently demonstrated that PTHrP140–173 has growth-regulatory actions *(5,12)*. These bioactive peptides can be derived through processing of native PTHrP at the many endoproteolytic processing sites *(11,13)*. In fact, the multiple processing sites in PTHrP predict over 90 peptides *(1,3,11)*. Enzymes have been recently identified from mammalian tissues that seem to serve this function, including the prohormone/proprotein convertases (PCs), although their roles in PTHrP processing have not been established *(1,13)*. Among its structural motifs, PTHrP also contains both classical and nonclassical nuclear localization sequences (NLSs) that have important implications for its mechanisms of action and biological effects *(9)*. All of these processed PTHrP peptides can have a non-amino-terminal (NTP) counterpart, likely through processing at arginine 36 *(3,11)*.

1.3. PTHrP and Growth Regulation

Parathyroid hormone-related protein regulates growth and differentiation in virtually every cell and tissue studied, including, as detailed subsequently, prostate and lung cancer *(1–5)*. Transgenic mouse models have shown that PTHrP is required for normal mammary development *(14)*, normal chondrocyte maturation and differentiation in the epiphyseal growth plate *(15)*, and normal epidermal and hair follicle development *(16)*. Targeted overexpression of PTHrP in pancreatic islets results in increased pancreatic, cell mass *(17)*. PTHrP also regulates the growth of vascular smooth muscle cells *(18)*, osteoblasts *(19)*, and chondrocytes *(12)*. More relevant to this proposal, PTHrP regulates the growth of many cancers, including prostate *(3)*, breast *(20,21)*, lung *(22,23)*, Leydig tumor cells *(24)*, renal carcinoma *(25)*, and, as we have recently reported, pancreatic adenocarcinoma *(26)*. PTHrPs proliferation effects can be dependent on cell type and PTHrP-derived peptide *(1,2)*. Although PTHrP stimulates cell proliferation, decreased proliferation in most cells has been observed in some cell types with some PTHrP species *(1–5,18,27–36)*.

1.4. Molecular Mechanisms of PTHrP's Biological Effects Signaling, Cell Cycle, and Apoptosis

The biological effects of PTHrP are mediated, at least in part, through the cell surface receptor that it shares with PTH and which is a member of the seven-membrane-spanning and G protein-coupled cell surface receptors *(1,10)*. Like PTH, the amino terminus of PTHrP signals through this receptor by the activation of adenylate cyclase and phospholipase C, especially the former, with the resulting accumulation of several signal transducers, including cAMP and inositol triphosphates, activation of protein kinase A (PKA) and C (PKC), and a transient increase in intracellular calcium *(10)*. In addition to its amino-terminus, there is accumulating and compelling evidence that non-amino-terminal forms of PTHrP, also generated through processing of the native isoforms, can exert biological effects; there is also evidence for receptors to these other regions of PTHrP, but none has been cloned *(1,10)*. Although multiple, the functions of PTHrP in malignant and normal tissues seem to be growth and proliferation related *(1–3)*. There are reports that PTHrP interacts in its growth-regulating properties with other cytokines and oncogenes *(3,27)*. Furthermore, there is considerable evidence that PTHrP has direct and/or indirect growth-regulating activities in a variety of malignant cells and tissues and in bone *(2,3,26)*. These biological effects interact in bone and cancer cells *(4–7,27)*.

In addition to its classical receptor-mediated biological effects, PTHrP has recently joined the family of growth regulators that also signal by translocation to the nucleus or nucleolus to act in an intracrine fashion *(9,27,28)*. Several investigators have shown that all three PTHrP translation products contain clusters of basic amino acids in the 87–107 region of the peptide that resemble the bipartite nuclear/nucleolar localization signal observed in a number of transcription factors *(28–34)*. Analogous to some studies of fibroblast growth factor, such PTHrP nuclear localization has been demonstrated for osteoblasts, chondrocytes, keratinocytes, PTHrP-transfected COS cells, and, most recently, vascular cells, where nuclear targeting was associated with dividing cells *(27–37)*. Furthermore, nuclear targeting of PTHrP seems to regulate growth by inhibiting apoptosis in some cells *(31,35)*. In certain cells, PTHrP exerts opposing mitogenic and antimitogenic effects *(18)*. Nuclear localization of PTHrP in chondrocytes requires an human immunodeficiency virus (HIV) Tat-like 87–107 domain, and nuclear phosphorylation of threonine 85 by cyclic-dependent kinase CDK2 can regulate PTHrP nuclear transport *(37)*. More recently, a region for importin β binding and nuclear targeting was mapped to an SV40 large T-antigen-like domain at PTHrP residues 66–94, which can be transported by the GTP-binding protein Ran in a cell-cycle-dependent manner *(30)*. Furthermore, it was also demonstrated that both endogenous and transfected PTHrP bind poly-(G) homopolymeric RNA, GC-rich double-stranded RNA (dsRNA), and total cellular RNA, thereby predicting a role for PTHrP in the processing of rRNA *(37)*. This interaction is mediated via a core motif localized within the NLS that is shared by other RNA-binding proteins that are targeted to the nucleolus. Because the nucleolus is the major site for biogenesis of ribosomes, nucleolar PTHrP could influence cellular functions by modulating ribosomal RNA synthesis, either by affecting RNA polymerase I activity or by altering ribosome assembly and/or function *(32,37)*. Adding further complexity, recent studies report that a PTHrP peptide containing the classical NLS could be localized to the nucleus independent of the PTHrP receptor *(9,32)*, whereas other studies have demonstrated the translocation of the PTHrP receptor to the nucleus *(9,33,34)*. Recent studies have also shown that PTHrP can exert differential effects on cell growth, depending on its mechanism of action *(9,18)*: When cells were treated with amino-terminus-containing PTHrP peptides, which act through cell surface receptors, cell proliferation was inhibited; by contrast, when the same peptides were introduced into the cells by PTHrP transfectants that also contained the nuclear targeting site, cell growth was stimulated. Deletion of either of the two sites within the NLS, PTHrP88–91 and PTHrP102–106, abrogated the effect.

Our own studies, along with those of other investigators, have also demonstrated novel growth-regulatory effects of PTHrP through its peptides *(1–5,12,27)*. We, like other investigators, have recently observed that PTHrP transfection (intracrine) and treatment (endocrine) of cancer cells have different effects on the expression of cytokines that regulate cancer cell growth *(12,27)*. Furthermore, we found that these differences can be the result of the intracrine effects of PTHrP but independent of the classical amino-terminal moieties of the oncoprotein and rather dependent on a novel non-amino-terminal forms *(1,3,4,27)*. Molecular interactions with bone cells through these novel molecular pathways that underlie PTHrP's nonclassical mechanism of growth regulation and skeletal tumor progression.

2. PTHrP IN PROSTATE AND PROSTATE CANCER

2.1. PTHrP and Prostate Cancer

Studies of PTHrP in prostate cancer demonstrate that PTHrP expression regulates prostate cancer progression and metastasis in bone. We *(3–5,27,38–47)*, along with other investigators *(48–67)*, have demonstrated that PTHrP is robustly expressed by prostate cancers. PTHrP levels are greater in malignant tissue than in hyperplastic and normal prostate *(48,49)*. Furthermore, mRNA levels and intensity of PTHrP immunostaining correlate with increasing tumor grade *(48,49,61)*. PTHrP expression in malignant prostate cell lines also correlates with tumor invasiveness and metastatic potential: PC-3 cells, derived from a prostatic bone metastasis, produce greater levels of PTHrP than LNCaP or DU 145 cells, derived from lymph node and brain metastases, respectively *(62–64)*. In the prostate, as in other tissues, PTHrP is processed into distinct peptides that have unique biological effects *(54–57)*. Sizing studies indicate that PC-3 cells and LNCaP cells process PTHrP into smaller forms, likely those that respectively stimulate and inhibit osteoclast activity *(54,55)*. As detailed subsequently, prostatic expression of PTHrP is associated with regulatory effects and interactions (e.g., with cytokines and oncoproteins) that are important in the development and progression of prostate cancer *(27,65–74)*. Some studies have also demonstrated that PTHrP and related measurements might have diagnostic and prognostic value for the tumor *(3,60,75)*.

Although it is well established that PTHrP regulates prostate cell cancer growth, some controversy remains about the nature of this biological effect *(56–59)*. This is likely the result of the differential processing and resulting heterogeneity of the expression of PTHrP and its receptor, PTHrPR, in different experimental preparations of prostate cells *(2–4,10,11)*. Consequently, we have come to appreciate that there are laboratory-to-laboratory differences in PTHrPR phenotype even among established prostate cell lines in the hands of experienced investigators *(27,58,59,76,77)*. Furthermore, for reasons beyond technical, these differences could be related to the recent demonstration, discussed elsewhere, that PTHrP might mediate its effects through nonclassical pathways *(3–5)*. Appreciating and invoking these pathways is now essential in order to fully elucidate the molecular mechanisms that PTHrP uses to exert its biological and growth regulatory effects in well-defined systems *(see* Table 1).

2.1.1. PROSTATE CANCER METASTASES

Although prostate cancer can spread to many organs, the tumor commonly spreads to bone *(2,3,78–80)*. Although prostate cancer is characterized by osteoblastic metastases, the lesions also cause osteolysis *(7,27,59,72,79)*. Also, although osteoblastosis is the common phenotype of prostate cancer metastases, osteolysis seems to be a necessary precursor for prostate cells to colonize bone, because metastatic cells would be less able to invade and grow in mineralized tissue without bone resorption *(78–81)*. A variety of factors produced by cancer cells can stimulate osteoclastic bone resorption, including

Table 1
Summary of PTHrPa and Cytokine Expression by Prostate Cancer Cells

Cell Preparation	PTHrP (pg/μg)[a]	IL-8 (pg/μg)[a]	IL-6 (pg/μg)[a]
1. PC-3	372	45	28
2. PPC-1	11	8	13
3. DuPro-1	7	6	13
4. LNCaP	114	3	22
5. PNT1-A[b]	3	NT	NT
6. 267B1[c]	12–17	2	32
7. DU145	9	11	31
8. Primary Culture	1	NT	NT

Note: NT, not yet tested.

[a] Media concentration/cell protein/72h. Measured by an immunoassay based on PTHrP1–34 and confirmed by assays based on PTHrP38–64 and PTHrP109–141. All cells also expressed PTHrP receptor mRNA as assessed by nucleic acid hybridization and/or immunocytology. Receptor negative cells are DuPro-1.

[b] SV-40 transformed.

[c] SV-40 transformed, also available as radiation transformed.

Literature citation for cell preparation:
1. Kaighn M, Narayan K, Ohnuki Y, Lechner J, Jones L. Establishment and characterization of a human prostatic line (PC-3). *Invest Urol* 1979; 17: 16–23.
2. Brothman A, Lesho L, Somers K, Wright G. Phenotypic and cytogenic characterization of a cell line derived from primary prostatic carcinoma. *Int J Cancer* 1989; 44:898–903.
3. Gingrich J, Tucker J, Walther P, Day J, Poulton S, Webb K. Establishment and characterization of a new human prostatic cell line (DuPro-1). *J Urol* 1991; 146:915–919.
4. Horoszewicz J, Leong S, Chu T, Wajsman Z, Friedman M, Papsidero L, et al. The LNCaP cell line - a new model for studies on human prostate carcinoma. *Prog Clin Biol Res* 1980; 37:115–132.
5. Cussenot O, Berthon P, Berger R, Mowszowicz A, Faille A, Hojman F, et al. Immortalization of human adult normal prostatic epithelial cells by liposome containing large T-SV40 gene. *J Urol* 1991; 143:881–886.
6. Lee M, Garkovenko E, Yun J, Weijerman P, Peehl D, Chen L, Rhim J. Characterization of adult human prostatic epithelial cells immortalized by polybrene-induced DNA transfection with a plasmid containing an origin-defective SV40 genome. *Int J Oncol* 1994; 4:821–830.
7. Stone K, Mickey D, Wunderli H, Mickey G, Paulson D. Isolation of a human prostate carcinoma cell line (DU145). *Int J Cancer* 1978; 21: 274–281.
8. Peehl, DM. Growth of prostate epithelial and stromal cells in vitro. Methods in molecular medicine. 2003; 81:41–57.

transforming growth factors, epidermal growth factors, interleukins, tumor necrosis factors, prostaglandins, cytokines, and, importantly, PTHrP *(3,27,65–74)*. Although there is clinical and experimental evidence from several cancers that PTHrP expression is related to the development and progression of bone metastases, this association has been, until recently, best established for breast cancer *(21)*. However, corresponding studies, including our own, are beginning to appear for prostate cancer and bone metastases

(20,21,48–59,64,77). Because PTHrP contains peptides that might differentially regulate both osteoblasts (e.g., PTHrP1–34) and osteoclasts (e.g., osteostatin), the processing of prostatic PTHrP can affect the tumor's development, type, and progression of bone metastases *(1–5,54–56).*

Although prostate cancers that express high levels of PTHrP produce more skeletal metastases than those that do not, essentially all of these studies have focused on the amino-terminus of PTHrP, which signals through the receptor shared with PTH *(3,4,7,46).* Our preliminary studies demonstrate a role for non-amino-terminal peptides of PTHrP on prostate cancer progression in the skeleton *(1–5).*

2.1.2. RANKL, RANK, AND OPG

The recent elucidation of a novel pathway of molecular regulation in bone by these three osteokines has provided both a physiologic link among bone cell functions and a pathogenetic link among cancer cells, the immune system, and bone cells in the regulation of the osteoclastic bone resorption, a key cellular mediator of skeletal tumor progression *(82).* The molecular participants in this pathway are the membrane-associated protein named RANKL (receptor activator of nuclear factor κB ligand), a member of the tumor necrosis factor family of cytokines, its cognate receptor, RANK, and OPG (osteoprotegerin), a soluble "decoy" receptor for RANKL *(5,82–85).* In the physiology of bone metabolism, RANKL is expressed on the surface of osteoblastic stromal cells. By binding to RANK, its receptor, on osteoclast precursors, RANKL enhances their recruitment into the osteoclastogenesis pathway. RANKL also activates mature osteoclasts to resorb bone. In the pathophysiology of bone metastases and hypercalcemia, many of the tumor cell types that are associated with cancer-stimulated bone resorption express a soluble form of RANKL (sRANKL). Furthermore, during the inflammation, which can be associated with infection as well as malignancy, activated T-lymphocytes also express increased amounts of RANKL which can stimulate osteoclasts. The activated lymphocytes also expresses interferon-γ (INF-γ), which opposes the effect of RANKL on osteoclast-mediated bone resorption. The osteoclastic effects of RANKL can also be attenuated by its soluble decoy receptor, OPG, also produced by osteoblasts and tumor cells. Hypercalcemia results when these opposing regulatory interactions of RANKL, RANK, OPG, and INF-γ allow osteoclastic activation to predominate *(82)* (*see* Fig. 1).

We, along with other investigators, have demonstrated that prostate cancer cells express OPG, RANKL, and RANK and that PTHrP, including nonamino-terminal peptides (NTPs), regulates their expression in this cancer *(3,5).* We evaluated several prostate cancer cell lines, including 267 B1, 267 B1-XR, DU 145, DuPro-1, PC-3, LNCaP, and PPC-1, for the expression of OPG/RANK/RANKL. All cell lines were shown to express these genes by RT-PCR. We next studied the effect of various PTHrP peptides (1–34, 38–64, 107–139, and 140–173) on the OPG/RANK/RANKL cascade. Using RT-PCR and immunoassays, we demonstrated that PTHrP1–34 and PTHrP140–173 treatment increased OPG expression in 267 B1-XR and PPC-1 cells. PTHrP38–64 treatment increased OPG expression in PPC-1 cells only. No significant effects on OPG levels by PTHrP peptides were observed in 267 B1, PC-3, DU 145, and Dupro-1 cells. Based on RT-PCR, RANKL expression was increased in PC-3 and 267B1-XR cells with PTHrP1–34 and PTHrP107–139 treatments, respectively. RANKL expression was decreased by PTHrP1–34 in 267 B1, 267B1–XR, PPC-1, and Dupro-1 cells. No PTHrP peptide treat-

Tumor and Skeletal Interactions

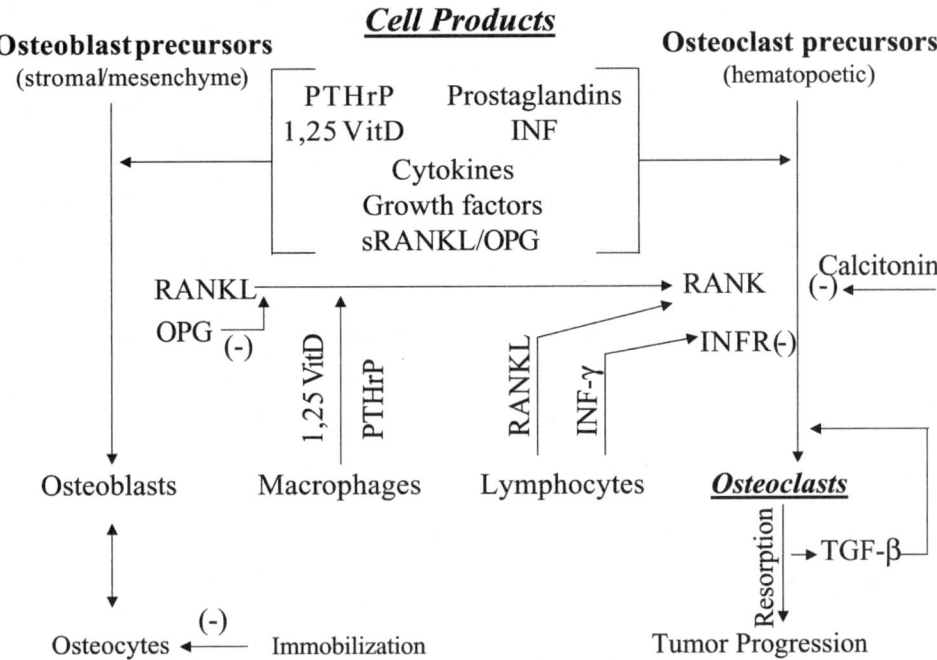

Fig. 1. Schematic representation of tumor and bone cell molecular interactions in PTHrP-producing cancer. Tumor and bone cells can express several cell products (in brackets) that initiate osteoclastogenesis and the osteolytic cascade (**right**). They include PTHrP, 1,25VitD (1,25-dihydroxyvitamin D), prostaglandins, especially of the PGE2 series, cytokines, especially interleukin (IL)-1, IL-6, and IL-8, growth factors, especially TGF-β, RANKL (receptor activator of nuclear factor κB ligand), a cell membrane-associated member of the tumor necrosis factor family of cytokines; soluble RANKL (sRANKL), and their cognate receptor, RANK, and OPG, a soluble "decoy" receptor for RANKL. The latter group is also expressed by osteoblast precursors as they develop into osteoblasts (**left**). In addition to OPG, the stimulation of osteoclastic bone resorption by RANKL is opposed by activation of the γ-interferon receptor (INF-γR) by INF-γ production by activated lymphocytes and by the peptide hormone, calcitonin. The relative activity of the osteoclast stimulatory effects of RANKL and sRANKL and the inhibitory effects of OPG and INF-γ determine the extent of osteolysis. Arrows indicate a positive (stimulatory) effect except where indicated by the negative sign. Several growth factors in addition to TGF-β (illustrated, right bottom) reside in the bone matrix and can be released upon resorption to exert their biological effects, often osteoclast stimulation. They include BMP (bone morphogenetic proteins, especially BMP-2), FGF (fibroblast growth factor), PDGF (platelet-derived growth factor), and IGFs (insulin-like growth factors) *(82)*.

ment effect was demonstrated on RANKL in the other cell lines. RANK expression did not appear to be regulated by PTHrP in the prostate cell lines, with the exception of PTHrP140–173, which decreased RANK mRNA in 267 B1 cells as measured by RT-PCR. In conclusion, these results suggest that PTHrP promotes prostate cancer to spread to bone by regulating the OPG/RANK/RANKL pathway *(1–5)*.

2.2. Effects of PTHrP and Its Peptides in Prostate Cancer

Many studies have demonstrated that PTHrP and its derived peptides regulate the pathobiology biology of prostate cancer *(1–5)*. The production of PTHrP and its biologic effects were investigated using the human prostate cancer cell lines PC-3, LNCaP, and DU 145 *(44–47)*. A synthetic peptide, PTHrP1–34, stimulated thymidine uptake in PC-3 and DU 145 cells more than threefold over the control under serum-free and steroid-free conditions, whereas LNCaP cells were not affected. However, in the presence of dihydrotestosterone, DNA synthesis of LNCaP cells was stimulated by PTHrP in a dose-dependent manner. Additionally, this PTHrP-induced DNA synthesis was completely neutralized by a validated mouse monoclonal antibody (8B12) raised against PTHrP1–34. Our data suggest that PTHrP might play a significant role in the growth of prostate cancer by acting locally in an autocrine fashion. However, in primary cultures, we were unable to identify growth-regulatory activity of synthetic and endogenous PTHrP peptides on normal prostatic epithelial cells *(45)*. These studies demonstrate the complexity of the biological effects of PTHrP and suggest that different mechanisms might be extant in normal and malignant prostate cells.

The complexity of PTHrP's growth effects in the prostate was demonstrated by our studies of peptide treatments that included non-amino-terminal forms *(3–5,27,30)*. Notably, treatment with the human-specific peptide, PTHrP140–173, caused a marked decrease in cell number in all prostate cell lines studied, with the most dramatic effect observed in the 267 B1 cells *(3,39)*. These data again demonstrate differential effects of PTHrP peptides on prostate cell growth. Most recently, we have demonstrated that several PTHrP-processed peptides regulate prostate cell growth *(3,39)*.

We confirmed that the biological effects of PTHrP are mediated, at least in part, through the cell surface receptor that it shares with PTH and which is a member of the seven-membrane-spanning and G protein-coupled cell surface receptors *(1,3)*. However, in addition to its classical receptor-mediated biological effects, we also discovered that PTHrP signals by translocation to the nucleus or nucleolus and thus acts in an intracrine fashion *(27,28)*. In fact, nuclear targeting of PTHrP seems to regulate apoptosis in some cells *(28–31)*.

2.3. PTHrP Receptor in Prostate Cancer

Although there have been no systematic studies of the PTHrP receptor in human prostate cancer, preliminary studies demonstrate paired expression of PTHrP and its receptor in the tumor and its bone metstases *(79)*. We studied in human prostate tissue and cell lines, including normal, normal-transformed (267 B1, PNT1A, PNT1B, and PNT2), and malignant prostate cell lines (DU 145, DuPro-1, LNCaP, PPC-1, PC-3, 267B1-XR, and 267 B1-Ki/ras), the expression of the PTHrP receptor by immunocytology and by RT-PCR. Using antibodies to the PTHrP receptor, we found PTHrP receptor expression in most prostate cells *(39,43)*. Prostate cancers and their derived cell lines demonstrated more intense immunostaining compared to normal and hyperplastic tissue. The cell lines and the staining patterns demonstrated colocalization between PTHrP and its receptor. The most intense immunostaining was observed in the 267 B1- K-ras, DuPro-1, LNCaP, and PC-3 cells. Oligonucleotides specific for human PTHrP receptor demonstrated a specific 415-bp band using RT-PCR in several cell lines *(43)*. In contrast to studies in animal models, several studies show that human normal, hyperplastic, and malignant prostate cells and cell lines commonly express both PTHrP and the PTHrP receptor *(3,39,43)*.

2.4. PTHrP and Bone-Regulatory Interactions in Prostate Cancer

2.4.1. PTHrP AND CYTOKINES/LYMPHOKINES

In addition to the interactions described earlier with OPG, RANK, and RANKL, several cytokines and lymphokines mediate the biological effects of PTHrP in cancer, notably IL-6 and IL-8 *(1–3,65–79,86–93)*. IL-6 is a prostate cancer product that mediates tumor morbidity in patients with metastatic disease and is associated with poor prognosis in several cancers *(86)*. IL-6 has unique and important effects on bone cells and serves as a mediator of bone resorption by promoting osteoclast formation *(66,67)*. IL-6 has been shown in vitro and in vivo to stimulate osteoclastic bone resorption *(3,67,68)*. IL-6 in concert with PTHrP seems to play a role in the development of bone metastasis of prostate cancer *(87)*. In an in vivo study, neutralizing antibodies to IL-6 were found to lower the blood calcium in the nude mice carrying the squamous cell carcinoma of the maxilla associated with IL-6 production *(88)*. However, in another similar study, IL-6 secreted by renal cell carcinomas did not contribute directly to hypercalcemia but stimulated the tumor growth of a subpopulation of PTHrP producing cells *(89)*.

PTHrP1–34 is known to stimulate IL-6 production in vitro as well as in vivo in osteoblasts cells *(1–3,27)*. In some studies, IL-6 seems an enhancer/helper factor rather than a primary bone resorbing factor in pathological conditions associated with increased bone resorption *(70,86,90)*. IL-6 was also found to potentiate the effects of PTHrP by acting at an earlier stages of osteoclast lineage than PTHrP; in contrast, PTHrP, a potent bone-resorbing factor, acts on cells in the later stages of osteoclastogenesis *(70,92)*.

Interleukin-8, a regulator of angiogenesis, is expressed by prostate cells *(27,65,71)*. Angiogenesis plays an important role in the metastasis of variety of tumors *(92,93)*. Both normal and malignant human prostate cells express IL-8, and IL-8 is expressed at higher levels in metastatic prostate cells compared with benign prostatic hyperplasia *(2,65,72)*. A role for IL-8 in tumor growth and metastasis is becoming established: A nonmetastatic and IL-8-negative melanoma cell line after transfection with the IL-8 gene was found to be highly tumorigenic and metastatic in nude mice *(94)*. Although PTHrP stimulates IL-8 production by prostate cancer cells in vitro, the molecular mechanism by which PTHrP modulates growth of prostate cells via cytokines is not clear *(2,27)*.

We have studied the regulatory interactions of PTHrP with cytokines that can play a role in the development of prostate cancer skeletal metastases *(28,53,57,59)*. Six prostate cancer cell lines exhibited constitutive expression of PTHrP and IL-8 that were significantly correlated ($r = 0.91$, $p < 0.01$). Because PC-3 cells demonstrated the highest levels of both PTHrP and IL-8 expression, we transfected wild-type and mutant PTHrP into these cells. Wild-type PTHrP1–173 and PTHrP 33–173, lacking the PTHrP receptor-binding domain, induced a threefold stimulation of IL-8 production in PC-3 and PPC-1 cells and a twofold stimulation of IL-8 in DuPro-1, DU 145, and PC-3 cells. Intracellular PTHrP in PC-3 and DuPro-1 cells selectively activated mitogen-activated protein (MAP) kinase (MAPK) ERK1/ERK2, a pathway known to relay signals for growth. Transfection of the C-terminal truncation mutant PTHrP1–87 induced a fivefold simulation of IL-8. In contrast, exogenous PTHrP1–34 and PTHrP1–86 did not significantly affect IL-8 production; moreover, PTHrP-neutralizing antibodies did not inhibit the production of IL-8 by PTHrP. Additional transfection studies with progressively C-terminally truncated PTHrP1–87 defined a 23-amino-acid sequence, PTHrP65–87, required for PTHrP1–87 to stimulate IL-8 in prostate cancer cells. We also showed that PTHrP mutant plasmids that blocked the processing of PTHrP at 147–150 (the amino acids KKKK at 147–150 were changed to GQKG) stimulated the production of IL-8 in the PC-3 cell line *(53)*. Corresponding studies were conducted with IL-6. When given exogenously, various PTHrP peptides (1–34, 38–64, and 1–86) did not show an effect on IL-8 or IL-6 production in PC-3, 267 B1-XR, and DU 145 cells. However, PTHrP140–173 (10 nM), which we have shown to inhibit prostate cell growth, inhibited IL-6 as well as IL-8 expression by 50% in 267B1 cells *(57)*. Our results demonstrate that PTHrP acts to induce IL-8 production in prostate cancer cells via an intracrine pathway independent of its NLS. Cells transfected with PTHrP1–87 and PTHrP1–173 also showed increased cell proliferation. Thus, PTHrP exerts these effects in prostate cancer through a nonclassical NLS that might mediate its effects on the progression of prostate cancer *(57)*.

Our results and those of other investigators demonstrate that PTHrP acts to regulate growth and cytokine production in prostate cancer cells via intracrine pathways independent of its amino-terminal domain. These observations identify novel molecular mechanisms for PTHrP that stimulates bone-active cytokine expression and might contribute to the progression in bone of prostate cancer *(57,58)*.

2.4.2. NOVEL MOLECULAR PATHWAYS OF PTHrP REGULATION: NON-AMINO-TERMINAL PEPTIDES OF PTHrP

We, and others, have demonstrated PTHrP effects in cancer cells of bioactive peptides derived through processing of native PTHrP at its many endoproteolytic-processing sites *(1–5,16)*. Enzymes have been recently identified from mammalian tissues that seem to serve this function *(16)*. In our own studies, we have demonstrated biological effects for several NTPs *(16,39,95–97)*. We have recently demonstrated in cartilage cells that the tetrabasic site within PTHrP140–173 determines intracrine regulatory effects of PTHrP1–173 *(12)*. We have also demonstrated effects of NTPs in pancreatic cells *(95–97)*. Eight cancer cell lines exhibited constitutive expression of PTHrP and IL-8, four of which also show overexpression of IL-6. The effects of PTHrP1–34, PTHrP67–86, PTHrP107–138, PTHrP140–173, and PTHrP140–173 scrambled (negative control) were investigated on interleukin production. The cell lines were treated with each of these different PTHrP peptides at 1, 10, and 100 nM concentrations. After 48 h of incubation, the media were collected and immunoassayed for IL-8 and IL-6. PTHrP1–34 significantly stimulated IL-8 secretion in a dose-dependent manner. However, PTHrP140–173 inhibited the secretion of IL-6 and stimulated the expression of IL-8 more than twofold in a dose-dependent manner that was significant at all concentrations ($p < 0.01$). The effect of PTHrP140–173 in these cells is another example of the biological relevance of this carboxy-terminal peptide of PTHrP1–173.

In prostate cells, PTHrP can also exert its biological actions through molecular mechanisms in addition to effects mediated by its amino-terminus through the PTHrP receptor. Using a nonmetastatic human prostate epithelial cell line (267 B1) and its tumorigenic derivative (267 B1-XR), we studied the effects on cell proliferation of various PTHrP-derived peptide fragments and transfected PTHrP1–87, PTHrP1–173, and a pre-pro PTHrP33–173 mutant that does not contain an intact 1–34 region *(39,76)*. Exogenous PTHrP1–34 had no effect on these cell lines, PTHrP107–139 was stimulatory only in 267

B1-XR cells and PTHrP140–173 was inhibitory in both cell lines. Transfected PTHrP1–87, PTHrP1–173, and PTHrP33–173 significantly increased cell number in the 267 B1-XR cells and had no effects in the nontumorigenic cell line, 267 B1. The mitotic effect of PTHrP33–173 confirms a role for non-amino-terminal PTHrP fragments in prostate cells. These studies demonstrate that, in addition to mediating its biological effects by interacting with classical cell surface receptors, PTHrP can mediate its growth regulatory effects by intracrine mechanisms in cancer cells. These mechanisms might involve the NLS domains of PTHrP or other unique downstream pathways *(2,3)*.

2.4.3. PTHrP AND APOPTOSIS

We have demonstrated in several cell types, including prostate, that PTHrP can mediate its growth regulation through the apoptotic pathway, as have other investigators *(37,45)*. We observed that both PTHrP1–34 and PTHrP107–138 decreased apoptosis of RPMI 1788 cells in a dose-dependent fashion by measuring the activity of caspase-3, a central, downstream component of the Fas- and tumor necrosis factor (TNF)-mediated apoptotic pathways *(55)*. PTHrP could regulate caspase-3 by interfering with upstream signaling, by blocking CD95 (FasR) or TNF receptor, by inhibiting other critical components of these two pathways, or by altering the level of bcl-2 (or related factors) that can regulate caspase-3 activity *(55,56)*. Although we did not see changes in cell cycle factors in these studies, the investigations of others, discussed earlier, support a systematic study of this molecular pathway. In studies of MAPK, we demonstrated that PTHrP increased the level of phosphorylation of p38 MAPK *(56)*. As detailed subsequently, we propose experiments to further dissect the molecular components of the apoptotic pathway through which PTHrP exerts growth regulatory effects.

In the prostate, we performed apoptosis studies using wild-type DU 145 cells, prostate carcinoma cells and DU 145 cells stably transformed to express various PTHrP peptides *(97)*. We evaluated PTHrP's effect on survival with clonogenic cell survival assays. Suspended cells were exposed to γ-irradiation (4 Gy) and replated in triplicate into 60-mm dishes: colonies (>50 cells) were counted after 14 d in culture. Multiple clones of DU 145 PTHrP1–173-expressing cells demonstrated a twofold increase in colony formation compared to the vector control transformed cells ($p < 0.01$). Conversely, DU 145 PTHrP1–87 and PTHrP1–141 expressing cells demonstrated a 50% and 30% decrease, respectively, in colony formation after γ-irradiation compared to the vector control cells. Studies of PTHrP's effect on staurosporine-induced apoptosis as measured by nuclear condensation and caspases-3 and caspases-9 activities showed in the DU 145 PTHrP1–173-expressing cells a reduction in nuclear condensation and caspases-3 and -9 activities compared to the vector control cells. DU 145 PTHrP1–87- and PTHrP1–141-expressing cells increased caspases-3 and caspases-9 activities slightly compared to vector control cells. The effects of PTHrP peptides on staurosporine-induced apoptosis were studied in wild-type DU 145 cells. PTHrP140–173 peptide treatment decreased caspases-3 and caspases-9 activities and nuclear condensation compared to vehicle-treated cells. No significant effects on nuclear condensation and caspases-3 or caspases-9 were observed with treatment with PTHrP1–34 or scrambled PTHrP140–173 peptide. Because protective effects on apoptosis were not observed for PTHrP1–34 peptide or PTHrP1–87 and PTHrP1–141 gene transfer, the human-specific PTHrP140–173 region appears responsible for the antiapoptotic properties of PTHrP in prostate cancer cells through a paracrine mechanism. The proapoptotic effects of PTHrP1–87 and PTHrP1–141 could result from an intracrine, nuclear targeting pathway *(28,98)*.

2.4.4. Androgens and PTHrP

Several recent studies have provided evidence for androgen regulation of the PTHrP axis in prostate cancer *(61,99)*. A study designed to assess the ability of androgens to regulate PTHrP production was conducted in androgen-insensitive human prostate cancer cells PC-3 and cells transfected with androgen receptor (PC-3T). Androgen responsiveness caused a marked decrease in PC-3T cell growth, and treatment of these cells with dihydrotestosterone led to inhibition of PTHrP production, an effect readily reversed by the androgen receptor antagonist flutamide. Animals inoculated with PC-3 and PC-3T cells developed palpable tumors. Inoculation of the PC-3T cells into castrated animals resulted in rapid tumor growth in PC-3T tumors, effects that were reversed in PC-3T tumors grown in castrated hosts. A PTHrP promoter luciferase reporter showed a 30% decrease in luciferase activity following treatment with dihydrotestosterone (DHT). These results indicate that PC-3 cell growth correlates inversely with androgen sensitivity and directly with PTHrP production in vitro and in vivo. Androgens can regulate PTHrP production in prostate cancer cells, and the androgen effect on PTHrP is mediated at least in part by transcriptional regulation via the androgen receptor. Another study evaluated the effects of PTHrP and/or DHT treatment on DNA synthesis in the androgen-dependent (LnCaP) and androgen-independent (PC-3) human prostate adenocarcinoma cell lines. The effect of PTHrP on prostate cancer cell proliferation was mediated through ornithine decarboxylase gene expression.

2.4.5. Adhesion Molecules

The role of adhesion molecules in cancer progression is well documented *(2,3)*. Corresponding studies have emerged in prostate cancer demonstrating PTHrP regulation of this family of cell surface proteins *(100,101)*. We and other investigators have shown that a cancer-facilitating adhesion molecule can be regulated by PTHrP. Overexpression of the oncoprotein increases adhesion of the human prostate cancer cell line PC-3 to the ECM molecules collagen type I, fibronectin, and laminin. Increased adhesion is accompanied by upregulation in the expression of $\alpha 1$, $\alpha 5$, $\alpha 6$, and $\beta 4$ integrin subunits. Mutation of the classical nuclear localization sequence negated the effects of PTHrP on $\alpha 1$, $\alpha 5$, $\alpha 6$, and $\beta 4$ integrin expression, indicating that these effects are mediated via an intracrine pathway requiring nuclear localization. Expression of the $\alpha 2$, $\alpha 3$, αv, and $\beta 1$ integrin subunits were comparable in wild-type and NLS-mutated PTHrP transfectants. The cells overexpressing PTHrP showed significantly higher adhesion to collagen type 1, fibronectin, and laminin. PTHrP overexpressing cells also exhibited higher expression of the $\alpha 1$, $\alpha 5$, $\alpha 6$, and $\beta 4$ integrin subunits. These findings support a role for PTHrP in prostate tumor invasion and metastasis through regulation of specific integrin subunits via an intracrine pathway.

Our studies in pancreatic cancer support this hypothesis *(102)*. Using the fast-growing (FG) variant of the COLO 357 metastatic pancreactic adenocarcinoma cell line, we demonstrate that the cells express PTHrP and the PTHrP receptor. In cell culture on either type I collagen or fibronectin, type I collagen increased the expression of the PTHrP receptor compared to fibronectin or tissue culture plastic. These observations suggest unique functional interactions among ECM proteins and PTHrP and its receptor and might have important implications in our understanding of the complex mechanisms responsible for the progression of cancer and its metastases *(103)*.

2.4.6. CALCIUM, VITAMIN D, AND THE CALCIUM-SENSING RECEPTOR

Ambient calcium and its regulators and mediator also play a role in prostate cancer progression *(74,77)*. Vitamin D seems to exert a protective effect against prostate cancer through its antiproliferative actions. Studies with 1,25-dihydroxyvitamin D showed inhibition of PTHrP mRNA and secreted protein levels though a transcriptional mechanism. By contrast, epidermal growth factor (EGF), which is normally secreted by prostate cancer cells, increased PTHrP gene expression. Corresponding studies demonstrated expression of the calcium-sensing receptor (CaR) in prostate cancer cells. Elevated extracellular calcium concentrations stimulate PTHrP. In addition, adenovirus-mediated infection of PC-3 cells with a dominant negative CaR construct attenuated calcium-induced PTHrP secretion, and pretreating the prostate cancer cells with transforming growth factor augmented both basal and high calcium stimulated PTHrP secretion. Thus, in PTHrP-secreting prostate cancers, especially those metastatic to bone, interactions among ambient calcium, vitamin D metabolites, and the CaR could establish a regulatory cycle for tumor progression.

3. PROSTATE CANCER AND SKELETAL PROGRESSION

As reviewed in the chapter, there is substantial in vitro data and indirect in vivo data to support the hypothesis that PTHrP expression promotes the progression of prostate cancer in the skeleton. In order to directly test this hypothesis in vivo, we studied the DU 145 cell line in a mouse model for prostate cancer *(2,3)*. The DU 145 cell line was selected because it has a low constitutive PTHrP expression and does not grow well in mouse tumor models. We studied four types of DU 145 cell: (1) wild-type cells, (2) vector (pCineo) transformed cells, (3) PTHrP1–87 transformed cells, and (4) PTHrP1–173 transformed cells. The PC-3 cell line (group 5) was also used as a known prostate cancer cell line that produces extensive bone lesions in immunocompromised mice. The cells were directly injected into the femurs of severe combined immunodeficiency (SCID) mice and the mice were evaluated 60 d later for biochemical changes in the sera and skeletal abnormalities by X-ray.

The DU 145 cell lines secreted PTHrP into the media culture at amounts ranging from 101 to 4337 pg PTHrP/mL/10^6 cells when cultured for 96 h at 37°C. The amount of PTHrP measured in the sera of the mice after femoral bone marrow injections was detected in only the DU 145-PTHrP1–87, DU 145–PTHrP1–173, and PC-3 mice. The mice skeletons were evaluated for abnormalities radiographically and demonstrated significant differences between the DU 145 wild-type and vector control mice and the DU 145–PTHrP1–173 and DU 145–PTHrP1–87 mice. The radiographs were generally normal for the DU 145 wild-type and vector control mice. Conversely, the radiographs of the DU 145–PTHrP1–87 and DU 145–PTHrP1–173 mice showed numerous lesions throughout the femurs, with multiple osteolytic and osteoblastic features. The PC-3 mice radiographs demonstrated severe osteolytic lesions. No abnormalities were observed for the control femurs or other areas of the skeleton for each group. Quantitation of the radiographic images of the mouse femurs showed progression of tumor in bone that correlated with PTHrP production by the tumor. The DU 145–PTHrP-transformed groups demonstrated increased bone lesions, serum calcium, and PTHrP. The PTHrP produced by the DU 145–PTHrP1–173 cells was less than the DU 145–PTHrP1–87, but the femur radiographs nevertheless showed more tumor damage in the DU 145–PTHrP1–173 mice.

Our results provide more evidence that PTHrP expression by prostate cancer cells promotes the development of skeletal lesions by the prostate cancer. Furthermore, PTHrP secreted into the blood of tumor-bearing animals served as a tumor biomarker by correlating with the primary prostate tumor volume and the degree of tumor burden in the bone. This animal model can be used to elucidate the role of PTHrP in human prostate cancer progression in bone. In addition to providing information about pathogenesis, such studies can also identify PTHrP-based diagnostic and therapeutic targets for prostate cancer *(104–110)*.

4. PTHrP IN LUNG AND LUNG CANCER

Parathyroid hormone-related protein was discovered as the mediator of humoral hypercalcemia of malignancy in a squamous cell bronchial carcinoma, but it is also made by normal fetal and adult lung. The source of PTHrP in those organs is alveolar type II epithelial cells. Type II cells are the cells that make pulmonary surfactant. They also express ion pumps that assist in keeping the air spaces dry, and they are pluripotential cells that proliferate in settings of lung injury and help repair damage to the alveolar epithelium. PTHrP is an important mediator in lung biology because of roles in lung development, homeostasis in normal adult lung, and pathophysiology of lung injury and lung cancer.

4.1. PTHrP in Fetal Lung

Parathyroid hormone-related protein regulates branching morphogenesis and type II cell maturation in fetal lung development. PTHrP or gene knockout results in hypoplastic lungs with arrested canalicular development *(111)*. Type II cell function is impaired with reduced capacity to synthesize disaturated phosphatidylcholine, the major phospholipid in surfactant, and reduced expression of surfactant apoproteins. PTHrP-null and PTHrPR-null animals die from respiratory failure in the acute neonatal period as a result of the pulmonary structural and functional abnormalities as well as skeletal defects that limit ventilation *(112)*. Overexpression of PTHrP during fetal development also causes pulmonary abnormalities. PTHrP excess causes pulmonary cysts *(113)*, similar to those seen in a developmental abnormality called congenital cystic adenomatoid malformation of the lung. Interestingly, overexpression of PTHrPR causes no structural abnormalities, suggesting that the action of PTHrP on pulmonary development can work through intracrine pathways or through effects of portions of the molecule other than PTHrP1–34 *(114)*. On the other hand, type II cell maturation is a function of amino-terminal PTHrP. PTHrPR is expressed in fetal lung but is restricted to the fetal fibroblasts *(115)*. Thus, the distribution of the ligand and receptor follows a hand-in-glove pattern, supporting a role for epithelial–mesenchymal interactions in the development of pulmonary cellular functions. PTHrP1–34 derived from fetal type II cells is involved in a bidirectional paracrine axis, involving stimulation of mediator release from fetal lung fibroblasts, that leads to development of the synthetic function for surfactant phospholipids. It has no effects on type II cells by themselves, but stimulates disaturated phosphatidylcholine (DSPC) production in mixed populations of epithelial cells and fibroblasts *(116,117)*.

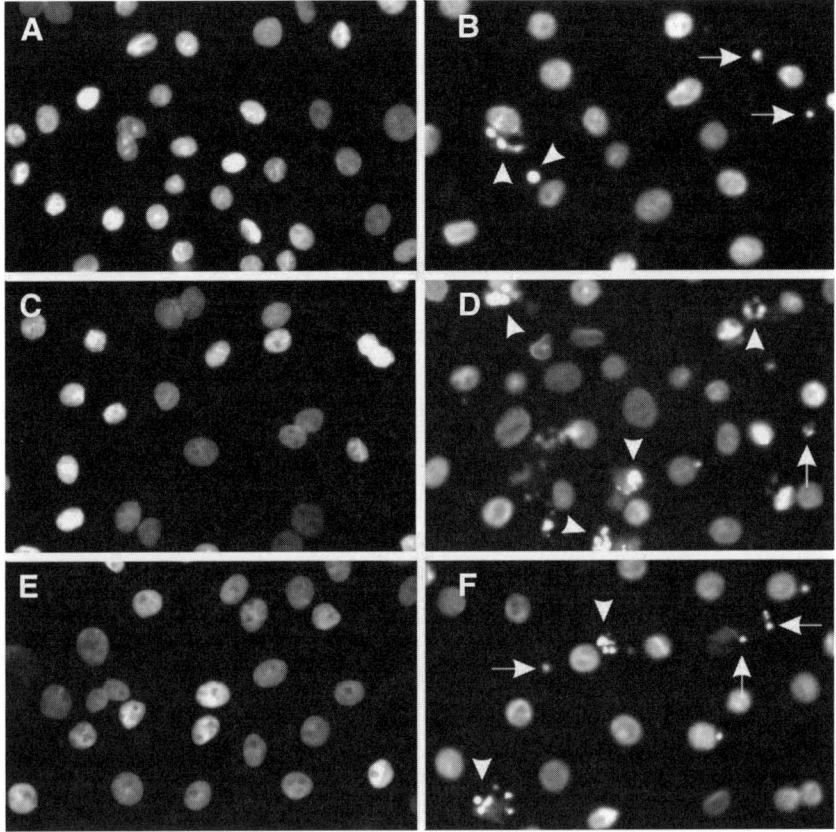

Fig. 2. PTHrP1–34 and PTHrP67–86 augment apoptosis after ultraviolet (UV) in alveolar type II cells. The figure shows micrographs of nonirradiated (**A, C, E**) and irradiated (**B, D, F**) type II epithelial cell nuclei stained with Hoescht 33342. The three rows show cells with no treatment (**A, B**), PTHrP1–34 treatment (**C, D**), and PTHrP67–86 treatment (**E, F**). Apoptotic bodies and cells with condensed and/or fragmented nuclei, indicating apoptosis, are present after UV exposure and are increased in cells treated with either PTHrP peptide. Arrowheads mark representative condensed nuclei and arrows denote representative apoptotic bodies. (From ref. *119*, with permission.)

4.2. PTHrP in Adult Lung

In contrast to the situation in fetal lung, PTHrP is an autocrine factor for adult type II cells. The adult cells express both PTHrP and PTHrPR and respond to PTHrP1–34 with increases in DSPC secretion and alkaline phosphatase expression, hallmarks of the differentiated type II cell phenotype *(21)*. PTHrP1–34 is also a type II cell growth inhibitor. Neutralizing its effects with antibodies stimulates type II cell division in cultured cells and also in lung in vivo *(22)*. A midmolecule peptide, PTHrP67–86, affects type II cells in much the same way as PTHrP1–34. It stimulates surfactant secretion and inhibits growth *(118,119)*. Both portions of the molecule augment inositol phosphate levels in cultured type II cells *(119)*, suggesting that PTHrP67–86 might act through a G protein-coupled receptor, similar to PTHrPR. Finally, both PTHrP1–34 and PTHrP67–86 have effects on type II cells *(119)*. Each peptide sensitizes type II cells to the apoptotic effects of ultraviolet radiation (Fig. 2).

4.3. PTHrP and Lung Injury

Because PTHrP is made by type II cells, it could be valuable as a marker for injury. In neonates, tracheal levels of PTHrP do bear a relation with acute neonatal lung injury, also called respiratory distress syndrome (RDS), and chronic injury, known as bronchopulmonary dysplasia (BPD). Tracheal levels of PTHrP are depressed in situations associated with RDS, such as low birth weight, prematurity, need for artificial surfactant administration, and male gender, but they are increased with maternal steroid administration, a treatment that promotes type II cell maturity *(120)*. In a baboon model of BPD, lung PTHrP levels fail to rise in newborn animals with BPD to the levels that they do in animals without injury *(121)*. Low PTHrP levels have also been associated with increased risk of lung injury in adults. Adults undergoing pulmonary thromboendarterectomy, an operation to treat chronic pulmonary emboli, can develop lung injury as a result of reperfusion of previously obstructed pulmonary vessels. Low levels of PTHrP in airway liquid obtained by bronchopulmonary lavage (BAL) indicate patients with increased risk of developing the injury *(122)*. Interestingly, the predictive capability holds for BAL obtained before the operation. In patients with acute respiratory distress syndrome, BAL PTHrP levels are inversely related to lung injury score, severity of infiltrates on chest radiographs, and BAL fluid albumin concentration *(120)*. The inverse relationship between PTHrP levels and risk of injury in the neonatal and adult studies indicate that PTHrP might reflect the strength of type II cell numbers of function in the lung. The results also open the possibility that PTHrP might play an active role in how the lung protects itself or responds to injury.

Because PTHrP has effects on type II function and growth, it could regulate the pulmonary response to damage. Several studies have shown that lung PTHrP levels are diminished in adult and newborn animals during the period of lung injury in which type II cells proliferate *(118,123–125)* (Fig. 3). Because PTHrP is a type II cell growth inhibitor, changes in its levels could regulate the proliferative response in an inverse fashion, reducing PTHrP decreases the level of growth inhibition and might contribute to proliferation in conjunction with other influences. In fact, restoring PTHrP levels toward normal values by instilling exogenous PTHrP1–34 or PTHrP67–86 into injured lungs reduces type II cell BrdU incorporation (Fig. 4) and expression of proliferating cell nuclear antigen, a growth marker in hyperoxic lung injury and silica injury *(123,126)*. Thus, these peptides do appear to have an inverse regulatory role in the type II cell response to injury.

4.4. PTHrP in Lung Cancer

4.4.1. PTHRP EXPRESSION

Parathyroid hormone-related protein was discovered in squamous lung carcinomas and is common in all types of lung cancer *(127,128)*. Roughly two-thirds of lung cancer express PTHrP *(127,129–132)*, although it might be more common in squamous cell carcinomas than adenocarcinomas *(130,132)*. Because it is commonly in expressed lung cancer, PTHrP could be a useful biomarker diagnosing the disease or following the response to therapy. Indeed, serum and urinary levels of PTHrP are elevated in lung cancer patients compared to normal subjects *(132,133)*. In addition to aiding in diagnosis, PTHrP levels could also be valuable in judging the response to therapy, but no studies are available. Further studies of the role of PTHrP as a lung cancer biomarker are warranted.

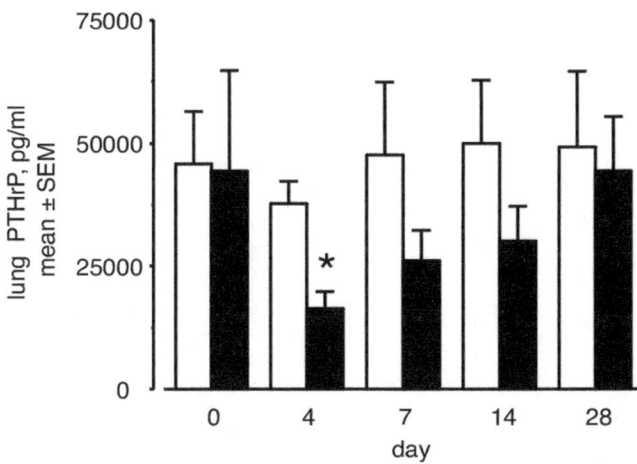

Fig. 3. Lung PTHrP expression after silica injury. Sprague Dawley rats were instilled with 10 mg silica/1 mL phosphate-buffered saline (PBS) (closed bars) or PBS alone (open bars) and followed for the time shown. Lungs were homogenized in a 3:1 (w/v) ratio of PBS with protease inhibitors and PTHrP was measured by radioimmunoassay in the supernatant. Lung PTHrP levels decreased from 43,111 ± 9685 pg/mL in control animals to 16,468 ± 3281 pg/mL 4 d after silica, a 60% decline. Levels rose progressively after 4 d and were not significantly different from control at 7, 14, and 28 d. Lung PTHrP levels did not change over this same period in animals instilled with PBS. The results of the analysis were unchanged by normalizing total lung PTHrP to lung weight. At 4 d, the silica-injured lungs contained 62,613 ± 12,690 pg PTHrP/g lung compared to 12,6526 ± 17,253 in control uninjured lung (*$p < 0.05$). (From ref. *118,* with permission.)

4.4.2. IMPORTANCE FOR PATHOPHYSIOLOGY

Much of the work on PTHrP in lung cancer has focused on its role in mediating humoral hypercalcemia of malignancy *(134,135)*. Hypercalcemia results from systemic levels of PTHrP acting on PTHrPR in bone and kidney. The protein also regulates cancer cell growth and could affect cancer progression, metastasis, and outcome. For example, PTHrP1–34 is an autocrine growth factor for BEN squamous lung cancer cells *(136)*, and PTHrP140–173 is antiapoptotic *(137)*. The effects of PTHrP on apoptosis have been examined after ultraviolet (UV) irradiation, Fas ligation, or staurosporine treatment (Fig. 5). PTHrP140–173 decreases apoptosis after UV as measured by caspase activities, cell mass, morphologic changes, and clonal survival. The peptide also reduces apoptosis after Fas ligation by activating the antibody. Because PTHrP decreases caspase-8 activity, it might have effects on death receptor-mediated apoptosis *(138)*. Consistent with this hypothesis, PTHrP does not protect against apoptosis after staurosporine, a stimulus that activates apoptosis through mitochondrial pathways rather than death receptors. However, the mitochondrial pathway can activate caspase-8, as well, through the action of caspase-6 *(139)*. Thus, the apoptosis pathways affected by PTHrP and the mechanism of the antiapoptotic effect are not known for sure. PTHrP has other effects that could affect a cancer's aggresiveness or invasiveness. For example, it stimulates matrix adhesion, augments angiogenesis, and induces expression of *(140–142)*. These actions could contribute to invasiveness or metastatic potential.

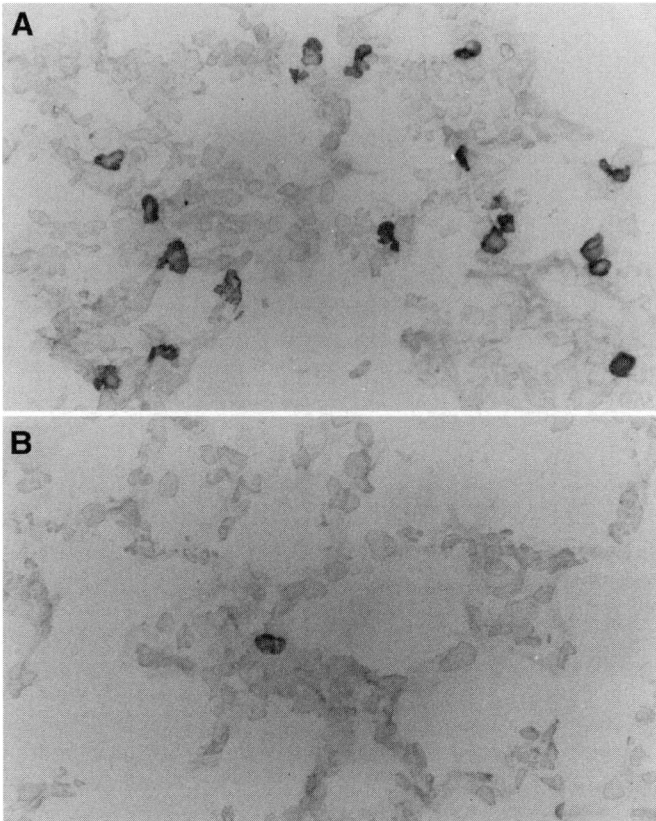

Fig. 4. Effects of PTHrP1–34 on alveolar cell proliferation in hyperoxic lung. After 4 d of exposure to 85% oxygen, 1 mL of PBS or 1 mL of PBS containing 7.5 μg/mL PTHrP1–34 was instilled into rat lungs. BrdU was given intraperitoneally 6 h later to label proliferating cells, and lungs were processed for immunohistology 8 h after PTHrP treatment. (**A**) Lungs instilled with PBS took up BrdU; (**B**) in contrast, PTHrP-instilled lungs showed little BrdU immunoreactivity. The number of BrdU-positive cells per high-power field was sixfold greater in lungs instilled with PBS and in lungs instilled with PTHrP, 3.2 ± 0.4 vs 0.5 ± 0.2, respectively ($p < 0.01$). Magnification, ×260. (From ref. *123*, with permission.)

4.4.3. PTHrP and Prognosis

PTHrP expression portends a poor prognosis sign in cancer. When tumors produce PTHrP, patients tend to have increased or earlier mortality and a higher rate of metastasis *(143–145)*. In one study, patients with high serum PTHrP levels survived 33 d after developing hypercalcemia compared to 66 d for patients with low PTHrP. Their tumor stage was greater than they showed a poorer response to bisphosphonates *(145)*. A relationship between PTHrP and mortality has been observed for lung cancer as well *(143)*. Median survival of lung cancer patients whose PTHrP levels were greater than 150 pmol/L was 1.4 mo compared to 5.4 mo in those with lower PTHrP levels.

Parathyroid hormone-related protein might be an indicator of poor prognosis because of associated hypercalcemia and because of its effects on tumor cell growth, angiogen-

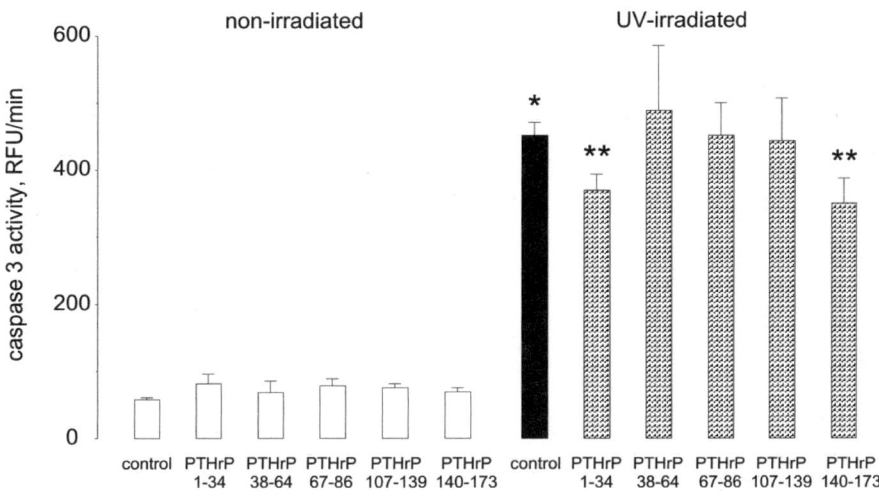

Fig. 5. Effect of PTHrP peptides on caspase-3 activity after UV irradiation in lung cancer cells. UV caused a sixfold increase in caspase-3 activity in BEN squamous lung carcinoma cells compared to nonirradiated cells (*$p < 0.01$). Pretreatment with 100 nM PTHrP1–34 or PTHrP140–173 for 24 h before irradiation reduced caspase-3 activity approx 25% (**$p < 0.05$). Other PTHrP peptides did not have significant effects had no effect on nonirradiated cells. Data are mean± SEM for seven separate experiments. (From ref. *137*, with permssion.)

esis, and invasiveness. The pulmonary tumors make PTHrP appear to be more aggressive than those that do not. For example, in two small cell lung cancer lines isolated at different times from the same patient, the line harvested at the more advanced stage produced much greater levels of PTHrP than the earlier line *(146)*. In an animal model study, PTHrP was related to metastasis of HARA lung cancer cells, a PTHrP-expressing line. Rats received an intraventricular administration of HARA cells and were then treated with systemic PTHrP antibody or isotype antibody *(147)*. Fewer bone metastases developed after PTHrP antibody treatment, implying that tumor-derived PTHrP might increase the propensity to metastasize, as is the case in animal models of breast *(148)*. In addition, 71% of patients with elevated serum PTHrP levels in a previously mentioned study had bone metastases vs 12.5% for patients with low PTHrP *(143)*. To summarize, advanced stage, aggressive tumors, more metastases, and earlier mortality appear associated with PTHrP expression in lung cancer. The biologic effects of PTHrP suggest that PTHrP could be a causal agent, but has not been established; further work is necessary to test this point.

Although the forgoing discussion suggests that PTHrP is an unfavorable marker, other studies provide evidence that PTHrP is favorable for patients with lung cancer and possibly breast cancer, although the assertion is controversial for breast cancer. A study in immunocompromised mice found that PTHrP antibody treatment reduced lung PTHrP levels and increased growth of orthotopic lung carcinomas (Figs. 6 and 7) *(149)*, suggesting that PTHrP inhibited lung tumor growth. Some studies suggest that PTHrP might increase mortality in breast cancer, whereas other studies report conflicting results. On the favorable side, Henderson and colleagues reported that patients with

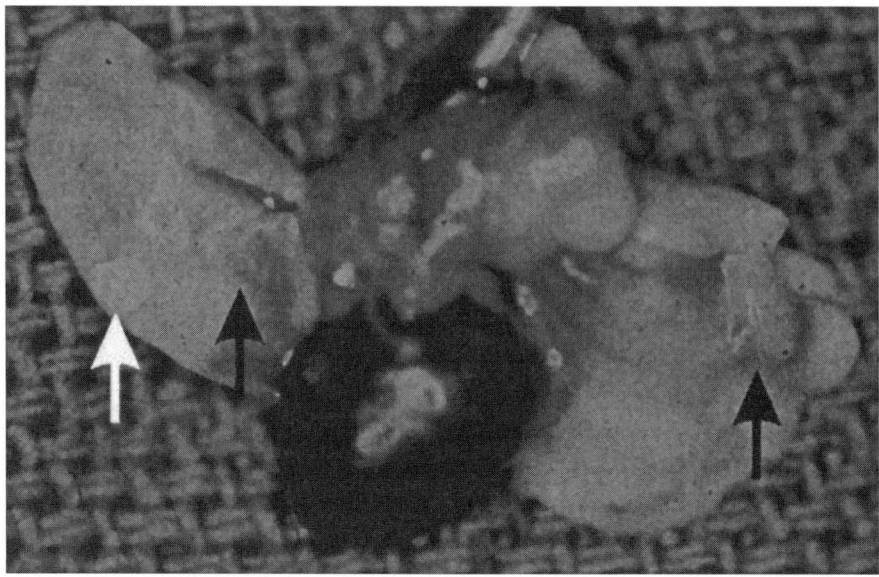

Fig. 6. Macroscopic appearance of orthotopic tumor nodules in athymic mice. This mouse was instilled with 3×10^6 BEN–green fluorescent protein (GFP) cells 30 d earlier and treated with biweekly injections of the neutralizing PTHrP antibodies, 8B12 and 1A5. Several small orthotopic carcinoma nodules were visible on the surface of the lungs (arrows). Six of the 10 mice that were treated with 8B12/1A5 had obvious tumors.

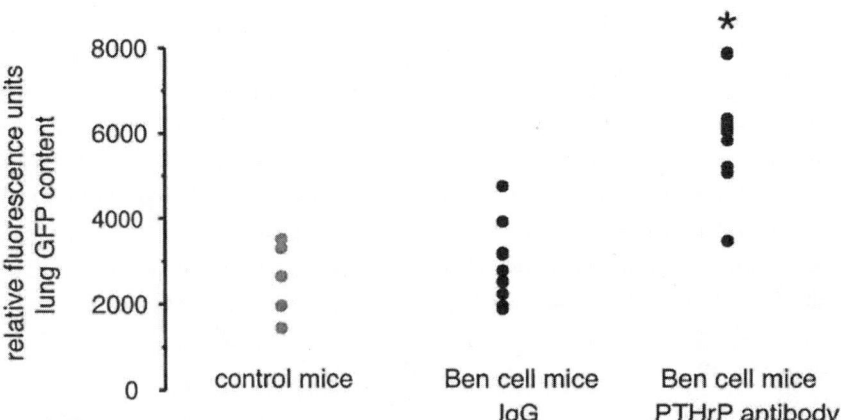

Fig. 7. Effect of PTHrP antibody treatment on orthotopic carcinoma growth. Tumor burden was estimated by measuring the fluorescence of green fluorescent protein (GFP) in homogenates of mouse lung. Each point represents the fluorescence of 125 L of lung homogenate. Lungs were homogenized with a standard volume of tissue lysis buffer (3 mL/g lung). Background fluorescence in the lungs of mice that were not instilled with the BEN–GFP cells was 2576±395 relative fluorescent units (RFU). GFP fluorescence was 331 ± 282 RFU higher than the background in tumor mice treated with irrelevant mouse immunoglobulin (Ig) G compared with 3430±411 RFU higher than the background in mice treated with 8B12/1A5 (*$p < 0.001$). (From ref. *149*, with permission.)

breast carcinomas that were immunoreactive for PTHrP1–14 had a 87% 5-yr survival and only a 13% risk of bone metastasis vs a 73% 5-yr survival and 26% metastasis rate compared to women with PTHrP-negative tumors *(150)*. Surowiak and colleagues found similar results using an antibody to PTHrP38–64 *(151)*. In contrast, PTHrP1–34 and PTHrPR were negative prognostic factors for breast cancer *(152)*. These paradoxical results could result from several factors. First, many of these studies measure only one part of the PTHrP molecule, yet the different parts can exert a variety of actions, sometimes in opposite directions. For example, the intracrine effect of PTHrP stimulates smooth muscle cell growth, whereas the paracrine effects inhibit cell division *(17)*. Thus, the results of antibody studies apply only to the epitope involved and cannot be extended to PTHrP in general or all actions of the protein. The high degree of variability in the effects of PTHrP in different tissues is another factor. PTHrP has both positive and negative effects on proliferation, apoptosis, or angiogenesis, depending on the tissue *(22,119,137,140)*. In fact, PTHrP inhibits growth in some clones of breast cancer cells and stimulates it in others *(153)*. A final factor might be interactions of PTHrP with the particular cancer, interactions that could vary with stage, patient comorbidities, or heterogeneity within the cancer. PTHrP is a complex, multifunctional protein that can activate multiple regulatory pathways, affect many cellular processes, and interact with numerous targets. Comprehensive studies will be needed to develop a complete understanding how PTHrP affects the pathophysiology of cancer.

In summary, PTHrP has many functions in pulmonary physiology. It might play a role in lung development, homeostasis in the aloveolar space, alveolar epithelial growth, the response to lung injury, and the pathophysiology of lung cancer. Based on effects on pulmonary cellular physiology and organ function, the protein could be useful as a marker of lung maturity, risk of lung injury, or presence of lung cancer. The protein is likely to have important effects in pulmonary carcinogenesis, lung cancer progression, metastasis, and outcome. Many studies have concentrated on the role of PTHrP in hypercalcemia of malignancy, but its role in the malignant nature of lung cancer is a relatively untouched, potentially fruitful area for investigation.

5. CURRENT CONCEPTS

Several mechanisms regulate the development and progression of cancer metastases to the skeleton, and they can be generally considered under the classical seed and soil paradigm. They included (1) exodus of the tumor from its primary site, (2) homing of the tumor to the skeleton, (3) invasion of the skeleton by the tumor, (4) the genesis of blood supply, and (5) osteolysis accompanied by a reactive but defective osteoblastosis. Each of these mechanisms is mediated by a variety of molecular factors. For example, exodus of the tumor from its primary site involves the expression enzymes like the matrix metalloproteinases (MMPs) that free the tumor from its site and adhesion molecules like the integrins that allow the tumor to migrate. These proteinases can also degrade vascular basement membranes and, thus, provide access to the vascular and lymphatic systems. The homing is mediated by tumor and target receptors like the chemokine receptor CXCR4 and by the PTHrP receptor that can attract and attach the tumor to skeleton and marrow cells. Invasion of the skeleton is also mediated by proteolytic enzmes that destroy target structures, such as MMP-2 and MMP-9. Angiogenesis is mediated by a variety of angiogenic factors such as vascular endothelial growth factor (VEGF) and connective tissue growth factor (CTGF). Also, osteolysis is mediated by the family of osteokines that include M-CSF, osteopontin RANK, RANKL, TRAIL, and OPG. The factors that mediate the reactive, perhaps compensatory, osteoblastosis that accompanies osteolysis are not well known, but likely include endothelin and bone morphogenetic proteins.

Once in bone, the tumor amplifies the metastatic process by releasing several growth factors from the resorbed bone that establish a cycle of tumor progression. These include TFG-β, TNF, insulin-like growth factor, and platelet-derived growth factor. The metastatic process is also amplified by tumor-derived growth factors, notably IL-1, IL-6, IL-8, and IL-11. In addition to bone and tumor cells, stromal interaction play an important role in tumor progression *(104)*.

Parathyroid hormone-related protein exerts a central regulatory role among these molecular interactions. This oncoprotein influences the production of essentially all of the tumor regulatory factors and stimulates most of them. In addition, PTHrP promotes osteoclastic activity by enhance the entry of precursor cells into the osteoclastogenic pathway.

Contemporary analytical procedures are identifying cancer regulating genes on a frequent basis, with new regulators molecules continuing to be identified *(105,106)*. In addition to PTHrP, these metastases-mediating molecules might be targeted for therapeutic intervention using antibodies, antagonists, antitransducers, aptamers, antireceptors, and antitranscriptional modalities.

ACKNOWLEDGMENTS

This work was supported by VA Merit Review awards, The National Institutes of Health (ES09227, DK60588, and AR47347), the California Tobacco-Related Disease Research Program, and the Flight Attendants Medical Research Institute.

REFERENCES

1. Rabbani SA. Molecular mechanism of action of parathyroid hormone related peptide in hypercalcemia of malignancy: therapeutic strategies (review). *Int J Oncol* 2000; 16:197–206.
2. Rabbani SA, Gladu J, Harakidas P, Jamison B, Goltzman D. Over-production of parathyroid hormone-related peptide results in increased osteolytic skeletal metastasis by prostate cancer cells in vivo. *Int J Cancer* 1999; 80:257–264.
3. Deftos, LJ. Prostate carcinoma: Production of bioactive factors. *Cancer* 2000; 88:3002–3008.
4. Deftos LJ. PTHrP regulates prostate cancer progression in bone. *J Invest Med* 2003; 51.S1.A154.
5. Ahmadpour OA, Burton DW, Tu S, Deftos LJ. Regulation of OPG/RANK/RANKL by PTHrP peptides in human prostate cancer cells. *J Bone Miner Res* 2002; 17:S286.
6. Jans Da, Thomas RJ, Gillespie MT. Parathyroid hormone-related protein (PTHrP): nucleocytoplasmic shuttling protein with distinct paracrine and intracrine roles. *Vitam Horm* 2003; 66:345–384.
7. Corey E, Quinn JE, Bladou F, Brown LG, Roudier MO, Brown JM, et al. Establishment and characterization of osseous prostate cancer models: intra-tibial injection of human prostate cancer cells. *Prostate* 2002; 52:20–33.
8. Xu M, Jiang P, Yang M, Burton D, Deftos LJ, Hoffman RM. PTHrP expression promotes prostate cancer metastases in orthotopic models. *Tumor Cell Biol* 2002; 43:378,379.
9. Lam MHC, Thomas RJ, Martin TJ, Gillespie MT, Jans DA. Nuclear and nucleolar localization of parathyroid hormone-related protein. *Immunol Cell Biol* 2000; 78:395–402.
10. Goltzman D. Interactions of PTH and PTHrP with the PTH/PTHrP receptor and with downstream signaling pathways: Exceptions that provide the rules. *J Bone Min Res* 1999; 14:173–177.
11. Yang KH, Stewart AF. PTHrP: The gene, its mRNA species, and protein products. In: Bilezikian JP, Raisy LG, Rodan GA, eds. *Principles of Bone Biology*. 4th ed. New York: Academic, 1996:Chap. 26.

12. Goomer RS, Johnson KA, Burton DW, Amiel D, Maris TM, Gurjal A, Deftos LJ, et al. The tetrabasic KKKK147-150 motif determines intracrine regulatory effects of PTHrP 1-173 on Chondrocyte Ppi metabolism and matrix synthesis. *Endocrinology* 2000; 141:4613–4622.

13. Deftos LJ, Burton D, Hastings RH, Terkeltaub R, Hook VY. Comparative tissue distribution of the processing enzyme "prohormone thiol protease," and prohormone convertase 1 and 2, in human PTHrP-producing cell lines and mammalian neuroendocrine tissues. *Endocrine* 2001; 15:217–224.

14. Wysolmerski JJ, Philbrick WM, Dunbar ME, Lanske B, Kronenberg H, Broadus AE. Rescue of the parathyroid hormone-related protein knockout mouse demonstrates that parathyroid hormone-related protein is essential for mammary gland development. *Development* 1998; 125:1285–1294.

15. Karaplis AC, Luz A, Glowacki J, Bronson RT, Tybulewicz VLJ, Kronenberg HM, et al. Lethal skeletal dysplasia from targeted disruption of the parathyroid hormone-related peptide gene. *Genes Dev* 1994; 8:277–289.

16. Wysolmerski JJ, Broadus AE, Zhou J, Fuchs E, Milstone LM, Philbrick WM. Overexpression of parathyroid hormone related protein in the skin of transgenic mice interferes with hair follicle development. *Proc Natl Acad Sci* 1994; 91:1133–1137.

17. Vasavada R, Cavalieri C, E'Ercole AJ, Dapp P, Burtis WJ, Madlener AL, et al. Overexpression of parathyroid hormone-related protein in the pancreatic islets of transgenic mice causes islet hyperplasia, hyperinsulinemia, and hypoglycemia. *J Biol Chem* 1998; 271:1200–1208.

18. Massfelder T, Dann P, Wu TL, Vasavada R, Helwig J-J, Stewart AF. Opposing mitogenic and antimitogenic actions of parathyroid hormone-related protein in vascular smooth muscle cells: A critical role for nuclear targeting. *PNAS* 1997; 94:13,630–13,635.

19. Kano J, Slugimoto T, Fukase M, Fujita. The activation of cyclic AMP-dependent protein kinase is directly linked to the inhibition of osteoblast proliferation (UMR-106) by parathyroid hormone-related protein. *Biochem Biophys Res Commun* 1991; 179:97–101.

20. Iezzoni JC, Bruns ME, Frierson HF, Scott MG, Pence RA, Deftos LJ, et al. Co-expression of parathyroid hormone-related protein and its receptor in breast carcinoma: A potential autocrine effector system. *Modern Pathology* 1998; 11:265–270.

21. Bucht E, Rong H, Sandberg Nordqvist A-C, Eriksson E, von Schoultz E, et al. Parathyroid Hormone-Related Protein in patients with breast cancer and eucalcemia. *Cancer Res* 1998; 58:4113–4116.

22. Hastings RH, Summers-Torres D, Cheung TC, Ditmer LS, Burton DW, et al. Parathyroid hormone-related protein, an autocrine regulatory factor in alveolar epithelial cells. *Am J Physiol* 1996; 278: 353–361.

23. Hastings RH, Summers-Torres S, Yaszay B, LeSeure J, Burton DW, Deftos LJ. Parathyroid hormone-related protein, autocrine growth inhibitor of alveolar type II epithelial cells. *Am J Physiol* 1997; 272: 394–399.

24. Rabbini SA, Gladu J, Liu B, Goltzman D. Regulation in vivo of the growth of Leydig tumors by antisense ribonucleic acid for parathyroid hormone-related peptide. *Endocrinolgy* 1995; 136:5416–5422.

25. Burton PBJ, Moniz C, Knight DE. Parathyroid hormone related peptide can function as an autocrine growth factor in human renal cell carcinoma. *Biochem Biophys Res Commun* 1990; 167: 11,234–11,238.

27. Gujral A, Burton DW, Terkeltaub R, Deftos LJ. PTHrP induces IL-8 production by prostate cancer cells via a novel intracrine mechanism not mediated by its classical nuclear localizing sequence. *Cancer Res* 2001; 61:2282–2288.

28. Logan A. Intracrine regulation at the nucleusBa further mechanism of growth factor activity. *J Endocrinol* 1990; 125:339–343.

29. Lam MHC, House CM, Tiganis T, Mitchelhill KI, Sarcevic B, Cures A, et al. Phosphorylation at the Cyclin-dependent Kinases site (Thr85) of parathyroid hormone-related protein negatively regulates its nuclear localization. *J Biol Chem* 1999; 274:18,559–18,566.

30. Lam MHC, Briggs LJ, Hu W, Martin TJ, Gillespie MT, Jans DA. Importin â recognized parathyroid hormone-related protein with high affinity and mediates its nuclear import in the absence of Importin á. *J Biol Chem* 1999; 274:7391–7398.

31. Henderson JE, Amizuka N, Warshawsky H, Biasotto D, Lanske BM, Goltzman D, Karaplis AC. Nucleolar localization of parathyroid hormone-related peptide enhances survival of chondrocytes under conditions that promote apoptotic cell death. *Mol Cell Biol* 1995; 115:4064–4075.

32. Aarts MM, Rix A, Guo K, Bringhurst R, Henderson JE. The nucleolar targeting signal (NTS) of parathyroid hormone related protein mediates endocytosis and nucleolar translocation. *J Bone Min Res* 1999; 14:1493–1503.

33. Watson PH, Fraher LJ, Natale BV, Kisiel M, Hendy GN, Hodsman AB. Nuclear localization of the type 1 parathyroid hormone/parathyroid hormone-related peptide receptor in MC3T3-E1 cells: Association with serum-induced cell proliferation. *Bone* 2000; 2626:221–225.

34. Watson PH, Fraher LJ, Hendy GN, Chung U-I, Kisiel M, Natale BV, Hodsman AB. Nuclear localization of the type 1 PTH/PTHrP peceptor in rat tissues. *J Bone Miner Res* 2000; 15:1033–1044.

35. Kaiser SM, Sebag M, Rhim JS, Kremer R, Goltzman D. Antisense-medication inhibition of parathyroid hormone related peptide production in a keratinocyte cell line impedes differentiation. *Mol Endocrinol* 1994; 8:139–147.

36. Kaiser SM, Laneuville P, Bernier SM, Rhim JS, Kremer R, Goltzman D. Enhanced growth of a human keratinocyte cell line induced by antisense RNA for parathyroid hormone-related peptide. *J Biol Chem* 1992; 267:13,623–13,628.

26. Bouvet M, Nardin SR, Burton DW, Lee NC, Yang M, Wang X, et al. Parathyroid hormone-related protein as a novel tumor marker in pancreatic adenocarcinoma. *Pancreas* 2002; 24:284–290.

37. Aarts MM, Levy D, He B, Stregger S, Chen T, Richard Sand Henderson JE. Parathyroid hormone related protein interacts with RNA. *J Biol Chem* 1999; 274:4832–4838.

38. Peehl DM, Edgar MG, Cramer SD, Deftos LJ. Parathyroid hormone-related protein (PTHrP) is not an autocrine growth factor for normal prostatic epithelial cells. *Prostate* 1997; 31:47–52.

39. Burton DW, Tu S, Smith KC, Ho TP, Rhim JS, Deftos LJ. PTHrP processed peptides regulate prostate cell growth. *Bone* 1998; 23:142.

40. Wu G, Iwamura M, di Sant-Agnese PA, Deftos LJ, Cockett ATK, Gershagen S. Characterization of the cell-specific expression of parathyroid hormone-related protein in normal and neoplastic prostate tissue. *Urology* 1998; 51:110–120.

41. Iwamura M, Wu G, di Sant 'Agnese PA, Cockett ATK, Deftos LJ, Abrahamsson P-A. Immunohistochemical localization of parathyroid hormone-related protein in human prostate cancer. *Cancer Res* 1993; 53:1724–1726.

42. Brandt DW, Wachsman W, Deftos LJ. Parathyroid hormone-like protein alternative mRNA splicing pathways in human cancer cell lines. *Cancer Res* 1994; 54:850–853.

43. Deftos LJ, Gujral A, Rhim JS, Bruns DE, Burton DW. Co-expression of the PTHrP Receptor and PTHrP peptides in human prostate cells. *Proceedings of the 81st Annual Meeting of the Endocrine Society* 1999; 413:626.

44. Iwamura M, Abrahamsson P-A, Foss KA, Wu G, Cockett ATK, Deftos LJ. PTHrP: A potential autocrine growth factor in human prostate cancer cell lines. *Urology* 1994; 43:675–679.

45. Cramer SC, Peehl DM, Edger MG, Wong ST, Deftos LJ, Feldman D. Parathyroid hormone-related protein (PTHrP) is an epidermal growth factor-regulated secretory product of human prostatic epithelial cells. *Prostate* 1996; 29:20–29.

46. Deftos, LJ. Granin-A, parathyroid hormone related protein, and calcitonin gene products in neuroendocrine prostate cancer. *Prostate* 1996; 8:23–31.

47. Gujral A, Burton DW, Arrington LS, Terkeltaub RA, Deftos LJ. PTHrP mediates its effects on prostate carcinoma cells via an intracrine pathway that stimulates IL-6, IL-8 expression and MAP kinase signaling. *J Bone Min Res* 1999; 14:210.

48. Asadi F, Farraj M, Sharifi R, Malakouti S, Antar S, Kukreja S. Enhanced expression of parathyroid hormone-related protein in prostate cancer as compared with benign prostatic hyperplasia. *Human Pathol* 1996; 27:1319–1323.

49. Goltzman D, Henderson J, Kaiser S, Kremer R, Rabbani SA, Hendy GN. Studies of the molecular biology of parathyroid hormone-like peptide. *J Endocrinol Invest* 1992; 15:43–49.

50. Dougherty KM, Blomme EA, Koh AJ, Henderson JE, Pienta KJ, Rosol TJ, McCauley LK. Parathyroid hormone-related protein as a growth regulator of prostate carcinoma. *Cancer Res* 1999; 59:6015–6022.

51. Blomme EA, Dougherty KM, Pienta KJ, Capen CC, Rosol TH, McCauley LK. Skeletal metastasis of prostate adenocarcinoma in rats: morphometric analysis and role of parathyroid hormone-related protein. *Prostate* 1999; 39:187–197.

52. Kremer R, Goltzman D, Amizuka N, Webber MM, Rhim JS. Ras activation of human prostate epithelial cells induces overexpression of parathyroid hormone-related peptide. *Clin Cancer Res* 1997; 3:855–859.

53. Blomme EA, Sugimoto Y, McCauley LK, Lin YC, Capen CC, Rosol TJ. Stromal and epithelial cells of the canine prostate express parathyroid hormone-related protein, but not the PTH/PTHrP receptor. *Prostate* 1998; 36:110–120.

54. Iwamura M, Hellman J, Cockett AT, Lilja H, Gershagen S. Alteration of the hormonal bioactivity of parathyroid hormone-related protein (PTHrP) as a result of limited proteolysis by prostate-specific antigen. *Urology* 1996; 48:317–325.

55. Cramer SD, Chen Z, Peehl DM. Prostate specific antigen cleaves parathyroid hormone-related protein in the like domain: inactivation of PTHrP-stimulated cAMP accumulation in mouse osteoblasts. *J Urol* 1996; 156:526–531.

56. Perez-Stable C, Altman NH, Mehta PP, Deftos LJ, Roos BA. Prostate cancer progression, metastasis, and gene expression in transgenic mice. *Cancer Res* 1997; 57:900–906.

57. Dougherty KM, Blomme EAG, Koh AJ, Pienta KJ, Henderson JE, Rosol TJ, McCauley LK. PTHrP as a regulator of growth and apoptosis in prostate carcinoma. *Cancer Res* 2000; 59:6015–6022.

58. Iddon J, Bundred NJ, Hoyland J, Downey SE, Baird P, Salter D, et al. Expression of parathyroid hormone-related protein and its receptor in bone metastases from prostate cancer. *J Pathol* 2000; 191:170–174.

59. Tovar Sepulveda VA, Falzon M. Parathyroid hormone-related protein enhances PC-3 prostate cancer cell growth via both autocrine/paracrine and intracrine pathways. *Regul Pept* 2002; 105:109–120.

60. Wachsman W, Burton DW, Chang H-S, Deftos LJ. PTHrP regulates B-cell proliferation through apoptosis. *J Bone Mineral Res* 1998; 23:W196.

61. Asadi F, Faraj M, Malakouti S, Kukreja SC. Effect of PTHrP and dihydrotestosterone on proliferation and ornithine decarboxylase mRNA in human prostate cancer cell lines. *Int Urol Nephrol* 2001; 33: 417–422.

62. Gleave ME, Jer-Tsong Hsieh. Animal models in prostate cancer. In: Raghavan, Scher, Leibel, Lange, eds. *Principles and Practice of Genitourinary Oncology.* 1996:367–378.

63. Thalman G, Anezinis P, Chung LWK, Devoll R, Farach-Carson C. Experimental approaches to skeletal metastasis of human prostate cancer. In: Raghavan, Scher, Leibel, Lange, eds. *Principles and Practice of Genitourinary Oncology.* 1996:409–416.

64. Shevrin DH, Kukreja SC, Ghosh L, Lad TE. Development of skeletal metastasis by human prostate cancer in athymic nude mice. *Clin Expl Metastasis* 1988; 6:401–409.

65. Veltri RW, Miller MC, Zhao G, NG A, Marley GM, Wright GL Jr, Vassela RL D. Interleukin-8 serum levels in patients with big benign prostatic hyperplasia and prostate cancer. *Urology* 1999; 53:139–147.

66. Chung TD, Yu JJ, Spiotto M T, Bartkowski M, Simons JW. Characterization of the role of IL-6 in the progression of prostate cancer. *Prostate* 1999; 15:199–207.

67. Sugihara A, Maeda O, Tsuji M, Tsujimura T, Nakata Y, Akedo H, et al. Expression of cytokines enhancing the osteoclast activity, and parathyroid hormone-related protein in prostatic cancers before and after endocrine therapy an immunohistochemical study. *Oncol Rep* 1998; 5:1389–1394.

68. Grey A, Mitnich MA, Masiukiewicz U, Sun BH, Rudikoff S, Jilka RL, et al. A role for interleukin-6 in parathyroid hornome-induced bone resorption in vivo. *Endocrinology* 1999; 140:4683–4690.

69. Hobisch A, Eder IE, Putz T, Horninger W, Bartsch G, Klocker H, Culig Z. IL-6 regulates PSA expression in prostate carcinoma cells by activation of the androgen receptor. *Cancer Res* 1998; 58:4640–4645.

70. De La Mata J, Un HL, Guise TA, Story B, Boyce BF, Mundy GR, et al. IL-6 enhances hypercalcemia and bone resorption mediated by parathyroid hormone related protein in vivo. *J Clin Invest* 1995; 95:2846–2852.

71. De Miguel, Martines-Fernandez P, Guillén C, Valin A, Rodrigo A, Martinez ME, Esbrit P. Parathyroid hormone-related protein (107-139) stimulates interleukin-6 expression in human osteoblastic cells. *J Am Soc Nephrol* 1999; 10:796–803.

72. Koeneman KS, Yeung F, Chung LWK. Osteomimetic properties of prostate cancer cells: A hypothesis supporting the predilection of prostate cancer metastasis and growth in the bone environment. *Prostate* 1999; 39:246–261.

73. Correale P, Micheli L, Vicchio MT, Sabatino M, Petrioli R, Pozzesser D, et al. A PTH-rP specific cytotoxic T cell response induced by in vitro stimulation of tumour-infiltrating lymphocytes derived from prostate cancer metastases, with epitope peptideBloaded autologous dendritic cells and low-dose IL-2. *Br J Cancer* 2001; 85:1722–1730.

74. Sanders JL, Chattopadhyay N, Kifor O, Yamaguchi T, Brown EM. Ca(2+)-sensing receeotpr expression and PTHrP secretion in PC-3 human prostate cancer cells. *Am J Physiol Endocrinol Metab* 2001; 281:E267–274.

75. Kao PC, Klee GG, Taylor RL, Heath H III. PTHrP in plasma of patients with hypercalcemia and malignant lesions. *Mayo Clin Proc* 1990; 65:1399–1407.

76. Burton DW, Deftos LJ. Co-expression of the PTHrP Receptor and PTHrP Peptides in Human Prostate Cells. *Proceedings of the 81st Annual Meeting of the Endocrine Society* 1999.

77. Tovar Sepulveda VA, Falzon M. Regulation of PTH-related protein gene expression by vitamin D in PC-3 prostate cancer cells. *Mol Cell Endocrinol* 2002; 1990:115–124.

78. Mundy GR. Mechanisms of bone metastases. *Cancer* 1997; 80:1546–1556.

79. Bryden AA, Hoyland JA, Freemont AJ, Clarke NW, George NJ. PTHrP and receptor expression in paired primary prostate cancer and bone metastases. *Br J Cancer* 2002; 86:322–325.

80. Goltzman D, Karaplis AC, Kremer R, Rabbani SA. Molecular basis of the spectrum of skeletal complications of neoplasia. *Cancer* 2000; 88:2903–2908.

81. Guise TA. Parathyroid hormone-related protein and bone metastases. *Cancer* 1997; 80:1546–1556.

82. Deftos LJ. Hypercalcemia in malignant and inflammatory diseases. *Endocrinol Metab Clin North Am* 2002; 31:141–158.

83. Hofbauer LC, Khosla S, Dunstan CR, Lacey DL, Boyle WJ, Riggs BL. The roles of osteoprotegerin and osteoprotegerin ligand in the paracrine regulation of bone resorption. *J Bone Miner Res* 2000; 15: 2–12.

84. Mancini L, Moradi-Bidhendi N, Brandi ML, Brandi ML, Perretti M, MacIntyre I. Modulation of the effects of osteoprotegerin (OPG) ligand in human leukemic cell line by OPG and calcitonin. *Biochem Biophys Res Commun* 2000; 279:391–397.

85. Nagai M, Kyakumoto S, Sato N. Cancer cells responsible for humoral hypercalcemia express mRNA encoding a secreted form of ODF/TRANCE that induces osteoclast formation. *Biochem Biophys Res Commun* 2000; 269:532–536.

86. Chung TD, Yu JJ, Spiotto MT, Bartkowski M, Simons JW. Characterization of the role of IL-6 in the progression of prostate cancer. *Prostate* 1999; 15:199–207.

87. Nagai Y, Yamato H, Akaogi K, Hirose K, Ueyma Y, Ikeda K, et al. Role of interleukins-6 in uncoupling of bone in vivo in a human squamous carcinoma coproducing parathyroid hormone-related peptide and interleukin-6. *J Bone Miner Res* 1998; 13:664–672

88. Yoneda T, Nakai M, Moriyama K, Scott L, Ida N, Kunitomo T, Mundy GR. Neutralizing antibodies to human IL-6 reverse hypercalcemia associated with a human squamous carcinoma. *Cancer Res* 1993; 53:737–740.

89. Weissglas M, Schamhart D, Lowik C, Papapoulos S, Vos P, Kurth KH. Hypercalcemia and osteosecretion of IL-6 and Parathyroid hormone related peptide by a human renal cell carcinioma implanted in nude mice. *J Urol* 1995; 153:854–857.

90. de la Mata J, Un HL, Guise TA, Story B, Boyce BF, Mundy GR, Roodman GD. IL-6 enhances hypercalcemia and bone resorption mediated by parathyroid hormone related protein in vivo. *J Clin Invest* 1995; 95:2846–2852.

91. Roodman GD. Interleukin-6 - an osteotropic factor. *J Bone Miner Res* 1992; 7:475–478.

92. Ferrer FA, Miller LJ, Andrawis RI, Kurtzman SH, Albertsen PC, Laudone VP, Kreutzer DL. Angiogenesis and prostate cancer: in vivo and in vitro expression of angiogenesis factors by prostate cancer cells. *Urology* 1998; 51:161–167.

93. Bar-Eli M. Role of IL-8 in tumor growth and metastases of melanoma. *Pathobiology* 1999; 67:12–18.

94. Bakre MM, Zhu Y, Yin H, Burton DW, Terkeltaub R, Deftos LJ, Varner A. Parathyroid hormone-related peptide is a naturally occurring, protein knase A-dependent angiognesis inhibitor. *Nature Med* 2002; 8:995–1003.

95. Bouvet M, Nardin SR, Burton DW, Gujral A, Behling C, Carethers JM, Deftos LJ. Growth regulating properties of PTHrP in pancreatic adenocarcinoma. *J Bone Mineral Res* 2000; 15:S254.

96. Bouvet M, SR Nardin, DW Burotn, C Behling, JM Carethers, RM Hoffman, AR Moossa, and LJ Deftos. Parathyroid hormone-related protein expression in human pancreatic adenocarcinoma. *Gastroenterology* 2000; 118:A1043.

97. Bouvet M, Burton DW, Nardin SR, Moossa AR, Deftos LJ. Parathroid hormone related protein regulates cytokine expression in pancreatic adenocarcinoma. *Proceedings of the 83rd Annual Meeting of the Endocrine Society* 2001;1–223.

98. Maheshwari VV, Burton DW, Hastings RH, Aguilera JA, Pardo FS, Deftos LJ. Apoptotic Effects of Parathyroid Hormone Related Protein in Prostate Cancer Cells. *J Bone Mineral Res* 2003; 18:S199.

99. Pizzi H, Gladu J, Carpio L, Miao D, Goltzman D, Rabbani SA. Androgen regulation of parathyroid hormone-related peptide production in human prostate cancer cells. *Endocrinology* 2003; 144:858–867.

100. Shen X, Falzon M. Parathyroid hormone-related protein upregulates integrin expression via an intracrine pathway in PC-3 prostate cancer cells. *Regul Pept* 2003; 13:17–29.

101. Shen X, Falzon M.PTH-related protein modulates PC-3 prostate cancer cell adhesion and integrin subunit profile. *Mol Cell Endocrinol* 2003; 199:165–177.
102. Grzesiak JJ, Chalberg C, Smith K, Burton DW, Silletti S, Moossa AR, Deftos LJ, Bouvet M. The extracellular matrix differentially regulates the expression of the PTH/PTHrP receptor in pancreatic cancer. *J Bone Miner Res* 2003; 18:309.
103. Keller ET, Zhang J, Cooper CR, Smith PC, McCauley LK, Pienta KJ, et al. Prostate carcinoma skeletal metastases: cross-talk between tumor and bone. *Cancer Metastasis Rev* 2001; 20:333–349.
104. Chung, L, et al. New targets for therapy in prostate cancer: Modulation of stromal-epithelial interactions. *Urology* 2003; 62:44–54.
105. Liang P, Pardee AB. Analyzing differential gene expression in cancer. *Nature Rev Cancer* 2003; 3: 869–873.
106. Shukeir N, Arakelian A, Kadhim S, Garde S, Rabbani SA. Prostate secretory protein PSP-94 decreases tumor growth and hypercalcemia of malignancy in a syngenic in vivo model of prostate cancer. *Cancer Res* 2003; 63:2072–2078.
107. Clark PE, Torti FM. Prostate cancer and bone metastases. *Clin Orthoped Rel Res* 2003; 415S:148–157.
108. Mohammad KS, Guise TA. Mechanisms of Osteoblastic Metastases. *Clin Orthoped Rel Res* 415S: 148–157.
109. Carano RAD, Filvaroff. Angiogenesis and bone repair. *Drug Discovery Today* 2003; 8:980–989.
110. Beer TM. Development of a weekly high-dose calcitriol based therapy for prostate cancer. *Urol Oncol* 2003; 21:399–405.
111. Rubin LP, Keyes CA, Tsai S-W, Pinar H, Torday JS, Kronenberg HM. The parathyroid hormone-related protein (PTHrP) knockout mouse shows delayed lung development. *Pediatric Res* 1997; 41:266a.
112. Lanske B, Karaplis AC, Lee K, et al. PTH/PTHrP receptor in early development and Indian Hedgehog-regulated bone growth. *Science* 1996; 2273:663–666.
113. Billis WM, Dreyer BE, Homer RJ, Philbrick WM. Regulation of branching morphogenesis in the lung by parathyroid hormone-related protein. *Bone* 1998; 23:S359.
114. Ramirez MI, Chung U-I, Williams MC. Aquaporin-5 expression, but not other peripheral lung marker genes, is reduced in PTH/PTHrP receptor null mutant fetal mice. *Am J Respir Cell Mol Biol* 1999; 22:367–372.
115. Lee K, Deeds JD, Segre GV. Expression of parathyroid hormone-related peptide and its receptor messenger ribonucleic acids during fetal development of rats. *Endocrinology* 1995; 136:453–463.
116. Rubin LP, Kifor O, Hua J, Brown EM, Torday JS. Parathyroid hormone (PTH) and PTH-related protein stimulate surfactant phospholipid synthesis in rat fetal lung, apparently by a mesenchymal-epithelial mechanism. *Biochim Biophys Acta* 1994; 1223:91–100.
117. Rubin LP, Torday JS Parathyroid hormone-related protein. In: Mendelson CR, ed. *Contemporatry Endocrinology: Endocrinology of the Lung: Development and Surfactant Synthesis.* Totowa, NJ: Humana, 2000: 269–297.
118. Hastings RH, Sandoval R, Quintana R, Burton DW, Deftos LJ. Amino-terminal and mid-molecule parathyroid hormone-related protein, phosphatidylcholine,and type II cell proliferation in silica lung injury. *Am J Physiol* 2003; 285:L1312–L1322.
119. Hastings RH, Quintana RA, Sandoval R, et al. Pro-apoptotic effects of parathyroid hormone-related protein in type II pneumocytes. *Am J Respir Cell Mol Biol* 2003; 29:733–742.
120. Speziale MV, Mannino FL, Berlin C, Hastings RH. Parathyroid hormone-related protein (PTHrP) is decreased in immature neonatal lung. *J Bone Mineral Res* 1997; 12:S214.
121. Torday JS, Torres E, Rehan VK. The role of fibroblast transdifferentiation in lung epithelial cell proliferation, differentiation, and repair in vitro. *Pediatr Pathol Mol Med* 2003; 22:189–207.
122. Hastings RH, Auger WR, Kerr KM, Quintana RA, Deftos LJ. Parathyroid hormone-related protein and lung injury after pulmonary thromboendarterectomy. *Regul Pept* 2001; 102:1–7.
123. Hastings RH, Berg JT, Summers-Torres D, Burton DW, Deftos LJ. Parathyroid hormone-related protein reduces alveolar epithelial cell proliferation during lung injury in rats. *Am J Physiol* 2000; 279:L194–L200.
124. Hastings RH, Asirvatham A, Quintana R, et al. Parathyroid hormone-related protein-(38-64) regulates lung cell proliferation after silica injury. *Am J Physiol* 2002; 283:L12–L21.
125. Hastings RH, Ryan RM, D'Angio CT, et al. Parathyroid hormone-related protein response to hyperoxic lung injury. *Am J Physiol Lung Cell Mol Physiol* 2002; 282:L1198–L1208.

126. Hastings RH, Araiza F, Burton DW, Deftos LJ. Role of parathyroid hormone-related protein in lung cancer cell survival. *Chest* 2003.

127. Brandt DW, Burton DW, Gazdar AF, Oie HE, Deftos LJ. All major lung cancer cell types produce parathyroid hormone-like protein: Heterogeneity assessed by high performance liquid chromatography. *Endocrinology* 1991; 129:2466–2470.

128. Moseley JM, Kubota M, Diefenbach-Jagger H, et al. Parathyroid hormone-related protein purified from a human lung cancer cell line. *Proc Natl Acad Sci USA* 1987; 84:5084–5052.

129. Asa SL, Henderson J, Goltzman D, Drucker DJ. Parathyroid hormone-like peptide in normal and neoplastic human endocrine tissues. *J Clin Endocrinol* 1990; 71:1112–1118.

130. Davidson LA, Black M, Carey FA, Lugue F, McNicol AM. Lung tumors immunoreactive for parathyroid hormone related peptide: analysis of serum calcium levels and tumour type. *J Pathology* 1996; 178:398–401.

131. Kitazawa S, Fukase M, Kitazawa R, et al. Immunohistologic evaluation of parathyroid hormone-related protein in human lung cancer and normal tissue with newly developed monoclonal antibody. *Cancer* 1991; 67:984–989.

132. Nishigaki Y, Ohsaki Y, Toyoshima E, Kikuchi K. Increased serum and urinary levels of a parathyroid hormone-related protein COOH terminus in non-small cell lung cancer patients. *Clin Cancer Res* 1999; 5:1473–1481.

133. Truong NU, deB Edwards MD, Papavasiliou V, Goltzman D, Kremer R. Parathyroid hormone-related peptide and survival of patients with cancer and hypercalcemia. *Am J Med* 2003; 115:115–121.

134. Burtis WJ, Brady TG, Orloff JJ, et al. Immunochemical characterization of circulating parathyroid hormone-related protein in patients with humoral hypercalcemia of cancer: PTHrP and PTHrP peptides. *J Med* 1990; 322:1106–1112.

135. Suva LJ, Winslow GA, Wettenhall RE, et al. A parathyroid hormone-related protein implicated in malignant hypercalcemia: cloning and expression. *Science* 1987; 237:896–896.

136. Burton PBJ, Knight DE. Parathyroid hormone-related peptide can regulate the growth of human lung cancer cells, and may form part of an autocrine TGF-_ loop. *FEBS Lett.* 1992; 305:228–232.

137. Hastings RH, Araiza F, Burton DW, Zhang L, Bedley M, Deftos LJ. Parathyroid hormone-related protein ameliorates death receptor-mediated apoptosis in lung cancer cells. *Am J Physiol Cell Physiol* 2003; 285:C1429–C1436.

138. Muzio M, Chinnaiyan AM, Kischkel FC, et al. FLICE, a novel FADD-homologous ICE/CED-3-like protease, is recruited to the CD95 (Fas/APO-1) death—inducing signaling complex. *Cell Mol Life Sci* 1996; 85:817–827.

139. Cowling V, Downward J. Caspase-6 is the direct activator of caspase-8 in the cytochrome c-induced apoptosis pathway: absolute requirement for removal of caspase-6 prodomain. *Cell Death Differ* 2002; 9:1046–1056.

140. Akino K, Ohtsuru A, Kanda K, et al. Parathyroid hormone-related peptide is a potent tumor angiogenic factor. *Endocrinology* 2000; 141:4313–4316.

141. Luparello C, Sirchia R, Pupello D. PTHrP [67-86] regulates the expression of stress proteins in breast cancer cells inducing modifications in urokinase-plasminogen activator and MMP-1 expression. *J Cell Sci* 2003; 116:2421–2430.

142. Ye Y, Seitz PK, Cooper CW. Parathyroid hormone-related protein overexpression in the human colon cancer cell line HT-29 enhances adhesion of the cells to collagen type I. *Regul Pept* 2001; 101:19–23.

143. Hiraki A, Ueoka H, Bessho A, et al. Parathyroid hormone-related protein measured at the time of first visit is an indicator of bone metastases and survival in lung carcinoma patients with hypercalcemia. *Cancer* 2002; 95:1706–1713.

144. Hutchesson AC, Bundred NJ, Ratcliffe WA. Survival in hypercalcaemic patients with cancer and co-existing primary hyperparathyroidism. *Postgrad Med J* 1995; 71:28–31.

145. Pecherstorfer M, Schilling T, Blind E, et al. Parathyroid hormone-related protein and life expectancy in hypercalcemic cancer patients. *J Clin Endocr Metab* 1994; 78:1268–1270.

146. Hidaka N, Nishimura M, Nagao K. Establishment of two human small cell lung cancer cell lines: the evidence of accelerated production of parathyroid hormone-related protein with tumor progression. *Cancer Lett* 1998; 125:149–155.

147. Iguchi H, Tanaka S, Ozawa Y, et al. An experimental model of bone metastasis by human lung cancer cells: the role of parathyroid hormone-related protein in bone metastasis. *Cancer Res* 1996; 56:4040–4043.

148. Guise TA, Yin JJ, Taylor SD, et al. Evidence for a causal role of parathyroid hormone-related protein in the pathogenesis of human breast cancer-mediated osteolysis. *J Clin Invest* 1996; 98:1544–1549.

149. Hastings RH, Burton DW, Quintana RA. Biederman E, Gujral A, Deftos LJ. Parathyroid hormone-related protein regulates the growth of orthotopic human lung tumors in athymic mice. *Cancer* 2001; 15:1402–1410.

150. Henderson MA, Danks JA, Moseley JM, et al. Parathyroid hormone-related protein production by breast cancers, improved survival and reduced bone metastases. *J Natl Cancer Inst* 2001; 93:234–237.

151. Surowiak P, DDziegiel P, Matkowski R, et al. Prognostic value of immunocytochemical determination of parathyroid hormone-related peptide expression in cells of mammary ductal carcinoma. Analysis of 7 years of the disease course. *Virchows Arch* 2003; 442:245–251.

152. Linforth R, Anderson N, Hoey R, et al. Coexpression of parathyroid hormone related protein and its receptor in early breast cancer predicts poor patient survival. *Clin Cancer Res* 2002; 8:3172–3177.

153. Luparello C, Birch MA, Gallagher JA, Burtis WJ. Clonal heterogeneity of the growth and invasive response of a human breast carcinoma cell line to parathyroid hormone-related peptide fragments. *Carcinogenesis* 1997; 18:23–29.

11 Antithrombotics in Tumor Growth and Metastasis

Shaker A. Mousa, PhD, MBA, FACC, FACB

Contents

1. INTRODUCTION

Metastasis of cancer cells from a primary site involves a sequence of events, including the extravasation of the tumor cells into circulation and the interactions with platelets and other components of the hemostatic system *(1,2)*. These interactions, in turn, result in the adhesion and penetration of these metastatic cells and subsequent intravasation into the tissue. Several studies demonstrated that tumor cells form complexes with platelets, fibrin, and leukocytes in the vasculature, forming microemboli *(3,4)*. Thrombin is a key final common pathway that plays a significant role in activating platelets and generating fibrin for enhanced tumor metastasis.

There are numerous reports in the literature that suggest the progression of cancer is associated with changes in cell surface glycosylation. More specifically, it has been noted that carcinomas expressing high levels of sialylated, fucosylated mucins have a poorer prognosis because of greater extent of metastasis. This metastatic process is facilitated by the coating of the mucin-expressing tumor cells with platelets, an interaction that is mediated by tumor cell mucin and platelet P-selectin *(5–7)*. The progression of cancer

From: *Cancer Drug Discovery and Development*
Bone Metastasis: Experimental and Clinical Therapeutics
Edited by: G. Singh and S. A. Rabbani © Humana Press Inc., Totowa, NJ

consists of a series of sequential steps, and its outcome depends on interactions between malignant cells and various host factors.

2. COAGULATION AND CANCER

The association between coagulation system activation and systemic thrombosis in human cancers has been recognized for over a century. It was first shown in Trousseau's original description of migratory thrombophlebitis complicating gastrointestinal malignancy *(8)*. Greater appreciation in recent years of the interdependency of the coagulation system and malignant behavior has led to an understanding of how an activated coagulation system could, in turn, enhance cancer cell growth *(9)*. Although this does not establish causality or even a biologic association, it is of interest that a recent Danish study showed that patients with cancer who developed venous thrombosis during the course of their disease had significantly shorter cancer-related survival than similar patients who remained thrombosis-free *(10)*. More convincingly, several studies have shown, conversely, that cancer-related survival is improved in patients treated with anticoagulants compared to those not receiving anticoagulants *(11–14)*. Fibrin(ogen) is a critical determinant of metastatic potential, but thrombin appears to contribute to tumor cell dissemination through at least one fibrinogen-independent mechanism. These findings suggest that therapeutic strategies directed at several hemostatic factors might be useful in the suppression of metastasis.

3. PLATELETS AND CANCER

Activated platelets release angiogenic growth factors and have, therefore, been proposed to contribute to tumor angiogenesis *(15–17)*. Growth factors dervied from platelets could include the following: vascular endothelial growth factor (VEGF), basic fibroblast growth factor (bFGF), and platelet-derived growth factor (PDGF) *(15–17)*. The role of platelets in tumor biology has been suggested *(18)*. Serum levels of VEGF have been shown to correlate with platelet counts during chemotherapy *(19)*. Platelet–tumor cell interactions are believed to be important in tumor metastasis. Tumor cell tissue factor (TF) expression enhances metastasis and angiogenesis and is primarily responsible for tumor-induced thrombin generation and the formation of tumor cell–platelet aggregates. Activated platelets express and release CD40 ligand (CD40L), which induces endothelial TF expression by binding to CD40. It has been shown that, in malignancy, the increase in cellular TF activity via CD40 (tumor cell)–CD40L (platelet) interaction might enhance intravascular coagulation and hematogenous metastasis *(20)*. Inhibition of experimental metastasis and tumor growth was demonstrated in animals by thrombocytopenia and antiplatelet therapies *(21,22)*.

Cancer disturbs cellular activities that maintain multicellular organisms, namely growth, differentiation, apoptosis, and tissue integrity. There are numerous clinical and experimental observations showing that invasion results from the crosstalk between cancer cells and host cells, comprising platelet, myofibroblasts, endothelial cells, and leukocytes, all of which are themselves invasive. In bone metastasis, host osteoclasts serve as targets for therapy. The molecular analysis of invasion-associated cellular activities (namely homotypic and heterotypic cell–cell adhesion, cell–matrix interactions, and ectopic survival, migration, and proteolysis) reveal branching signal transduction pathways with extensive networks between individual pathways. Cellular responses to invasion-stimulatory molecules (such as scatter factor, chemokines, leptin, trefoil factors, and bile acids) or inhibitory factors (such as platelet-activating factor and thrombin) depend on activation of trimeric G proteins, phosphoinositide 3-kinase, and the Rac and Rho family of small GTPases. The role of proteolysis in invasion is not limited to breakdown of extracellular matrix but also to the cleavage of proinvasive fragments from cell surface glycoproteins.

In vivo, tumor cells interact with a variety of host cells such as endothelial cells and platelets, and these interactions are mediated by integrins GPIIb/IIIa and $\alpha v\beta 3$. In a xenograft model, m7E3 Fab'2 binds to both human tumor and host platelet GPIIb/IIIa and endothelial $\alpha v\beta 3$ integrins, thus participating as an antiangiogenic agent and an antitumor agent. Data suggested that combined blockade of GPIIb/IIIa and $\alpha v\beta 3$ affords significant antiangiogenic and antitumor benefit *(23)*. Classic studies indicate that the formation of tumor cell–platelet complexes in the bloodstream is important in facilitating the metastatic process. Metastasis in animal models can be inhibited by heparin, and retrospective analyses of heparin use in human cancer have supported this idea *(24)*.

The activation of coagulation, angiogenesis, and inflammatory cytokines are considered to be related to tumor growth and metastasis. A recent study demonstrated that the plasma levels of platelet microparticles (PMP), VEGF, interleukin (IL)-6, and regulated on activation, normal T-cell expressed and secreted (RANTES) were markedly increased in patients with stage IV disease and that these increased plasma levels of IL-6, RANTES, and especially PMP might be useful for identifying metastatic gastric patients *(25)*.

A recent preclinical study demonstrated a critical role for platelet αIIβ3 in tumor entry into bone and suggested a mechanism by which antiplatelet therapy might be beneficial in preventing the metastasis of solid tumors *(26)*.

4. COAGULATION IN TUMOR GROWTH AND METASTASIS

Thrombin generation and fibrin formation are constantly detectable in patients with malignancy, who are at increased risk of thromboembolic complications. Most importantly, fibrin formation is also involved in the processes of tumor spread and metastasis. Activation of blood coagulation in cancer is a complex phenomenon, involving many different pathways of the hemostatic system and numerous interactions of the tumor cell with other blood cells, including platelets, monocytes, and endothelial cells. Tumor cells possess the capacity to interact with all parts of the hemostatic system. They can directly activate the coagulation cascade by producing their own procoagulant factors or they can stimulate the prothrombotic properties of other blood cell components. The etiology of thrombosis in malignancy is multifactorial, and mechanisms include release of procoagulants by tumor cells in addition to other hypercoaguable state predisposing factors, such as chemotherapeutic and radiotherapeutic agents *(27–31)*. Unexplained thromboembolism might be an early indicator of the presence of a malignant tumor before signs and symptoms of the tumor itself become obvious.

Hemostatic abnormalities are present in a majority of patients with metastatic cancer. These abnormalities can be categorized as (1) increased platelet aggregation and activation, (2) abnormal activation of coagulation cascade, (3) release of plasminogen activator inhibitor (PAI)-1, and (4) decreased hepatic synthesis of anticoagulant proteins like Protein C and antithrombin III. Activation of the coagulation cascade is mediated through release of TF and other procoagulants from the plasma membrane vesicles of tumor cells *(28,31)*. Hemostatic mechanisms regulate blood flow by controlling platelet adhesion and fibrin deposition. A number of hemostatic proteins have been shown to regulate angiogenesis, either directly, by interacting with endothelial cells themselves, or indirectly, by interacting with other regulators of angiogenesis. The polypeptide fibrinogen is the central protein in the hemostasis pathway and is found deposited in the majority of human and experimental animal tumors. The ability of fibrinogen and various protein/peptide fragment derivatives to modulate angiogenic mechanisms in vitro and to affect tumor growth and metastasis has been demonstrated *(32)*.

Increasing evidence suggests that thrombotic episodes might also precede the diagnosis of cancer by months or years, thus representing a potential marker for occult malignancy *(27)*. Recently, emphasis has been given to the potential risk of cancer therapy (both surgery and chemotherapy) in enhancing the risk for thromboembolic disease *(28,31)*. Postoperative deep-vein thrombosis (DVT) is, indeed, more frequent in patients operated on for malignant diseases than for other disorders. On the other hand, both chemotherapy and hormone therapy are associated with an increased thrombotic risk, which can be prevented by low-molecular-weight heparin (LMWH) *(33)*. In particular, procoagulant activities of tumor cells have been extensively studied; one of these specific tumor procoagulants could represent a novel marker of malignancy. Clearly, tumor-induced coagulation is intrinsically involved with tumor growth, angiogenesis, and metastasis.

5. TREATMENT OF VENOUS THROMBOEMBOLISM IN CANCER PATIENTS

The management of DVT and pulmonary embolism (PE) in patients with cancer can be a clinical dilemma. Comorbid conditions, warfarin failure, difficult venous access, and a high bleeding risk are some of the factors that often complicate anticoagulant therapy in these patients. In addition, the use of central venous access devices is increasing, but the optimal treatment of catheter-related thrombosis remains controversial. Unfractionated heparin (UFH) is the traditional standard for the initial treatment of venous thromboembolism (VTE) but LMWH has been shown to be equally safe and effective in hemodynamically stable patients. For long-term treatment or secondary prophylaxis, vitamin K antagonists remain the mainstay treatment. However, the inconvenience and narrow therapeutic window of oral anticoagulants make extended therapy unattractive and problematic. As a result, LMWHs are being evaluated as an alternative for long-term therapy *(34,35)*. The role of inferior vena cava filters in cancer patients remains ill-defined, but these devices remain the treatment of choice in patients with contraindications for anticoagulant therapy.

Clinical investigations of various LMWHs (including enoxaparin, dalteparin, certoparin, and tinzaparin) demonstrated survival benefits as compared to UFH in cancer patients, with certain tumor types at early stages *(36–38)*. Additionally, the efficacy and safety profile for LMWH was also shown to be superior as compared to UFH or another anticoagulant such as warfarin *(38)*.

A growing body of evidence supports the existence of a tumor-mediated hypercoagulation state and a strong association between cancer and VTE. Patients with cancer are at a remarkably higher risk of VTE than patients free from malignant disorders during prolonged immobilization from any cause and following surgical interventions. In cancer patients affected by DVT, the treatment with LMWH has been reported to lower mortality to a greater extent compared to standard heparin therapy. Such an observation suggests that these agents might modify tumor growth progression directly or indirectly.

Studies have found an increase in the incidence of newly diagnosed malignancy among patients with unexplained VTE during the first 6–12 mo after the thromboembolic event *(39–42)*. A positive feedback loop between tumor and clot has been demonstrated *(1)*. Tumor fibrin is a consistent feature of tumor stroma and is deposited shortly after tumor cell inoculation *(1,43)*. Because fibrin might be beneficial to tumor growth, it is possible that the ability of normal or malignant tissue to generate fibrin might influence metastasis *(43)*.

6. HEPARIN AND LMWH IN THROMBOSIS AND CANCER

Heparin and its fractionated derivative, LMWH, are glycosaminoglycans (GAGs) *(44,45)*. Each residue is heavily polysulfated, thus giving the biopolymer a highly negative charge *(46,47)*. This anionic property is responsible for heparin's inhibitory effect on malignant processes, including angiogenesis and tumor cell adhesion, and malignant cell transformations. The antithrombotic effect of heparin is another effective countermeasure against malignancy, chemotherapy, radiation, catheter, or surgery-induced thrombosis. Because heparin was discovered over a half of a century ago, our knowledge of the chemical structure and molecular interactions of this fascinating poly-component was limited at the early stages of its development. Through the efforts of multidisciplinary groups of researchers and clinicians, it is now well recognized that heparin has multiple sites of actions and can be used in multiple indications. In the not too distant in the future, we might witness the impact of heparin derivatives or LMWH in the management of various diseases.

LMWHs vary in their affinity for ATIII, presumably as a result of production method *(48)*. Such differences have been cited as explaining, in part, the differences in LMWH pharmacodynamics as assessed by anti-Xa activity and one reason why they cannot be used interchangeably. In contrast, tissue factor pathway inhibitor (TFPI), a vascular endothelial biomarker that is ATIII independent, might represent a greater potential for elucidating the role of LMWH in various diseases *(49)*. Tinzaparin is an LMWH produced by controlled enzymatic depolymerization of conventional, unfractionated porcine heparin *(48)*. In clinical trials, tinzaparin is more effective than UFH as treatment for DVT and is effective in the treatment of PE *(32,49)*.

7. TUMOR FACTORS PREDICTING SENSITIVITY TO ANTICOAGULANTS

The various tumor types differ in the nature of their interactions with the coagulation system. In this regard, there are two types of tumor: (1.) those that activate the coagulation system directly and (2.) those that mediate coagulation activation indirectly via a paracrine mechanism. Tumors in the first group include renal cell cancer (RCC), melanoma, and ovarian and small cell lung cancers. These tumors overexpress procoagulant molecules such as TF, cancer procoagulant, or, in the case of RCC, hepsin on cell surfaces. The entire coagulation pathway is assembled on the surface of these tumor cells, leading to fibrin formation in close proximity to the tumors. This, at least partly, explains the occasional finding in RCC of a clot emanating from the tumor and extending into the renal vein and inferior vena cava. Tumors in the second group, on the other hand, tend to activate systemic coagulation by releasing cytokines (e.g., tumor necrosis factor [TNF-α], IL-1β) that in turn stimulate the production procoagulant molecules on the surface of circulating monocytes. Examples of these tumor types include breast, colorectal, and non-small-cell lung cancers. Based on this difference in the biology of coagulation activation, one would predict that tumors in the first group might be more likely to respond to an anticoagulant that interferes with TF/VIIa than tumors in the second group. In support of this hypothesis, anticoagulants have had significant activity in melanoma and small cell lung cancer but not in breast, colorectal, and non-small-cell lung cancers in prospective trials *(11–14,50)*.

8. ANGIOGENESIS

The coagulation system, which is activated in most cancer patients, has an important role in tumor biology. It can make a substantial contribution to tumor angiogenesis, which represents an imbalance in the normal mechanisms that allow organized healing after injury. The steadily growing knowledge of the relationship between the coagulation and angiogenesis pathways has important research and clinical implications. Manipulation of these systems can minimize both the neoangiogenesis essential for tumor growth and associated thromboembolic complications.

Angiogenesis is a process that is dependent on the coordinated production of angiogenesis stimulatory and inhibitory (angiostatic) molecules, and any imbalance in this regulatory circuit might lead to the development of a number of angiogenesis-mediated diseases. Angiogenesis is a multistep process, including activation, adhesion, migration, proliferation, and transmigration of endothelial cells across cell matrices to form new capillaries from existing vessels. Angiogenesis is a process that involves the formation of new vessels by sprouting from pre-existing vessels. A combined defect in the overproduction of positive regulators of angiogenesis and a deficiency in endogenous angiostatic mediators are features documented in tumor angiogenesis, psoriasis, rheumatoid arthritis (RA), and other neovascularization-mediated disorders *(51)*.

9. ACTIVATION OF COAGULATION AND ANGIOGENESIS IN CANCER

Many cancer patients have hemostatic abnormalities that predispose them to develop platelet activation and fibrin formation leading to clinical or subclinical thrombosis *(52,53)*. Thus, cancer leads to thrombosis, which, in turn, enhances the metastatic spread of tumor cells. Heparin therapy is effective and safe for thromboprophylaxis, and LMWH works just as well or better compared to UFH. Its antithrombotic action is another method by which heparin exhibits an inhibitory effect on malignant processes.

TF has been implicated in the upregulation of proangiogenic factors such as VEGF by tumor cells. This is the result of a complex interaction among tumor cells, macrophages, and endothelial cells leading to TF expression, fibrin formation, and tumor angiogenesis *(54)*.

A recent study has suggested that thrombin generation occurs via the extrinsic (TF dependent) coagulation pathway on cell surfaces and that some chemotherapeutic agents are able to upregulate TF mRNA and protein expression in cancer cells *(55)*.

10. ROLE OF THE COAGULATION SYSTEM IN ANGIOGENESIS

The processes of blood coagulation and the generation of new blood vessels both play crucial roles in wound healing. Platelets, for example, are the first line of defense during vascular injury and contain at least a dozen promoters of angiogenesis, which can be induced to secrete into the surrounding vasculature upon activation by thrombin *(22)*. It follows that these pathways are also intricately linked within human tumors. Targeting both the coagulation and angiogenesis pathways might provide more potent antitumor effect than targeting either pathway alone. Elucidation of the TF signaling pathway using tumor cells as a model system should provide new insights into the cellular biology of TF that might be applied to signaling in endothelial cells, smooth muscle cells, and fibroblasts. Also, because new classes of anticoagulant molecules have been developed over the past several years *(23,24,56)* that selectively target TF and/or the TF-VIIa complex, an understanding of this pathway might provide the rational basis for the development of new agents to prevent and treat angiogenesis-related disorders, tumor-associated thrombosis, and the positive feedback loop between thrombosis and cancer *(4)*.

Activation of the blood coagulation system stimulates the growth and dissemination of cancer cells through multiple mechanisms. Because of this, anticoagulant drugs inhibit the progression of certain cancers. Laboratory data on the effects of anticoagulants in various tumors suggest that this treatment approach has considerable potential in some cancers but not others. For example, RCC is one of a small number of human tumor types in which the tumor cell contains an intact coagulation pathway leading to thrombin generation and conversion of fibrinogen to fibrin immediately adjacent to viable tumor cells (57). Similar observations have been made in melanoma, ovarian, and small cell lung cancers, but not in breast, colorectal, and non-small-cell lung cancers *(58)*. This is of considerable relevance to the finding that growth of melanoma and small cell lung cancer is inhibited by anticoagulants, but that no such effect has been observed in those other tumor types *(11)*. Based on the relatively unique features of the interaction of the coagulation system with RCC, RCC might respond to anticoagulation therapy in a way that is similar to that for small cell lung cancer and melanoma. Hence, an anticoagulant that inhibit at the TF/VIIa level might have an improved efficacy and safety in inhibiting tumor-associated thrombosis, angiogenesis, and metastasis.

11. ANTICOAGULANTS IN THE MODULATION OF ANGIOGENESIS

TF, FGF2, VEGF, and IL-8, a chemokine, are also proangiogenic *(59)*. Heparin counters these factors, although the inhibitory effect occurs through different actions. The natural inhibitor of TF is known as TFPI. In the presence of heparin, Zhang et al. showed that TFPI activity is enhanced and the stimulatory effects of TF on angiogenesis is reduced *(59)*. Chemokines have positively charged domains *(60)*. Heparin might exhibit its inhibitory effect on IL-8 by binding these positive domains. In addition to angiogenesis, another key component of metastasis is the adhesion of cells to areas away from primary tumor growth. Selectins and integrins are families of cellular components that mediate cell adhesion and are involved in a complex cascade of events following endothelial cell activation. Tumor cells act as a ligand for the activation of these cellular elements. Studies have shown that heparin inhibited selectin and integrin-mediated interactions with tumor cells *(61)*.

The effects of LMWH tinzaparin, anti-VIIa, and r-TFPI on the modulation of angiogenesis-related processes, including in vitro endothelial tube formation and in vivo angiogenesis mediated by angiogenic factors and cancer cells, were demonstrated. Data demonstrated significant and comparable inhibitory effects of the LMWH tinzaparin, anti-VIIa, or r-TFPI in a concentration-dependent manner on endothelial cell tube formation. Tinzaparin, anti-VIIa, or r-TFPI blocked FGF2-induced angiogenesis in the chick chorioallantioc membrane model. Additionally, a significant inhibition of colon or lung carcinoma-induced angiogenesis, tumor growth, and regression was demonstrated with tinzaparin, anti-VIIa, and r-TFPI (62). These studies demonstrated a significant role for tinzaparin, anti-VIIa, and tinzaparin-releasable TFPI on the regulation of angiogenesis and tumor growth (62).

12. LMWH, TFPI, AND TUMOR METASTASIS

Using the experimental metastasis B16 melanoma-injectable model in mice, subcutaneous injection of tinzaparin (10 mg/kg) 4 h before intravenous injection of 2.5×10^5 melanoma cells reduced lung tumor formation in experimental mice (63). Similarly, intravenous injection of TFPI (700 ng) 5 min prior to tumor cell injection also reduced B16 lung metastasis and abolished tumor-cell-induced thrombocytopenia. These results support the potential role of the LMWH and its releasable TFPI in tumor growth and metastasis (64).

13. CONCLUSION

Many cancer patients reportedly exhibit a hypecoaguable state, with recurrent thrombosis as a result of the impact of cancer cells and chemotherapy, radiation, immobility, and catheter on further activation of coagulation cascade. Several experimental studies have demonstrated that UFH or LMWH interferes with various processes involved in tumor growth and metastasis that still need to be clinically documented. These processes might include fibrin formation, binding of heparin to angiogenic growth factors such as FGF2 and VEGF, modulation of TF, TFPI release, inhibition of matrix-degrading enzymes, and other mechanisms. Clinical trials have suggested a clinically relevant effect of LMWH, as compared to UFH on the survival of cancer patients with DVT that needs to be further documented in a large multicenter trial in cancer patients with defined tumor types and tumor stage. Recent studies from our laboratory defined the role of the LMWH, anti-factor VIIa, and recombinant TFPI in the modulation of angiogenesis, tumor growth, and metastasis. Additionally, antiplatelet agents such as aspirin and platelet GPIIb/IIIa antagonists might be a useful adjunct to standard cancer therapies in limiting platelet–tumor cell interactions.

REFERENCES

1. Mousa SA. Anticoagulants in thrombosis and cancer: the missing link. *Semin Thromb Haemost* 2002; 28:45–52.
2. Mousa SA, Fareed JW. Advances in anticoagulant, antithrombotic and thrombolytic drugs. *Exp Opin Invest Drugs* 2001; 10:157–162.
3. Chambers AF. The metastatic process: basic research and clinical implications. *Oncol Res* 1999; 11:161–168.
4. Chambers AF, MacDonald IC, Schmidt EE, Koop S, Morris VL, Khokha R, et al.. Steps in tumor metastasis: new concepts from intra-vital video microscopy. *Cancer Metastasis Rev* 1995; 14:279–301.

5. Borsig L, Wong R, Feramisco J, Nadeau DR, Varki NM, Varki A. Heparin and cancer revisited: mechanistic connections involving platelets, P-selectin, carcinoma mucins, and tumor metastasis. *PNAS* 2001; 98:3352–3357.

6. Koenig A, Norgard-Sumnicht K, Linhardt R, Varki A. Differential interactions of heparin and heparin sulfate glycosaminoglycans with the selectins. *J Clin Invest* 1998; 101:877–889.

7. Varki A, Varki NM. P-selectin, carcinoma metastasis and heparin: novel mechanistic connections with therapeutic implications. *Braz J Med Biol Res* 2001; 34:711–717.

8. Trousseau A. Phlegmasia alba dolens. *Clinique medicale de l'hotel-dieu de Paris.* London: New Sydenham Society, 1865:3:94.

9. Schiller H, Bartscht T, Arlt A, Zahn MO, Seifert A, Bruhn T, Bruhn HD, et al. Thrombin as a survival factor for cancer cells: thrombin activation in malignant effusions in vivo and inhibition of idarubicin-induced cell death in vitro. *Int J Clin Pharmacol Ther* 2002; 40(8):329–335.

10. Sorensen H, Mellemkjaer L, Olsen J, Baron J. Prognosis of cancers associated with venous thromboembolism. *N Engl J Med* 2000; 343:1846–1850.

11. Caine GJ, Lip GY. Anticoagulants as anticancer agents? *Lancet Oncol* 2002; 3(10):591,592.

12. Lebeau B, Chastang C, Brechot J-M, et al. Subcutaneous heparin treatment increases survival in small cell lung cancer. *Cancer* 1994; 74:38–45.

13. Chahinian A, Propert K, Ware J, et al. A randomized trial of anticoagulation with warfarin and of alternating chemotherapy in extensive small-cell lung cancer by the Cancer and Leukemia Group B. *J Clin Oncol* 1989; 7:993–1002.

14. Thornes R. Coumarins, melanoma and cellular immunity. In: McBrien D, Slator T, eds. *Protective Agents in Cancer.* London: Academic Press, 1983:43–56.

15. Pintucci G, Froum S, Pinnell J, Mignatti P, Rafii S, Green D. Trophic effects of platelets on cultured endothelial cells are mediated by platelet-associated fibroblast growth factor-2 (FGF-2) and vascular endothelial growth factor (VEGF). *Thromb Haemost* 2002; 88(5):834–842.

16. Manegold PC, Hutter J, Pahernik SA, Messmer K, Dellian M. Platelet-endothelial interaction in tumor angiogenesis and microcirculation. *Blood* 2003; 101(5):1970–1976

17. Werther K, Christensen IJ, Nielsen HJ. Determination of vascular endothelial growth factor (VEGF) in circulating blood: significance of VEGF in various leucocytes and platelets. *Scand J Clin Lab Invest* 2002; 62(5):343–350.

18. Verheul HM, Pinedo HM. Tumor growth: a putative role for platelets? *Oncologist* 1998; 3(2):II.

19. Verheul HM, Hoekman K, Luykx-de Bakker S, Eekman CA, Folman CC, Broxterman HJ, et al. Platelet: transporter of vascular endothelial growth factor. *Clin Cancer Res* 1997; 3(12 Pt 1):2187–2190.

20. Amirkhosravi A, Amaya M, Desai H, Francis JL. Platelet-CD40 ligand interaction with melanoma cell and monocyte CD40 enhances cellular procoagulant activity. *Blood Coagul Fibrinolysis* 2002; 13(6):505–512.

21. Gasic GJ, Gasic TB, Stewart CC. Anti-metastatic effect associated with platelet reduction. *Pathology* 1998; 61:46–52.

22. Amirkhosravi A, Mousa SA, Amaya M, Blaydes S, Desai H, Meyer T, et al. Inhibition of tumor cell-induced platelet aggregation and lung metastasis by the oral GPIIb/IIIa antagonist XV454. *Thromb Haemost* 2003; 90(3):549–554.

23. Trikha M, Zhou Z, Timar J, Raso E, Kennel M, Emmell E, Nakada MT. Multiple roles for platelet GPIIb/IIIa and alphavbeta3 integrins in tumor growth, angiogenesis, and metastasis. *Cancer Res* 2002; 62(10):2824–2833.

24. Varki NM, Varki A. Heparin inhibition of selectin-mediated interactions during the hematogenous phase of carcinoma metastasis: rationale for clinical studies in humans. *Semin Thromb Hemost* 2002; 28(1):53–66.

25. Kim HK, Song KS, Park YS, Kang YH, Lee YJ, Lee KR, et al. Elevated levels of circulating platelet microparticles, VEGF, IL-6 and RANTES in patients with gastric cancer: possible role of a metastasis predictor. *Eur J Cancer* 2003; 39(2):184–191.

26. Bakewell SJ, Nestor P, Prasad S, Tomasson MH, Dowland N, Mehrotra M, et al. Platelet and osteoclast beta3 integrins are critical for bone metastasis. *Proc Natl Acad Sci* 2003;100(24):14,205–14,210.

27. Baron JA, Gridley G, Weiderpass E, Nyren O, Linet M. Venous thromboembolism and cancer. *Lancet* 1998; 351:1077–1080.

28. Rickles FR, Edwards RL. Activation of blood coagulation in cancer: Trousseau's syndrome revisited. *Blood* 1982; 62:14–31.

29. Levine MN. Prevention of thrombotic disorders in cancer patients undergoing chemotherapy. *Thromb Haemost* 1997; 78:133–136.

30. Falanga A. Mechanisms of hypercoagulation in malignancy and during chemotherapy. *Haemostasis* 1998; 28:50–60.

31. Kakkar AJ, De Ruvo N, Tebbutt S, Williamson RCN. Extrinsic pathway activation with elevated tissue factor and factor VIIa in patients with cancer. *Lancet* 1995; 346:1004,1005.

32. Staton CA, Brown NJ, Lewis CE. The role of fibrinogen and related fragments in tumor angiogenesis and metastasis. *Exp Opin Biol Ther* 2003; 3(7):1105–1120.

33. Koopman MMW, Prandoni P, Piovella F, et al. Treatment of venous thrombosis with intravenous unfractionated heparin administered in the hospital as compared with subcutaneous low-molecular-weight heparin administered at home. *N Engl J Med* 1996; 334:682–687.

34. Kakkar AJ, Williamson RC. Prevention of venous thromboembolism in cancer using low molecular weight heparin. *Haemostasis* 1997; 27(Suppl 1):32–37.

35. Zacharski LR, Ornstein DL. Heparin and cancer. *Thromb Haemost* 1998; 80:10–23.

36. von Tempelhoff GF, Harenberg J, Neimann F, et al. Effect of low molecular weight heparin (Certoparin) versus unfractionated heparin on cancer survival following breast and pelvic cancer surgery: a prospective randomized double-blind trial. *Int Oncol* 2000; 16:815–824.

37. Zacharski LR. Anticoagulant in cancer treatment: malignancy as a solid phase coagulopathy. *Cancer Lett* 2002; 186:1–9.

38. Meyers G, Marjanovic Z, Valcke J, et al. Comparison of LMWH and wafarin for the secondary prevention of venous thromboembolism in patients with cancer. *Arch Intern Med* 2002; 162:1729–1735.

39. Trousseau A. Plegmasia alba dolens. In: Baillier JB, ed. *Clinique de l'Hotel-Dieu de Paris*, 2nd ed. 1865:3:654–712.

40. Howard W. Phlebitis and thrombosis. *Lancet* 1906; 1:650–655.

41. Dvorak HF. Thrombosis and cancer. *Human Pathol* 1987; 18:275–284.

42. Kakkar AK, Levine MN, Prandoni P, Lee AY, Rasmussen MS, Kuter D. What is the role for antithrombotics in cancer care? Interactive session with panel discussion. *Cancer Treat Rev* 2002; 28(3):157–159.

43. Dvorak HF, Senger DR, Dvorak AM. Fibrin as a component of the tumor stroma: origins and biological significance. *Cancer Metastasis Rev* 1983; 2:41–73.

44. Hirsh J, Levine MN. Low molecular weight heparin. *Blood* 1992; 79(1):1–17.

45. Nielsen JI, Ostergaard P. Chemistry of heparin and low molecular weight heparin. *Acta Chir Scand Suppl* 1988; 543:52–56.

46. Engelberg H. Actions of heparin that may affect the malignant process. *Cancer* 1999; 85:257–272.

47. Linhardt RJ and Gunay NS. Production and chemical processing of low molecular weight heparins. *Semin Thromb Haemost* 1999; 25(3):5–16.

48. Mousa SA, Bozarth J, Larnkjaer A, Johanson K. Vascular effects of heparin molecular weight fractions and LMWH on the release of TFPI from human endothelial cells. *Blood* 2000; 16 (11):59.

49. Hull RD, Raskob GE, Pineo GF, et al. Subcutaneous low-molecular weight heparin compared with continuous intravenous heparin in the treatment of proximal-vein thrombosis. *N Engl J Med* 1992; 326:975–982.

50. Levine M, Hirsh J, Gent M, et al. Double-blind randomized trial of a very-low-dose warfarin for prevention of thromboembolism in stage IV breast cancer. *Lancet* 1994; 343:886–889.

51. Mousa SA. Mechanisms of angiogenesis in vascular disorders: potential therapeutic targets. In: Mousa SA, ed. *Angiogenesis Inhibitors and Stimulators: Potential Therapeutic Implications*. Gorgtown, TX: Landes, 2000.

52. Falanga A, Rickles FR. Pathophysiology of the thrombophilic state in the cancer patient. *Semin Thromb Hemost* 1999; 25(2):173–182.

53. Markus G. The role of haemostasis and fibrinolysis in the metastatic spread of cancer. *Thromb Hemost* 1984; 10:61–72.

54. Ruf W, Mueller BM. Tissue factor in cancer angiogenesis and metastasis. *Cur Opin Haematol* 1996; 3:379–384.

55. Paredes N, Xu L, Berry LR, Chan AK. The effects of chemotherapeutic agents on the regulation of thrombin on cell surfaces. *Br J Haematol* 2003; 120(2):315–324.

56. Pinedo H, Verheul H, D'Amato R, Folkman J. Involvement of platelets in tumor angiogenesis? *Lancet* 1998; 352:1775–1777.

57. Wojtukiewicz M, Zacharski L, Memoli V, et al. Fibrinogen-fibrin transformation in situ in renal cell carcinoma. *Anticancer Res* 1990; 10:579–582.

58. Zacharski L, Wojtukiewicz M, Costantini V, et al. Pathways of coagulation/fibrinolysis activation in malignancy. *Sem Thromb Hemostas* 1992; 18:104–116.

59. Zhang Y, Deng Y, Luther T, et al. Tissue factor controls the balance of angiogenic and anti-angiogenic properties of tumor cells in mice. *J Clin Invest* 1994; 94:1320–1327.

60. Engelberg H. Actions of heparin in the atherosclerotic process. *Pharmacol Rev* 1996; 48:327–352.

61. Nelson RM, Ceccioni D, Roberts WG, et al. Heparin oligosaccharides bind L- and P- selectins and inhibit acute inflammation. *Blood* 1993; 82:3253–3258.

62. Mousa SA, Mohamed S. Anti-angiogenic mechanisms and efficacy of the low-molecular-weight heparin: anti-cancer efficacy. *Oncol Rep* 2004; 12:683–688.

63. Amirkhosravi A, Mousa SA, Amaya M, Francis JL. Antimetastatic effect of tinzaparin, a low-molecular-weight heparin. *J Thromb Haemost* 2003; 1(9):1972–1976.

64. Mousa, SA. Anticoagulants in thrombosis and cancer: the missing link. *Exp Rev Anticancer Ther* 2002; 2(2):227–233.

II THERAPEUTIC STRATEGIES

12

Challenges and Strategies in the Analysis of Multiple Events in Oncology

Pierre P. Major, MD, FRCPC,
and Richard J. Cook, PhD

CONTENTS

INTRODUCTION
A CLINICAL TRIAL
SKELETAL-RELATED EVENTS AS A COMPOSITE END POINT
HISTORICAL METHODS OF ANALYSIS AND THEIR SHORTCOMINGS
ROBUST METHODS FOR RECURRENT EVENTS
CONCLUSION
REFERENCES

1. INTRODUCTION

Patients with bone metastases are at risk for a variety of skeletal complications *(1)*, each of which can lead to a significant reduction in patient quality of life and considerable expense to the health care system. Skeletal complications are multifactorial in nature and typically include vertebral fractures, nonvertebral fractures, spinal cord compression, episodes of bone pain requiring radiation therapy, and surgery for the prevention or treatment of fractures. Each of these complications can occur repeatedly over time. The mechanisms causing skeletal complications are complex biological processes. The objective of this chapter is to discuss some statistical concepts for the analysis of the clinical complications resulting from metastases to bone and some basic methods of analysis. Concepts to be discussed include the use of composite end points, the analysis of recurrent clinical events, heterogeneity in the clinical course of bone complications, and the need to address the link between the propensity for bone complications and survival time.

2. A CLINICAL TRIAL

Bisphosphonates have well-documented efficacy for the treatment of bone metastases *(2)*. To provide a basis for discussion and graphical illustration, we draw from a

From: *Cancer Drug Discovery and Development*
Bone Metastasis: Experimental and Clinical Therapeutics
Edited by: G. Singh and S. A. Rabbani © Humana Press Inc., Totowa, NJ

multicenter randomized trial by Hortobagyi et al. *(3)* designed to investigate the effect of pamidronate vs placebo on the development of skeletal complications in breast cancer patients with bone metastases. In this study, patients were accrued between January 1991 and March 1994 from 97 study sites in the United States, Canada, Australia and New Zealand. Patients with stage IV breast cancer receiving cytotoxic chemotherapy with at least one predominantly lytic bone lesion ≥ 1 cm in diameter were randomized within strata defined by ECOG status. A total of 382 women were enrolled in the study; 185 were randomized to receive pamidronate and 197 placebo. Two patients randomized to placebo did not have bone metastases and were, therefore, excluded from subsequent analyses. Patients randomized to the pamidronate arm received 90 mg of pamidronate disodium via a 2-h infusion every 4 wk, whereas patients randomized to the placebo received dextrose infusions. Patients on a 3-wk chemotherapy regimen were permitted to receive the study drug every 3 wk. After completion of the planned 1 yr follow-up, the observation was extended for an additional year *(4)*. Each patient was followed until death, the last date of contact or loss to follow-up, or February 1, 1996.

At monthly visits, patients were assessed and the occurrence of skeletal complications was recorded. The skeletal complications of interest include pathologic fractures, spinal cord compression with vertebral fracture, the need for surgery to treat or prevent fractures, and the need for radiation for the treatment of bone pain.

Figure 1 displays the duration of observation and the occurrence of skeletal complications for the control patients in the Hortobagyi trial *(3,4)*. Each patient is represented by a horizontal line, the length of which represents the time on study. In most patients, early termination of follow-up was because of death. The dots on the lines represent the occurrence of skeletal complications; multiple episodes recorded on the same day are represented by adjacent dots. The different types of clinical event are not distinguished in Fig. 1. Because death precludes the occurence of future skeletal complications, simply counting the number of skeletal complications is not sensible. For example, patients dying skeletal-related even (SRE)-free shortly after randomization would be treated as having had a favorable outcome. It is therefore important for the analysis to summarize the occurrence of clinical events while dealing appropriately with patients whose process terminates early because of death, after which no complications can occur, and patients who terminate early as a result of study withdrawal, after which skeletal complications may occur.

3. SKELETAL-RELATED EVENT AS A COMPOSITE END POINT

In settings where patients might experience a range of adverse clinical outcomes, it is common to base treatment comparisons on a composite end point. A composite endpoint is one that is said to have occurred if any one of a set of particular clinical events occurs. Composite end points are used in studies of a wide range of chronic diseases. In neurovascular diseases, the composite end point might include fatal stroke, nonfatal stroke, and transient ischemic attacks (TIAs); in studies of aquired immunodeficiency syndrome (AIDS), the composite end point might include opportunistic infections, decline in CD4 cell counts below a threshold, and death. Relapse-free survival used for evaluating adjuvant chemotherapies in oncology is another example of a composite end point. In this case, a treatment failure is considered to have occurred if a patient experiences a relapse in any body organ or dies.

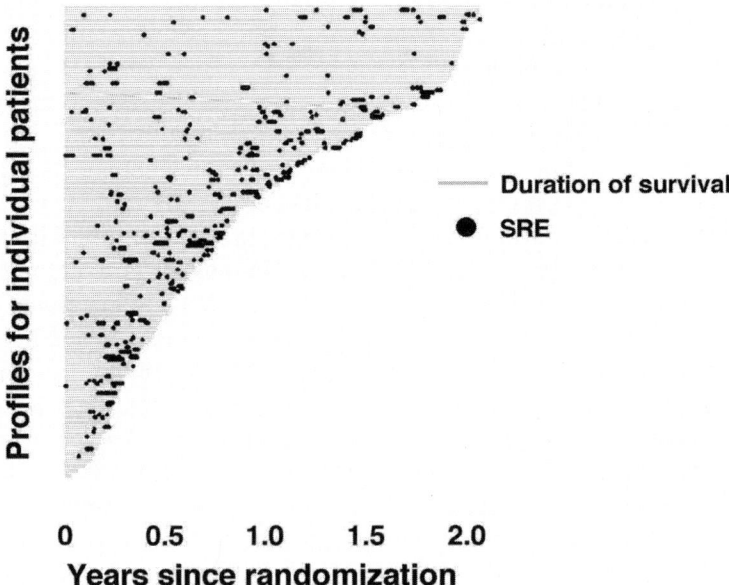

Fig. 1. The duration of survival (or trial participation) is given for the 185 patients of the placebo arm. Each dot represents a skeletal complication. The data are from the trial of Hortobagyi et al. *(4)*.

Various rationales have been put forward to support the use of composite end point, including increased efficiency or power of clinical trials *(5)*. Care must be exercised, however, when interpreting estimates of treatment effect based on these outcomes *(6)*. Presumably, each component of the composite end point represents the occurrence of an undesirable clinical event. If a treatment can be shown to delay the onset of the first of these events, then it might be favorably viewed because these events are all reflections of temporal progression of the underlying disease process. However, each component of the composite end point has a different clinical burden for both the patient and the health care system. Difficulties arise when interest lies in making conclusions regarding particular components of the composite end point because studies based on composite end points are typically not powered to demonstrate treatment effects on a particular component and analyses focusing on any one end point will not typically yield significant effects. Qualitative explorations of particular components are warranted to gain insight into the effect of treatment on each component of the composite end point; if the treatment effects are consistently in the same direction, inferences on the individual components of the composite end point might be more plausible. We now proceed with the assumption that the composite end point SRE is clinically meaningful and consider issued related to their recurrence.

4. HISTORICAL METHODS OF ANALYSIS AND THEIR SHORTCOMINGS

Clinical trials in oncology most often evaluate a simple dichotomous response such as whether or not a patient responded successfully to treatment (i.e., whether a skeletal-related event was prevented by 1 yr). In previous work we have discussed the difficulties in interpreting analyses based on such dichotomous outcomes when follow-up is variable because of death or study withdrawal (7–9).

Another strategy is to assess the effect of treatment on the time to the first skeletal-related event. Unfortunately, when applying standard methods for survival analysis to events that might not ultimately occur, one must distinguish between subjects who die and those who withdraw without having experienced the clinical event of interest. In the former case, the event will not occur with certainty, and in the latter, it might or might not occur eventually. In the SRE analyses, one must effectively address the fact that patients experience "competing risks" for death and skeletal-related events. This must be contrasted with survival analyses (i.e., the occurrence of death), where death is a certainty for all individuals. Naive application of the Kaplan–Meier method gives biased estimates (overestimates) of the proportion of patients experiencing an SRE because patients are typically treated as being at risk for SREs even after death. It is therefore impossible to give clinical meaning to median times to events estimated from these curves. Fortunately, estimates of relative risk based on Cox regression models are valid and are clinically interpretable; their computation is based only on those subjects observed to be at risk and not on extrapolations beyond death, provided risk sets are appropriately defined (10).

One approach for dealing with the competing risk issue for the time to the first SRE is to examine treatment effects on SRE-free survival. This is another example of a composite end point in which the response is the minimum of the time to first SRE and death. This solves the conceptual problem by changing the question from one based on SREs alone to one that incorporates both the end point and death. For example, when there is no treatment effect on survival, one should be able to detect a treatment effect on the occurrence of SREs. If treatment prolongs survival, this is a beneficial effect of treatment and, hence, the analyses based on SRE-free survival would be more powerful. If, on the other hand, the treatment reduces survival, this would be reflected by reducing the evidence of treatment benefit in an SRE-free analysis.

If one wishes to restrict attention to end points based solely on the first SRE, the cumulative incidence function gives the proportion of patients who have actually experienced their first SRE, accounting for the fact that none will occur after death (10). This can be viewed as a generalization of the Kaplan–Meier estimate for the competing risk setting. Estimates of the cumulative incidence function are, therefore, interpretable and offer a useful graphical approach in this setting.

Skeletal complications might recur many times during follow-up, and while neglecting all but the first event allows the use of familiar statistical techniques, this approach ignores the majority of the clinical events. From Fig. 1, it is readily apparent that analyzing only the first event fails to capture the complexity of the pathological process. Moreover, if cost-effectiveness analyses are intended, it is important to consider the overall burden of disease for health policy reasons by counting each event, because each one might incur a cost to the health care system. Table 1 summarizes the advantages and shortcoming of different methods of statistical analysis. In the following paragraphs, we make some remarks on methods for the analysis of multiple events.

The first approach that naturally comes to mind is to compute an event rate. For a particular treatment arm, this is the total number of events for all patients in that arm divided by the total time under observation for all patients in that arm. This can be

Table 1

Summary of the Advantages and Shortcomings of Different Methods of Analyzing SRE Data

	Advantage	Shortcoming	Complexity
Proportion of patients having an event	Simple; analyses typically based on crude comparison of proportions	Neglects the time of the first event and the number of events per patient	Minimal, but overly simplistic: YES or NO
Time to occurrence of the first event	More informative; captures timing of events	Neglects the number of events per patient (what happens after)	More complex: YES or NO; WHEN?
Multiple-event analysis	More informative; reflects the effect of treatment on the entire course of the disease	Considers the number and timing of events	Complex methods less wellknown. Anderson–Gill (1982): YES or NO; HOW MANY?; WHEN?

computed for the patients in the control arm and then compared to corresponding rate for the treatment arm based on Poisson regression models to asses treatment effects. This analysis, although intuitively appealing, is based on the premise that the events experienced by each patient are independent of each other; that is, the occurrence of one event does not alter the risk of subsequent events *(11,12)*. This assumption is often overlooked and can lead to mistaken claims of positive results *(8,9,11,12)*. Moreover, the competing risk issue (i.e., that deaths preclude subsequent SREs) must also be addressed to obtain clinically meaningful estimates of treatment effect. It is the need to incorporate the features, (1) variation in susceptibility and (2) the competing risk of death, that mandates the use of the techniques we will discuss.

5. ROBUST METHODS FOR RECURRENT EVENTS

Statistical techniques for analyzing multiple events occurring over a period of observation have received considerable attention during the past 20 yr. The purpose of these different methods vary from providing a comprehensive and accurate representation of the disease process to providing a simple basis for comparing two or more groups of patients with respect to overall disease burden. Regardless of the precise objective, any suitable methods for analyzing SREs must reflect the heterogeneity in the time-course of bone complications and variation in survival. This will ensure reliable estimates of treatment effects and ensure valid scientific inferences through use of appropriate measures of variablity.

Examination of Fig. 1 suggests several approaches for modeling these data and comparing placebo and treatment arms. The time between events in both arms of the trial could be compared. Alternatively, the time to the first, second, and subsequent events could also be compared *(13)*. We limit the discussion to a method that is intuitive and lends itself to graphical presentation. We rely on the cumulative mean function (CMF), which provides a convenient interpretable summary of the data. Several publications are available on multiple event analysis *(13–16)*. However, only more recently has the issue of competing risks been addressed and methods for calculating measures of variability of the data being developed *(17,18)*.

The CMF is simply a weighed sum of the average number of SREs per patient over time.

Data from Fig. 1 are used to illustrate these computations, which are detailed in Table 2. The event rate is estimated on each day of follow-up by dividing the number of events occurring on that day by the number of patients under observation at that time. On days with no events, the estimated rates are zero. These daily event rates also represent estimates of the average number of events occurring on each day for patients still at risk of events. It is convenient to synthesize these average numbers (or estimated rates) by accumulating their values over time. A straightforward approach is to simply compute a sum of these the daily averages over an interval of interest; the result can be interpreted as an estimate of the cumulative number of events (CMF) over this interval. This approach is valid if there is no risk of patients dying over the interval during which computations are conducted. If death can occur over this interval, then a weighted sum must be computed in which the weights associated with each day's rates are simply the probabilities of surviving to that day. Weighting by the probability of survival ensures that the resulting sum is interpretable as an estimate of the average number of events over time, per patient in the population of patients receiving the corresponding treat-

Table 2
Calculation of the CMF Values for d 365–375
of the Placebo and Treatment Arms of the
Hortobagyi Trial in Patients With Breast Cancer

t	r(t)	S(t)	r(t)S(t)	CMF
365	0	0.556623	0	2.054810
366	0	0.556623	0	2.054810
367	0	0.556623	0	2.054810
368	0.009524	0.546219	0.005202	2.060013
369	0.009615	0.541017	0.005202	2.065215
370	0.019231	0.541017	0.010404	2.075619
371	0.019417	0.535815	0.010404	2.086023
372	0	0.535815	0	2.086023
373	0.029412	0.535815	0.015759	2.101782
374	0.039216	0.535815	0.021012	2.122795
375	0.009804	0.535815	0.005253'	2.128048

Note: Data for the placebo arm from ref. *4* and corresponds with the steps in Fig. 2.

ment, and accounting for the fact that events cannot occur in patients who are not alive. For rare events, it is often convenient to express these estimates per 100 patients; this avoids excessively small estimated cumulative expected numbers of events, which are not readily interpretable clinically (i.e., 0.1 event/patient is expressed more meaning fully as 10 events per 100 patients). The CMF for the data from Fig. 1 is displayed in Fig. 2 and the inset in Fig. 2 is an expansion of the graph for d 365–375 for the control patients. We also show the CMF for the pamidronate (AREDIA) treatment arm.

The above computation is described symbolically as follows. Let $r(t)$ denote the rate of events on day t among subjects at risk of events (i.e., still under observation) and let $S(t)$ denote the probability of survival beyond day t. As stated earlier, the estimate of the rate on day t is also an estimate of the average number of events on day t among those alive. The average number of events on day t among all randomized patients is the product $r(t)S(t)$, because to contribute to this average, one must survive to this time. The average cumulative number of events over a 2-yr interval (730 d) is then computed as $r(t_1)S(t_1) + r(t_2)S(t_2) + \cdots + r(t_{730}) \times S(t_{730})$. The estimate of this quantity is obtained by replacing $r(t)$ and $S(t)$ with their corresponding estimates. Table 2 shows the results of calculations for d 365–375 of the placebo and treatment arms of the Hortobagyi data *(4)*.

The cumulative mean functions for both the pamidronate and control arms can be compared using confidence intervals that appropriately reflect the variability of the clinical data *(17)*. Results of these analyses show that treatment with pamidronate delays the onset of complications from bone metastases at 1 and 10 yr.

The precision of the CMF in this setting is determined by the degree of dependence in the event process (i.e., how correlated the events are), the mortality rate, and the association between the event rate and mortality. The formulas for variance computations are too complex for presentation here, but Ghosh and Lin *(18)* provide the technical details for variance estimation of the CMF and associated test statistics.

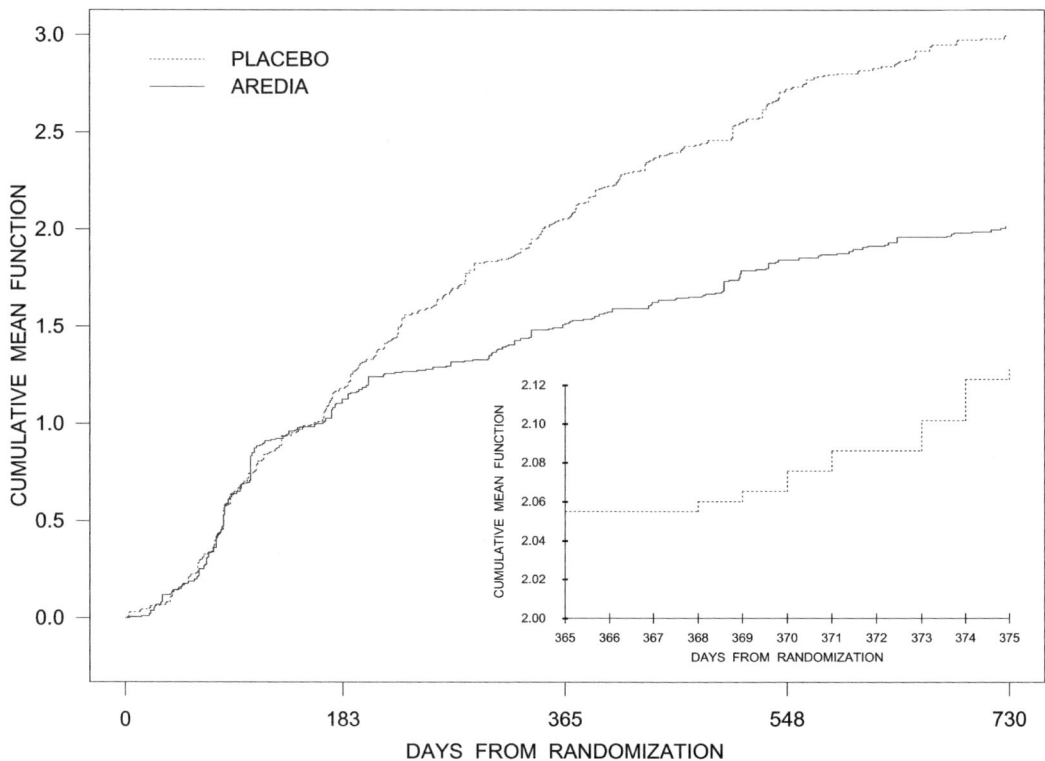

Fig. 2. Cumulative mean functions for the treatment (—) and the placebo (- - -) arms of the Hortobagyi data are displayed. The curves are significantly different. The inset an expansion of placebo arm curve for d 365–375. The steps in the function are clearly seen. The corresponding calculations are shown in Table 2.

6. CONCLUSION

The above-outlined computation is, conceptually, reasonably straightforward. The methods are suitable when interest lies in characterizing disease burden in a population of patients or in assessing the impact of different treatment strategies for health policy-makers. There has been some reluctance to adopt analyses of this sort, as the primary analyses of clinical trials and alternative methods based on SRE-free survival, for example, are more familiar. Models to gain insight into the effect of treatments on different aspects of the recurrent event process are available and their selection requires careful exploration of available data *(19–21)*.

In previously reported exploratory analyses of the Hortobagyi trial, we showed that SRE rates were not independent within patients and that they also varied with length of observation. Failure to reflect this biological variability in the statistical model could lead to spurious results *(8,11,12)*. The concepts of the CMF method for displaying recurrent event data enables one to proceed from the complex data displayed in Fig. 1 to the more intuitive display in Fig. 2. The CMF for the placebo and control arms of the Hortobabyi trial *(4)* can be computed and compared statistically to determine the impact of treatment on the risk of developing SRE using appropriate tests or significance

(18). Such analyses are best done in collaborations between statistical and clinical scientists. Through such collaborations, maximum information can be extracted from available trial data and used to guide clinical practice.

REFERENCES

1. Coleman RE, Rubin RD. The clinical course of bone metastases from breast cancer. *Br J Cancer* 1987; 55:61–66.
2. Ross, JR, Saunders Y, Edmonds PM, Patel S, Broadley KE, Johnston SRD. Systemic review of role of bisphosphonates on skeletal morbidity in metastatic cancer. *Br Med J* 2003; 327:1–6.
3. Hortobagyi GN, Theriault RL, Porter L, Blayney D, Lipton A, Sinoff C, et al. Efficacy of pamidronate in reducing skeletal complications in patients with breast cancer and lytic bone metastases. *N Engl J Med* 1996; 335:1785–1791.
4. Hortobagyi GN, Theriault RL, Lipton A, Porter L, Blayney D, Sinoff C, et al. Long-term prevention of skeletal complications of metastatic breast cancer with pamidronate. *J Clin Oncol* 1998; 16:2038–2044.
5. Fremandtlke N, Calvert M, Wood, J, Eastaugh J, Griffin C. Composite outcomes in randomized trial: Greater precision but with greater uncertainty? *JAMA* 2003; 289(19):2554–2559.
6. Lauer MS, Topol EJ. Clinical trials – multiple treatments, multiple end points, and multiple lessons. *JAMA* 2003; 289(19):2575.
7. Major PP; Cook RJ, Tozer R, Hirte H. Bisphosphonates for bone metastases in breast cancer patients. Trial design issues and evaluation of published studies. *Curr Oncol* 1998; 5:181–187.
8. Cook RJ, Major PP. Methodology for treatment evaluation in patients with cancer metastatic to bone. *J Nat Cancer Inst* 2001; 93:7:534–538.
9. Major P, Cook RJ. Efficacy of bisphosphonates in the management of skeletal complications of bone metastases and selection of clinical endpoints. *Am J Clin Oncol* 2002;2 (5 Suppl.):S1–S9.
10. Crowder M. *Classical Competing Risks*. London: Chapman & Hall/CRC, 2001.
11. Glynn RJ, Buring JE. Ways of measuring rates of recurrent events. *Br Med J* 1996; 312:364–367.
12. Windeler J, Lange S, Events per person year—a dubious concept. *Br Med J* 1995; 310:454–456.
13. Therneau TM, Grambsch PM. *Modeling Survival Data: Extending the Cox Model*, 2nd ed. New York: Springer-Verlag, 2001.
14. Anderson PK, Borgan O, Gill RD, Keiding N. *Statistical Models Based on Counting Processes*. New York: Springer-Verlag, 1993.
15. Hougaard P. *Analysis of Multivariate Survival Data*. New York: Springer-Verlag, 2000.
16. Nelson, WB. *Recurrent Events Data Analysis for Product Repairs, Disease Recurrences, and Other Applications*. American Statistical Association and Society for Industrial Applied Mathematics 2003.
17. Diggle, PJ, Heagerty P, Liang KY, Zeger SL. *Analysis of Longitudinal Data*, 2nd ed. Oxford: Oxford University Press, 2003.
18. Ghosh D, Lin DY. Nonparemetric analysis of recurrent events and death. *Biometrics* 2002; 56:554–562.
19. Cook RJ, Major P. Marginal analysis of point processes with competing risks. In: *Handbook of Statistics*, vol 23. Amsterdam: Elsevier Science, 2004.
20. Cook RJ, Lawless JF, Lee KA. Cumulative processes related to event histories. *SORT 27* 2003; 1: 13–30.
21. Chen BE, Cook RJ. Tests for multivariate recurrent events in the presence of a terminal event. *Biostatistics* 2004; 5(1):129–143.

13 Integrins

Novel Targets for the Treatment of Bone Metastasis

Graham C. Parry, PhD, Fernando Doñate, PhD,
Marian L. Plunkett, PhD, David E. Shaw, PhD,
Steven Pirie-Shepherd, PhD,
and Andrew P. Mazar, PhD

CONTENTS

1. INTRODUCTION

Metastasis to bone is a major complication of advanced cancer and occurs in more than 400,000 cancer patients each year. Bone metastasis can arise from many different tumor types, including breast, prostate, lung, renal cell, thyroid, and bladder cancer, and in patients with melanoma and myeloma. The development of bone metastasis in cancer patients contributes significantly to the morbidity and mortality associated with the disease and leads to increased bone pain, increased bone fragility and fracture, and sometimes death. Metastatic tumor cells in the bone co-opt normal processes involved in bone resorption and bone formation and stimulate the formation of either osteolytic (dependent on the lytic, bone-resorptive activities of osteoclasts) or osteoblastic (dependent on the bone-forming activities of osteoblasts) metastatic lesions. Most tumor types form predominantly osteolytic lesions, with the exception of prostate cancer, which can lead to metastatic lesions of both the osteoblastic and the osteolytic phenotype.

Despite its prevalence in cancer patients, there are few therapeutic options available for the treatment of bone metastasis. In general, most available interventions are palliative and attempt to decrease bone pain and minimize the destruction of bone often asso-

From: *Cancer Drug Discovery and Development*
Bone Metastasis: Experimental and Clinical Therapeutics
Edited by: G. Singh and S. A. Rabbani © Humana Press Inc., Totowa, NJ

ciated with the progression of bone metastasis. Nevertheless, there has been significant advancement in the understanding of bone biology and how it pertains to the progression of bone metastasis in recent years, with a concomitant acceleration of discovery efforts targeting the treatment of bone metastasis. A significant body of data has now identified integrins as being central to many of the processes involved in the pathobiology of bone metastasis. In this chapter, we provide a survey of the recent integrin literature with respect to structure, signaling, and expression in cancer and summarize the most recent advances in the therapeutic targeting of bone metastasis. In addition, we review opportunities for the development of therapeutic approaches, including the targeting of integrins, for the treatment of bone metastasis in the future.

2. INTEGRIN STRUCTURE

Integrins are heterodimeric, membrane-bound cell surface molecules that mediate binding to a variety of ligands involved in cell attachment, migration, proliferation, differentiation, and survival. As such, integrins play a role in development, angiogenesis, wound healing, neoplastic transformation, and thrombosis (1).

Each integrin heterodimer consists of an α-subunit and a β-subunit. There are 18 known α-subunits and 8 known β-subunits in humans (2). Available human genome data have not indicated the presence of any novel α- or β-subunits not already identified. The α subunits of integrins are approx 150–180 kDa. and the β-subunits are smaller at approx 90–115 kDa (3). The overall dimensions of integrins have been determined by electron microscopy, and recent studies have provided crystal structures of two integrins, $\alpha_v\beta_3$ $(3,4)$ and $\alpha_{IIb}\beta_3$ (5). Based on these two sets of data, it has been inferred that integrin heterodimers form an 8×12-nm globular head with two 18-nm flexible tails that extend into and across the plasma membrane.

Sequence analysis of α-subunits reveals an N-terminal region comprised of seven 60-amino-acid repeats that are similar in sequence. These repeats form a seven-bladed "β-propeller" domain in available crystal structures, with each blade being formed from a four-stranded antiparallel β-sheet (3). The inner channel of this propeller is lined predominantly with amide and carbonyl groups, with few side chains projecting into the cavity. Four Ca^{2+} binding sites are found in blades 4–7 of this domain, and the calcium-binding region of blade 7 is hypothesized to stabilize the interaction of the β-propeller with the "thigh" domain, which resides at the carboxyl-terminal end of the propeller. The thigh domain extends into two calf domains (calf-1 and calf-2) (3). A recent three-dimentional (3-D) structure based on electron microscopy (EM) analysis coupled with X-ray crystallographic data suggests that the calf domains extend into α-helical domains that span the plasma membrane (5). The β-subunit of integrins is comprised of the βA domain (an essential requirement for ligand binding) located at the "head" of the subunit, followed by a PSI domain (plexins, semaphorins, and integrins), four endothelial growth factor (EGF) domains and a β-tail domain. Although it is assumed that the membrane-spanning regions of both the α- and β-subunits are α-helical, this remains to be proven (26).

The α-subunits are subdivided into two groups based on some structural differences. The first group is formed by $\alpha_1, \alpha_2, \alpha_{10}, \alpha_{11}, \alpha_D, \alpha_L, \alpha_M,$ and α_X. These α-subunits have an extra approx 180-residue domain inserted between repeats 2 and 3 of the β-propeller domain. This αA domain (also referred to as the I or inserted domain) resembles a domain found in von Willebrand factor that mediates binding to collagen and is necessary and sufficient for the divalent cation-dependent binding of these integrins to their physiologic ligands *(2)*. The second group is formed by the αA-lacking integrins α_3, α_5, α_6, α_7, α_8, α_{IIb}, α_V, and α_{IEL}. These integrins are formed by a posttranslational cleavage of their precursor chains into a heavy chain and light chain that are held together by a disulfide bond. The light chain is comprised of the entire cytoplasmic domain, the transmembrane region, and a small portion of the extracellular domain, whereas the heavy chain comprises the majority of the extracellular domain (approx 120 kDa) of the integrin α-chain. In heterodimers containing subunits from this second group of α integrins, ligand recognition requires the αA-like domain (βA) present in all integrin β-subunits *(3)*.

The midsegment of integrin β-subunits contains a metal cation-dependent adhesion site (MIDAS). This MIDAS site is also present in the αA domain of those integrins that possess such a domain. The MIDAS site contains a motif (DXSXS) that provides three of the five metal cation coordination sites. In the recently published crystal structure of the β_3-subunit , the MIDAS site is unoccupied in the absence of a ligand *(4)*. In the unligated structure, the side chain of a glutamine residue intrudes into the MIDAS site and prevents cation binding. However, in the ligated structure, this side chain is rotated out of the MIDAS domain, allowing occupancy of this site by a cation. In addition, the Asp residue of the Arg-Gly-Asp (RGD) adhesion sequence that mediates ligand binding to integrins contacts this cation as well and is thought to stabilize the activated conformation of the integrin. Furthermore, recent crystallography data have also revealed a secondary cation-binding site located 6 Å from the MIDAS domain *(4)*. Occupancy of this secondary site also requires the integrin to be ligated, because in the unligated state, the secondary cation coordination space does not exist *(4)*. Mutational studies on integrins have also revealed the presence of an additional cation-binding site in the βA domain, but the proposed coordination sites were not entirely consistent with data derived from crystallographic studies *(7)*. Nevertheless, the existence of different conformers of integrins stabilized by differential binding to cations and leading to different activation states cannot be ruled out.

The ligand-binding site is hypothesized to comprise sections of both the α- and β-subunits. Recent data show that the prototypic integrin ligand, the peptide RGD (described in detail in Section 4), inserts into a crevice between these two domains *(4)*. This interaction requires eight divalent metal ions, such as Mn^{2+} or Ca^{2+}. Each residue in RGD makes extensive contact with the integrin, and this binding causes extensive tertiary and quaternary changes in the conformation of the β-subunit and the relationship of the subunits to each other. The α- and β-subunits move closer together at the RGD-binding site, and the propeller domain of the α-subunit undergoes a small rotation, with the βA domain of the β-subunit moving in concert. Natural protein ligands, being larger than the simple RGD, might cause larger changes. Further, the simultaneous or sequential binding of two ligands, such as the RGD and the synergy sequence of fibronectin, could cause even more pronounced conformational changes *(4)*.

Based on data obtained from electron cryomicroscopy studies *(5)*, it has been suggested that the compact conformation depicted in Fig. 1 represents the inactive state of the integrin and that, upon activation, the entire integrin structure will straighten and extend. Activation might be induced by ligand binding and could result in changes in divalent metal coordination and the previously discussed tertiary and quaternary changes.

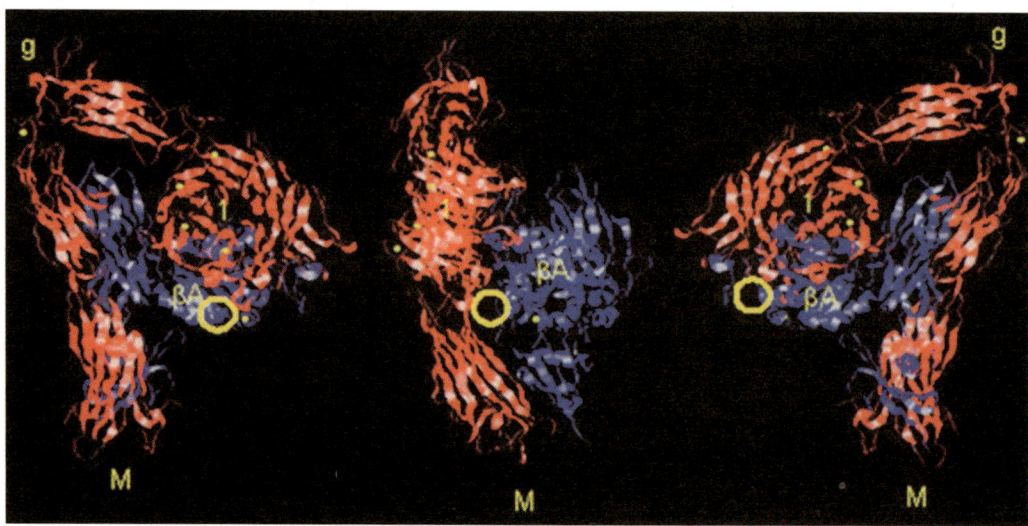

Fig. 1. Crystal structure of $\alpha_v\beta_3$. The α-subunit is colored red, the β-subunit is colored blue. Metal ions are represented by yellow spheres. The image is generated using RasMol and pdb file 1M1X.pdb. The image is shown in three planes, each rotated 90° with respect to each other. The portion of the molecule that will extend into the plasma membrane is at the bottom of the image (M). Area 1 is the seven-bladed β-propeller domain. Area g represents the genu region, around which the integrin might straighten upon activation. The RGD ligand will bind to a region composed of portions of the propeller domain (1) and the A domain of the β-subunit (βA) as approximately indicated by the yellow circle. (From refs. *8* [PDB ID: IL6G] and *9*.)

However, it is not clear how such changes in the extracellular domains of the integrin heterodimer could be transmitted to the α-helical transmembrane stalks of the α- and β-subunits, eventually resulting in changes being transmitted to the cytoplasmic domains of the two subunits. Sequence analysis data and modeling studies suggests that the two α-helical transmembrane segments might be capable of undergoing helix–coil transitions such as helical rotation or scissoring. The α-helical extension of the β-tail could then serve as a lever to facilitate cytoplasmic conformational changes *(5)*. Conformational change induced by ligand-mediated integrin activation is proposed to dissociate the cytoplasmic tails of the α- and β-subunits, which are otherwise clustered in the unactivated integrin *(10)*. This process, also referred to as outside-in signaling (Fig. 2), would allow for the cytoplasmic tails of each integrin subunit to interact with intracellular effector molecules to transduce ligand-induced signaling events. Integrin signaling is discussed in greater detail in Section 3.

The cytoplasmic tails from various α-subunits share little sequence similarity except in the membrane-proximal region, suggesting that the α-tails play a unique role in the activation of each integrin. Each α-subunit is highly conserved across species, suggesting that these α-tails are important for specific heterodimer function. Each α-tail can regulate function by directly initiating signaling events, by modulating β-subunit signaling or regulating β-tail ligand binding. The cytoplasmic tails of the α-subunits do have a conserved membrane-proximal region. Experiments that delete the entire α-tail result in constitutive activation of the integrin, suggesting that the α-tail is a negative regulator of

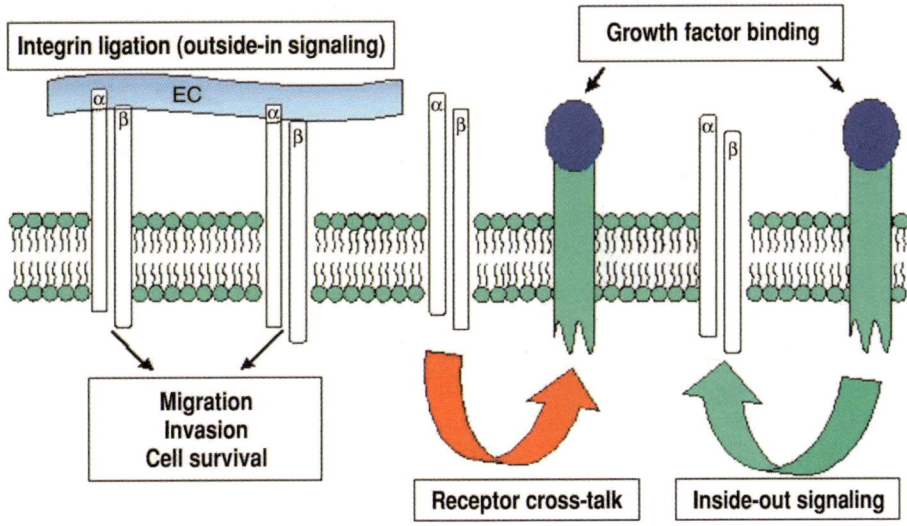

Fig. 2. Schematic representation of integrin signaling.

integrin function *(6)*. Structure analysis of the α-tail by nuclear magnetic resonance (NMR) reveals a conformation whereby the N-terminal membrane-proximal region forms an α-helix followed by a turn, allowing the C-terminal end of the tail to loop back and form an association with the membrane-proximal section of the tail *(11)*. Mutation of the highly conserved membrane-proximal region, such that this association is abolished, also results in a constitutively activated integrin.

2.1. Structural Aspects of Integrin Activation

In quiescent cells, integrins have low binding affinity for their ligands. In response to certain stimuli, integrins can switch to a state of high ligand binding affinity *(12–15)*. Conformational changes are responsible for the switch to a high-affinity state in the extracellular domain of integrins and are triggered by signaling from the cytoplasm (inside-out signaling; Fig. 2) *(13)*. Ligand binding also increases affinity for the ligand by inducing the clustering of integrins, which induces signaling back to the cytoplasm (outside-in signaling; Fig. 2) *(14)*. The conformational changes induced by ligand binding manifest themselves by the appearance of neo-epitopes within the integrin, called ligand-induced binding sites (LIBS). Antibodies against these LIBS mimic inside-out signaling by endowing integrins with a higher binding affinity for their ligands *(12–14)*. Activation of integrins in a purified state or on the surface of cells can also be achieved by the addition of Mn^{2+} or dithiothreitol (DTT) *(16)*. The activation by DTT suggests a role for cysteine (Cys) residues in the mechanism of integrin activation. The role of Cys residues in integrin activation has only been studied in detail for the activation of $\alpha_{IIb}\beta_3$ *(17–22)*. However, the participation of Cys residues might be part of a general mechanism of activation for other integrins as well. The β-subunits of integrins contain 56 highly conserved cysteine residues, some of which have recently been discovered to be unpaired in $\alpha_{IIb}\beta_3$ *(23)*. It has been proposed that $\alpha_{IIb}\beta_3$ integrin has a different arrangement of free and paired cysteine residues in the activated and resting states, suggesting a link between the redox state of the integrin and its activation state *(17–21)*. Several lines of experimental evidence in the literature support this hypothesis. For example, selective blockage of free cysteine residues in $\alpha_{IIb}\beta_3$ has been demonstrated to abrogate the binding of this integrin to fibrinogen, collagen, and fibronectin *(22)*. Substitutions of certain Cys residues constitutively activate $\alpha_{IIb}\beta_3$ *(20,24)*. In addition, $\alpha_{IIb}\beta_3$, as well as $\alpha_v\beta_3$ and $\alpha_5\beta_1$, have endogenous thiol isomerase activity comparable to that of protein disulfide isomerase (PDI) *(23)*. PDI is present on the surface of platelets and has been postulated to possibly play a role in activating $\alpha_{IIb}\beta_3$ by catalyzing disulfide bond rearrangement *(25)*. Alternatively, or complementary to the activity of PDI, activated $\alpha_{IIb}\beta_3$ might induce self-activation or the activation of a neighboring molecule of $\alpha_{IIb}\beta_3$ through its PDI-like activity. A corollary to these observations is that Mn^{2+}, an integrin activator, stimulates the thiol isomerase activity of $\alpha_{IIb}\beta_3$ *(26)*. In addition, manipulating the redox state of integrins with exogenously added agents such as glutathione might result in blocking the transition of the integrin to its high-affinity state. These observations have led to the hypothesis that one way to therapeutically target integrins involved in disease progression (e.g., those integrins involved in cancer progression) is to manipulate their redox state and prevent the transition of the integrin to its activated conformation. Alternatively, agents that bind to and inhibit only the activated state of the integrin (i.e., that target a particular redox state of the integrin) could provide a higher level of selectivity for integrin targeted therapeutics.

3. INTEGRIN SIGNALING AND THE CYTOSKELETON

Integrins associate with many protein ligands on the outside of cells that regulate integrin function and cellular activity *(27,28)*. Integrin clustering is a prerequisite for integrin signaling and can be mediated by association of the integrin extracellular domains with extracellular ligands. For example, the major platelet integrin $\alpha_{IIb}\beta_3$ binds to fibrinogen once it has been activated during the process of coagulation. Members of the β_2 integrin family are responsible for activated leukocytes binding to counterreceptors such as inflammatory cell adhesion molecules (ICAMs) on endothelial cells. This attachment of leukocytes is essential for phenomena such as phagocytosis and T-cell-mediated cytotoxicity *(6)*. The integrin $\alpha_5\beta_1$ binds the RGD and synergy sequences in fibronectin, facilitating the attachment and migration of cells on the extracellular matrix (ECM).

The cytoplasmic tails of both the α- and β-subunits are short (less than 60 residues generally) and devoid of any enzymatic activity. However, the cytoplasmic domains of integrins also play a vital role in integrin function. Recent data suggest that in addition to ligand binding on the outside of the cells, the cytoplasmic tails of integrins also play a critical role in clustering integrins, thereby generating a binding site for cytoskeletal components and signaling molecules *(29)*. Early studies of integrins showed that the β_1-subunit co-localized with cytoskeletal components in addition to colocalizing with fibronectin. Specifically, talin and α-actinin (both actin binding proteins) bind to the cytoplasmic tail of β_1. Talin and α-actinin can further associate with proteins such as zyxin, paxillin, and vinculin *(28)*. Thus, integrins provide a link between the exterior of the cell and the cytoskeleton of the cell, controlling attachment, which, in turn, regulates cell shape and cell spreading.

The interaction of integrins with cytoskeletal components also leads to the binding of signaling molecules. Integrins can activate protein kinases, including focal adhesion kinase (FAK) (27,28). This can be facilitated when FAK interacts with integrins through talin and paxillin. Activated FAK undergoes autophosphorylation, which creates a binding site for the Src homology 2 (SH2) domain of Src or Fyn, two kinases involved in cell survival and migration. Src can, in turn, phosphorylate a number of focal adhesion components. FAK can also activate phosphatidylinositol (PI)-3 kinase (either directly or through Src kinase). Src will also phosphorylate FAK, creating additional SH2 binding sites. These sites can then bind several molecules, including Src kinases, PTEN, PI-3 kinase, Grb2, and Grb7. These various protein interactions result in cascades of protein activations transducing signals to downstream pathways including those mediated by RAS, RAF, MEK, and ERK. These pathways are known to be involved in cell survival and motility. Integrins can also regulate members of the Rho family of GTPases (30). These enzymes control the dynamics and structure of actin-based processes, including formation of filopodia and lamellipodia, as well as the assembly of stress fibers. In tumor cells, integrins and many of the above-listed pathways are often constitutively activated and probably contribute to tumor progression.

3.1. Integrin Signaling, Control of the Cell Cycle, and Proliferation

Attachment of normal cells to the ECM is a requirement for proliferation, and integrins can activate growth-promoting signaling pathways (27,28,31). Integrins can also synergize with growth factors to activate extracellular signal regulated kinase (ERK). ERK phosphorylates factors that are responsible for the transcription of c-fos, a transcription factor. Furthermore, integrins can activate c-jun N-terminal kinase (JNK), which regulates progression of a cell through the G_1 phase of the cell cycle. Activated JNK enter the nucleus, and activate the transcription factor c-jun, which combines with c-fos to form the AP-1 complex. AP-1 regulates the expression of multiple genes that are important for cell proliferation such as cyclins (32). JNK is poorly activated by growth factors alone, thus explaining why proliferation of cells requires integrin-mediated attachment. Cells that are not attached to the ECM (via integrins) do not show a sustained, robust activation of ERK, which is a requirement for the initiation of the cell cycle. Integrins synergize with growth factors to control the entry and exit from cell cycle phases, but the specific coordination of growth factor and integrin very much depends on the cell type and substrate. For example, FGF-2 and $\alpha_v\beta_3$ signaling is required for proliferation of endothelial cells, whereas in fibroblasts FGF-2 synergizes with β_1 integrins.

3.2. Integrin-Growth Factor Crosstalk

The requirement for both growth-factor-mediated and integrin-mediated signaling for many cellular processes is described as integrin-growth factor crosstalk. Integrins transduce outside-in signals upon ligation of extracellular proteins that regulate several aspects of cell behavior such as migration and survival, but they also respond to inside-out signals from a variety of stimuli. In migrating or invading tumor cells, these processes can be dysregulated and contribute to the malignant phenotype. Integrins are often constitutively activated in tumor cells as well as angiogenic tumor-associated endothelial cells and may mediate outside-in signaling through aberrant phosphorylation and activation of FAK and RHO kinases as well as integrin downstream signaling mediators (33).

These same cells can also have aberrant inside-out signaling leading to changes in integrin affinity (activation), avidity (clustering) *(33)*, and signals that mediate translocation of integrins to migratory structures *(34,35)*. At least four different mechanisms for integrin-growth factor crosstalk have been described:

1. Binding of a growth factor to its receptor can activate integrins by increasing the affinity, avidity or level of expression of the integrin: VEGF has been described to activate $\alpha_v\beta_3$, $\alpha_v\beta_5$, $\alpha_2\beta_1$, and $\alpha_5\beta_1$ integrins in tumor cells via a paracrine loop involving PI-3 kinase, Akt, and PTEN signaling, leading to increased migratory activity *(36)*.
2. Ligation of an integrin results in the enhancement of growth factor response: EGF, PDGF-BB, and FGF-2 mediated signaling is enhanced by integrin ligation *(37)*.
3. Signaling through a growth factor receptor is amplified by an unligated integrin: Hepatocyte growth factor (HGF)-induced invasion of tumour cells requires both c-Met and integrin $\alpha_6\beta_4$. Binding of HGF to its receptor triggers the ligand-independent phosphorylation of the β_4-subunit, which is physically associated with c-Met. Phosphorylated $\alpha_6\beta_4$ activates Sch and PI-3 kinases *(38)*. Similarly, the $\alpha_6\beta_4$ integrin also associates with and amplifies signals from the ErbB-2 receptor independently of ligation of the integrin extracellular domain *(39)*.
4. Ligation of an integrin results in growth-factor-independent activation of a receptor: $\alpha_v\beta_3$ and β_1 integrins associate with the EGF receptor and ligation of the integrins resulted in growth-factor-independent activation of the receptor, which is different than that resulting from the activation of the receptor upon binding of EGF *(40)*.

3.3. Integrin Signaling and Apoptosis

Apoptosis (programmed cell death) might be induced by signaling through death receptors or by the release of cytochrome-*c* from the mitochondria *(6,30,31)*. Apoptosis can also be initiated by cell detachment from the ECM (a process termed anoikis). Integrin signaling can prevent the induction of apoptosis, leading to increased survival. For examples, the ligation of integrin $\alpha_5\beta_1$ (which binds to fibronectin) can induce expression of Bcl-2, protecting cells from stress-induced apoptosis caused by the absence of growth factors. Furthermore, ligation of $\alpha_v\beta_3$ promotes survival of endothelial cells by suppressing the induction of the p53 pathway and activating necrosis factor (NF)-κB. $\alpha_5\beta_1$ is also capable of activating Shc, which also mediates survival. Integrin ligation also promotes survival by activating PI-3-K, ILK, Erk, and JNK. Integrin-mediated activation of PI-3-K produces PI(3,4,5)P3 and PI(3,4)P2, which promote the relocation of Akt to the plasma membrane and stimulate its phosphorylation. Akt blocks apoptosis by inactivating a number of pro-apoptotic molecules, including Bad, caspase-9, and transcription factors of the forkhead family. Akt can also phosphorylate IκB, causing the disruption of the IκB- NF-κB complex and leading to the activation of NF-κB. NF-κB activation leads to the expression of numerous survival factors. Depending on the cell type, these can include vascular endothial growth factor (VEGF), fibroblast growth factor (FGF)-2, interleukin (IL)-6, IL-8, and others.

In contrast, unligated or inappropriately ligated integrins in cells can transmit apoptosis-stimulating signals. For example, ligation of integrins $\alpha_v\beta_3$ and $\alpha_5\beta_1$ in angiogenic endothelial cells by antagonists induces apoptosis in those cells *(41–43)*. A recent study demonstrated that when cells attach to specific matrix-exposing integrins that are unligated, the cells enter the apoptotic pathway mediated by activated caspase-8 which binds to $\alpha_v\beta_3$ *(44)* through a mechanism termed "integrin-mediated death" (IMD). IMD can provide the cell with a mechanism to sense its surroundings. Thus, when a cell is in the wrong environment (characterized by an absence of ligand for a particular integrin), IMD is triggered. The exception can be tumor cells, which are known to be capable of anchorage-independent growth most likely supported by the fact that integrins are often constitutively activated (mimicking the ligated state) in tumor cells and do not require the presence of ligand for activation.

3.4. Integrin Signaling and Cell Motility

Cell migration is essential for normal physiological processes such as leukocyte extravasation as well as dysregulated processes such as tumor metastasis and pathological angiogenesis. Membrane protrusions at the leading edge of the cell (formed by rearrangements of the cytoskeleton) are fixed to components of the ECM by integrins, which trigger the signaling cascades described previously. Integrins can then stimulate cell contraction, allowing the cell to move along the ECM *(43)*. Inactivation of integrins at the trailing edge of the cell allows for detachment from the substratum and the disassembly of the focal adhesion complex. Integrins can also activate ECM-degrading proteases such as metalloproteinases. Matrix remodeling by these proteases alters integrin ligation and further promotes motility.

4. INTEGRIN LIGANDS AND CANCER

A characteristic of the integrin family of proteins is their ability to bind multiple ligands *(46)*. Selectivity for a particular ligand is determined by a number of factors, including the activation state of the integrin, the relative affinity for a particular ligand, and the conformational state of the ligand that determines the exposure of particular integrin recognition sequences. Table 1 provides a list of ligands for some of the members of the integrin family of proteins. The types of ligand represented include a number of ECM proteins (collagen, fibronectin, fibrinogen, laminin, vitronectin, von Willebrand factor, thrombospondin, bone sialoprotein, and osteopontin) consistent with the primary role of integrins in mediating cell adhesion to the extracellular matrix. Integrins also play an essential role in the formation of cell–cell contacts and many counterreceptors are, therefore, also integrin ligands. Of particular importance to tumor cell biology are recent observations describing the interactions of integrins with other cell surface proteins with well-defined roles in tumor cell invasion and metastasis, such as matrix metalloproteinase-2 (MMP-2) and the urokinase plasminogen-activated receptor (uPAR).

A large body of work has defined the minimal recognition sequences required for the interaction of many of these extracellular ligands with specific integrins *(47)*. The prototypic example of these recognition sequences is the RGD sequence, which was originally identified as the sequence within fibronectin that bound integrin to $\alpha_5\beta_1$. The RGD sequence has subsequently been shown to be present in multiple ligands with specificity for a number of integrins *(47)*. Importantly, RGD-containing peptides are able to inhibit ligand binding to integrins with RGD recognition specificity. Integrins are able to discriminate between particular RGD-containing ligands based on a number of criteria, including the amino acid residues flanking the RGD sequence, three-dimensional presentation of the sequence and specific features of the integrin binding pocket *(48)*.

The complexity of integrin–ligand interactions can be illustrated by considering the binding of various integrins to the RGD-containing ECM protein fibronectin (FN).

Table 1
Extracellular Protein Ligands of Selected Integrin Heterodimeric Complexes

Integrin	Integrin extracellular ligand(s)
$\alpha_2\beta_1$	Collagens, fibronectin, laminin
$\alpha_3\beta_1$	Fibronectin, thrombospondin, epiligrin, invasin, uPAR
$\alpha_4\beta_1$	Fibronectin, invasin, VCAM-1
$\alpha_5\beta_1$	Fibronectin, fibrinogen, invasin, uPAR
$\alpha_6\beta_1$	Laminin, invasin, uPAR
$\alpha_6\beta_4$	Laminin
$\alpha_v\beta_3$	Bone sialoprotein, fibronectin, fibrinogen, laminin, osteopontin, thrombospondin, vitronectin, von Willebrand factor, disintegrins, MMP-2, uPAR
$\alpha_v\beta_5$	Bone sialoprotein, fibronectin, vitronectin

Fibronectin is a ligand for 12 members of the integrin family of proteins *(46,49)*, including the prototypic FN receptor $\alpha_5\beta_1$. The RGD peptide sequence is found in the 10th type III repeat of FN (FN-III$_{10}$) and, as described earlier, binding is complex. A second peptide sequence, PHSRN or the synergy site, found in FN-III$_9$, promotes specific binding of FN to $\alpha_5\beta_1$ apparently through interaction with the α_5-subunit *(50)*. A peptide, PHSCN, based on this sequence has been shown to inhibit tumor growth and metastasis in preclinical models and has served as the basis for a novel integrin antagonist, ATN-161, that is currently in early clinical development *(51,52)*. Binding of integrin $\alpha_5\beta_1$ to a N-terminal fragment of FN containing type I repeats 1–9 and type II repeats 1,2 can also support cell adhesion. This interaction activates signaling pathways distinct from those activated by binding to RGD-containing fragments. Cell recognition sequences leucine-asparic acid-valine (LDV) and arginine-glutamic acid-aspartic acid-valine (REDV) were originally identified in the alternatively spliced V region of FN and are recognized by both integrin $\alpha_4\beta_1$ and $\alpha_4\beta_7$ *(53,54)*. The sequences IDAPS (present in FN-III$_{14}$) and KLDAPT (present in FN-III$_5$) are also recognized by integrin $\alpha_4\beta_1$ *(55)*. Taken together, these examples illustrate that, although there is considerable diversity associated with ligand recognition by integrins, the specific interaction of integrins with extracellular proteins can be reduced in many cases to small peptide sequences.

4.1. Fibronectin

Fibronectin (FN) is the principle ligand for integrin $\alpha_5\beta_1$. This prototypic integrin–ligand pair is functionally important because it mediates fibronectin fibril formation and regulates ECM assembly, which is essential for cell function in vivo *(49)*. Furthermore, the interaction between integrin $\alpha_5\beta_1$ and FN is essential for vertebrate development. Targeted disruption of the FN gene results is an early embryonic lethal phenotype *(56)*. FN typically consists of a dimer of two subunits of approx 250 kDa each, covalently linked by a pair of disulfide bonds. FN is an abundant soluble plasma protein (approx 300 μg/mL) as well as an essential component of the insoluble ECM. Plasma fibronectin is synthesized predominantly by liver hepatocytes, but many other cell types also express FN. Alternative splicing of the single FN gene results in the expression of many diverse isoforms of FN with unique cell-adhesive, ligand-binding, and solubility properties *(49)*.

This complex pattern of expression enables cells to precisely regulate the composition of the ECM in a developmental and tissue-specific manner. Recent work from Kim et al. *(57)* has more precisely defined the role of fibronectin and its principle receptor, integrin $\alpha_5\beta_1$, in angiogenesis and demonstrated, for the first time, a role for an ECM protein in the promotion of angiogenesis. As noted earlier, expression of integrin $\alpha_5\beta_1$ and fibronectin are significantly enhanced on blood vessels of primary human tumors but not on vessels of normal tissues. Similarly, fibronectin and integrin $\alpha_5\beta_1$ expression is coordinately regulated on growth-factor-stimulated blood vessels, and the functional role of integrin $\alpha_5\beta_1$ and fibronectin in angiogenesis appears to be a direct consequence of their growth-factor-induced expression. Antibodies directed against the central cell-binding fragment (CBD) of fibronectin, which contains the PHSRN and RGDS integrin-binding sites, inhibited angiogenesis, suggesting that integrin ligation by fibronectin and downstream signal transduction events are important for angiogenesis *(57)*. The distribution of fibronectin in areas of skeletogenesis suggests that it may also be involved in the differentiation of osteoblasts and the early stages of bone formation. Indeed, using in vitro models of osteoblast differentiation, it has been demonstrated that antifibronectin antibodies can inhibit the formation of mineralized nodules and the expression of genes characteristic of the osteoblast phenotype *(58)*. Furthermore, fragments of fibronectin containing the RGD sequence, as well as an RGD-containing peptide GRGDSPK, also inhibited osteoblast differentiation. The effects of the peptide GRGDSPK were distinct from those of larger fragments of fibronectin tested (e.g., FN-III$_{6-10}$), suggesting that other sequences might contribute to the overall process of differentiation *(58)*.

4.2. Vitronectin

Vitronectin (VN) is a mixture of two monomeric glycoproteins of 65 and 75 kDa found both in the circulation and in the ECM. Synthesized primarily by the liver, VN is involved in a number of physiological processes, including blood coagulation and fibrinolysis, cellular immunity, and tumor metastasis *(59,60)*. VN contains an RGD motif and regulates cellular functions via integrins $\alpha_v\beta_3$ and $\alpha_v\beta_5$. In addition to the integrin mediated functions of VN, the protein can interact with other ligands including PAI-1, urokinase (uPA), uPAR, glycosaminoglycans (such as heparin), other ECM components (such as collagen), and complement complexes (such as C5b-9a) to mediate a diverse array of biological effects *(61)*. Binding of VN to some of these ligands, including PAI-1 and complement components, causes conformational changes in VN that alter certain functions of the protein *(62)*.

4.3. Collagen

The major structural protein of the extracellular matrix is collagen. The collagens are a large family of proteins, containing at least 19 different members. They are characterized by the formation of triple helices in which three polypeptide chains are wound tightly around one another to form a ropelike structure. The most abundant type of collagen (type I collagen) is one of the fibril-forming collagens and is a basic structural components of skin, tendon, bone, ligaments, dentin, and interstitial tissues. Collagen type I in its native form can be bound by two integrins, $\alpha_1\beta_1$ and $\alpha_2\beta_1$, through interactions with the tetrapeptide RGDA. In contrast, denaturation of collagen I results in exposure of cryptic RGD sites that bind to integrin $\alpha_v\beta_3$. This ability to recognize different forms of collagen might allow the cell to bind this substrate under different circumstances such as tissue remodeling or metastatic dissemination. Recent work has demonstrated that expression of integrin $\alpha_v\beta_3$ in tumor cells increases their propensity to metastasize to bone *(63)*. Moreover, integrin $\alpha_v\beta_3$ over-expression increases tumor cell invasion, migration, and adhesion to mineralized bone and bone matrix proteins, including type I collagen, but does not affect tumor cell proliferation.

4.4. Laminin

The major glycoprotein of the basement membrane is laminin, which is involved in the attachment, spreading, migration, and differentiation of normal and neoplastic cells *(64)*. Interaction between cancer cells and laminin is a prerequisite for basement membrane invasion and metastasis *(65)*. In addition, laminin regulates interactions between malignant cells and the immune system *(66)*. Several cell surface laminin-binding proteins have been described, including integrins $\alpha_2\beta_1$, $\alpha_6\beta_1$, $\alpha_6\beta_4$, and $\alpha_v\beta_3$ *(46)* as well as nonintegrin laminin receptors *(67)*. Laminin does not contain an RGD sequence and binding to integrins occurs primarily via the amino acid sequence YIGSR. A synthetic peptide containing this sequence has been demonstrated to inhibit the formation of osteolytic bone metastases in a mouse model *(68)*.

4.5. Osteopontin

Osteopontin (OPN) is a phosphorylated glycoprotein expressed by a number of cell types, including activated macrophages and leucocytes, and is found at sites of inflammation as well as in the ECM of mineralized tissues *(69)*. OPN contains an RGD sequence (amino acids 166–168) and regulates cell responses, including adhesion and migration, through several integrin receptors. OPN facilitates the attachment of osteoclasts to the bone matrix via integrin $\alpha_v\beta_3$ *(70)*. Furthermore, it has been suggested that the subsequent remodeling of the bone matrix is also dependent on this interaction. Other sequences within OPN have also been shown to mediate cell adherence. For example, cleavage of human OPN by thrombin exposes the SVVYGLR sequence, promoting the adherence of cells expressing integrins α_9 and α_4 *(71)*. OPN is also a ligand for the CD44 receptor, through which it acts as a chemoattractant *(72)*. Increased OPN expression is often associated with malignant transformation *(73)*, and in animal models, this increased expression is associated with increased metastatic potential *(74)*. A study in breast cancer patients demonstrated that increased tumor cell expression of OPN was a marker of poor prognosis for patients with this disease *(75)*.

4.6. Bone Sialoprotein

Bone sialoprotein (BSP) is a noncollagenous, acidic bone matrix glycoprotein synthesized by both osteoclasts and osteoblasts *(76)* that plays an important role in mineralization and in the adhesion of osteoclasts to the bone surface *(77)*. BSP contains an RGD sequence near its carboxy-terminus and is a ligand for the integrin $\alpha_v\beta_3$ *(78)*. BSP expression is upregulated in carcinomas that exhibit microcalcifications and that metastasize to bone with high frequency *(79)*. In a study of patients with primary breast cancer, serum BSP levels were found to be the most important prognostic factor for the development of skeletal metastasis *(80)*. The interaction of integrins $\alpha_v\beta_3$ and $\alpha_v\beta_5$ with BSP has been shown to support human breast cancer cell adhesion, proliferation, and migration *(81)*. More recently, it has been demonstrated that BSP, through interaction with integrin $\alpha_v\beta_3$, can promote both adhesion and chemotactic migration of endothelial cells *(82)*. This study also demonstrated that BSP stimulates angiogenesis in a CAM assay, with activity comparable to that observed with FGF-2 *(82)*.

4.7. uPAR

Degradation of the ECM plays an essential role in a number of pathological processes, including tumor cell invasion, metastasis, and angiogenesis. The high-affinity, glycolipid-anchored receptor for the serine protease urokinase (uPAR) is often upregulated on invading tumor cells *(83)* and spatially restricted degradation of the ECM, via uPA catalyzed plasminogen activation, is thought to be a prerequisite for metastasis from many solid tumors *(84)*. More recent work has focused on the physical association of uPAR with various integrins on the surface of highly migratory tumor cells *(85–87)*. uPAR is able to form a complex with activated integrins when attached to specific ECM proteins. These uPAR–integrin complexes both inhibit the integrin adhesive function and promote the chemotaxis and adhesion to vitronectin via a ligand-binding site on uPAR *(86)*. Recent work also suggests that uPAR binds to unique non-ligand-binding sites in repeat 4 of several integrin α-subunits *(88)* and, importantly, several peptides have been identified that disrupt the uPAR–integrin interaction *(86,88)*. These peptides inhibit uPAR-mediated adhesion to vitronectin, β_1-integrin-dependent cell spreading, and migration on various substrates. The role of these uPAR–integrin complexes has also been studied in an in vivo bone xenograft model *(89)*. MDA-MB-231 cells overexpressing the inhibitory peptide p25 showed a significant reduction in tumor progression in bone. More importantly, systemic delivery of the p25 peptide had a similar effect on MDA-MB-231 tumor progression in bone *(89)*. Taken together, these data suggest that uPAR physically associates with integrins and that disruption of this interaction regulates integrin function in a variety of cellular processes.

4.8. Metastasis is Facilitated by Integrins

Metastasis to bone and other tissues involves dissemination of tumor cells via the bloodstream and the lymphatic system. This multistep process depends on the ability of the tumor cell to complete a program of steps that includes tumor cell intravasation, adhesion to the vessel wall, extravasation at the metastatic site, infiltration, and proliferation of the tumor cell within the target tissue. Many of these steps involve the participation of integrin receptors. The role of a particular integrin in these processes is dependent not only on its pattern of expression but also its activation state. The activation state of an integrin determines its affinity for a particular ligand and, in general, controls cell adhesion *(90)*. This is particularly important within the vasculature, where cell attachment is physically opposed by blood flow. For example, the integrin $\alpha_v\beta_3$ has been shown to play an essential role in the process of tumor cell arrest within the vasculature by binding to soluble ligands that crosslink tumor cells to activated platelets bound to endothelium, and only the activated form of $\alpha_v\beta_3$ can mediate this tumor cell arrest *(91–93)*. Furthermore, the growth of new blood vessels, angiogenesis, is essential for tumor growth and provides the conduit by which tumor cells disseminate to distant sites. Although the role of growth factors (e.g., vascular endothelial growth factor [VEGF] and basic fibroblast growth factor [FGF-2]) has been clearly established in pathological angiogenesis associated with solid tumor growth, diabetic retinopathy, and rheumatoid arthritis, it is also apparent that interactions with the ECM play a vital role in this process. The ECM provides precise, spatially restricted signals to guide the process of angiogenesis. These signals include matrix-associated growth factors, cytokines, and proteases, as well as the ECM proteins themselves, including laminins, collagens, and fibronectin. Integrins $\alpha_v\beta_3$, $\alpha_v\beta_5$, and $\alpha_5\beta_1$ are highly expressed in angiogenic endothelial cells and are essential to this process *(94,95)*. In addition, metastasis can also occur via the lymphatic system and the interaction of metastatic cells with lymphatic tissue is facilitated by integrins. Breast cancer cells have been observed to attach to fibronectin through $\alpha_3\beta_1$ *(96)* and melanoma cells are known to bind to vitronectin *(97)* within the milieu of a lymph node. High-expression levels of integrin α_3 have also been shown to predict for the risk of lymph node metastasis in oral squamous cell carcinoma *(98)* and the integrin $\alpha_6\beta_1$ is upregulated in prostate cancer that has metastasized to lymph node *(99)*.

4.9. Integrins Can Regulate Proteolysis of Invasive Carcinoma

The contribution of proteases to tumor invasion has long been appreciated and represents a target for clinical intervention. Integrins and proteases are known to be involved in regulating each other's activity. As such, adhesive and proteolytic events can be interdependent in invasive carcinoma. For example, proMMP2 (gelatinase A) is activated on the cell surface by a complex that includes membrane type 1 MMP (MT1-MMP), tissue inhibitor of metalloproteinase 2 (TIMP2), and $\alpha_v\beta_3$ *(7)*. Therefore, the $\alpha_v\beta_3$ integrin is not only an adhesion/migration receptor but also controls remodeling of the basement membrane through the formation of the MMP complex. In addition, the receptor (uPAR) for the protease uPA physically associates with integrins and disruption of that interaction inhibits progression of breast cancer growth in bone *(89)*. The binding of uPA to uPAR also induces the association of uPAR to $\alpha_5\beta_1$ and the activation of this integrin *(100)*. Formation of the uPA/uPAR/$\alpha_5\beta_1$ complex triggered migration of Chinese hamster ovary (CHO) cells.

4.10. Integrin Expression in Cancer Tissue

Primary tumor growth is often associated with changes in integrin expression relative to the normal tissue or cell type from which the tumor is derived. These changes include *de novo* expression of specific integrin subunits, changes in the level of integrin expression, and, in some cases, changes in the pattern or cellular distribution of integrins. Characterization of the pattern of integrin expression in tumor biopsies can have utility in determining the stage of a tumor or provide a useful prognostic marker, especially with regard to tumor metastasis. Immunohistochemistry provides a valuable tool in the evaluation of integrin expression in tumor biopsies and data for three tumor types commonly associated with bone metastasis are summarized in Table 2. Changes in the level or pattern of integrin expression are unique for each tumor type and can be complex, as discussed in the following. In general, the loss or gain of integrin expression is not associated with malignant transformation but is associated with tumor progression and metastasis *(101)*.

Some tumors are characterized by potentially specific changes in integrin expression. In renal cell carcinoma, the promiscuous $\alpha_2\beta_1$ integrin is expressed on metastatic tumor cells but is not expressed by the primary lesion *(109)*, suggesting that $\alpha_2\beta_1$ is involved in metastasis or the colonization of the metastatic site. Strong expression of $\alpha_6\beta_1$ and weak expression of $\alpha_5\beta_1$ integrin expression has been reported as being a good prognostic indicator for ductal adenocarcinoma of the pancreas and correlates well with the risk of metastasis *(110)*. It is important to note that expression of particular integrin subunits,

Table 2
Expression of Integrin Heterodimeric Complexes in Selected
Tumor Tissues as Determined by Immunohistochemistry

Tumor tissue	Lesion	$\alpha_2\beta_1$	$\alpha_3\beta_1$	$\alpha_4\beta_1$	$\alpha_5\beta_1$	$\alpha_6\beta_1$	$\alpha_6\beta_4$	$\alpha_v\beta_3$	$\alpha_v\beta_5$
Breast	Primary	±	±	−	+	±	±	+	
	Metastatic	±	±	−		+	+	+	±
Kidney	Primary	−	+	+	±	±		±	±
	Metastatic	+	±	+	+				±
Prostate	Primary	±	+		+	±	±	+	
	Metastatic	+			+			+	

Note: Data extracted and compiled from ref. 101 (and references therein), and 102–108. Scoring system adapted from ref. 101. (+) = increase in the level of integrin expression; (—) = decrease in the level of integrin expression; (±) = change in the pattern of integrin expression and/or reduced expression; (blank) = insufficient data.

or heterodimer complexes, is only one measure of the complex interactions of a tumor cell with its environment. Application of antibodies specific for activated integrin conformations can reveal significant differences between normal and tumor tissues, even if the expression level of a particular integrin remains constant. For example, it has been reported that the expression level of activated integrin $\alpha_5\beta_1$ is critical to the process of metastasis and that this is particularly important in the kidney, where tumor cells adhere to fibronectin associated with glomeruli (103).

Integrin $\alpha_6\beta_4$, a laminin receptor, has been implicated in the invasive phenotype of many carcinomas and represents a potential therapeutic target. However, the expression of integrin $\alpha_6\beta_4$ also provides a good illustration of the complexity associated with integrin profiling in general. For example, integrin $\alpha_6\beta_4$ is found at the basolateral aspect of the epithelium in normal breast tissue and in benign lesions. Primary breast tumors express either reduced levels of $\alpha_6\beta_4$ or show a significant change in the cellular distribution of the integrin. In contrast, metastatic lesions generally express normal levels of the integrin (104). Integrin β_4 expression is also elevated on the most invasive pancreatic cell lines. Recently, Lipscomb et al. (111) demonstrated that small interfering (si)RNA directed against either integrin subunit significantly reduced the invasive potential of MDA-MB-231 breast carcinoma cells. Similarly, the expression of integrin $\alpha_6\beta_1$, also a laminin receptor, is elevated in metastatic lesions (101).

A number of studies have reported that integrin $\alpha_5\beta_1$ expression correlates with tumor progression. A survey of lung cancer cell lines and node-negative non-small-cell lung cancers (NSCLCs) revealed a high frequency of integrin $\alpha_5\beta_1$ expression (112). The overall survival rate of patients with integrin $\alpha_5\beta_1$ overexpressing tumors was significantly worse than for individuals whose tumors had normal levels of integrin $\alpha_5\beta_1$ expression (112). Similar results have been reported for primary bladder cancers, as well as bladder cancer cell lines (113). A more recent study evaluated the expression of integrin $\alpha_5\beta_1$ in frozen sections taken from human colon, breast, ovarian, and pancreatic carcinoma (105). These studies revealed that integrin $\alpha_5\beta_1$ expression colocalized with CD31-positive endothelial cells of the tumor vasculature. Importantly, CD31-positive blood vessels found in sections of normal human colon and breast, as well as other normal adult tissues, were negative for integrin $\alpha_5\beta_1$. Similar results were obtained when tumor blood vessels were stained for fibronectin expression, suggesting a functional interaction between the two proteins in the formation and/or maintenance of the tumor vasculature.

Metastases show an organ-specific pattern of spread, and this can be determined, in part, by the pattern of integrin expression. A survey of integrin expression in orbital metastatic lesions from prostate carcinoma, malignant melanoma, and breast carcinoma revealed elevated expression of integrin subunits α_2, α_4, and β_3 when compared to normal tissue (106). The authors further suggest that these changes in integrin expression may be responsible for the tendency of these tumors to metastasize to the orbit and prostate tumors to metastasize to bone.

Loss or reduction in integrin expression by the primary tumor could result in less adhesive cells more likely to migrate to distant sites. Characterization of primary breast tumors demonstrated that loss of β_1-subunit containing integrins as well as $\alpha_v\beta_5$ integrin was related to the presence of metastasis (107). Although the expression level of each integrin alone was not predictive of metastatic disease, multivariate analysis including all of the integrins tested predicted metastatic disease with approx 97% accuracy. A recent survey of integrin expression in effusions, primary tumors, and solid metastases of ovarian carcinoma patients showed that the α_v- and β_1-integrin subunits are frequently expressed in ovarian carcinoma cells and that the α_v-integrin subunit is a diagnostic marker for these cells (114). Expression of the α_v-integrin subunit correlated with expression of matrix metalloproteinase-9 (MMP-9). Expression of the β_1-integrin subunit was not exclusive to tumor cells but could also be detected on endothelial and stromal cells. Indeed, the authors detected reduced expression of the β_1-integrin subunit in primary tumors and suggested that other integrin subunits, such as β_3 as part of the $\alpha_v\beta_3$-vitronectin receptor, compensate for the loss of β_1 expression in these lesions.

A role for integrins in angiogenesis was originally established by the observation that integrin $\alpha_v\beta_3$ is overexpressed in the vasculature of some tumors (115) and provides survival signals to activated endothelial cells (41,108). These studies have since been extended to show that antibody and small peptide inhibitors of integrin $\alpha_v\beta_3$, and the related integrin $\alpha_v\beta_5$, block angiogenesis in models of both tumor and retinal angiogenesis (41). Similarly, expression of integrin $\alpha_5\beta_1$ and its ligand fibronectin are significantly enhanced on blood vessels of primary human tumors but not on vessels of normal tissues. The role of integrin $\alpha_5\beta_1$ and its ligand fibronectin in vascular development and angiogenesis is strongly supported by studies of knockout mice (116) and recent work from Kim et al. (105) has precisely defined the role of integrin $\alpha_5\beta_1$ in angiogenesis and demonstrated, for the first time, a role for an ECM protein in the promotion of angiogenesis.

The roles of $\alpha_v\beta_3$ and $\alpha_v\beta_5$ in angiogenesis have recently been called into question (117). Mice null for either β_3 or β_5 do not have reduced angiogenesis and, in fact, display enhanced pathological angiogenesis and tumor growth (118,119). It is presently not clear how to reconcile these results with the extensive literature demonstrating the ability of $\alpha_v\beta_3$ and $\alpha_v\beta_5$ antagonists to inhibit angiogenesis and tumor growth. One possibility is that in the null mice, compensatory mechanisms arise that overcome the lack of β_3 or β_5 integrins and, as a result, lead to enhanced angiogenesis and tumor growth. However, regardless of the role of these integrins in angiogenesis, they remain important targets for the inhibition of tumor growth and metastasis.

Expression of integrin $\alpha_v\beta_3$ correlates with tumor progression in melanoma, glioma, ovarian, and breast cancer *(120)*. Importantly, $\alpha_v\beta_3$ expression characterizes the metastatic phenotype and, for example, is abundant in breast cancer cells that metastasize to bone *(121)*. In addition, the expression of integrin subunits α_5 and α_1 are also significantly correlated with metastasis associated with some tumor types, such as lung cancer *(122)*. Mechanistically, expression of $\alpha_v\beta_3$ supports breast cancer cell attachment under flow conditions in an activation-dependent manner *(123)*. This same study also established that the metastatic phenotype of MDA-MB-435 human breast cancer cells, as well as primary metastatic cells from patients, correlated with the expression of activated $\alpha_v\beta_3$. These data have led to the suggestion that expression of $\alpha_v\beta_3$ is necessary but not sufficient for breast cancer metastasis and that additional factors controlling the state of integrin activation are required for metastatic dissemination. For example, a recent study demonstrated that activated $\alpha_v\beta_3$ integrin cooperates with MMP-9 to regulate the migration of metastatic breast carcinoma cells *(124)*.

4.11. Integrins in Bone Metastasis

Recent studies have also established a clear role for $\alpha_v\beta_3$ in bone metastasis *(92,125–127)*. In general, there are two types of metastatic lesion formed in bone: those that promote bone growth (osteblastic) and those that promote bone destruction (osteolytic). Patients with prostate cancer metastasis and some patients with breast cancer metastasis are the most likely to have osteoblastic lesions. However, most patients with breast cancer as well as lung cancer, renal cell cancer, and myeloma develop primarily osteolytic lesions, which appear to depend on the presence of $\alpha_v\beta_3$ on tumor cells and osteoclasts.

In preclinical studies, the expression of $\alpha_v\beta_3$ in CHO cells increased the incidence, number, and area of osteolytic lesions in a mouse model by increasing tumor cell invasion and adhesion to mineralized bone and bone matrix proteins, in particular type I collagen, an important ligand for $\alpha_v\beta_3$ *(128)*. Cells expressing a functionally inactive mutant of $\alpha_v\beta_3$ had a significantly reduced ability to form osteolytic lesions. Similar results were obtained with the breast cancer line B02 which expresses $\alpha_v\beta_3$ at a high level. More recently, the role of $\alpha_v\beta_3$ expressed by cells native to the bone in the growth and pathogenesis of prostate cancer bone metastases was evaluated *(116)*. Using $\alpha_v\beta_3$-negative tumor cells, this study demonstrated that inhibition of $\alpha_v\beta_3$ significantly reduced the amount of angiogenesis within tumor bearing bone implants and, as a consequence, reduced the proliferation of $\alpha_v\beta_3$-negative tumor cells. Furthermore, the inhibition of $\alpha_v\beta_3$ significantly reduced the recruitment of osteoclasts in response to tumor cells and the degradation of calcified bone tissue.

The relevance of the integrin $\alpha_v\beta_3$ for metastasis to the bone and its importance as a clinical target is further supported by several studies that demonstrate the ability of therapies directed against this integrin to inhibit metastasis *(92,125–127)*. Integrin $\alpha_v\beta_3$ binds a number of ECM and serum proteins *(46)* and also mediates the binding of tumor cells to the RGD-containing protein BSP, which is a bone-specific protein known to play an important role in metastasis *(129,130)*. A number of invasive breast carcinoma cells express constitutively active $\alpha_v\beta_3$, which endows these cells with the capacity to adhere and migrate to BSP *(129)*. Finally, SPARC (secreted protein acidic and rich in cysteine), also known as osteonectin or BM-40, is a component of the bone matrix, contains a functional RGD motif and binds to the $\alpha_v\beta_3$ integrin *(131)*. The role of SPARC in supporting migration of highly metastatic prostate cancer lines was recently demonstrated and showed that increased migration to SPARC was mediated by VEGF-activated $\alpha_v\beta_3$ and $\alpha_v\beta_5$ integrins *(132)*. Integrin engagement of SPARC also enhanced VEGF expression, establishing an autocrine loop of integrin activation. Thus, SPARC, through binding to activated $\alpha_v\beta_3$ and $\alpha_v\beta_5$, promoted migration, localization to bone, and VEGF-mediated survival of the tumor cells within the bone environment *(132)*.

5. THERAPEUTIC APPROACHES TARGETING BONE METASTASIS

Bone metastases, like metastases to other organs, are often treated using systemic or in some cases localized therapies. Bone metastases that are localized to a few isolated bones can be treated with external beam radiation or, in some cases, with surgery as a palliative measure. For metastases from hormone-sensitive cancers such as prostate and breast cancer, hormone therapy might be indicated. Unfortunately, by the time prostate or breast cancer metastasizes to the bone, it is usually hormone refractory and will no longer respond to hormonal agents. Metastron (strontium-89) has been used in men with diffuse bone metastasis resulting from advanced prostate cancer but has not been used as frequently to treat metastases resulting from other cancer types. Metastron deposits in bone because of its similarity to calcium but is only approved as a palliative agent and has not led to reduction of tumor burden in the bone, even when combined with chemotherapeutic agents such as gemcitabine *(133)*. Finally, despite a multitude of chemotherapeutic approaches to treat patients with bone metastasis, most of these approaches remain palliative in hormone refractory breast and prostate cancer patients and are generally not recommended for bone metastases arising from chemoresistant tumors such as lung cancer. Thus, there is a tremendous need to identify alternative approaches for the treatment of bone metastasis.

5.1. Drugs That Inhibit Bone Resorption

Although there are several drugs currently approved for the treatment of bone metastasis, none of these drugs were actually developed for this indication. Approved drugs for the treatment of bone metastasis fall into the class of bisphophonates, which were originally developed for the treatment of osteoporosis. Bisphosphonates bind to bone surfaces that are undergoing active remodeling, inhibit osteoclast maturation and recruitment, and induce osteoclast apoptosis. This reduces osteoclast activity as well as the production of cytokines and growth factors that induce bone resorption. Preclinical studies in vitro have demonstrated the ability of bisphosphonates to prevent tumor cell adhesion and invasion to bone, inhibit MMP activity generated by tumor cells, reduce the growth or induce apoptosis of tumor cells, and inhibit tumor angiogenesis *(134,135)*. Further, preclinical as well as clinical results suggest that bisphosphonates lower tumor burden in bone and enhance survival *(136)*. To date, pamidronate (Aredia) has been the most often used Food and Drug Administration (FDA)-approved bisphosphonate to treat patients with multiple myeloma or breast cancer bone metastases. Pamidronate is also effective in reducing osteoporosis in men with prostate cancer during androgen withdrawal but has not been effective in palliating bone pain in men with prostate cancer metastases *(137)*. However, a more potent third-generation bisphosphonate, zoledronate (Zometa), has been demonstrated to be effective for the palliation of bone pain in men with metastatic prostate cancer and has recently been approved by the FDA for the treatment of bone metastases from all solid tumors as well as the osteolytic lesions associated with multiple myeloma *(138)*. Zoledronate also reduces the osteoporosis often associated with bone metastasis in addition to its palliative effects. Additional studies to explore whether bisphosphonates are capable of lessening the incidence, delaying the appearance, or inducing the regression of bone metastasis are currently under way.

5.2. Drugs That Stimulate Bone Formation

The identification of drugs that stimulate bone formation is desirable for the treatment of metastasis-related osteoporosis in patients with osteolytic metastases or lesions. Currently, there are no drugs that stimulate bone formation approved for this indication although teriparatide (Forteo) was approved in 2002 for the treatment of osteoporosis. Forteo is a 34-amino acid fragment of parathyroid hormone (PTH) that was approved despite concerns over the tumor-promoting activity of Forteo (Forteo induced osteosarcoma in rats in preclinical studies) (139). Thus, it is unlikely that this drug will be tested in cancer patients any time in the near future. In addition, there would be concern over using a drug that stimulates bone formation in patients with an osteoblastic component to their bone metastasis, such as in prostate cancer.

5.3. Drugs in Development Targeting Bone Metastasis

There are only a few drugs aside from the bisphosphonates currently under development for the treatment of bone metastasis. One of these compounds, Atrasentan (ABT-627) is an endothelin-1 (ET-1; endothelin-A) antagonist currently in phase III trials sponsored by Abbott Laboratories. ET-1 can mediate pathological bone remodeling by tumors, producing ET-1-stimulated osteoblastic lesion progression in preclinical studies in vivo. The inhibition of ET-1 binding to its receptor significantly reduced osteoblastic bone metastasis and tumor burden in these preclinical studies (140,141). Thus, targeting the ET-1 pathway with an antagonist such as Atrasentan holds tremendous potential for the treatment of bone metastasis. A second drug that is currently in development for the treatment of bone metastasis is a humanized monoclonal antibody called CAL. This antibody, under development by Chugai Pharmaceuticals, targets parathyroid hormone related peptide (PTHrP) and is currently in several phase II studies. PTHrP is expressed by tumor cells from cancers that metastasize to the bone (such as breast and lung) and generates osteolytic lesions. Neutralizing antibodies against PTHrP have been demonstrated to inhibit the progression of osteolytic metastasis and decrease the hypercalcemia often associated with osteolytic bone metastasis in preclinical studies thus emphasizing the promise of this therapeutic approach (142).

Finally, osteoprotegerin, which behaves as a receptor decoy and binds to receptor activator of NF-κB ligand (RANK-L) is currently in phase I trials for the treatment of bone metastasis. The RANK-L target are discussed in the following section.

5.4. Future Targets for the Treatment of Bone Metastasis

Although there is some effort underway in the area of osteoblast inhibition, many of the current approaches for targeting bone metastasis are still focused on the osteoclast because the majority of bone metastases are osteolytic in nature. This is true even for prostate cancer patients whose metastases are often characterized as being osteoblastic but, nevertheless, have an underlying osteoclastic component (143). There are a number of potential osteoclast processes that are amenable to intervention, including osteoclast differentiation, osteoclast binding to bone, and osteoclast enzymatic activity. Targets involved in these processes include transforming growth factor (TGF)-β and its receptor(s), CXCR4, RANK-L, cathepsin K, CD44, c-Src-tyrosine kinase, and integrins such as $\alpha_v\beta_3$. Many of these targets are in fact interrelated and part of the same pathways mediating osteoclastogenesis and osteoclast differentiation. For example, RANK-L expression is upregulated in bone endothelial cells by TGF-β *(144)*. RANK-L mediates osteoclastogenesis and osteoclast differentiation by increasing osteoclast adhesion and fusion through the upregulation of $\alpha_v\beta_3$ *(145)* and the expression of bone remodeling proteases such as MMPs *(146)*. $\alpha_v\beta_3$ signaling is thought to occur through c-Src and TGF-β expression may be regulated through CD44-mediated adhesion *(147)*. Thus, there might be multiple points for therapeutic intervention in the same pathway and decisions on where to intervene will need to involve an analysis of the druggability of the target as well as the specificity of that target for osteoclast driven metastasis vs other physiologic functions. Currently, Pfizer has a discovery program to identify small-molecule antagonists of CXCR4 and Schering-Plough has an antibody targeting RANK-L. Both of these efforts are still in the preclinical stage and are focused on inflammation rather than on the treatment of bone metastasis.

Recent studies also suggest that cancer cell metastasis is mediated by signature sets of genes for poor-prognosis *(148)* and for bone-specific metastasis *(149)*. Elevated expression of bone-metastasis-enhancing factors from breast cancer cells include the chemokine CXCR4, MMP-1, a disintegrin and metalloprotease with thrombospondin motifs-1 (ADAMTS-1), FGF-5, connective tissue growth factor (CTGF), IL-11, follistatin, and proteoglycan-1. Functional assays suggest a causal role for IL-11, CTGF, and CXCR4, along with OPN in osteolytic metastasis formation. Overexpression of IL-11 and OPN combined with either CXCR4 or CTGF in breast cancer cells led to the formation of aggressive bone lesions *(149)*. The identification of CTGF and OPN as bone metastasis signature genes is also consistent with the proposed role of TGF-β in promoting bone metastasis. OPN is a ligand for CD44, and OPN itself is up-egulated by TGF-β *(150)*. In addition, TGF-β has been demonstrated to regulate CTGF expression and activity in cell types other than bone suggesting the possibility that a similar situation could also exist in osteoclasts although this remains to be investigated *(151)*. Thus, both biochemical and genetic data implicate the TGF-β axis in the progression of bone metastasis and provide a set of targets for the development of therapeutics to treat bone metastasis.

5.5. Integrin-Targeting Drugs in Development

Although changes in integrin expression were not observed in the signature set for bone metastasis of breast cancer cells, there is nevertheless overwhelming data supporting integrin targeting as a viable therapeutic strategy for targeting bone metastasis (*see* Section 4.10.). In addition, integrin activation and integrin-mediated adhesion are downstream of many of the genes identified in the signature set as well as through biochemical techniques. For example, CXCR4 has been demonstrated to mediate integrin activation and adhesion on various cell types *(152,153)*. Similarly, IL-11 and CTGF have both been demonstrated to increase the adhesion of cells to fibronectin through the activation of $\alpha_5\beta_1$ *(154,155)*. Finally, OPN is a ligand for integrins and integrins such as $\alpha_v\beta_3$ potentiate the malignancy-inducing effects of OPN *(156)*.

In the integrin antagonist category, several companies are in phase I or early phase II trials with monoclonal antibodies or peptides targeting $\alpha_v\beta_3$, $\alpha_v\beta_5$, or $\alpha_5\beta_1$ (Table 3).

Table 3
Integrin Antagonists in Clinical Development

Candidate	Sponsor	Type of molecule	Target	Clinical trial phase
MEDI-522	Medimmune	Humanized mAb	$\alpha_v\beta_3$	Phase II
EMD12197 (Cilengitide)	Merck KGa	Cyclic pentapeptide	$\alpha_v\beta_3$, $\alpha_v\beta_5$	Phase II
CNTO95	Centocor/Johnson & Johnson	Human mAb	$\alpha_v\beta_3$, $\alpha_v\beta_5$	Phase I
ATN-161	Attenuon, LLC	Capped, 5-mer peptide	$\alpha_5\beta_1$, $\alpha_v\beta_5$, $\alpha_v\beta_3$	Phase I/II
Osteoprotegerin	Amgen	Protein	RANK-L, attenuates β_3 expression	Phase I
EOS 200-4	Protein Design Labs	mAb	$\alpha_5\beta_1$	Phase I

Vitaxin (MEDI-523), one of the first integrin antagonists to be entered into clinical trials for the treatment of cancer, has been replaced by a newer version monoclonal antibody (MEDI-522), which is currently in phase II trials. The only integrin-related therapeutic currently in clinical trials for bone metastasis is osteoprotegerin. Unfortunately, all of the agents targeting integrins for cancer treatment are still early in development and it is, therefore, too early to assess whether the preclinical promise of these agents will be translated into the clinic.

6. CONCLUSION

Bone metastasis continues to be a major therapeutic challenge in oncology and the underlying cause of the morbidity and mortality observed in numerous cancer patients. Thus, there is a tremendous need to develop agents that can be used to intervene in this patient population. Recent advances in understanding the pathobiology of bone metastasis have led to the identification of integrins and, specifically, integrin $\alpha_v\beta_3$ as targets for the development of novel therapeutic approaches for this indication. Several integrin antagonists are currently in early clinical development and will hopefully be evaluated in patients with bone metastasis as they advance into later-stage clinical trials.

REFERENCES

1. Humphries, MJ. Integrin structure. *Biochem Soc Trans* 2000; 28:311–339.
2. Whittaker CA, Hynes RO. Distribution and evolution of von Willebrand/integrin A domains: widely dispersed domains with roles in cell adhesion and elsewhere. *Mol Biol Cell* 2002; 13:3369–3387.
3. Xiong JP, Stehle T, Diefenbach B, Zhang R, Dunker R, Scott DL, et al. Crystal structure of the extracellular segment of integrin $\alpha_V\beta_3$. *Science* 2001; 294:339–345
4. Xiong JP, Stehle T, Zhang R, Joachimiak A, Frech M, Goodman SL, et al. Crystal structure of the extracellular segment of integrin $\alpha_V\beta_3$ in complex with an Arg-Gly-Asp ligand. *Science* 2002; 296: 151–155.
5. Adair BD, Yeager M. Three-dimensional model of the human platelet integrin alpha IIb beta 3 based on electron cryomicroscopy and x-ray crystallography. *Proc Natl Acad Sci USA* 2002; 99:14,059–14,064.

6. Hynes, RO. Integrins: bidirectional allosteric signaling machines. *Cell* 2002; 110:673–687.
7. Cierniewska-Cieslak A, Cierniewski CS, Blecka K, Papierak M, Michalec L, Zhang L, et al. Identification and characterization of two cation binding sites in the integrin β_3 subunit. *J Biol Chem* 2002; 277:11,126–11,134.
8. Xiong J-P, Stehle T, Zhang R, Joachimiak A, Frech M, Goodman SL, et al. Crystal structure of the extracellular segment of integrin $\alpha_V\beta_3$ in complex with an Arg-Gly-Asp ligand. *Science* 2002; 296: 151–155.
9. Berman HM, Westbrook J, Feng Z, Gilliland G, Bhat TN, Weissig H, et al. The protein data bank. *Nucleic Acids Res* 2000; 28:235–242.
10. Vinogradova O, Velyvis A, Velyviene A, Hu B, Haas T, Plow E, Qin J. A structural mechanism of integrin $\alpha_{IIb}\beta_3$ "inside-out" activation as regulated by its cytoplasmic face. *Cell* 2002; 110:587–597.
11. Vinogradova O, Haas T, Plow EF, Qin J. A structural basis for integrin activation by the cytoplasmic tail of the α_{IIb}-subunit. *Proc Natl Acad Sci USA* 2000; 97:1450–1455.
12. Hughes PE, Pfaff M. Integrin affinity modulation. *Trends Cell Biol* 1998; 8:359–364.
13. Ginsberg MH, Du X, Plow EF. Inside-out integrin signalling. *Curr Opin Cell Biol* 1992 ; 4:766–771.
14. Shattil SJ, Kashiwagi H, Pampori N. Integrin signaling: the platelet paradigm. *Blood* 1998; 91: 2645–2657.
15. Schwartz MA. Integrin signaling revisited. *Trends Cell Biol* 2001; 11:466–470.
16. Ni H, Li A, Simonsen N, Wilkins JA. Integrin activation by dithiothreitol or Mn2+ induces a ligand-occupied conformation and exposure of a novel NH2-terminal regulatory site on the beta1 integrin chain. *J Biol Chem* 1998; 273:7981–7987.
17. Yan B, Smith JW. A redox site involved in integrin activation. *J Biol Chem* 2000; 275:39,964–39,972.
18. Yan B, Hu DD, Knowles SK, Smith JW. Probing chemical and conformational differences in the resting and active conformers of platelet integrin $\alpha_{IIb}\beta_3$. *J Biol Chem* 2000; 275:7249–7260.
19. Yan B, Smith JW. Mechanism of integrin activation by disulfide bond reduction. *Biochemistry* 2001; 40:8861–8867.
20. Chen P, Melchior C, Brons NH, Schlegel N, Caen J, Kieffer N. Probing conformational changes in the I-like domain and the cysteine-rich repeat of human β_3 integrins following disulfide bond disruption by cysteine mutations: identification of cysteine 598 involved in $\alpha_{IIb}\beta_3$ activation. *J Biol Chem* 2001; 276:38,628–38,635.
21. Essex DW, Li M. Redox control of platelet aggregation. *Biochemistry* 2003; 42:129–136.
22. Lahav J, Gofer-Dadosh N, Luboshitz J, Hess O, Shaklai M. Protein disulfide isomerase mediates integrin-dependent adhesion. *FEBS Lett* 2000; 475:89–92.
23. O'Neill S, Robinson A, Deering A, Ryan M, Fitzgerald DJ, Moran N. The platelet integrin $\alpha_{IIb}\beta_3$ has an endogenous thiol isomerase activity. *J Biol Chem* 2000; 275:36,984–36,990.
24. Niewiarowski S, Kornecki E, Hershock D, Tuszynski GP, Bennett JS, Soria C, et al. Aggregation of chymotrypsin-treated thrombasthenic platelets is mediated by fibrinogen binding to glycoproteins IIb and IIIa. *J Lab Clin Med* 1985; 106:651–660.
25. Essex DW, Li M. Protein disulphide isomerase mediates platelet aggregation and secretion. *Br J Haematol* 1999; 104:448–454.
26. Walsh, GM, Sheehan, D, Kinsella, A, Moran, N and O'Neill, S. Redox modulation of integrin $\alpha_{IIb}\beta_3$ involves a novel allosteric regulation of its thiol isomerase activity. *Biochemistry* 2004; 43:473–480.
27. Giancotti, FG and Ruoslahti, E. Integrin signaling. *Science* 1999; 285:1028–1032.
28. Miranti, CK, and Brugge, JS. Sensing the environment: a historical perspective on integrin signaling. *Nature Cell Biol* 2002; 4:83-90.
30. Martin, KH, Slack, JK, Boerner, SA, Martin, CC, Parsons, JT. Integrin connections map:to infinity and beyond. *Science* 2002; 296:1652,1653.
31. Brakebusch C, Bouvard D, Stanchi F, Sakai T, Fassler R. Integrins in invasive growth. *J Clin Invest* 2002; 109:999–1006.
32. Giancotti FG, Ruoslahti E. Integrin signaling. *Science* 1999; 285:1028–1032.
33. Eliceiri BP. Integrin and growth factor receptor crosstalk. *Circ Res* 2001; 89:1104–1110.
34. Mercurio AM, Rabinovitz I. Towards a mechanistic understanding of tumour invasion—lessons from the alpha6beta4 integrin. *Semin Cancer Biol* 2001; 11:129–141.
35. Rabinovitz I, Toker A, Mercurio AM. Protein kinase C-dependent mobilization of the alpha6beta4 integrin from hemidesmosomes and its association with actin-rich cell protrusions drive the chemotactic migration of carcinoma cells. *J Cell Biol* 1999; 146:1147–1160.

36. Byzova TV, Goldman CK, Pampori N, Thomas KA, Bett A, Shattil SJ, et al. A mechanism for modulation of cellular responses to VEGF: activation of the integrins. *Mol Cell* 2000; 6:851–860.

37. Miyamoto S, Teramoto H, Gutkind JS, Yamada KM. Integrins can collaborate with growth factors for phosphorylation of receptor tyrosine kinases and MAP kinase activation: roles of integrin aggregation and occupancy of receptors. *J Cell Biol* 1996; 135:1633–1642.

38. Trusolino L, Bertotti A, Comoglio PM. A signaling adapter function for $\alpha_6\beta_4$ integrin in the control of HGF-dependent invasive growth. *Cell* 2001; 107:643–654.

39. Gambaletta D, Marchetti A, Benedetti L, Mercurio AM, Sacchi A, Falcioni R. Cooperative signaling between $\alpha_6\beta_4$ integrin and ErbB-2 receptor is required to promote phosphatidylinositol 3-kinase-dependent invasion. *J Biol Chem* 2000; 275:10,604–10,610.

40. Moro L, Dolce L, Cabodi S, Bergatto E, Erba EB, Smeriglio M, et al. Integrin-induced epidermal growth factor (EGF) receptor activation requires c-Src and p130Cas and leads to phosphorylation of specific EGF receptor tyrosines. *J Biol Chem* 2002; 277:9405–9414.

41. Brooks PC, Montgomery AM, Rosenfeld M, Reisfeld RA, Hu T, Klier G, et al. Integrin $\alpha_V\beta_3$ antagonists promote tumour regression by inducing apoptosis of angiogenic blood vessels. *Cell* 1994; 79: 1157–1164.

42. Kim S, Bell K, Mousa SA, Varner JA. Regulation of angiogenesis in vivo by ligation of integrin $\alpha_5\beta_1$ with the central cell-binding domain of fibronectin. *Am J Pathol* 2000; 156:1345–1362.

43. Kim S, Bakre M, Yin H, Varner JA. Inhibition of endothelial cell survival and angiogenesis by protein kinase A. *J Clin Invest* 2002; 110:933–941.

44. Stupack DG, Puente XS, Boutsaboualoy S, Storgard CM, Cheresh DA. Apoptosis of adherent cells by recruitment of caspase-8 to unligated integrins. J *Cell Biol* 2001; 155:459–470.

45. Brakebusch C, Bouvard D, Stanchi F, Sakai T, Fassler R. Integrins in invasive growth. *J Clin Invest* 2002; 109:999–1006.

46. Plow EF, Haas TA, Zhang L, Loftus J, Smith JW. Ligand binding to integrins. *J Biol Chem* 2000; 275:21,785–21,788.

47. Naglich JG, Jure-Kunkel M, Gupta E, Fargnoli J, Henderson AJ, Lewin AC, et al. Inhibition of angiogenesis and metastasis in two murine models by the matrix metalloproteinase inhibitor, BMS-275291. *Cancer Res* 2001; 61:8480–8485.

48. Haas TA, Plow EF. Integrin-ligand interactions: a year in review. *Curr Opin Cell Biol* 1994; 6:656–662.

49. Pankov R, Yamada KM. Fibronectin at a glance. *J Cell Sci* 2002; 115:3861–3863.

50. Aota,S, Nomizu,M, Yamada,KM. The short amino acid sequence Pro-His-Ser-Arg-Asn in human fibronectin enhances cell-adhesive function. *J Biol Chem* 1994; 269:24,756–24,761.

51. Livant DL, Brabec RK, Pienta KJ, Allen DL, Kurachi K, Markwart S, et al. Anti-invasive, antitumourigenic, and antimetastatic activities of the PHSCN sequence in prostate carcinoma. *Cancer Res* 2000; 60:309–320.

52. Stoeltzing O, Liu W, Reinmuth N, Fan F, Parry GC, Parikh AA, et al. Inhibition of integrin $\alpha_5\beta_1$ function with a small peptide (ATN-161) plus continuous 5-FU infusion reduces colorectal liver metastases and improves survival in mice. *Int J Cancer* 2003; 104:496–503.

53. Mould AP, Komoriya A, Yamada KM, Humphries MJ. The CS5 peptide is a second site in the IIICS region of fibronectin recognized by the integrin $\alpha_4\beta_1$. Inhibition of $\alpha_4\beta_1$ function by RGD peptide homologues. *J Biol Chem* 1991; 266:3579–3585.

54. Komoriya A, Green LJ, Mervic M, Yamada SS, Yamada KM, Humphries MJ. The minimal essential sequence for a major cell type-specific adhesion site (CS1) within the alternatively spliced type III connecting segment domain of fibronectin is leucine-aspartic acid-valine. *J Biol Chem* 1991; 266:15,075–15,079.

55. Moyano JV, Carnemolla B, Dominguez-Jimenez C, Garcia-Gila M, Albar JP, Sanchez-Aparicio P, et al. Fibronectin type III5 repeat contains a novel cell adhesion sequence, KLDAPT, which binds activated alpha4beta1 and alpha4beta7 integrins. *J Biol Chem* 1997; 272:24,832–24,836.

56. George EL, Georges-Labouesse EN, Patel-King RS, Rayburn H, Hynes RO. Defects in mesoderm, neural tube and vascular development in mouse embryos lacking fibronectin. *Development* 1993; 119:1079–1091.

57. Kim S, Bell K, Mousa SA, Varner JA. Regulation of angiogenesis *in vivo* by ligation of integrin $\alpha_5\beta_1$ with the central cell-binding domain of fibronectin. *Am J Pathol* 2000; 156:1345–1362.

58. Moursi AM, Damsky CH, Lull J, Zimmerman D, Doty SB, Aota S, et al. Fibronectin regulates calvarial osteoblast differentiation. *J Cell Sci* 1996; 109:1369–1380.

59. Preissner KT, Jenne D. Structure of vitronectin and its biological role in haemostasis. *Thromb Haemost* 1991; 66:123–132.

60. Preissner KT, Jenne D. Vitronectin: a new molecular connection in haemostasis. *Thromb Haemost* 1991; 66:189–194.

61. Minor KH, Peterson CB. Plasminogen activator inhibitor type 1 promotes the self-association of vitronectin into complexes exhibiting altered incorporation into the extracellular matrix. *J Biol Chem* 2002; 277:10,337–10,345.

62. Podor TJ, Shaughnessy SG, Blackburn MN, Peterson CB. New insights into the size and stoichiometry of the plasminogen activator inhibitor type-1 vitronectin complex. *J Biol Chem* 2000; 275:25,402–25,410.

63. Pecheur I, Peyruchaud O, Serre CM, Guglielmi J, Voland C, Bourre F, et al. Integrin $\alpha_V\beta_3$ expression confers on tumour cells a greater propensity to metastasize to bone. *FASEB J* 2002; 16:1266–1268.

64. Liotta LA, Stetler-Stevenson WG. Tumour invasion and metastasis:an imbalance of positive and negative regulation. *Cancer Res* 1991; 51:5054s–5059s.

65. Ziober BL, Lin CS, Kramer RH. Laminin-binding integrins in tumour progression and metastasis. *Semin Cancer Biol* 1997; 7:119–128.

66. Hunt G. The role of laminin in cancer invasion and metastasis. *Exp Cell Biol* 1989; 57:165–176.

67. Mercurio AM. Laminin: multiple forms, multiple receptors. *Curr Opin Cell Biol* 1990; 2:845–849.

68. Nakai M, Mundy GR, Williams PJ, Boyce B, Yoneda T. A synthetic antagonist to laminin inhibits the formation of osteolytic metastases by human melanoma cells in nude mice. *Cancer Res* 1992; 52:5395–5399.

69. Denhardt DT, Noda M. Osteopontin expression and function: role in bone remodeling. *J Cell Biochem* 1998; 30–31(Suppl):92–102.

70. Ross FP, Chappel J, Alvarez JI, Sander D, Butler WT, Farach-Carson MC, et al. Interactions between the bone matrix proteins osteopontin and bone sialoprotein and the osteoclast integrin $\alpha_V\beta_3$ potentiate bone resorption. *J Biol Chem* 1993; 268:9901–9907.

71. Yokosaki Y, Matsuura N, Sasaki T, Murakami I, Schneider H, Higashiyama S, et al. The integrin $\alpha_9\beta_1$ binds to a novel recognition sequence (SVVYGLR) in the thrombin-cleaved amino-terminal fragment of osteopontin. *J Biol Chem* 1999; 274:36,328–36,334.

72. Sodek J, Zhu B, Huynh MH, Brown TJ, Ringuette M. Novel functions of the matricellular proteins osteopontin and osteonectin/SPARC. *Connect Tissue Res* 2002; 43:308–319.

73. Senger DR, Perruzzi CA. Secreted phosphoprotein markers for neoplastic transformation of human epithelial and fibroblastic cells. *Cancer Res* 1985; 45:5818–5823.

74. Craig AM, Bowden GT, Chambers AF, Spearman MA, Greenberg AH, Wright JA, et al. Secreted phosphoprotein mRNA is induced during multi-stage carcinogenesis in mouse skin and correlates with the metastatic potential of murine fibroblasts. *Int J Cancer* 1990; 46:133–137.

75. Rudland PS, Platt-Higgins A, El Tanani M, De Silva RS, Barraclough R, Winstanley JH, et al. Prognostic significance of the metastasis-associated protein osteopontin in human breast cancer. *Cancer Res* 2002; 62:3417–3427.

76. Bianco P, Fisher LW, Young MF, Termine JD, Robey PG. Expression of bone sialoprotein (BSP) in developing human tissues. *Calcif Tissue Int* 1991; 49:421–426.

77. Roach HI. Why does bone matrix contain non-collagenous proteins? The possible roles of osteocalcin, osteonectin, osteopontin and bone sialoprotein in bone mineralisation and resorption. *Cell Biol Int* 1994; 18:617–628.

78. Oldberg A, Franzen A, Heinegard D. The primary structure of a cell-binding bone sialoprotein. *J Biol Chem* 1988; 263:19,430–19,432.

79. Waltregny D, Bellahcene A, Van RI, Fisher LW, Young M, Fernandez P, et al. Prognostic value of bone sialoprotein expression in clinically localized human prostate cancer. *J Natl Cancer Inst* 1998; 90:1000–1008.

80. Diel IJ, Solomayer EF, Seibel MJ, Pfeilschifter J, Maisenbacher H, Gollan C, et al. Serum bone sialoprotein in patients with primary breast cancer is a prognostic marker for subsequent bone metastasis. *Clin Cancer Res* 1999; 5:3914–3919.

81. Sung V, Stubbs JT, III, Fisher L, Aaron AD, Thompson EW. Bone sialoprotein supports breast cancer cell adhesion proliferation and migration through differential usage of the $\alpha_V\beta_3$ and $\alpha_V\beta_5$ integrins. *J Cell Physiol* 1998; 176:482–494.

82. Bellahcene A, Bonjean K, Fohr B, Fedarko NS, Robey FA, Young MF, et al. Bone sialoprotein mediates human endothelial cell attachment and migration and promotes angiogenesis. *Circ Res* 2000; 86:885–891.

83. Mazar AP, Henkin J, Goldfarb RH. The urokinase plasminogen activator system in cancer: implications for tumour angiogenesis and metastasis. *Angiogenesis* 1999; 3:15–332.

84. Ploug M. Structure-function relationships in the interaction between the urokinase-type plasminogen activator and its receptor. *Curr Pharm Des* 2003; 9:1499–1528.

85. Xue W, Mizukami I, Todd RF, III, Petty HR. Urokinase-type plasminogen activator receptors associate with β_1 and β_3 integrins of fibrosarcoma cells: dependence on extracellular matrix components. *Cancer Res* 1997; 57:1682–1689.

86. Wei Y, Lukashev M, Simon DI, Bodary SC, Rosenberg S, Doyle MV, et al. Regulation of integrin function by the urokinase receptor. *Science* 1996; 273:1551–1555.

87. Sitrin RG, Todd RF, III, Albrecht E, Gyetko MR. The urokinase receptor (CD87) facilitates CD11b/CD18-mediated adhesion of human monocytes. *J Clin Invest* 1996; 97:1942–1951.

88. Simon DI, Wei Y, Zhang L, Rao NK, Xu H, Chen Z, et al. Identification of a urokinase receptor-integrin interaction site. Promiscuous regulator of integrin function. *J Biol Chem* 2000; 275:10,228–10,234.

89. van der PG, Sijmons B, Vloedgraven H, van der BC, Drijfhout JW, Verheijen J, et al. Urokinase-receptor/integrin complexes are functionally involved in adhesion and progression of human breast cancer in vivo. *Am J Pathol* 2000; 159:971–982.

90. Ruoslahti E. Fibronectin and its integrin receptors in cancer. *Adv Cancer Res* 1999; 76:1–20.

91. Felding-Habermann B. Integrin adhesion receptors in tumour metastasis. *Clin Exp Metastasis* 2003; 20:203–213.

92. Felding-Habermann B, O'Toole TE, Smith JW, Fransvea E, Ruggeri ZM, Ginsberg MH, et al. Integrin activation controls metastasis in human breast cancer. *Proc Natl Acad Sci USA* 2001; 98(4):1853–1858.

93. Pilch J, Habermann R, Felding-Habermann B. Unique ability of integrin $\alpha_V\beta_3$ to support tumour cell arrest under dynamic flow conditions. *J Biol Chem* 2002; 277:21,930–21,938.

94. Folkman J. Angiogenesis and apoptosis. *Semin Cancer Biol* 2003; 13:159–167.

95. Bergers G, Benjamin LE. Tumourigenesis and the angiogenic switch. *Nat Rev Cancer* 2003; 3:401–410.

96. Tawil NJ, Gowri V, Djoneidi M, Nip J, Carbonetto S, Brodt P. Integrin $\alpha_3\beta_1$ can promote adhesion and spreading of metastatic breast carcinoma cells on the lymph node stroma. *Int J Cancer* 1996; 66:703–710.

97. Nip J, Shibata H, Loskutoff DJ, Cheresh DA, Brodt P. Human melanoma cells derived from lymphatic metastases use integrin alpha v beta 3 to adhere to lymph node vitronectin. *J Clin Invest* 1992; 90:1406–1413.

98. Nagata M, Fujita H, Ida H, Hoshina H, Inoue T, Seki Y, et al. Identification of potential biomarkers of lymph node metastasis in oral squamous cell carcinoma by cDNA microarray analysis. *Int J Cancer* 2003; 106:683–689.

99. Fornaro M, Manes T, Languino LR. Integrins and prostate cancer metastases. *Cancer Metastasis Rev* 2001; 20:321–331.

100. Tarui T, Andronicos N, Czekay RP, Mazar AP, Bdeir K, Parry GC, et al. Critical role of integrin $\alpha_5\beta_1$ in urokinase (uPA)/urokinase receptor (uPAR, CD87) signaling. *J Biol Chem* 2003; 278:29,863–29,872.

101. Mizejewski GJ. Role of integrins in cancer: survey of expression patterns. *Proc Soc Exp Biol Med* 1999; 222:124–138.

102. Anastassiou G, Duensing S, Steinhoff G, Kirchner H, Ganser A, Atzpodien J. In vivo distribution of integrins in renal cell carcinoma:integrin-phenotype alteration in different degrees of tumour differentiation and VLA-2 involvement in tumour metastasis. *Cancer Biother* 1995; 10:287–292.

103. Tani N, Higashiyama S, Kawaguchi N, Madarame J, Ota I, Ito Y, et al. Expression level of integrin $\alpha 5$ on tumour cells affects the rate of metastasis to the kidney. *Br J Cancer* 2003; 88:327–333.

104. Natali PG, Nicotra MR, Botti C, Mottolese M, Bigotti A, Segatto O. Changes in expression of α_6/β_4 integrin heterodimer in primary and metastatic breast cancer. *Br J Cancer* 1992; 66:318–322.

105. Kim S, Bell K, Mousa SA, Varner JA. Regulation of angiogenesis *in vivo* by ligation of integrin $\alpha_5\beta_1$ with the central cell-binding domain of fibronectin. *Am J Pathol* 2000; 156:1345–1362.

106. Hartstein ME, Grove AS, Jr, Woog JJ. The role of the integrin family of adhesion molecules in the development of tumours metastatic to the orbit. *Ophthal Plast Reconstr Surg* 1997; 13:227–238.

107. Gui GP, Wells CA, Browne PD, Yeomans P, Jordan S, Puddefoot JR, et al. Integrin expression in primary breast cancer and its relation to axillary nodal status. *Surgery* 1995; 117:102–108.

108. Stromblad S, Becker JC, Yebra M, Brooks PC, Cheresh DA. Suppression of p53 activity and p21WAF1/CIP1 expression by vascular cell integrin $\alpha_V\beta_3$ during angiogenesis. *J Clin Invest* 1996; 98:426–433.

109. Anastassiou G, Duensing S, Steinhoff G, Kirchner H, Ganser A, Atzpodien J. In vivo distribution of integrins in renal cell carcinoma:integrin-phenotype alteration in different degrees of tumour differentiation and VLA-2 involvement in tumour metastasis. *Cancer Biother* 1995; 10:287–292.

110. Sawai H, Funahashi H, Matsuo Y, Yamamoto M, Okada Y, Hayakawa T, et al. Expression and prognostic roles of integrins and interleukin-1 receptor type I in patients with ductal adenocarcinoma of the pancreas. *Dig Dis Sci* 2003; 48:1241–1250.

111. Lipscomb EA, Dugan AS, Rabinovitz I, Mercurio AM. Use of RNA interference to inhibit integrin $\alpha_6\beta_4$-mediated invasion and migration of breast carcinoma cells. *Clin Exp Metastasis* 2003; 20: 569–576.

112. Adachi M, Taki T, Higashiyama M, Kohno N, Inufusa H, Miyake M. Significance of integrin α_5 gene expression as a prognostic factor in node-negative non-small cell lung cancer. *Clin Cancer Res* 2000; 6:96–101.

113. Saito T, Kimura M, Kawasaki T, Sato S, Tomita Y. Correlation between integrin α_5 expression and the malignant phenotype of transitional cell carcinoma. *Br J Cancer* 1996; 73:327–331.

114. Davidson B, Goldberg I, Reich R, Tell L, Dong HP, Trope CG, et al. α_V- and β_1-integrin subunits are commonly expressed in malignant effusions from ovarian carcinoma patients. *Gynecol Oncol* 2003; 90:248–257.

115. Brooks PC, Clark RA, Cheresh DA. Requirement of vascular integrin $\alpha_V\beta_3$ for angiogenesis. *Science* 1994; 264:569–571.

116. Nemeth JA, Cher ML, Zhou Z, Mullins C, Bhagat S, Trikha M. Inhibition of $\alpha_V\beta_3$ integrin reduces angiogenesis, bone turnover, and tumour cell proliferation in experimental prostate cancer bone metastases. *Clin Exp Metastasis* 2003; 20:413–420.

117. Hynes RO. A reevaluation of integrins as regulators of angiogenesis. *Nature Med* 2002; 8:918–921.

118. Reynolds LE, Wyder L, Lively JC, Taverna D, Robinson SD, Huang X, et al. Enhanced pathological angiogenesis in mice lacking β_3 integrin or β_3 and β_5 integrins. *Nature Med* 2002; 8(1):27–34.

119. Taverna D, Moher H, Crowley D, Borsig L, Varki A, Hynes RO. Increased primary tumour growth in mice null for β_3- or β_3/β_5-integrins or selectins. *Proc Natl Acad Sci USA* 2004; 101:763–768.

120. Gasparini G, Brooks PC, Biganzoli E, Vermeulen PB, Bonoldi E, Dirix LY, et al. Vascular integrin $\alpha_V\beta_3$: a new prognostic indicator in breast cancer. *Clin Cancer Res* 1998; 4:2625–2634.

121. Liapis H, Flath A, Kitazawa S. Integrin $\alpha_V\beta_3$ expression by bone-residing breast cancer metastases. *Diagn Mol Pathol* 1996; 5:127–135.

122. Han JY, Kim HS, Lee SH, Park WS, Lee JY, Yoo NJ. Immunohistochemical expression of integrins and extracellular matrix proteins in non-small cell lung cancer: correlation with lymph node metastasis. *Lung Cancer* 2003; 41:65–70.

123. Felding-Habermann B, O'Toole TE, Smith JW, Fransvea E, Ruggeri ZM, Ginsberg MH, et al. Integrin activation controls metastasis in human breast cancer. *Proc Natl Acad Sci USA* 2001; 98:1853–1858.

124. Rolli M, Fransvea E, Pilch J, Saven A, Felding-Habermann B. Activated integrin $\alpha_V\beta_3$ cooperates with metalloproteinase MMP-9 in regulating migration of metastatic breast cancer cells. *Proc Natl Acad Sci USA* 2003; 100:9482–9487.

125. Trikha M, Zhou Z, Timar J, Raso E, Kennel M, Emmell E, et al. Multiple roles for platelet GPIIb/IIIa and $\alpha_V\beta_3$ integrins in tumour growth, angiogenesis, and metastasis. *Cancer Res* 2002; 62:2824–2833.

126. Posey JA, Khazaeli MB, DelGrosso A, Saleh MN, Lin CY, Huse W, et al. A pilot trial of Vitaxin, a humanized anti-vitronectin receptor (anti-$\alpha_V\beta_3$) antibody in patients with metastatic cancer. *Cancer Biother Radiopharm* 2001; 16:125–132.

127. Tucker GC. Inhibitors of integrins. *Curr Opin Pharmacol* 2002; 2:394–402.

128. Pecheur I, Peyruchaud O, Serre CM, Guglielmi J, Voland C, Bourre F, et al. Integrin $\alpha_V\beta_3$ expression confers on tumour cells a greater propensity to metastasize to bone. *FASEB J* 220; 16:1266–1268.

129. Byzova TV, Kim W, Midura RJ, Plow EF. Activation of integrin $\alpha_V\beta_3$ regulates cell adhesion and migration to bone sialoprotein. *Exp Cell Res* 2000; 254:299–308.

130. Ganss B, Kim RH, Sodek J. Bone sialoprotein. *Crit Rev Oral Biol Med* 1999; 10:79–98.

131. Brekken RA, Sage EH. SPARC, a matricellular protein:at the crossroads of cell-matrix communication. *Matrix Biol* 2001; 19:816–827.

132. De S, Chen J, Narizhneva NV, Heston W, Brainard J, Sage EH, et al. Molecular pathway for cancer metastasis to bone. *J Biol Chem* 2003; 278:39,044–39,050.

134. Boissier S, Magnetto S, Frappart L, Cuzin B, Ebetino FH, Delmas PD, et al. Bisphosphonates inhibit prostate and breast carcinoma cell adhesion to unmineralized and mineralized bone extracellular matrices. *Cancer Res* 1997; 57:3890–3894.

135. Boissier S, Ferreras M, Peyruchaud O, Magnetto S, Ebetino FH, Colombel M, et al. Bisphosphonates inhibit breast and prostate carcinoma cell invasion, an early event in the formation of bone metastases. *Cancer Res* 2000; 60:2949–2954.

136. Powles T, Paterson S, Kanis JA, McCloskey E, Ashley S, Tidy A, et al. Randomized, placebo-controlled trial of clodronate in patients with primary operable breast cancer. *J Clin Oncol* 2002; 20: 3219–3224.

133. Pagliaro LC, Delpassand ES, Williams D, Millikan RE, Tu SM, Logothetis CJ. A Phase I/II study of strontium-89 combined with gemcitabine in the treatment of patients with androgen independent prostate carcinoma and bone metastases. *Cancer* 2003; 97:2988–2994.

137. Small EJ, Smith MR, Seaman JJ, Petrone S, Kowalski MO. Combined analysis of two multicenter, randomized, placebo-controlled studies of pamidronate disodium for the palliation of bone pain in men with metastatic prostate cancer. *J Clin Oncol* 2003; 21:4277–4284.

138. Neville-Webbe H, Coleman RE. The use of zoledronic acid in the management of metastatic bone disease and hypercalcaemia. *Palliat Med* 2003; 17:539–553.

139. Whitfield JF. The bone growth-stimulating PTH and osteosarcoma. *Medscape Womens Health* 2001; 6:7.

140. Yin JJ, Mohammad KS, Kakonen SM, Harris S, Wu-Wong JR, Wessale JL, et al. A causal role for endothelin-1 in the pathogenesis of osteoblastic bone metastases. *Proc Natl Acad Sci USA* 2003; 100: 10,954–10,959.

141. Mohammad KS, Guise TA. Mechanisms of osteoblastic metastases: role of endothelin-1. *Clin Ortop* 2003; 415(Suppl):S67–74.

142. Bendre M, Gaddy D, Nicholas RW, Suva LJ. Parathyroid hormone-related protein (PTHrP) is responsible for production of bone metastasis, but not visceral metastasis, by human small cell lung cancer SBC-5 cells in natural killer cell-depleted SCID mice. *Int J Cancer* 2004; 108:511–515.

143. Keller ET. The role of osteoclastic activity in prostate cancer skeletal metastases. *Drugs Today* (Barc) 2002; 38:91–102.

144. Ishida A, Fujita N, Kitazawa R, Tsuruo T. Transforming growth factor-beta induces expression of receptor activator of NF-κB ligand in vascular endothelial cells derived from bone. *J Biol Chem* 2002; 277:26,217–26,224.

146. Ohshiba T, Miyaura C, Inada M, Ito A. Role of RANKL-induced osteoclast formation and MMP-dependent matrix degradation in bone destruction by breast cancer metastasis. *Br J Cancer* 2003; 88: 1318–1326.

145. Kim HH, Chung WJ, Lee SW, Chung PJ, You JW, Kwon HJ, et al. Association of sustained ERK activity with integrin β3 induction during receptor activator of nuclear factor κB ligand (RANKL)-directed osteoclast differentiation. *Exp Cell Res* 2003; 289:368–377.

147. Rameshwar P, Chang VT, Gascon P. Implication of CD44 in adhesion-mediated overproduction of TGF-beta and IL-1 in monocytes from patients with bone marrow fibrosis. *Br J Haematol* 1996; 93:22–29.

148. Ramaswamy S, Ross KN, Lander ES, Golub TR. A molecular signature of metastasis in primary solid tumours. *Nature Genet* 2003; 33:49–54.

149. Kang Y, Siegel PM, Shu W, Drobnjak M, Kakonen SM, Cordon-Cardo C, et al. A multigenic program mediating breast cancer metastasis to bone. *Cancer Cell* 2003; 3:537–549.

150. Sodek J, Chen J, Nagata T, Kasugai S, Todescan R Jr, Li IW, et al. Regulation of osteopontin expression in osteoblasts. *Ann NY Acad Sci* 1995; 760:223–241.

151. Denton CP, Abraham DJ. Transforming growth factor-beta and connective tissue growth factor: key cytokines in scleroderma pathogenesis. *Curr Opin Rheumatol* 2001; 13:505–511.

152. Burger M, Glodek A, Hartmann T, Schmitt-Graff A, Silberstein LE, Fujii N, et al. Functional expression of CXCR4 (CD184) on small-cell lung cancer cells mediates migration, integrin activation, and adhesion to stromal cells. *Oncogene* 2003; 22:8093–8101

153. Cardones AR, Murakami T, Hwang ST. CXCR4 enhances adhesion of B16 tumour cells to endothelial cells in vitro and in vivo via β1 integrin. *Cancer Res* 2003; 63:6751–6757.

154. Wang LS, Liu HJ, Broxmeyer HE, Lu L. Interleukin-11 enhancement of VLA-5 mediated adhesion of CD34+ cells from cord blood to fibronectin is associated with the PI-3 kinase pathway. *In Vivo* 2000; 14:331–337.

155. Weston BS, Wahab NA, Mason RM. CTGF mediates TGF-beta-induced fibronectin matrix deposition by upregulating active $\alpha_5\beta_1$ integrin in human mesangial cells. *J Am Soc Nephrol* 2003; 14:601–610.

156. Furger KA, Allan AL, Wilson SM, Hota C, Vantyghem SA, Postenka CO, et al. β3 integrin expression increases breast carcinoma cell responsiveness to the malignancy-enhancing effects of osteopontin. *Mol Cancer Res* 2003; 1:810–819.

14 Bone Metastasis and Pathological Fractures

Bone Tissue Engineering as a Novel Therapy

Laurie A. McDuffee, PhD, DVM, DACVS, Nigel Colterjohn, MD, and Gurmit Singh, PhD

CONTENTS

1. INTRODUCTION

1.1. Occurrence and Location of Bone Metastasis in Cancer Patients

Bone metastasis commonly occurs in association with solid malignant tumors such as breast, prostate, lung, and renal cancers *(1–5)*. Thirty to seventy percent of cancer patients have skeletal metastasis *(6)*, making the axial skeleton the third most common site for metastasis after lung and liver. Because all of these cancers (breast, prostate, lung, and renal) are common, metastatic bone lesions actually outnumber primary bone malignancies. The spine is affected in approximately half of all patients with bone metastasis *(5,6)*, and involvement of the appendicular skeleton, primarily the femur and humerus, is also common. Metastatic bone lesions can be classified as osteolytic, osteoblastic, mixed, or intertrabecular type based on histology *(3,4,7)*. Bone metastases secondary to breast cancer are typically osteolytic in nature, and these lesions are of particular interest as bone resorption at these sites often leads to pathological fracture. Thus, breast cancer is also the most common cause of pathological fracture *(7)*.

In addition to causing significant bone pain, pathological fractures associated with bone metastasis also lead to loss of function in the affected region *(1,2,8,9)*. For example,

From: *Cancer Drug Discovery and Development*
Bone Metastasis: Experimental and Clinical Therapeutics
Edited by: G. Singh and S. A. Rabbani © Humana Press Inc., Totowa, NJ

fractures within the vertebral bodies of the spinal column can lead to spinal cord compression *(1,2,8)*, pelvic and femoral fractures limit ambulation if not surgically treated, and humeral fractures can limit function of the arm and hand *(10)*. All of these outcomes limit function for everyday activities and lead to decreased quality of life and loss of independence for the patient.

During the last decade, the philosophy of management of bone metastasis has changed from one of simply providing comfort in anticipation of an early demise to providing pain-free maintenance of normal daily function so that the patient will have the best quality of life for their remaining life-span, whether it be months or years *(11)*. Much research has been conducted into the mechanisms of bone metastasis and pathological fractures. This knowledge has lead to advances in treatment and advances in achieving the goal of maintaining a good quality of life and independence. However, there are still complications that could be improved upon with novel therapies.

1.2. Current Treatment

The current treatment of bone metastasis is both anti-neoplastic and bone supportive, and remains palliative *(1,12)*. Many such treatments are aimed at "freezing" or slowing down the spread of the metastatic tumors, inhibiting osteoclastic bone resorption, decreasing or eliminating bone pain, and surgically repairing pathological fractures. A variety of approaches have been used with variable success, including (1) analgesics—both nonsteroidal agents and opioids, individually or in combination with other agents, (2) specific inhibitors of biochemical mediators of pain such as bisphosphonates, mithramycin, or calcitonin, (3) radiation therapy—including external beam radiation therapy (EBRT), hemibody or magna field radiation, and systemic radioisotope therapy using radio pharmaceuticals, (4) hormonal therapy—in breast and prostate cancer patients, and (5) chemotherapy *(1,13)*. Additional novel therapies are also under investigation, and promising agents include lumiracoxib (a novel COX–2 enzyme inhibitor) *(14)* and doxycycline (a member of the tetracycline family of antibiotics) *(15)*.

Although all of these treatment options play a role in treating cancer patients with bone pain and bone metastasis, there are many instances in which surgical intervention is required *(1)*. For instance, approx 10% of prostate cancer patients develop spinal cord compression, which then requires surgical decompression and stabilization. Similarly, although bisphosphonates might reduce the risk of pathological fracture, once a pathological fracture occurs, medical management will not result in healing or return to function.

1.3. Surgical Treatment of Metastatic Bone Tumors

Surgery is an important aspect of antineoplastic treatment of bone tumors. Metastatic tumors of the axial and appendicular skeleton often require surgical intervention to relieve bone pain and allow return to function. The goal of surgery should be to have an independent, ambulatory, pain-controlled patient.

1.4. Spinal Metastasis

Tumors of the vertebral column might be located in the cervical, thoracic, lumbar or sacral vertebral bodies. Tumor invasion results in painful microfractures or vertebral body collapse that can be associated with vertebral instability and kyphosis *(6)* and, possibly, spinal cord compression. Surgery is indicated when there is neural compression, pathological fracture, instability, progressive deformity, and for nursing reasons *(5)*. A wide excision might be necessary for the treatment of some vertebral tumors *(16)*; however, this might result in instability. Reconstruction might be required to maintain stability as well as to facilitate early mobilization, ambulation, and return to normal activities. When reconstruction is required, various methods have been used, including spinal instrumentation to support the spine and bone graft to promote fusion. When bony fusion is part of the surgical plan, "massive" autogenous bone graft material might be required *(16)*. This could be difficult to obtain in elderly patients with osteoporotic bone.

Because patients with vertebral metastasis are often in advanced stages of cancer *(16)* and could be in a reduced state of health, surgical intervention under general anesthesia is somewhat risky. In addition, surgery might be undesirable because hospitalization could take up too much of the patients' remaining life *(17)*. In these cases, vertebroplasty (VP) is used as an alternative to surgery that restores spinal stability, relieves pain, and decreases thromboembolic and cardiopulmonary comorbidity *(6,17,18)*.

Vertebroplasty consists of image-guided injection of polymethylmethacrylate (PMMA) bone cement into the collapsing vertebral body, and in patients with bone metastases, the goal of this treatment is to provide permanent, partial, or complete pain relief and stabilization of the anterior column *(6)*. This procedure is indicated in patients for whom radiation therapy and conservative management have not reduced pain in a short period of time and surgical intervention is undesirable *(17)*. Importantly, the patient's health must tolerate only sedation and local anesthesia. VP can be used in combination with radiation therapy, or in the case of neurocompressive lesions, VP can be combined with a decompressive surgery *(6)*. VP will relieve bone pain in 80–90% of patients with spinal metastasis, and the complication rate has been reported in the range of 1–10% *(6,18)*, with cement extrusion into the spinal canal and neuroforamen representing the most critical complications.

1.5. Appendicular Metastasis

With the progression of treatment of primary cancers, the prognosis for many cancer patients has improved greatly. With the improvement in prognosis, surgeons have moved from amputation of affected limbs toward limb-sparing procedures. With aggressive treatment of appendicular bone metastasis, function can be restored, pain diminished, and quality of life improved *(19)*.

1.6. Femoral Metastasis

Considering metastasis to the appendicular skeleton, the femur is the most common site of bone lesions *(20,21)*. When surgical treatment is indicated, removal of the tumor and reconstruction of the defect is carried out while bypassing all areas of weakened bone. Because of the shortened life-span of these patients, the aim of bone reconstruction should be to allow immediate weight bearing and easy return to function *(20)*. The surgical goal is to provide durable fixation that will last his/her remaining lifetime while minimizing morbidity associated with procedures. Surgical options are resection of the metastatic lesion or curettage with stabilization often including adjuvant bone cement *(20)*. Surgical reconstruction can vary depending on the location of the pathological fracture in the femur. Reconstruction techniques include cemented hemiarthroplasty, total hip arthroplasty, modular prosthesis, intramedullary reconstruction nails, statically locked intramedullary nails, intercallary metal spacers *(20,22–24)* and sometimes a construct of plate and screws. These implants are used in carefully chosen procedures to maximize quality of life while minimizing morbidity.

1.7. Humeral Metastasis

The proximal humerus is also a common site of bone metastasis. This results in bone destruction, instability of the upper extremity, and loss of functional capacity of the shoulder joint and joints below that *(25)*. Similar to treatment of femoral bone tumors, treatment of humeral tumors should include both removal of the tumor and preservation of limb function. In the past, amputation was conducted, leaving poor functional outcome. Tumor patients with poor general health tend to experience more difficulties using unaffected limbs to compensate for amputated or functionally impaired limbs *(26)*. Therefore, treatments should permit postoperative mobilization.

Currently, reconstructive techniques with mechanical devices such as intramedullary nails or prostheses, autogenous or allogenic bone graft, vascularized fibular graft, or arthrodesis are being conducted to achieve these goals *(10,25,26)*. With various prostheses, functional scores have been reported between 50% and 57%. These scores were highest in pain relief but lowest in emotional acceptance and functional outcome.

1.8. Complications With Surgical Treatment

Although the goal of reconstructive surgical treatment of metastatic lesions is to return the patient to ambulatory status with the use of all limbs, this can be challenging *(27)*. Surgical reconstruction of bones of the appendicular and axial skeleton in cancer patients suffers from lack of available donor tissue and donor-site morbidity. Therefore, mechanical devices such as implants or prostheses are often used to achieve this goal. The most common complication associated with implants in both the appendicular and axial skeleton is implant loosening and associated mechanical failure *(28)*. Loosening occurs when there is lack of bone formation and absence of integration of bone with the prosthesis. Bone cement is often used in combination with implants in attempt to improve stability; however, this can then place patients at increased risk of postoperative infection. Mechanical failure can also occur because there is a lack of bone healing in pathological fractures. When there is no bone healing, there is no load sharing between the implant and bone. This leaves the implant to withstand all of the forces placed on the limb and often results in fatigue failure *(29)*.

Because mechanical devices are limited by a finite durability and increased risk of infection *(28)*, biologically active constructs or living tissues are progressively replacing the world of inert medical devices *(30)*. Conventionally, living tissue used to promote bone healing has been in the form of autogenous cancellous bone graft, which has osteogenic (bone forming), osteoconductive (bone cell supportive), and osteoinductive (bone cell stimulating) properties. Cancellous bone graft has been the "gold standard" to promote bone healing for many years *(31–35)*. However, limitations include insufficient quantity of graft tissue, morbidity at the donor site, variable transfer of viable bone forming cells (osteoblasts), and requirement of a surgical procedure for each bone graft procedure *(31–36)*. These limitations are exacerbated in cancer patients, who are often elderly, and have osteoporotic bones in many areas of their skeleton, including bone graft donor sites, and who often cannot tolerate multiple surgical procedures for obtaining multiple bone grafts. More recently, the trend for replacement of mechanical devices with living tissue is being accomplished and investigated through selective cell transfer and tissue engineering methods *(27,28,37)*.

2. TISSUE ENGINEERING: A NOVEL THERAPY

Tissue engineering is an interdisciplinary field that applies the principles and methods of life sciences toward the development of biological substitutes that can restore, maintain, or improve tissue function *(28)*. Regeneration of skeletal tissues is among the most promising areas of biological tissue repair *(30,38)*. The first clinical successes have been recorded in the repair of structural tissues such as cartilage and bone *(30)*. Clinically, tissue engineering involving selective cell transplantation using autologous cultured chondrocytes is being used successfully to repair damaged articular cartilage in orthopedic patients *(38)*.

Bone tissue engineering focuses on restoration, maintenance, and improved bone tissue function. One of the primary goals for tissue engineering in oncology is to develop new methods of tissue replacement to restore posttreatment anatomical structures and their function *(28,30,39)*.

Three essential elements are required for successful bone tissue engineering: cells (osteogenic properties), growth factors (osteoinductive properties), and scaffold or matrix (osteoconductive properties). Therefore, three general approaches have been applied to the art of tissue engineering of bone: cell-based therapies, factor-based therapies, and matrix-based therapies *(28,40)*.

2.1. Cell-Based Therapy

Cell-based therapies in tissue engineering are based on transplantation of differentiated cells or progenitors of a certain lineage into the site of tissue defect. Cells used in tissue engineering can be derived from numerous sources, including primary tissues and cell lines. Ideally the cells should be nonimmunogenic, highly proliferative, and easy to harvest and have the ability to differentiate into a cell type with a specialized function *(28)*. Cells are responsible for the formation and maintenance of the integrity of the respective tissues. The proper cells will further contribute to the repair of tissues by a number of mechanisms, including the secretion of soluble signals and matrix molecules *(28,30)*. Therefore, it seems logical to provide additional cells, fully differentiated or progenitors, as building blocks for the repair of damaged tissues *(30)*. One way to do this is through cell-expansion technologies. With cell-expansion techniques only a small amount of donor tissue is required for isolation of cells compared to "massive" amounts of bone graft required with some conventional surgical techniques.

Cells can be obtained as autologous, allogenic, or xenogenic cell populations *(31,38,41–43)*. Autologous cells are still the first choice because they generally limit problems in terms of potential inflammatory reactions, immune reactions, and other issues related to transfer of potential pathogens *(30)*. Because only a small amount of donor tissue is required when expansion techniques are used, harvest of autologous cells can be achieved with minimal donor-site morbidity.

Reimplantation of cells or cell transplantation is central to tissue engineering *(39)*. Not only does this require harvesting donor tissue and isolating and expanding cells, but the cells might also be modified in vitro prior to implantation to restore tissue function. Cell transplantation can take the form of direct injection of dissociated cells or placement of cells onto natural extracellular matrix proteins such as collagen *(39)*. Tissue engineering can take it a step further to create three-dimentional (3-D) cultures on scaffolds prior to implantation *(44)*.

2.2. Factor-Based Therapies

Factor-based therapies involve the introduction of proliferative and differentiation factors into the bone defect site *(45–48)*. In bone tissue engineering, this might be accomplished using demineralized bone matrix, which is allogenic bone treated so that the bone morphogenetic proteins (BMP) and other osteoinductive factors present in the bone matrix are made available *(49)*, or purified growth factors *(50)*. Osteoinductive factors introduced into a defect site depend on a source of inducible, osteogenic cells available at that site for success *(51–54)*.

The direct application of purified growth factors in a bone defect has other limitations that diminish its usefulness clinically at this time. Rapid physical resorption of factors placed in the bone defect and lack of temporal and spatial control over local concentrations of the growth factors *(32,37)* might lead to a requirement of large quantities of osteoinductive factors for induction of bone formation in vivo *(48,55,56)*. This might be cost-prohibitive for widespread clinical use. Additionally, it has been difficult to translate experimental therapy in rodents through large-animal models to humans *(37,57,58)*, and optimum clinical dosages have not been determined for use in human patients. Use in cancer patients is controversial. Orthopedic oncologists have concerns that direct use of a growth factor that "turns on" many types of cells, including bone-forming cells, might also "turn on" quiescent cancer cells *(39,59)*. Although use of factor-based therapy alone has some drawbacks, a combination of cells and/or matrix with factor-based therapy might eliminate these shortcomings.

2.3. Matrix-Based Therapies

Matrix-based therapies in bone tissue engineering involve the use of synthetic osteoconductive materials or biomaterials such as titanium, bone cements, and ceramics. When there is a healthy source of osteogenic cells at the defect site, the macroporosity of the biomaterials facilitates the penetration of cells into the implant, allowing the osteogenic process to occur within the inner surfaces of the pores in order to potentiate bone healing and bone integration *(60)*. New biomaterials are required to serve as temporary implantable devices that can act as hollow molding chambers, porous tissue scaffolds, and bioactive material delivery devices *(39)*. Calcium phosphate (CaP) bone substitutes are currently used for bone replacement or augmentation in many different clinical applications such as repair of bone defects or coatings for metallic implants *(60)*. Recently percutaneous techniques for implanting bone substitutes have been developed including injectable CaP biomaterials for bone replacement.

Various materials have been used as bone substitutes, but many of them possess problems such as poor biocompatability and inferior mechanical strength *(31,61–64)*. Osteoconductive materials also lack osteogenic and osteoinductive properties that limits their usefulness *(57,61)*. A source of induced osteogenic cells must be present at the bone defect site for osteoconductive materials to be successful. Success with the use of biomaterials alone in cancer patients could be limited by a lack of healthy osteogenic cells at the defect site. However, combining cells and/or osteoinductive factors with biomaterials should improve the outcome of matrix-based therapy.

Ideally, bone tissue engineering would involve a combination of cell-, factor-, and matrix-based therapies that mimic the properties of autogenous cancellous bone grafts, the gold standard for promotion of bone healing, to the highest degree and lead to optimum results in bone healing. There are many places where selective cell transplantation and bone tissue engineering would benefit treatment of bone metastasis and pathological fracture. For instance, expanded cells and an injectable matrix could be useful in VP in place of bone cement, which has some complications. Cells and matrix could be used in combination with mechanical devices to promote bone healing and integration and prevent loosening and mechanical failure of the implants. In some instances, bone tissue engineering could be used to improve the strength of the bone and prevent pathological fracture.

3. DEVELOPING A NOVEL THERAPY

Considering complications that occur with conventional antineoplastic and bone-supportive therapies, there is a need for novel therapy in the treatment of bone metastasis and pathological fractures. Bone tissue engineering is a promising novel therapy for use in combination with conventional therapies.

The success of each product, and of tissue engineering in general, is dependent on the ability to demonstrate that products are both safe and effective *(57,65)*. This requires much research during the development of the tissue-engineered product prior to clinical use.

3.1. Cell and Tissue Sourcing

Although autogenous cells are considered the best source of cells for use in tissue engineering, allogenic and xenogenic cells are being investigated as cell sources as well. Regardless of the source of cells, relevant characteristics of the donor(s) should be specified, including species, age, and sex. Harvesting of tissues or cells from the donor should be performed under aseptic conditions, and cell culture operations should be carefully managed in terms of quality of materials, manufacturing controls, and equipment validation and monitoring *(65)*. Records should be kept detailing the components used in culture media, including their source and lot number.

The essential characteristics of the cultured cell population (phenotypic markers, functional properties, activity in bioassays) should be defined, and the stability of these characteristics established with respect to time in culture *(65)*.

3.2. Cell and Tissue Characterization

Cells or tissues used for tissue-engineered products need to function in a predictable and clinically relevant manner *(30,65)*. The development of in vitro assay systems that assess the consistency of cell differentiation and identity, purity, and potency might play a key role in ensuring the ultimate function of tissue-engineered products. When these assays are extended and validated in the context of an appropriate in vivo or other model, they might be predictive of clinical potency *(65)*.

In vitro assays to assure expression of the clinically desired phenotype in expanded cell strains might be needed to ensure appropriate function of the tissue-engineered product *(65)*. Because many isolated cell populations are heterogeneous, methods to assess whether the desired cells are present and in what proportion will be required for cell and tissue characterization.

3.3. Cell Identity

Production of tissue-engineered products requires the development and validation of specific methods for the positive identification of cells, which may include evaluation of cellular morphology, cell-specific antigen expression, or gene/gene product expression *(30,65)*. Each component of cell characterization can be monitored through the development of in vitro assay systems to ensure that the cells of interest are present and capable of performing the expected task.

3.4. Cell Potency

Cell potency is a measure of the ability of the cells to exhibit a desired phenotype or express appropriate levels of a therapeutic agent *(65)*. The potency of autogenous cells is based on cell viability and/or the expression of specific cellular markers that are associated with the desired phenotype.

3.5. Animal Models

Animal models for structural repair or physiological restoration are often preferred for the assessment of potency using tissue-engineered products *(65)*. If the development of an appropriate in vivo model is not possible, then in vitro models of cell differentiation on surrogate animal models, in which the appropriate cellular function can be demonstrated, can also be valuable.

4. OUR RESEARCH INTO SELECTIVE CELL TRANSPLANTATION AND BONE TISSUE ENGINEERING

In our research, we are conducting in vitro and in vivo experiments to develop suitable procedures for osteogenic cell expansion, stimulation, and transplantation into bone defects following the requirements outlined earlier. Our research program focuses on translational research, which will use previously determined techniques and information of in vitro mechanistic studies combined with in vivo experiments to move toward clinical use of this knowledge in promotion of bone healing in cancer patients.

4.1. Osteogenic Cells

We are isolating osteogenic cells from human and animal osteogenic donor tissues, including bone, periosteum, and bone marrow. Isolated osteogenic cell populations include a heterogenous population of cells such as fibroblasts, chondroblasts, and cells of the osteoblastic lineage *(66,67)*. Cells of the osteoblastic lineage include osteoprogenitors, which are the proliferative cells of the lineage known to differentiate into bone-forming osteoblasts *(66–68)*. The greater the number of osteoprogenitor cells at the bone defect site, the greater the amount of new bone will be formed *(51)*. For this reason, it is important to assess the proportion of osteoprogenitors in the total osteogenic cell population. We are determining this proportion using a well-accepted osteoprogenitor assay *(69)*.

Periosteal tissue and cancellous bone tissue are available as autogenous donor tissues; small amounts of these tissues could be readily collected at surgery with minimal morbidity *(33)*. We are evaluating human bone and equine periosteal tissue in parallel. This will allow us to evaluate two osteogenic cell donor tissues simultaneously and to evaluate the horse as a large animal model for bone tissue engineering.

4.2. Expansion Techniques

Autogenous osteogenic tissue from a donor will be limited in quantity. Therefore, culture methods that result in optimum expansion of osteogenic cells for use in cell-based therapy will be essential. The timeframe for expansion of bone cells is also an important issue. Clinical usefulness of transplanted bone cells for promotion of bone healing in fracture patients will require that large numbers of cells be available as early as 2 wk postsurgical stabilization of a fracture or resected tumor. Two main cell culture techniques are commonly used to isolate and expand osteogenic cells in vitro: explant cultures and enzyme-released cells *(31,43,56,70–72)*. Significant differences in cell proliferation *(40)* and ultimate cell number obtained have been shown with these methods. We are comparing these techniques with a dynamic cell culture system involving cells attached to micro carrier beads maintained in suspension within a spinner flask *(73)*. Although dynamic culture techniques are more complicated systems, a dynamic in vitro microenvironment for tissues might be an important aspect in guiding the formation of tissue with certain structural and functional characteristics *(28)*. The use of dynamic culture systems allows the investigator to control flow and mixing, which can enhance the mass transfer of nutrients, wastes, and regulatory molecules *(28)*. Some researchers have shown that stirred conditions improve the quality of cartilage produced in comparison to static cultures. Hydrodynamic stimulation of the cartilage resulted in the production of greater amounts of extracellular matrix components, such as GAGs, and collagen, leading to improved mechanical properties. We are comparing the number and proportion of expanded osteoprogenitor cells available for transplantation *(69)* between techniques.

4.3. Stimulatory Factors

Once we have determined the best culture technique to provide the highest numbers of the desired cell type (osteoprogenitors), we will attempt to modify the cells in vitro prior to transplantation in vivo. Various factors will be investigated for stimulating or "priming" the cells to differentiate and produce maximum amounts of new bone.

Inductive factors, including bone morphogenetic proteins (BMP) and insulin-like growth factors (IGF), have been investigated with osteogenic cells of different species and have been shown to increase production of bone matrix proteins.

Vascular endothelial growth factor (VEGF) has been shown to be expressed by osteoblasts *(74)*. Because angiogenesis is important for bone formation in vivo, we are investigating the effect of VEGF on osteogenic cells in vitro along with other factors that have been studied more extensively.

Other stimulatory factors including doxycycline will be investigated for their effect on differentiation and bone production. Research recently conducted by one coinvestigator (GS) at the Hamilton Regional Cancer Center (HRCC) showed that treatment with doxycycline significantly increased several parameters of bone formation in long bones of mice including osteoid volume, osteoid surface and number of osteoblasts/ bone surface *(15)*.

The factor that is most effective in stimulating the production of bone matrix will be used in the preparation of osteogenic cells prior to trasplantation in vivo. Because the cells are being primed with the stimulatory factor rather than local implantation of the factor at the bone lesion, the risk of stimulating quiescent cancer cells is eliminated.

Once appropriate in vitro studies have been completed, the isolated, expanded, and stimulated osteogenic cells will be mixed with a collagen gel that will provide a matrix for the osteogenic cells. A mixture of collagen gel with osteogenic cells will be able to be injected percutaneously into the bone defect site, thereby eliminating the need for an invasive surgical procedure.

5. TRANSLATIONAL RESEARCH

This research program uses translational research to move from mechanistic in vitro studies of bone physiology toward use in clinical bone defects. An important step in translational research is the in vivo investigation in appropriate animal models. We are focusing on the use of adult horses as a large animal model for promotion of human bone healing. Horses have been used as a large animal model for cartilage repair in humans for many years *(75)*. The horse will be a more appropriate large-animal model compared to small ruminants or dogs, which are often used *(63,76)*. Horse fractures are often large segmental defects, and they often have delayed union of fractures and other bone-healing-related problems similar to humans *(77)*. Dogs do not typically have bone-healing problems and can ambulate readily on three limbs after fracture repair. Small ruminants (sheep and goats) are known to have especially good bone-healing properties because of the formation of plexiform bone during bone healing. Therefore, the horse, an animal that has similar bone-healing problems as humans, who must bear weight to ambulate post-operatively, and an animal often required to perform athletically after the bone is healed, will be a good large animal model for use in investigations of human bone healing.

6. CONCLUSION

For tissue engineering to change clinical oncology practice, much progress still needs to be made *(39)*. A cooperative interdisciplinary effort among engineers, biological scientists, and clinicians is essential for this progress *(27,28,30,39)*. Once methods are derived to engineer tissues, methods must be discovered that yield marketable products in ways that can be scaled up for industry *(30,65)*. Products must pass regulatory standards and become acceptable to clinicians and patients. Many researchers are involved in various aspects of the development of tissue-engineered products for cancer patients. It is likely that this novel therapy will be instituted clinically in the near future as an important adjunct for treatment of bone metastasis and pathological fractures.

REFERENCES

1. Serafini AN. Therapy of metastatic bone pain. *J Nucl Med* 2001; 42:895–906.
2. Van Poznak CH. The use of bisphosphonate in patients with breast cancer. *Cancer Control* 2002; 9: 480–489.
3. Vukmirovic-Popovic S, Colterjohn N, Lhotak S, et al. Morphological, histolomorphometric, and micro-structural alterations in human bone metastsis from breast carcinoma. *Bone* 2002; 31:529–535.
4. Coleman RE. Skeletal complications of malignancy. *Cancer* 1997; 80:1588–1594.
5. Aebi M. Spinal metastases in the elderly. *Eur Spine J* 2003; 12(Suppl):S202–S213.
6. Wenger M. Vertebroplasty for metastasis. *Med Oncol* 2003; 20:203–209.
7. Vinholes J, Coleman R, Eastell R. Effects of bone metastases on bone metabolism: implications for diagnosis, imaging and assessment of response to cancer treatment. *Cancer Treat Rev* 1996; 22:289–331.

8. Domchek SM, Younger J, Finkelstein DM, et al. Predictors of skeletal complications in patients with metastatic breast carcinoma. *Cancer* 2000; 89:363–368.

9. Mastro AM, Gay Carol V, Welch DR, et al. Breast cancer cells induce osteoblast apoptosis: A posible contributor to bone degradation. *J Cell Biochem* 2004; 91:265–276.

10. Frassica FJ, Frassica DA. Evaluation and treatment of metastases to the humerus. *Clin Orthop Related Res* 2003; 415S:S212–S218.

11. Buggay D, Jaffe K. Metastatic bone tumors of the pelvis and lower extremity. *J Surg Orthop Adv* 2003; 12:192–199.

12. Campa JA, Payne R. The management of intractable bone pain: a clinicians perspective. *Semin Nucl Med* 1992; 22:3–10.

13. Maisano R, Pergoizzo S, Cascinu S. Novel therapeutic approaches to cancer patients with bone metastsis. *Crit Rev Oncol Hematol* 2001; 40:239–250.

14. Fox A, Medhurst S, Courade JP, et al. Anti-hyperalgesic activity of the cox-2 inhibitor lumiracoxib in a model of bone cancer pain in the rat. *Pain* 2004; 107:33–40.

15. Duivenvoorden WCM, Popovic SV, Lhotak S, et al. Doxycycline decreases tumor burden in a bone metastasis model of human breast cancer. *Cancer Res* 2002; 62:1588–1591.

16. Doita M, Harada T, Iguchi T, et al. Total sacrectomy and reconstruction for sacral tumors. *Spine* 2003; 28:E296–301.

17. Kaemmerlen P, Thiesse P, Jonas P, et al. Purcutaneous injection of orthopedic cement in metastatic vertebral lesions. *N Engl J Med* 1989; 321:121.

18. Mathis JM. Percutaneous vertebroplasty. *JBR-BTR* 2003; 86:299–301.

19. Faisham WI, Zulmi W, Biswal BM. Metastatic disease of the proximal femur. *Med J Malaysia* 2003; 58:120–124.

20. Weber KL, OConner MI. Operative treatment of long bone metastases. *Clin Orthop Related Res* 2003; 415S:S276–S278.

21. Dalgorf D, Borkhoff CM, Stephen JG, et al. Venting during prophylatic nailing for femoral metastases: current orthopedic practice. *Can J Surg* 2003; 46:427–431.

22. Ilyas L, Kurar A, Moreau PG, et al. Modular megaprosthesis for distal femoral tumors. *Int Orthop* 2001; 25:375–377.

23. Kawai A, Lin PP, Boland PJ, et al. Relationship between magnitude of resection, complications, and prosthetic survival after prosthetic knee reconstructions for distal femoral tumors. *J Surg Oncol* 1999; 70:109–115.

24. Shin DS, Choong PFM, Chao EYH, et al. Large tumor endoprostheses and extracortical bone bridging. *Acta Orthop Scand* 2000; 71:305–311.

25. Shin KH, Park HJ, Yoo JH, et al. Reconstructive surgery in primary malignant and aggressive benign bone tumor of the proximal humerus. *Yonsei Med J* 2000; 41:304–311.

26. Franck WM, Olivieri M, Jannasch O, et al. An expandable nailing system for the management of pathological humerus fractures. *Arch Orthop Trauma Surg* 2002; 122:400–405.

27. Jacofsky DJ, Papagelopoulos PJ, Sim FH. Advances and challenges in the surgical treatment of metastatic bone disease. *Clin Orthop Related Res* 2003; 415S:S14–S18.

28. Fuchs JR, Nasseri BA, Vacanti JP. Tissue engineering: A 21st century solution to surgical reconstruction. *Ann Thorac Surg* 2001; 72:577–91.

29. Ramkrishnan M, Prasad SS, Parkinson RW, et al. Management of subtrochanteric femoral fractures and metastases using long proximal femoral nail. *Injury* 2004; 35:184–190.

30. Luyton FP, Francesco DA, De Bari C. Skeletal tissue engineering; opportunities and challenges. *Best Pract Res Cl Rh* 2001; 15:759–770.

31. Yamanouchi K, Satomura K, Gotoh Y, et al. Bone formation by transplanted human osteoblasts cultured with collagen sponge with dexamethasone in vitro. *J Bone Miner Res* 2001; 16:857–867.

32. Oldham JB, Hefferan TE, Larson DR, et al. Biological activity of rhBMP-2 released from PLGA microspheres. *J Biomech Engin* 2000; 122:289–292.

33. Perka C, Schultz R, Lindenhayn K, et al. Segmental bone repair by tissue-engineered periosteal cell transplants with bioresorbable fleece and fibrin scaffolds in rabbits. *Biomaterials* 2000; 21:1145–1153.

34. Holy CE, Shoichet MS, Davies JE. Engineering three-dimensional bone tissue in vitro using biodegradable scaffolds: Investigating initial cell-seeding density and culture period. *J Biomed Mater Res* 2000; 51:376–382.

35. Stevenson S. Enhancement of fracture healing with autogenous and allogenic bone grafts. *Clin Orthop Related Res* 1998; 355S:S239–S246.

36. Lane JM, Tomin E, Bostrom MPG. Biosynthetic bone grafting. *Clin Orthop Related Res* 1999; 367S:S107–S117.
37. Boden SD. Bioactive factors for bone tissue engineering. *Clin Orthop Related Res* 1999; 367S:S84–S94.
38. Tamura S, Kataoka H, Matsui Y, et al. The effects of transplantation of osteoblastic cells with bone morphogenetic protein (BMP)/carrier complex on bone repair. *Bone* 2001; 29:169–175.
39. Miller MJ. Osseous tissue engineering in oncological surgery. *Semin Surg Oncol* 2000; 19:294–301.
40. Voegele TJ, Voegele- Kadletz M, Esposito V, et al. The effect of different techniques on human osteoblast-like cell growth. *Anticancer Res* 2000; 20:3575–3582.
41. De Bari C, Dell-Accio F, Tylzanowski P, et al. Multipotent mesenchymal stem cells from adult human synovial membrane. *Arthritis Rheumat* 2001; 44:1928–1942.
42. Martinez P, Moreno I, Miguel F, et al. Changes in osteocalcin response to 1,25-dihydroxyvitamin D3 stiulation and basal vitamin D receptor expression in human osteoblastic cells according to donor age and skeletal origin. *Bone* 2001; 29:35–41.
43. Hankey DP, McCabe RE, Doherty MJ, et al. Enhancement of human osteoblast proliferation and phenotypic expression when cultured in human serum. *Acta Orthop Scand* 2001; 72:395–403.
44. Kim WS, Vacanti CA, Upton J, et al. Bone defect repair with tissue- engineered cartilage. *Plast Reconstr Surg* 1994; 94:580–584.
45. Cook SD, Rueger DC. Osteogenic protein-1. Biology and Applications. *Clin Orthop Related Res* 1996; 324:29–38.
46. Sampath TK, Maliakal JC, Hauschka PV, et al. Recombinant human osteogenic protien-1 induces new bone formation in vivo with a specific activity comparable with natural bovine osteogenic protein and stimulates osteoblast proliferation and differentiation in vitro. *J Biol Chem* 1992; 267:20,352–20,362.
47. Baylink DJ, Finkelman RD, Mohan S. Growth factors to stimulate bone formation. *J Bone Miner Res* 1993; 8(Suppl 2):s565–s572.
48. Kirker-Head CA, Gerhart TN, Armstrong R, et al. Healing bone using recombinant human bone morphogenetic protein 2 and copolymer. *Clin Orthop* 1998; 349:205–217.
49. Harakas NK. Demineralized bone-matrix-induced osteogenesis. *Clin Orthop Related Res* 1983; 188: 239–251.
50. Khan SN, Tomin E, Lane JM. Clinical applications of bone graft substitutes. *Orthop Clin NA* 2000; 31:389–398.
51. Bassett CAL. Clinical Implications of Cell Function in Bone Grafting. *Clin Orthop Related Res* 1972; 87:49–55.
52. Friedlaender GE. Current concepts review: Bone grafts. The basic science rationale for clinical applications. *J Bone Joint Surg* 1987; 69A:786-790.
53. Kveiborg M, Flyvbjerg A, Eriksen EF, et al. Transforming growth factor-beta1 stimulates the production of insulin-like growth factor-1 and insulin-like growth factor-binding protein-3 in human bone marrow stromal osteoblast progenitors. *J Endocrin* 2001; 169:549–561.
54. Takagi K, Urist MR. The role of bone marrow in bone morphogenetic protein- induced repair of massive diaphyseal defects. *Clin Orthop Related Res* 1982; 171:224.
55. Moxham JP, Kibblewhite DJ, Dvorak M, et al. TGF-_1 forms fuctionally normal bone in a segmental sheep tibial diaphyseal defect. *J Otolarygology* 1996; 23:388–392.
56. Johnson EE, Urist MR, Finerman GA. Bone morphogenetic protein augmentation grafting of resistant femoral nonunions. *Clin Orthop Related Res* 1998; 230:257–265.
57. Bruder SP, Fox BS. Tissue engineering of bone. *Clin Orthop Related Res* 1999; 367S:S68–S83.
58. Wozney JM, Rosen V. Bone morphogenetic protein and bone morphogenetic protein gene family in bone formation and repair. *Clin Orthop Related Res* 1988; 346:26–37.
59. Guo W, Gorlick R, Ladanyi M, et al. Expression of bone morphogenetic proteins and receptors in sarcomas. *Clin Orthop Related Res* 1999; 365:175–183.
60. Gauthier O, Khairoun I, Bosco J, et al. Noninvasive bone replacement with a new injectable calcium phosphate biomaterial. *J Biomed Mater Res* 2003; 66A:47–54.
61. Kadiyala S, Young RG, Thiede MA, et al. Culture expanded canine mesenchymal stem cells possess osteochondrogenic potential in vivo and in vitro. *Cell Transplant* 1997; 6:125–134.
62. Khan SN, Tomin E, Lane JM. Clinical applications of bone graft substitutes. *Orthop Clin NA* 2000; 31:389–398.
63. Sciadini MF, Dawson JM, Johnson KD. Evaluation of bovine-derived bone protein with a natural coral carrier as a bone-graft substitute in a canine segmental defect model *J Orthop Res* 1997; 15: 844–857.

64. Moore DC, Chapman MW, Manske D. The evaluation of a biphasi calcium phosphate ceramic for use in grafting long-bone diaphyseal defects. *J Orthop Res* 1987; 5:356–365.

65. Omstead DR, Baird LG, Christienson L, et al. Voluntary guidance for the development of tissue-engineered products. *Tissue Engineer* 1998; 3:239–266.

66. Bellows CG, Aubin JE. Determination of numbers of osteoprogenitors present in isolated fetal rat calvaria cells in vitro. *Dev Biol* 1989; 133:8–13.

67. Aubin JE. Advances n the osteoblastic lineage. *Biochem Cell Biol* 1998; 76:899–910.

68. Jia D, Heersche JNM. Insulin-like growth factor -1 and -2 stimulate osteoprogenitor proliferation and differentiation and adipocyte formation in cell populations derived from adult rat bone *Bone* 2000; 27:785–794.

69. Bellows CG, Heersche JNM. The frequency of common progenitors for adipocytes and osteoblasts of committed and restricted adipocyte and osteoblast progenitors in fetal rat calvaria cell populations. *J Bone Miner Res* 2001; 16:1983–1993.

70. Beresford JN, Beresford JN, Graves SE, Smoothy CA. Formation of mineralized nodules by bone derived cells in vitro: A model of bone formation? *Am J Med Genet* 1993; 45:163–178.

71. Matsuyama T, Lau KHW, Wergedal JE. Monolayer cultures of normal human bone cells contain multiple subpopulations of alkaline phosphatase positive cells. *Calcif Tissue Int* 1990; 47:276–283.

72. Bellows CG, Aubin JN, Heersche JNM, Antosz ME. Mineralized bone nodules formed in vitro from enzymatically released rat calvarial cell populations. *Calcif Tissue Int* 1986; 38:143–154.

73. Harris-Hooker SA, Gajduek CM, Wight TN, et al. Neovascular responses induced by cultured aortic endothelial cells. *J Cell Physio* 1988; 14:302–310.

74. Deckers M, van der Plum G, Dooijewaard S, et al. Effect of angiogenic and antiangiogenic compounds on the outgrowth of capillary structures from fetal mouse bone explants. *Lab Invest* 2001; 81:5–15.

75. Hendrickson DA, Nixon AJ, Grande DA, et al. Chondrocyte- fibrin matrix transplants for resurfacing extensive articular cartilage defects. *J Orthop Res* 1994; 12:485–497.

76. Yamaji T, Ando K, Wolf S, et al. The effect of micromovement on callus formation. *J Orthop Sci* 2001; 6:571–575.

77. Ducharme NG, Nixon AJ. Delayed union, non union, and malunion, In: Nixon AJ, ed. *Equine Fracture Repair*. Philadelphia, PA: Saunders, 1996:354–358.

15 Role of Photodynamic Therapy for Bone Metastasis

Shane Burch, MD and Albert J. M. Yee, MD

CONTENTS

1. INTRODUCTION

Cancer spread to bone is a significant cause of morbidity in patients with metastatic spread. Metastatic bone disease is also the most common cause of destructive lesions in the adult skeleton. With improvements in adjuvant therapies and a decline in age-standardized cancer mortality, skeletal metastases are increasingly prevalent in advanced spread *(1)*. As such, there will be greater emphasis on the treatment of patients with metastatic spread. Breast, lung, prostate, and kidney are the carcinomas with the greatest propensity for bony metastatic spread. Common anatomic sites of such spread include the axial skeleton (vertebral bodies) and proximal limb girdles (humeri and femora).

Management of bone metastasis is palliative and is mostly directed toward positively influencing patient quality of life. Goals of treatment include pain relief, preservation of ambulation, and improvement of emotional and psychological well-being. Pain is the most common presenting symptom, and with increasing bony tumour burden, the risk of pathologic bony fracture imposes significant morbidity. The clinical sites of most significant consequence include weight-bearing long bones and the vertebral column. The consequences of pathologic fracture include acute pain from bony instability and tumor emboli causing respiratory complications relating to extensive bony tumor spread *(2,3)*. In the weight-bearing lower extremity, pathologic fracture impacts ambulatory capacity and, often, the femur is a site with the propensity for tumor emboli *(2–4)*. Treatment is directed toward providing the highest quality of life at acceptable risk and, often, surgical stabilization is recommending for pathologic fracture of weight-bearing long bones to assist in pain control, afford skeletal stability, and facilitate patient mobility.

From: *Cancer Drug Discovery and Development*
Bone Metastasis: Experimental and Clinical Therapeutics
Edited by: G. Singh and S. A. Rabbani © Humana Press Inc., Totowa, NJ

Involvement of the vertebral column can lead to pathologic burst fracture that contributes toward progressive spinal cord compression with resultant paralysis. Apart from analgesia and systemic strategies to deal with global tumor burden, local strategies include external-beam radiation therapy, vertebroplasty, and conventional spinal surgery. Each of these local strategies has limitations and potentially significant complications. There are radiation exposure limits prior to radiation-induced spinal cord damage. There is a threefold to fourfold increased risk of major wound complications in patients undergoing spinal surgery who have had previous local radiation *(5,6)*. Complication rates in conventional spine surgery are significant in what are often complex cases *(5–13)*. The complication rates of vertebroplasty in spinal metastases also appear to be greater than its use in osteoporosis *(14–17)*.

Although systemic strategies to deal with metastatic involvement are important in reducing overall tumor burden, the clinical issue of treatment for significant precritical bony lesions posing risk for pathologic fracture and complications is important. Ongoing research is required to develop efficacious local therapies with minimal side effects and associated patient morbidity. The approach of the early identification of clinically significant precritical bone metastatic lesions followed by early institution of treatment poses the most promise in patient palliation.

2. PHOTODYNAMIC THERAPY AND ITS MUSCULOSKELETAL APPLICATION

Photodynamic therapy (PDT) is a promising cancer treatment that induces targeted localized tumor destruction by the photochemical generation of cytotoxic singlet oxygen *(18–22)*. PDT employs wavelength-specific light in combination with a photosensitizing agent. The photosensitizing agent accumulates in neoplastic cells and is activated by light at low power, which does not cause thermal effects. Subsequent oxidative stress elicits direct local tumor cell death. Cellular mechanisms include microvascular injury inducing tissue hypoxia, complement-mediated infiltration of activated neutrophils, and induction of cell apoptosis *(18,23–27)*. Effects are governed by light energy applied, tissue oxygenation, and the optical properties of the tissues. Clinically, PDT has been used in breast cancer recurrences and other primary malignancies with encouraging early results *(27–35)*.

The use of PDT in musculoskeletal neoplasms has been limited and is an area of current development. In primary bone maligancies, the goal is often cure, with the modern-era treatment of primary sarcomas having improved dramatically through the use of multimodality therapy involving wide-resection surgery and neo-adjuvant or adjuvant chemotherapy/radiotherapy. However, there are many tumors that recur locally or occur in anatomical locations that make wide-resection difficult. PDT can be a useful adjuvant to current local strategies in such situations. The feasibility of such an approach was demonstrated by Nambisan et al. in a case series of 10 patients who had recurrent retroperitoneal sarcomas treated by repeat surgical resection and adjuvant intraoperative PDT of the tumor bed *(36)*. There were no complications reported from PDT using hematoporphyrin derivate (HPD) or dihematoporphyrin ether (DHE) at a total light dose of 30–288 J/cm^2 *(36)*. Because photosensitizer drugs are preferentially taken up by tumor cells, tumor-related red fluorescence was concluded to be clinically useful in identifying residual tumor areas *(36)*.

Knowledge is evolving in the use of PDT for the treatment of musculoskeletal neoplasms. In 1993, Hourigan et al. corroborated the in vitro sensitivity of primary human sarcomas to photodynamic tumoricidal therapy (37). The authors confirmed the presence of an energy dose-dependent effect for porphyrin-based PDT on three different human musculoskeletal neoplasms grown in vitro (37). When compared to human osteogenic sarcoma and dedifferentiated chondrosarcoma, a giant cell tumor exhibited the greatest cytotoxic response to therapy (37). There are also reports demonstrating in vivo efficacy of PDT in chondrosarcoma and fibrosarcoma in orthotopic rat and mouse models, respectively (38,39). There have also been reports on the use of PDT in a mouse osteosarcoma cell line (40,41). The clinical feasibility of PDT as an adjunct to surgical resection to treat recurrent sarcomas was demonstrated in the aforementioned study by Nambisan et al. (36).

Other musculoskeletal applications of PDT include evaluation of photodynamic synovectomy in an inflammatory arthritis model (42,43). There have been reports on the use of the therapy in extracorporeal photochemical purging of bone marrow constituents in transplantation (44–49). The use of PDT to directly treat structural bone lesions is limited (50). The ability of the therapy to treat bone relate, in part, to the ability to access lesions contained within bone and issues regarding light transmission and attenuation through human bone.

3. OPTICAL PROPERTIES OF BONE

Knowledge is evolving regarding the optical properties of bone (51–55). Takeuchi et al. evaluated the correlation between bone mineral density and light penetration in bovine cortical and trabecular bone. The investigators were able to demonstrate a correlation between bone mineral density and light-scattering properties corroborating the intuitive notion that light attenuation through cortical bone is greater than that through cancellous bone (52). Light transmittance and reflectance has also been evaluated between wavelengths of 630 and 950 nm in porcine cochlear and skull bone (51,55). Firbank et al. evaluated diffuse reflectance and transmittance and scattering phase function measurement in fresh adult porcine parietal skull bone samples (51). The authors described the porcine bone as a reasonable model in that the physical and chemical composition of bone in large mammals does not vary greatly (51,56). The authors concluded nonisotropic scattering properties of their bone samples that the authors inferred might be explained by conglomerations of hydroxy-apatite crystals, that have a greater scattering efficiency than individual crystals (51). The scattering coefficent of light demonstrated a linear fall with wavelength over the range investigated (650–950 nm), with no difference if samples were either parallel or perpendicular to the skull surface (51). The features of the absorption spectra analysis demonstrated the water peak above 900 nm and a rise below 700 nm together with a small ripple at 750 nm, which was believed attributable to residual deoxygenated hemoglobin (51). The authors estimated that water accounted for approx 90% of the absorption and hemoglobin accounted for 3–6% (51). The effects of other potentially significant variables on light attentuation and transmittance in bone (e.g., fluid flow) require further in vivo study. The ability of laser light as a therapeutic strategy directed toward cochlear dysfunction has been demonstrated in cadaveric and clinical studies (53,54). The ability of optical imaging to infer bony architecture and properties is another area that has contributed to our understanding on the optical properties of bone (57,58).

4. LOCAL MINIMALLY INVASIVE
SURGICAL TECHNIQUES TO ACCESS BONE

Minimally invasive surgical strategies have been at the forefront of current research and clinical use in the treatment of a variety of medical conditions. Specifically related to orthopaedic surgery, such strategies have allowed access to treat bone conditions through minimally invasive routes with lessened surgical morbidity. The use of endoscopic guided spinal surgery in the treatment of adult deformity and degenerative conditions of the spine has been described *(59–65)*. More recently, minimally invasive approaches for routine surgical lumbar decompression and instrumentation have been reported *(62,64,65)*.

Vertebroplasty, used clinically for the treatment of painful osteoporotic spinal compression fractures and spinal metastases, is gaining increasing acceptance and use *(14–17)*. This minimally invasive local technique employs percutaneous fluoroscopic placement of a spinal needle or trochar in the vertebral body to allow direct injection of PMMA (i.e., bone cement) to mechanically stabilize the vertebra. This technique can afford significant pain relief in patients with pathologic and osteoporotic vertebral fractures *(66–68)*. Vertebroplasty has become an important adjunct in the treatment of painful vertebral metastases, and, more recently, a similar technique has been used in our and other centers to treat periacetabular bony metastases (i.e., cementoplasty) (69–71).

By adapting such minimally invasive strategies to allow placement of optical fibers adjacent to osteolytic lesions, the feasibility and potential of photodynamic therapy to treat bone metastases is currently being investigated in the preclinical setting. Such an approach to adapt minimally invasive surgical techniques to access bone has also been demonstrated with other local adjuvants such as laser or radio-ablation *(63,72)*.

5. PRECLINICAL MODELS OF BONE METASTASES

There are a variety of strategies to study bone metastases in preclinical models. Several models of both osteolytic and osteoblastic metastasis have been reported *(73–81)*. Tumor cells can be injected locally adjacent to a bone surface, into the bone marrow, or onto the periosteal surface. Local injection methods, however, might not as accurately reflect the metastatic process and distortion to local tissue by the technique might confound interpretation of results. As such, systemic or orthotopic inoculation of tumor cells has been the more widely applied approach. A systemic approach by intracardiac injection of cancer cells has been described in both mouse and rat models *(73–80)*. Metastatic spread preferentially to bone is, in part, dependent on the particular cell line and animal species chosen. Engebraaten and Fodstad used two estrogen and progesterone receptor-negative human breast cancer cell lines (MA-11, MT-1) in nude rats with evaluation of site-specific growth and metastasis *(82)*. The authors demonstrated the MT-1 cell line to more predictably produce bone/bone marrow metastases when compared to selective neural tissue metastases observed using MA-11 cells. Our experiments using MDA-MB-231, MT-1, and other cell lines in rodent species have corroborated this previous work, demonstrating the MT-1 cell line, when inoculated into nude rats, to more predictably produce bony metastatic lesions *(82–84)*. The MDA-MB-435 human breast carcinoma cell line has also been recently reported to be more site specific to bone when inoculated intracardially into mice *(75)*. In our studies, we have used the human breast cancer cell line

MT-1 inoculated intracardially into 4- to 6-wk-old athymic *rnu/rnu* rats. The rat species was also chosen over mouse models of bone metastases because of animal size and the technical aspects behind the surgery that were anticipated to be required for laser light application to targeted bone lesions.

In our model, human breast cancer MT-1 cells are grown in RPMI media to 70–80% subconfluency, at which time they are refed with media 24 h prior to inoculation into *rnu/rnu* rats. Cell viability is determined by trypan blue exclusion, and cell suspensions with greater than 95% viability without cell clumping are used. An intracardiac injection of 0.2 mL free RPMI media with 2×10^6 MT-1 cells is then performed into the left heart ventricle of anesthetized 4- to 6-wk-old *rnu/rnu* female rats using techniques similar to that described by several investigators *(82,85,86)*. The spontaneous, pulsatile entrance of bright red oxygenated blood into the syringe determines appropriate positioning in the left ventricle of the heart. There is a learning curve with the intracardiac technique, and even with trained individuals, the success rate of a rat subsequently developing metastasis is approx 70 to 80%.

5.1. Quantification of Bone Metastatic Burden

There are a variety of strategies to quantify bone metastatic burden in the aforementioned preclinical models. Although fine-detail radiography can detect osteolytic lesions in certain models 3–4 wk after tumor cell inoculation, there is a balance between the identification of tumor lesions that can be targeted for local therapies so that treatment can be initiated and evaluation of treatment effects quantified prior to acceptable tumor end points for animal care *(78,80,81)*. Conventional radiographic imaging (fine-detail radiography, fluoroscopy, and micro-CT scanning) is limited in only identifying the extent of osteolytic involvement and has the limitation of not visualizing the viable tumor cell population. In vivo real-time imaging of viable metastatic tumor cells has recently been made possible, adapting strategies of gene transfection for fluorescence *(75,87)*. In the study by Harms et al., human breast carcinoma cell line MDA-MB-435 was transfected to constitutively express enhanced green fluorescent protein (GFP) *(75)*. In a mouse intracardiac inoculation bone metastases model using luciferase-transfected cells, Wetterwald et al. described the sensitivity of bioluminescent reporter imaging in detecting intramedullary tumor growth preceding the appearance of radiographic osteolysis by approx 2 wk *(87)*. As such, bioluminescent imaging enables continuous monitoring in the same animal of growth kinetics for each metastatic site and can provide end-point analysis of photodynamic treatment to osteolytic lesions affected by metastatic growth (Fig. 1). The technique, therefore, also facilitates the earlier identification of bone metastases that can be targeted for local therapies.

6. PHOTODYNAMIC THERAPY AND BONE METASTASES

Photosensitizer drugs have been previously shown to elicit efficacy in PDT through different mechanisms *(80,82,88,89)*. There are several photosensitizer drugs now available with minimal systemic side effects. 5-aminolevulinic acid (5-ALA) is a pro-drug that leads to endogenous synthesis of the photosensitizer protoporphyrin IX, PpIX. The drug possesses predominantly cellular effects on tumor activity and has the potential for high tumor-to-neural tissue selectivity *(88,90,91)*. Benzoporphyrin-derivative monoacid ring A (BPD-MA, Verteporfin®, QLT Inc., British Columbia) is a drug that can be used to

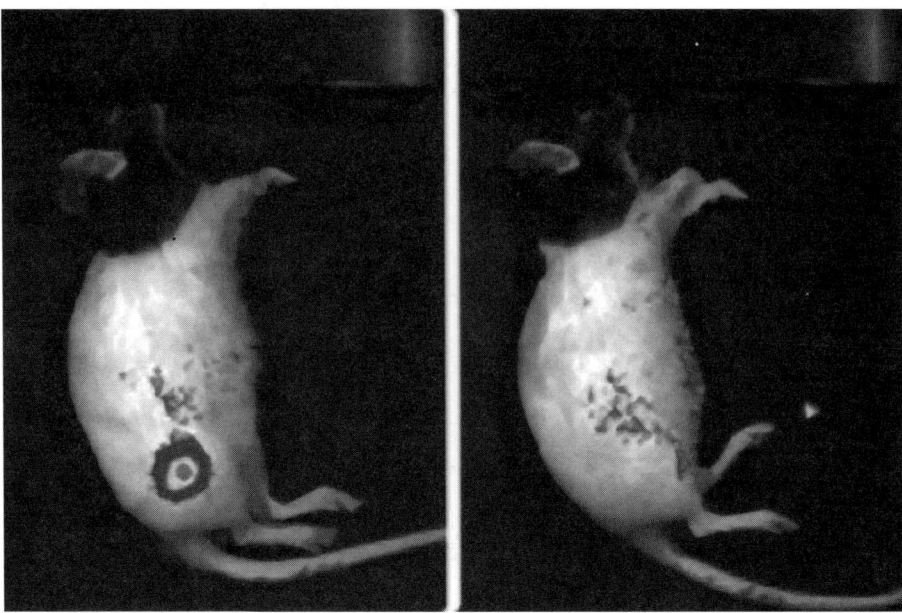

Fig. 1. Bioluminescent-targeted PDT of a femoral metastasis. The image on the left demonstrates pretreatment signal intensity of femoral lesion targeted for therapy. The image on the right demonstrated the same animal imaged 48 h post-PDT.

target either the neo-vasculature that provides the essential nutrients to the cells or the cells directly depending on the drug–light interval *(38,92–95)*. A short drug–light interval favors vascular targets as the photosensitizers are still circulating within the vasculature, however, with longer intervals the photosensitizer has time to extravasate and accumulate into the tumor cells *(38,94)*. Its absorption spectrum is stimulated by a longer wavelength of light, which might be desirable to achieve a greater depth of tissue penetration. The drug has been used clinically for ocular macular degeneration, demonstrating minimal systemic side effects *(96–102)*. The drug of choice for potential clinical utility in bone metastases will depend, in part, on the intrinsic sensitivity of the primary malignancy responsible for the metastasis and will likely vary on tumor type. The advantages of the rodent model of human breast carcinoma is the ability to evaluate the effect of PDT on human cells. Clinical experience of PDT in such primary cancers coupled with ongoing preclinical study using human cancer cell lines will assist in addressing the sensitivity of the therapy in influencing tumor growth kinetics. In directing treatment in bone, a drug that is stimulated by a longer wavelength of light might assist in achieving a greater depth of penetration of light dependent on the bone mineral density and particular bone that requires treatment. This would be important in bone, where significant attenuation of light might occur. Finally, drug pharmacokinetics will be important when defining the appropriate drug–light interval for treatment as this will impact the practicality of time required for the treatment to be administered.

There has been recent interest in the evaluation of PDT in the treatment of intraosseous tumors and bone metastases. Koudinova et al. recently evaluted the use of Pd–Bacterio-pheophorbide (TOOKAD) in the in vivo treatment of human prostatic small cell carcinoma xenografts *(50)*. TOOKAD is a novel bacteriochlorophyll-derived second-generation photosensitizer. The strong light absorbance in the near infrared region ($\lambda = 763$nm) facilitates deep tissue pentration. In this recent study, male CD-I nude mice were grafted with human SCCP (WISH-PC2) in three anatomic locations; subcutaneous (to represent tumor mass), intraosseous (direct injection representing bone metastases), and orthotopically within the prostate microenvironment *(50)*. PDT consisted of intravenous administration of 4 mg/kg TOOKAD followed by immediate illumination (650–800 nm) from a xenon light source or diode laser emitting at 770 nm. Tumor volume, human plasma chromogranin A levels, animal well-being, and survival were used as end points. Histopathology and immunohistochemistry were also used to define the tumor response. Subcutaneous tumors demonstrated complete healing within 28–40 d, reaching an overall long-term cure rate at 90 d following treatment of 69%. Intratibial lesions responded with a 50% rate of tumor elimination in treated mice at 70–90 d after therapy, as confirmed histologically. The feasibility of the therapy to treat structural bone lesions was demonstrated in their transcutaneous PDT approach to tibial lesions of WISH-PC2 enabled by the near-infrared absorption of the TOOKAD *(50)*.

In summary, PDT poses an interesting adjunct to locally treat bone metastases. Adapting current clinically utilized minimally invasive surgical techniques to place optical fibers adjacent to or within target bone lesions facilitates local treatment by PDT. Preclinical study using a human breast carcinoma cell line has confirmed the feasibility and efficacy of a single percutaneous treatment of PDT to elicit a significant reduction in tumor growth kinetics of bone metastasis as documented by bioluminescent reporter imaging (Fig. 1). The potential clinical utility of this approach as an adjunct to current local strategies in bone metastases is significant. There are no known contraindications to the use of photodynamic therapy preradiation or postradiation therapy or surgery. Unlike radiation therapy, where there are limits to the amount of spinal irradiation that can be administered and wound complications following subsequent conventional spinal surgery are significant, there are no limits to the extent of PDT that can be applied assuming that a safe and efficacious therapeutic window can be defined. PDT can also potentially be applied to radioresistant tumors. In considering vertebroplasty, the potential biologic benefits of PDT on tumor growth kinetics might be considered a neo-adjuvant potentially coupled during the same surgical setting by injection of PMMA to mechanically stabilize metastatically involved vertebrae. The selectivity of PDT in being able to locally target cancer cells is appealing in the spine, where conservation of healthy neural tissue (i.e., spinal cord) is critical. Ongoing preclinical study is required to closely define the therapeutic window for PDT to treat bone metastases. The potential need for fractionated treatments requires further study although the ability to percutaneously implant an optical fiber, which can be left *in situ*, would be a practical solution similar to the brachytherapy approach. Such a transdisciplinary approach encompassing tumor biology and minimally invasive surgical techniques may provide an important future adjunct to patient palliation.

REFERENCES

1. Wong DA, Fornasier VL, MacNab I. Spinal metastases: the obvious, the occult, and the impostors. *Spine* 1990; 15:1–4.
2. Choong PF. Cardiopulmonary complications of intramedullary fixation of long bone metastases. *Clin Orthop* 2003; S245–253.

3. Ahmed AA, Heller DS. Fatal pulmonary tumour embolism caused by chondroblastic osteosarcoma: report of a case and review of the literature. *Arch Pathol Lab Med* 1999; 123:437–440.

4. Peter RE, Schopfer A, Le Coultre B, Hoffmeyer P. Fat embolism and death during prophylactic osteosynthesis of a metastatic femur using an unreamed femoral nail. *J Orthop Trauma* 1997; 11: 233,234.

5. Ghogawala Z, Mansfield FL, Borges LF. Spinal radiation before surgical decompression adversely affects outcomes of surgery for symptomatic metastatic spinal cord compression. *Spine* 2001; 26: 818–824.

6. Wai EK, Finkelstein JA, Tangente RP, et al. Quality of life in surgical treatment of metastatic spine disease. *Spine* 2003; 28:508–512.

7. Wedin R, Bauer HC, Rutqvist LE. Surgical treatment for skeletal breast cancer metastases: a population-based study of 641 patients. *Cancer* 2001; 92:257–262.

8. Tomita K, Kawahara N, Kobayashi T, Yoshida A, Murakami H, Akamaru T. Surgical strategy for spinal metastases. *Spine* 2001; 26:298–306.

9. Hatrick NC, Lucas JD, Timothy AR, Smith MA. The surgical treatment of metastatic disease of the spine. *Radiother Oncol* 2000; 56:335–339.

10. Gerszten PC, Welch WC. Current surgical management of metastatic spinal disease. *Oncology* (Huntingt) 2000; 14:1013–1024; discussion 1024, 1029, 1030.

11. Weigel B, Maghsudi M, Neumann C, Kretschmer R, Muller FJ, Nerlich M. Surgical management of symptomatic spinal metastases. Postoperative outcome and quality of life. *Spine* 1999; 24:2240–2246.

12. Klekamp J, Samii H. Surgical results for spinal metastases. *Acta Neurochir (Wien)* 1998; 140:957–967.

13. Finkelstein J, Zaveri G, Wai E, Vidmar M, Kreder H, Chow E. A population-based study of surgery for spinal metastases: Survival rates and complications. *J Bone Joint Surg Br* 2003; 85-B:1045–1050.

14. Amar AP, Larsen DW, Esnaashari N, Albuquerque FC, Lavine SD, Teitelbaum GP. Percutaneous transpedicular polymethylmethacrylate vertebroplasty for the treatment of spinal compression fractures. *Neurosurgery* 2001; 49:1105–1114; discussion 1114,1115.

15. Mathis JM, Barr JD, Belkoff SM, Barr MS, Jensen ME, Deramond H. Percutaneous vertebroplasty: a developing standard of care for vertebral compression fractures. *AJNR Am J Neuroradiol* 2001; 22: 373–381.

16. Rodriguez-Catarino M. [Percutaneous vertebroplasty—a new method for alleviation of back pain]. *Lakartidningen* 2002; 99:882–890.

17. Ratliff J, Nguyen T, Heiss J. Root and spinal cord compression from methylmethacrylate vertebroplasty. *Spine* 2001; 26:E300–302.

18. Ferrario A, von Tiehl KF, Rucker N, Schwarz MA, Gill PS, Gomer CJ. Antiangiogenic treatment enhances photodynamic therapy responsiveness in a mouse mammary carcinoma. *Cancer Res* 2000; 60:4066–4069.

19. Luna MC, Ferrario A, Wong S, Fisher AM, Gomer CJ. Photodynamic therapy-mediated oxidative stress as a molecular switch for the temporal expression of genes ligated to the human heat shock promoter. *Cancer Res* 2000; 60:1637–1644.

20. Gomer CJ, Luna M, Ferrario A, Wong S, Fisher AM, Rucker N. Cellular targets and molecular responses associated with photodynamic therapy. *J Clin Laser Med Surg* 1996; 14:315–321.

21. Whitacre CM, Feyes DK, Satoh T, et al. Photodynamic therapy with the phthalocyanine photosensitizer Pc 4 of SW480 human colon cancer xenografts in athymic mice. *Clin Cancer Res* 2000; 6: 2021–2027.

22. Whitacre CM, Satoh TH, Xue L, Gordon NH, Oleinick NL. Photodynamic therapy of human breast cancer xenografts lacking caspase-3. *Cancer Lett* 2002; 179:43–49.

23. Korbelik M, Cecic I. Contribution of myeloid and lymphoid host cells to the curative outcome of mouse sarcoma treatment by photodynamic therapy. *Cancer Lett* 1999; 137:91–98.

24. Cecic I, Parkins CS, Korbelik M. Induction of systemic neutrophil response in mice by photodynamic therapy of solid tumours. *Photochem Photobiol* 2001; 74:712–720.

25. Ratkay LG, Chowdhary RK, Iamaroon A, et al. Amelioration of antigen-induced arthritis in rabbits by induction of apoptosis of inflammatory cells with local application of transdermal photodynamic therapy. *Arthritis Rheum* 1998; 41:525–534.

26. Xue LY, Chiu SM, Oleinick NL. Photochemical destruction of the Bcl-2 oncoprotein during photodynamic therapy with the phthalocyanine photosensitizer Pc 4. *Oncogene* 2001; 20:3420–3427.

27. Allison R, Mang T, Hewson G, Snider W, Dougherty D. Photodynamic therapy for chest wall progression from breast carcinoma is an underutilized treatment modality. *Cancer* 2001; 91:1–8.

28. Wyss P, Schwarz V, Dobler-Girdziunaite D, et al. Photodynamic therapy of locoregional breast cancer recurrences using a chlorin-type photosensitizer. *Int J Cancer* 2001; 93:720–724.

29. Fehr MK, Hornung R, Schwarz VA, Simeon R, Haller U, Wyss P. Photodynamic therapy of vulvar intraepithelial neoplasia III using topically applied 5-aminolevulinic acid. *Gynecol Oncol* 2001; 80:62–66.

30. Sutedja G, Risse R, Van Mourik JC, Postmus PE. Photodynamic therapy for treatment of bronchial carcinomas. *Thorax* 1994; 49:289,290.

31. Sutedja TG, Postmus PE. Photodynamic therapy in lung cancer. A review. *J Photochem Photobiol B* 1996; 36:199–204.

32. Waidelich R, Hofstetter A, Stepp H, Baumgartner R, Weninger E, Kriegmair M. Early clinical experience with 5-aminolevulinic acid for the photodynamic therapy of upper tract urothelial tumours. *J Urol* 1998; 159:401–404.

33. Nseyo UO. Photodynamic therapy in the management of bladder cancer. *J Clin Laser Med Surg* 1996; 14:271–280.

34. Walther MM, Delaney TF, Smith PD, et al. Phase I trial of photodynamic therapy in the treatment of recurrent superficial transitional cell carcinoma of the bladder. *Urology* 1997; 50:199–206.

35. Barr H, Dix AJ, Kendall C, Stone N. Review article: the potential role for photodynamic therapy in the management of upper gastrointestinal disease. *Aliment Pharmacol Ther* 2001; 15:311–321.

36. Nambisan RN, Karakousis CP, Holyoke ED, Dougherty TJ. Intraoperative photodynamic therapy for retroperitoneal sarcomas. *Cancer* 1988; 61:1248–1252.

37. Hourigan AJ, Kells AF, Schwartz HS. In vitro photodynamic therapy of musculoskeletal neoplasms. *J Orthop Res* 1993; 11:633–637.

38. Fingar VH, Kik PK, Haydon PS, et al. Analysis of acute vascular damage after photodynamic therapy using benzoporphyrin derivative (BPD). *Br J Cancer* 1999; 79:1702–1708.

39. Cincotta L, Szeto D, Lampros E, Hasan T, Cincotta AH. Benzophenothiazine and benzoporphyrin derivative combination phototherapy effectively eradicates large murine sarcomas. *Photochem Photobiol* 1996; 63:229–237.

40. Kusuzaki K, Minami G, Takeshita H, et al. Photodynamic inactivation with acridine orange on a multidrug-resistant mouse osteosarcoma cell line. *Jpn J Cancer Res* 2000; 91:439–445.

41. Kusuzaki K, Aomori K, Suginoshita T, et al. Total tumour cell elimination with minimum damage to normal tissues in musculoskeletal sarcomas following photodynamic therapy with acridine orange. *Oncology* 2000; 59:174–180.

42. Trauner KB, Gandour-Edwards R, Bamberg M, Shortkroff S, Sledge C, Hasan T. Photodynamic synovectomy using benzoporphyrin derivative in an antigen-induced arthritis model for rheumatoid arthritis. *Photochem Photobiol* 1998; 67:133–139.

43. Beischer AD, Bhathal P, de Steiger R, Penn D, Stylli S. Synovial ablation in a rabbit rheumatoid arthritis model using photodynamic therapy. *ANZ J Surg* 2002; 72:517–522.

44. Chen BJ, Cui X, Liu C, Chao NJ. Prevention of graft-versus-host disease while preserving graft-versus-leukemia effect after selective depletion of host-reactive T cells by photodynamic cell purging process. *Blood* 2002; 99:3083–3088.

45. Danilatou V, Lydaki E, Dimitriou H, Papazoglou T, Kalmanti M. Bone marrow purging by photodynamic treatment in children with acute leukemia: cytoprotective action of amifostine. *Leuk Res* 2000; 24:427–435.

46. Villeneuve L. Ex vivo photodynamic purging in chronic myelogenous leukaemia and other neoplasias with rhodamine derivatives. *Biotechnol Appl Biochem* 1999; 30(Pt 1):1–17.

47. Yamazaki T, Sieber F. Effect of hypothermia on the merocyanine 540-mediated purging of hematopoietic cells. *J Hematother* 1997; 6:31–39.

48. Mulroney CM, Gluck S, Ho AD. The use of photodynamic therapy in bone marrow purging. *Semin Oncol* 1994; 21:24–27.

49. Sieber F, Gaffney DK, Yamazaki T, Qiu K. Importance of cellular defense mechanisms in the photodynamic purging of autologous bone marrow grafts. *Prog Clin Biol Res* 1994; 389:147–154.

50. Koudinova NV, Pinthus JH, Brandis A, et al. Photodynamic therapy with Pd-Bacteriopheophorbide (TOOKAD): successful in vivo treatment of human prostatic small cell carcinoma xenografts. *Int J Cancer* 2003; 104:782–789.

51. Firbank M, Hiraoka M, Essenpreis M, Delpy DT. Measurement of the optical properties of the skull in the wavelength range 650–950 nm. *Phys Med Biol* 1993; 38:503–510.

52. Takeuchi A, Araki R, Proskurin SG, et al. A new method of bone tissue measurement based upon light scattering. *J Bone Miner Res* 1997; 12:261–266.

53. Tauber S, Baumgartner R, Schorn K, Beyer W. Lightdosimetric quantitative analysis of the human petrous bone: experimental study for laser irradiation of the cochlea. *Lasers Surg Med* 2001; 28:18–26.

54. Tauber S, Schorn K, Beyer W, Baumgartner R. Transmeatal cochlear laser (TCL) treatment of cochlear dysfunction: a feasibility study for chronic tinnitus. *Lasers Med Sci* 2003; 18:154–161.

55. Ugnell AO, Oberg PA. The optical properties of the cochlear bone. *Med Eng Phys* 1997; 19:630–636.

56. Hancox NM. *Biology of Bone.* Cambridge: Cambridge University Press, 1972.

57. Bamett AH, Culver JP, Sorensen AG, Dale A, Boas DA. Robust inference of baseline optical properties of the human head with three-dimensional segmentation from magnetic resonance imaging. *Appl Opt* 2003; 42:3095–3108.

58. Wang X, Pang Y, Ku G, Stoica G, Wang LV. Three-dimensional laser-induced photoacoustic tomography of mouse brain with the skin and skull intact. *Opt Lett* 2003; 28:1739–1741.

59. Holly LT, Foley KT. Three-dimensional fluoroscopy-guided percutaneous thoracolumbar pedicle screw placement. Technical note. *J Neurosurg* 2003; 99:324–329.

60. Krasna MJ, Jiao X, Eslami A, Rutter CM, Levine AM. Thoracoscopic approach for spine deformities. *J Am Coll Surg* 2003; 197:777–779.

61. Lieberman IH, Kuzhupilly RR, Reinhardt MK, Davros WJ. Three-dimensional computed tomographic volume rendering techniques in endoscopic thoracoplasty. *Spine J* 2001; 1:390–394.

62. Yeung AT, Yeung CA. Advances in endoscopic disc and spine surgery: foraminal approach. *Surg Technol Int* 2003; 11:253–261.

63. Hadjipavlou AG, Lander PH, Marchesi D, Katonis PG, Gaitanis IN. Minimally invasive surgery for ablation of osteoid osteoma of the spine. *Spine* 2003; 28:E472–477.

64. Fessler RG. Minimally invasive percutaneous posterior lumbar interbody fusion. *Neurosurgery* 2003; 52:1512.

65. Deen HG, Fenton DS, Lamer TJ. Minimally invasive procedures for disorders of the lumbar spine. *Mayo Clin Proc* 2003; 78:1249–1256.

66. Barr JD, Barr MS, Lemley TJ, McCann RM. Percutaneous vertebroplasty for pain relief and spinal stabilization. *Spine* 2000; 25:923–928.

67. Jensen ME, Evans AJ, Mathis JM, Kallmes DF, Cloft HJ, Dion JE. Percutaneous polymethylmethacrylate vertebroplasty in the treatment of osteoporotic vertebral body compression fractures: technical aspects. *AJNR Am J Neuroradiol* 1997; 18:1897–1904.

68. Lieberman I, Reinhardt MK. Vertebroplasty and kyphoplasty for osteolytic vertebral collapse. *Clin Orthop* 2003:S176–186.

69. Bresler F, Roche O, Chary-Valckenaire I, Blum A, Mole D, Schmitt D. [Femoral head osteonecrosis: original extra-articular cementoplasty technique. A series of 20 cases]. *Acta Orthop Belg* 1999; 65 (Suppl 1):95,96.

70. Hodge JC. Cementoplasty and the oncologic population. *Singapore Med J* 2000; 41:407–409.

71. Marcy PY, Palussiere J, Descamps B, et al. Percutaneous cementoplasty for pelvic bone metastasis. *Support Care Cancer* 2000; 8:500–503.

72. Cantwell CP, Obyrne J, Eustace S. Current trends in treatment of osteoid osteoma with an emphasis on radiofrequency ablation. *Eur Radiol* 2004; 14:607–617.

73. Blomme EA, Dougherty KM, Pienta KJ, Capen CC, Rosol TJ, McCauley LK. Skeletal metastasis of prostate adenocarcinoma in rats: morphometric analysis and role of parathyroid hormone-related protein. *Prostate* 1999; 39:187–197.

74. El-Abdaimi K, Ste-Marie LG, Papavasiliou V, et al. Pamidronate prevents the development of skeletal metastasis in nude mice transplanted with human breast cancer cells by reducing tumour burden within bone. *Int J Oncol* 2003; 22:883–890.

75. Harms JE, Welch DR. MDA-MB-435 human breast carcinoma metastasis to bone. *Clin Exp Metastasis* 2003; 20:327–334.

76. Michigami T, Hiraga T, Williams PJ, et al. The effect of the bisphosphonate ibandronate on breast cancer metastasis to visceral organs. *Breast Cancer Res Treat* 2002; 75:249–258.

77. Mundy G. Preclinical models of bone metastases. *Semin Oncol* 2001; 28:2–8.

78. Nakata A, Tsujimura T, Sugihara A, et al. Inhibition by interleukin 18 of osteolytic bone metastasis by human breast cancer cells. *Anticancer Res* 1999; 19:4131–4138.

79. Peyruchaud O, Winding B, Pecheur I, Serre CM, Delmas P, Clezardin P. Early detection of bone metastases in a murine model using fluorescent human breast cancer cells: application to the use of the bisphosphonate zoledronic acid in the treatment of osteolytic lesions. *J Bone Miner Res* 2001; 16:2027–2034.

80. Sasaki A, Boyce BF, Story B, et al. Bisphosphonate risedronate reduces metastatic human breast cancer burden in bone in nude mice. *Cancer Res* 1995; 55:3551–3557.
81. Yoneda T, Michigami T, Yi B, Williams PJ, Niewolna M, Hiraga T. Actions of bisphosphonate on bone metastasis in animal models of breast carcinoma. *Cancer* 2000; 88:2979–2988.
82. Engebraaten O, Fodstad O. Site-specific experimental metastasis patterns of two human breast cancer cell lines in nude rats. *Int J Cancer* 1999; 82:219–225.
83. Burch S, Bisland SK, Whyne CM, Finkelstein J, Wilson B, Yee A. The novel application of photodynamic therapy for spinal metastases: Evaluation in a preclinical athymic nude rat model. *Proceedings: North American Spine Society, Annual Meeting*, 2003.
84. Burch S, Wilson B, Bisland SK, Bogaards A, Whyne CM, Yee A. Percutaneous photodynamic therapy for the treatment of metastatic breast carcinoma to the spine. *CBCRA 3rd Scientific Conference Reasons for Hope*, 2003.
85. Ree AH, Tvermyr M, Engebraaten O, et al. Expression of a novel factor in human breast cancer cells with metastatic potential. *Cancer Res* 1999; 59:4675–4680.
86. Arguello F, Baggs RB, Frantz CN. A murine model of experimental metastasis to bone and bone marrow. *Cancer Res* 1988; 48:6876–6881.
87. Wetterwald A, van der Pluijm G, Que I, et al. Optical imaging of cancer metastasis to bone marrow: a mouse model of minimal residual disease. *Am J Pathol* 2002; 160:1143–1153.
88. Wilson BC, Olivo M, Singh G. Subcellular localization of Photofrin and aminolevulinic acid and photodynamic cross-resistance in vitro in radiation-induced fibrosarcoma cells sensitive or resistant to photofrin-mediated photodynamic therapy. *Photochem Photobiol* 1997; 65:166–176.
89. Hiraga T, Williams PJ, Mundy GR, Yoneda T. The bisphosphonate ibandronate promotes apoptosis in MDA-MB-231 human breast cancer cells in bone metastases. *Cancer Res* 2001; 61:4418–4424.
90. Lilge L, Wilson BC. Photodynamic therapy of intracranial tissues: a preclinical comparative study of four different photosensitizers. *J Clin Laser Med Surg* 1998; 16:81–91.
91. Lilge L, Portnoy M, Wilson BC. Apoptosis induced in vivo by photodynamic therapy in normal brain and intracranial tumour tissue. *Br J Cancer* 2000; 83:1110–1117.
92. Takeuchi Y, Kurohane K, Ichikawa K, Yonezawa S, Nango M, Oku N. Induction of intensive tumour suppression by antiangiogenic photodynamic therapy using polycation-modified liposomal photosensitizer. *Cancer* 2003; 97:2027–2034.
93. Gluck S, Chadderton A, Ho AD. The selective uptake of benzoporphyrin derivative mono-acid ring A results in differential cell kill of multiple myeloma cells in vitro. *Photochem Photobiol* 1996; 63: 846–853.
94. Kurohane K, Tominaga A, Sato K, North JR, Namba Y, Oku N. Photodynamic therapy targeted to tumour-induced angiogenic vessels. *Cancer Lett* 2001; 167:49–56.
95. Momma T, Hamblin MR, Wu HC, Hasan T. Photodynamic therapy of orthotopic prostate cancer with benzoporphyrin derivative: local control and distant metastasis. *Cancer Res* 1998; 58:5425–5431.
96. Houle JM, Strong HA. Duration of skin photosensitivity and incidence of photosensitivity reactions after administration of verteporfin. *Retina* 2002; 22:691–697.
97. Houle JM, Strong A. Clinical pharmacokinetics of verteporfin. *J Clin Pharmacol* 2002; 42:547–557.
98. Rubin GS, Bressler NM. Effects of verteporfin therapy on contrast on sensitivity: Results from the treatment of age-related macular degeneration with photodynamic therapy (TAP) investigation-TAP report No 4. *Retina* 2002; 22:536–544.
99. Bressler NM, Arnold J, Benchaboune M, et al. Verteporfin therapy of subfoveal choroidal neovascularization in patients with age-related macular degeneration: additional information regarding baseline lesion composition's impact on vision outcomes-TAP report No. 3. *Arch Ophthalmol* 2002; 120:1443–1454.
100. Blumenkranz MS, Bressler NM, Bressler SB, et al. Verteporfin therapy for subfoveal choroidal neovascularization in age-related macular degeneration: three-year results of an open-label extension of 2 randomized clinical trials—TAP Report no. 5. *Arch Ophthalmol* 2002; 120:1307–1314.
101. Woodburn KW, Engelman CJ, Blumenkranz MS. Photodynamic therapy for choroidal neovascularization: a review. *Retina* 2002; 22:391–405; quiz 527,528.
102. Sharma S, Hollands H, Brown GC, Brown MM, Shah GK, Sharma SM. Improvement in quality of life from photodynamic therapy: a Canadian perspective. *Can J Ophthalmol* 2001; 36:332–338.

16

Docetaxel for Metastatic Cancer and Its Role in Combination Therapies for Advanced Prostate Cancer

Ellen K. Wasan, RPh, PhD, Martin Gleave, MD, Karen Fang, BSc, Kim Chi, MD, Gwyn Bebb, BMBCh, PhD, Lincoln Edwards, BSc, and Marcel B. Bally, PhD

CONTENTS

INTRODUCTION
PHARMACOLOGY OF DOCETAXEL
OVERVIEW OF DOCETAXEL USE IN TREATMENT OF CANCERS OTHER
    THAN PROSTATE
DOCETAXEL IN HORMONE-REFRACTORY AND METASTATIC
    PROSTATE CANCER
TARGETED DRUG DELIVERY TO BONE METASTASES
CONCLUSIONS
REFERENCES

1. INTRODUCTION

Although strides have been made in the diagnosis and treatment of cancer in the past few decades, advanced, metastatic cancer remains extremely difficult to treat. Obviously, a major hurdle in improving survival is the treatment or prevention of metastatic disease, either to eliminate it completely or to contain it like other chronic diseases. To reach the metastatic stage, the cancer cells undergo many and various changes in the usual regulatory mechanisms governing cellular proliferation and apoptosis, resulting in great heterogeneity. Therein lies the challenge in developing appropriate and effective combination therapies for metastatic disease that utilize multiple mechanisms to overcome resistance to cell death. In this chapter, the relatively new cytotoxic taxane docetaxel will be discussed in the context of its current role in treating metastatic cancer and its future role in combination with novel, molecularly targeted chemotherapeutic agents.

From: *Cancer Drug Discovery and Development*
Bone Metastasis: Experimental and Clinical Therapeutics
Edited by: G. Singh and S. A. Rabbani © Humana Press Inc., Totowa, NJ

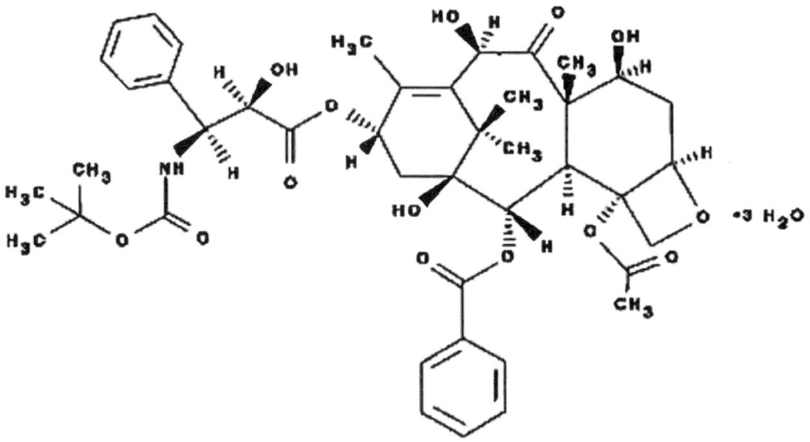

Fig. 1. Chemical structure of docetaxel.

Docetaxel (Taxotere®) is a semisynthetic taxoid compound derived from the needles of the European yew tree. It is similar to paclitaxel in its chemical structure (Fig. 1) and has a broad spectrum of antitumor activity. It has become an important drug used in a variety of combinations in the treatment of breast, prostate, small cell lung cancer, urologic cancers, solid tumors in children, and other tumor types. This chapter will focus on the use of docetaxel in metastatic cancers, with a special focus on advanced, hormone-refractory, and metastatic prostate cancer, including the use of docetaxel in combination with novel therapeutics.

Finally, a special section on targeting therapeutics to bony metastases explores different approaches to drug delivery to bone and to specifically targeted molecular therapy. From our perspective, targeted drug delivery encompasses concepts related to three distinct targeting approaches: (1) targeting molecular defects, which lead to the survival and progression of cancer cells that have already metastasized to the bone; (2) targeting normal bone elements and processes, which includes bone formation and resorption homeostasis, to improve delivery of drugs to bone, and (3) targeting to tumor-mediated changes in bone structure. These three approaches will be discussed in detail at the end of this chapter.

Prostate cancer is a particularly important target for therapies directed at advanced disease metastatic to bone. Prostate cancer progresses to an androgen-independent stage (hormone refractory prostate cancer [HRPC]), which responds poorly to current treatment and readily metastasizes to regional lymph nodes and to bone. Therapy is aimed at palliation to reduce bone pain and improve quality of life, which, until recently, did not include aggressive chemotherapy *(1)*. Once the hormone-refractory stage is reached, mean survival is approx 12–18 mo without chemotherapy, and few trials have yet demonstrated improved survival for HRPC with combination chemotherapy, although one such trials has recently been completed, such as with mitoxantrone/prednisone (Tax 327 [prednisone + docetaxel or mitoxantrone]) *(2)* or docetaxel/estramustine. These latter two trials are reporting survival advantages with the docetaxel based regimens and were presented at ASCO 2004 *(3,4)*. Breast cancer metastasizes to lymph nodes, lung, liver, brain and also to bone, and patients have a mean survival of approx 22 mo with first-line anthracycline or taxoid-based chemotherapy. When the patient relapses after anthracycline therapy, second-line agents such as vinca alkaloids can be used, and the mean survival is reduced to 12–15 mo. Non-small-cell lung cancer (NSCLC) and ovarian cancer have similar tendencies to be diagnosed at an advanced stage. NSCLC responds poorly to treatment with chemotherapy. Advanced ovarian cancer can respond well to first-line chemotherapy with platinum/taxane combinations, however, recurrent disease might be resistant to cisplatin or to paclitaxel. In that case, docetaxel has demonstrated antitumor activity as a second-line agent in both cisplatin-resistant and paclitaxel-resistant ovarian cancers, resulting in encouraging response rates in phase II trials.

The progression of prostate cancer from androgen responsive to hormone refractory is a highly negative prognostic factor. Androgen-independent prostate cancer is poorly responsive to treatment and uniformly fatal. Intense study has been focused on the factors that regulate the progression from hormone dependence to hormone independence, resulting in the identification of key biochemical pathways controlling proliferation, survival, and metastasis of prostate cancer. Work in this area has led to the exploration of novel therapies for androgen-independent and metastatic prostate cancer. Application of antisense molecules targeting Bcl-2 and clusterin will be discussed here as exciting examples of novel agents that should enhance the therapeutic effects achieved with currently used chemotherapy, such as docetaxel.

2. PHARMACOLOGY OF DOCETAXEL

Because of its broad spectrum of activity in a number of cancers, docetaxel has become one of the most widely used cytotoxic agents. In the most simplistic terms, this drug causes mitotic arrest and, subsequently, apoptosis because docetaxel binds microtubulin. Binding inhibits depolymerization of the microtubules. However, like all broad-spectrum anticancer drugs, the value associated with its use in treatment of epithelial cancers is not a consequence of a single defined action. The mechanism of action of docetaxel is multifactorial and involves a number of direct and indirect effects that combine to produce meaningful therapeutic responses. The broad-spectrum activity of docetaxel has been reviewed recently (5); therefore, this chapter highlights activities that are of particular interest when considering docetaxel use in combinations with molecularly targeted therapeutics for treatment of advanced metastatic disease. These include interactions that enhance apoptosis, inhibit angiogenesis, and stimulate the immune system.

2.1. Microtubular Stabilizer

Docetaxel binds to β-tubulin and stabilizes polymerized microtubules, thereby inducing cell cycle arrest at the G2/M-phase. By binding to free tubulin, as does paclitaxel, docetaxel promotes the formation of abnormal microtubules and prevents microtubule depolymerization. Mitotic and interphase functions are therefore disrupted and cellular apoptosis or cell lysis is induced (6). Docetaxel is more efficacious than paclitaxel for many tumor types, which is thought to be the result, at least in part, of its greater affinity for microtubules, higher drug levels within the tumor cells, and slower rate of drug efflux than paclitaxel (7).

2.2. Apoptosis Induction

Docetaxel anticancer activity appears to be associated with the phosphorylation and inactivation of Bcl-2 protein. *Bcl-2* is a proto-oncogene belonging to a growing family of regulatory proteins that can promote cell survival (Bcl-2, Bcl-XL, Bcl-w, Mcl-1, A1/Bfl-l) or cause cell death (Bak, Bad, Bid, Bik, Hrk, Bok, Bax) *(8–13)*. Most Bcl-2 family members associate with intracellular membranes such as the endoplasmic reticulum and the mitochondrial membrane. Despite structural similarities between Bcl-2 and other pro-apoptotic family members that determine their ability to interact with each other and ultimately decide the life or death of a cell, the mechanism by which Bcl-2 promotes cell survival is controversial *(14)*. It is presently thought that homodimerization or heterodimerization of Bcl-2 with pro-apoptotic family members and the relative proportions of these pro- or anti-apoptotic proteins leads to the initiation or inhibition of cell death or cell survival pathways *(11)*. The pro-apoptotic protein Bax appears to undergo a conformational change, which results in its translocation from the cytosol to the mitochondria *(15–18)*, where it forms pores releasing cytochrome-*c (19–21)*. Cytochrome-*c* release, in turn, leads to caspase activation and cell death *(22)*. Bcl-2 can interact with Bax, which can result in an antiapoptotic mechanism depending on the relative amounts of Bax and Bcl-2 *(23)*. However, Bcl-2 binding to Bax might not be all that is required for inhibition of a Bax-mediated apoptotic pathway. Bcl-2 might disrupt Bax/Bax homodimerization or abrogate Bax function, or Bax might disrupt the activity of a death-repressor-type Bcl-2 protein *(23)*. Hou et al. showed that transient Bcl-2 expression in vitro led to cell death independent of Bax *(24)*. Regardless of the mechanisms involved, a major role of Bcl-2 is antagonizing pro-apoptotic proteins such as Bax *(25)*.

Docetaxel promotes phosphorylation of serine 70 of the Bcl-2 protein, resulting in dissociation of the antiapoptotic Bax/Bcl-2 heterodimer and a pro-apoptotic signal transduction environment (Fig. 2). Highlighting the importance of this activity, Shitashige et al. demonstrated that human breast cancers sensitive to docetaxel possessed higher levels of pS70-BCL-2 expression than docetaxel-insensitive tumors *(26)*. Downstream effects associated with docetaxel mediated phosphorylation of BCL-2 include activation of jun N-terminal kinase (JNK) pathway and poly(ADP-ribose) polymerase-1 (PARP) *(27)*.

However, studies assessing docetaxel-induced lymphoma cell death have suggested that the drug caused cell lysis, rather than the typical features of programmed cell death *(28)*. This obviously indicates that docetaxel has more than one mechanism of action and might have differential effects, depending on the tumor cell type. These multiple actions contribute to the efficacy of combination therapies, which include docetaxel because this drug can promote apoptosis, and might limit the effect of tumor drug resistance attributed to overexpression of Bcl-2.

In an effort to capitalize on complementary mechanisms of action, docetaxel has been tested in combination with estramustine, which binds to nuclear matrix tubule-associated proteins and thereby stabilizes the microtubules *(29,30)*. This prevents cellular mitosis in prostate cancer cells, leading to cell death *(31)*. Cell death by non-Bcl-2-related mechanisms has also been demonstrated in the prostate cancer cell line DU-145, which has low levels of Bcl-2 expression but, nevertheless, is highly susceptible to docetaxel *(32)*. Recent studies have also indicated a possible role for diacylglycerol and phosphatidic acid signaling pathways, which, through cell signaling cascades, activate Raf-1 (and thereby MAP kinase pathway) and necrosis factor (NF)-κB *(33)*. The variety of effects of docetaxel might indicate its utility in a diverse range of combination therapies rationally designed to treat cancer.

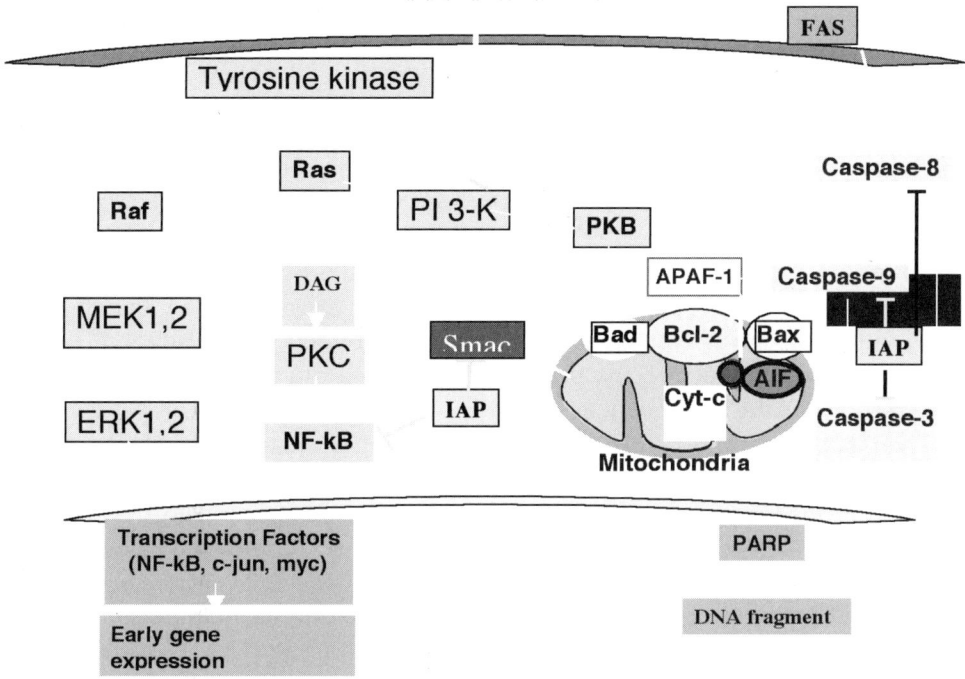

Fig. 2. BCL-2 and pathways of apoptosis.

2.3. Antiangiogenic Effects

Docetaxel has been shown to have antiangiogenic properties in many different cancer cell types *(34)*, including breast *(35)*, T-cell leukemia *(36)*, and colon cancer *(37)*. What is potentially most interesting is that, it appears that the antiangiogenic effects of docetaxel occur at noncytotoxic concentrations of the drug. In this context, it might be important to consider strategies put forward by Kerbel and colleagues, who suggest that metronomic low-dose chemotherapy regimens might be particularly promising for inhibiting angiogenesis *(38,39)*.

It is worth noting here that preclinical and clinical studies are evaluating the use of docetaxel in combination with angiogenesis inhibitors. In vivo, docetaxel showed an antiangiogenic effect in xenograft metastatic transitional cell in combination with the experimental antiangiogenic compound TNP-470, an analog of fumagillin *(40)*. Its role in antiangiogenesis in combination with other cytotoxic agents (or with Herceptin® in the case of breast cancer *[41]*) or antiangiogenic entities such as the vascular endothelial growth factor (VEGF) antagonists ZD6474 (Astra-Zeneca) or VEGF-Trap (Aventis), both in clinical trials, remains to be determined. Early studies have also been initiated using docetaxel in combination with bevacizumab (Avastin®, Genentech), a humanized monoclonal antibody targeting VEGF *(42)*. This combination might prove to be particularly interesting in the context of metastatic prostate cancer because it has recently been shown that VEGF released from prostate cancer cells might promote bone remodeling—in particular, osteosclerosis *(43)*.

2.4. Immunostimulatory Effects of Docetaxel

Immunomodulatory effects, such as the induction of cyclooxygenase (COX)-2, have been demonstrated in cell lines exposed to docetaxel (44) and might contribute nonspecifically to docetaxel's antitumor effects. In a study of 30 advanced breast cancer patients who received either paclitaxel or docetaxel, multiple changes in immune effector molecules were noted. Docetaxel raised serum levels of MLR, natural killer (NK), and lymphokine activated killer (LAK) activity and interferon (IFN)-γ, interleukin (IL)-2, IL-6, and, granulocyte colony stimulating factor (G-CSF) more than paclitaxel, while reducing levels of IL-1 and TNF (45). Another, smaller study of 10 patients with advanced cancers treated with paclitaxel or docetaxel also found docetaxel to have more of an impact on the immune system, but did not demonstrate the same changes as noted in the breast cancer study (46). For example, NK levels were decreased rather than increased, and LAK activity did not change. Clearly, the effects of taxanes on the immune system and the consequences for tumor progression are not clearly understood at this time but warrant further investigation (reviewed by Chan [47]), particularly given the important role of cytokines in the establishment and progression of cancer in the bone.

It should be noted that immune stimulation is also an important factor in docetaxel's toxicity profile, which includes hypersensitivity reactions and fluid retention/generalized edema. Hypersensitivity has been related to the solvent (polysorbate 80) used to solubilize docetaxel rather then the drug itself and patients are typically premedicated with corticosteroids to reduce these effects.

2.5. Pharmacokinetics of Docetaxel

Docetaxel is administered by short intravenous (iv) infusion. Very little is absorbed following oral administration. Following a dose of 100 mg/m² iv over 1 h, docetaxel has linear pharmacokinetics which fit a three-compartment pharmacokinetic model. The terminal half-life is approx 11 h (Table 1) (48,49). The drug is highly protein bound (>94%), primarily to α-1 acid glycoprotein (AAG). Elevated levels of AAG are associated with a reduced risk of docetaxel toxicity, such as neutropenia. Elimination is primarily via hepatic metabolism with biliary excretion. Only 5% is excreted unchanged in the urine, whereas 75% is excreted in the feces (49). There are at least four metabolites arising from cytochrome P450 activity. Cytochrome 3A4 is a primary metabolizing enzyme for docetaxel. The major metabolic product (cyclized oxazolidinedione) is not an active cytotoxic agent. Hepatic impairment leads to reduced drug clearance, with plasma levels elevated by approx 27% when AST and ALT are ≥1.5-fold elevated or when alkaline phosphatase is ≥2.5-fold elevated. Hepatic impairment increases the risk of toxicity, such as neutropenia (50), and dose reduction by 25% is recommended by the manufacturer in the case of hepatic impairment. Pharmacogenomic differences in CYP3A4 likely contribute to the wide interpatient variability in plasma drug and metabolite levels (51). Biodistribution studies in rats indicate that the drug is distributed in most tissues, but little, if any, crosses the blood–brain barrier (52). The favorable pharmacokinetics of the drug as well as its intracellular pharmacodynamics makes docetaxel less schedule dependent in combination chemotherapy than paclitaxel. It is typically given once every 3 wk.

Table 1
Pharmacokinetic Parameters for Docetaxel

	Following a 1-hinfusion of 100 mg/m^2 (48) *(Mean ± SD)*	*Summary data from phase I and phase II trials (48)* *(Mean ± SD)*
Half-Life		
t^1/$_2$ α (min)	5.0 ± 2.1	4
t^1/$_2$ β (min)	51 ± 6.2	36
t^1/$_2$ γ (h)	10.8 ± 14.1	11.1
C_{max} (mg/L)	2.6 ± 0.5	3.7
AUC 0→ (h·mg/L)	3.1 ± 0.9	4.6
Cl (L/h·m^2)	34.8 ± 9.3	21
Vd$_{ss}$ (L/m^2)	84 ± 86.1	67.3

2.6. Docetaxel Toxicities

The maximum tolerated dose of docetaxel is 80–115 mg/m^2, as determined in phase I trials, with grade 3 or 4 neutropenia as the main dose-limiting toxicity *(49)*. At least 70 to 80% of patients receiving the typical dose of 75–100 mg/m^2 every 3 wk experience grade 3 neutropenia (but not necessarily with a febrile episode). The manufacturer cites the neutropenia rate as 96% and severe neutropenia as 32% with a nadir at 8 d, and a mean duration of 7 d for severe neutropenia *(54)*. Additional adverse reactions associated with docetaxel include hematologic abnormalities (neutropenia, leukopenia, and thrombocytopenia) increased infections, fever, neurosensory problems, cutaneous eruptions, gastrointestinal toxicity and stomatitis, alopecia (as high as 97% incidence), asthenia (could be dose limiting in some cases), myalgia, and arthralgia *(53)*.

The hematologic toxicity of docetaxel is schedule dependent: In a phase II trial of 18 metastatic breast cancer patients receiving weekly docetaxel (36–40 mg/m^2) for second-line monotherapy after anthracycline failure, the incidence of neutropenia was 17%, and this was the only severe hematological toxicity. Asthenia, nail changes, and ocular and skin disorders (rash) were also noted but were not dose limiting *(53)*. Fatigue was dose limiting in the phase I trials of weekly docetaxel. A similarly designed phase II trial had 2/18 patients (11%) experiencing neutropenia after 40 mg/m^2 weekly docetaxel *(55)*.

Clinical trials are ongoing to determine the role of G-CSF in treatment regimens containing docetaxel, in order to minimize this dose-limiting toxicity and permit dose escalation *(56)*. The use of lower-dose docetaxel administered weekly compared to higher dose docetaxel administered every 3 wk is presently in clinical trials to determine not only relative efficacy but also the incidence and severity of neutropenia. Generally, the lower dose given weekly is tolerated better by patients; however, this must be balanced by the potential for a reduction in response.

Docetaxel is less neurotoxic than paclitaxel, but it still causes significant peripheral neuropathy, particularly sensory (both paresthesias and dysthesias) *(57)*. This effect is not ameliorated by the administration of corticosteriods and is dependent on cumulative dose and dose level *(58)*. The degeneration of peripheral nerves might also be involved in the nail changes observed in some patients treated with taxanes (59). The precise mechanism for docetaxel-induced neuropathy is not established, but it is important to recognize that neuropathy is an important side effect associated with a number of anti-cancer drugs, including cisplatin, vincristine, and suramin. This toxicity could, therefore, limit how docetaxel is used in combinations and it has been demonstrated that synergistic combinations of cisplatin/paclitaxel can cause greater neurotoxicity.

Hypersensitivity reactions, characterized by flushing and bronchospasm, are thought to be the result of mast cell degranulation and histamine release. As indicated earlier, this effect is thought to be the result of the solubilizing excipient polysorbate 80 (Tween-80). Presently, this adverse reaction is avoided by premedicating the patient with corticosteroids and by starting the infusion slowly, gradually increasing the rate. A typical premedication course is 5–8 mg dexamethasone twice daily starting at least 1 d before treatment and continuing for 3–5 d. Our institutional protocols require that three doses of corticosteroid be given prior to starting docetaxel. Some centers use prednisolone and the anti-histamine clemastine as the premedication. If a hypersensitivity reaction does occur, the docetaxel infusion can be stopped for 30 min and then resumed. Presumably, once the mast cell degranulation process is completed, the patient can then tolerate the drug with no further hypersensitivity response. Another significant and very common effect of docetaxel administration is edema, with significant weight gain. This side effect, which could be related to the solvent, could take 6–9 mo to fully resolve. A reduction in the incidence and severity of edema was noted upon introduction of standard premedication with corticosteroids, as mentioned earlier.

3. OVERVIEW OF DOCETAXEL USE IN TREATMENT OF CANCERS OTHER THAN PROSTATE

The intention of this chapter is to focus on emerging drug combinations that include docetaxel for treatment of advanced prostate cancer. It is understood that prostate cancer is unusual in that the vast majority of prostate cancer metastases may involve the bone, and targeted drug combinations against prostate cancer that has metastasized to the bone might have to be tailored to the disease. However, it is important to consider the successes and failures of chemotherapy regimes using docetaxel to manage other highly metastatic cancers that also involve bony metastases, albeit less frequently.

3.1. Metastatic Breast Cancer

Taxanes have been used in adjuvant chemotherapy for early-stage breast cancer (60) as well as locally advanced breast cancer after failure with prior chemotherapy (reviewed by Hutcheon [61]). They are used for adjuvant therapy and for advanced disease (local or metastatic). The overall response rate of metastatic breast cancer to docetaxel treatment as a first-line therapy is 59% (range: 52 to 68%, pooled from 5 early trials for a total of 180 patients) (62). Larger phase III clinical studies have assessed metastatic breast cancer treated with anthracycline–taxane combinations, selected because of the lack of overlap in their mechanism of action and their individual toxicity profiles (63) (Table 2) (64–70). The addition of docetaxel to anthracycline-based adjuvant chemotherapy (doxorubicin or epirubicine) produces a greater response rate, although longer study times might be required to determine whether long-term survival is improved consistently. There might be an advantage over paclitaxel-containing adjuvant therapy in that docetaxel

Table 2
Randomized Phase III Trials of Docetaxel for Metastatic Breast Cancer

No. of patients	Treatment (dose mg/m²/schedule)	Efficacy (p-value)			Main trial results of docetaxel or docetaxel-containing regime	Reference
		% Overall RR (CR + PR)	Median TTP	Median OS		
Single-agent						
326; failed prior alkylating agent CT; no previous anthracycline exposure	Docetaxel (100/ q3w) Doxorubicin (75/q3w)	47.8 33.3 (0.008)	26 w 21 w	15 m 14 m	Higher RR, CR, response time. Similar TTP, OS. Without clinically significant cardiotoxicity	Chan et al., 1999 (303 Study Group) (64)
392; previous anthracycline-containing CT	Docetaxel (100/q3w) Mitomycin (12/q6w) + vinblastine (6/q3w)	30.0 11.6 (<0.0001)	19 w 11 w (0.001)	11.4 m 8.7 m (0.0097)	Much higher RR, TTP, OS	Nabholtz et al., 1999 (304 Study Group) (65)
283; after anthracycline failure	Docetaxel (100/q3w) Methotrexate (200 + 5-fluorouracil (600/d1, 8/q3w)	42 21 (<0.001)	6.3 m 3.0 m (<0.001)	10.4 m 11.1 m (0.79)	Higher RR, TTP	Sjöstrom et al., 1999 (Scandinavian Breast Group) (66)
176; previous anthracycline-containing CT	Docetaxel (100/q3w) 5-Flurouracil (750/d1-5/q3w) + vinorelbine (d1,5/q3w)	43.0 38.9c (0.69)	6.5 m 5.1 m (0.34)	16.0 m 15.0 m	No significant difference	Bonneterre et al., 2002 (67)

(continued)

Table 2 (*continued*)

| No. of patients | Treatment (dose mg/m^2/schedule) | Efficacy (p-value) | | | Main trial results of docetaxel or docetaxel-containing regime | Reference |
		% Overall RR (CR + PR)	Median TTP	Median OS		
Combination						
484; 11% anthracycline exposure; 39% prior adjuvant CT	Docetaxel (75) + doxorubicin (50) + cyclophosphamide (500)/q3w	55	31 w	21 m	Higher RR, no significant difference in TTP, OS	Mackey, 2002 (68)
	5-Fluorouracil (500) + doxorubicin (50) + cyclophosphamide (500) q3w	44 (0.02)	29 w (0.51)	22 m (0.93)		
511; previous anthracycline-containing CT	Docetaxel (75/d1) + capecitabine (1250 × 2 d1–14) q3w	41.6	6.1 m	14.5 m	Higher TTP, OS in combination with Capecitabine	O'Shaugnessy et al., 2002 (69)
	Docetaxel (100/q3w)	29.7 (0.006)	4.2 m (0.0001)	11.5 m (0.0126)		
429; no previous anthracycline exposure[a]	Docetaxel (75/q3w) + doxorubicin (50/q3w)	59	37.3 w	22.5 m b	Higher RR, TTP. Similar OR	Nabholtz et al., 2003 (TAX 306 Study Group) (70)
	Doxorubicin (60/q3w) + cyclophosphamide (600/q3w)	47 (0.009)	31.9 w (0.014)	21.7 m		

Abbreviations: RR, response rate; TTP, time to progression; d, day; w, weeks; mo, months; pt, patient; OS, overall survival, q, every.
[a]No previous CT for metastatic disease, but adjuvant or neoadjuvant non-anthracycline-containg chemotherapy were eligible.
[b]Median survival when 79% died.

264

seems to be less dependent on the schedule and sequencing in relation to the anthracycline treatment and might be better tolerated *(71)*. However, this combination does raise some questions about cardiotoxicity that have not been fully investigated *(72)*. Combination therapy with gemcitabine and docetaxel has also been explored in breast cancer patients who have failed anthracycline therapy, where response rates have ranged from 36 to 54%, with median times to disease progression of 7–8 mo and median survival of 12.7–14 mo in phase II trials *(73)*. Another promising combination for metastatic breast cancer in clinical trials is capecitibine combined with docetaxel.

3.2. Non-Small-Cell Lung Cancer

Adenocarcinoma, squamous cell carcinoma, large cell carcinoma, and bronchoalveolar carcinoma (BAC) comprise the group of epithelial malignancies known as non-small-cell lung cancer (NSCLC). More than 80% are smoking related. Close to 80% of NSCLC patients have advanced or metastatic disease at the time of diagnosis and have a poor prognosis. In the setting of metastatic disease, the median survival with best supportive care (BSC) is 4–5 mo, with less than 10% alive at 1 yr. Changing the natural history of metastatic NSCLC has proved challenging. However, the introduction in the last decade and a half of platinum-based chemotherapy protocols that include the newer cytotoxic agents, paclitaxel, vinorelbine, gemcitabine, and docetaxel has consistently shown clinical benefit in terms of increased survival and improved quality of life for patients with good performance status (ECOG 0-1) *(74,75)*. Docetaxel has found an important role in this paradigm in the following settings: (1) first-line treatment in combination with cisplatin; (2) first-line treatment as a single agent; (3) second-line setting when used alone. Its use in combination with newer molecular targeted therapy is currently being explored (Table 3).

The standard pattern of practice for treating newly diagnosed patients with metastatic NSCLC is platinum-based doublet chemotherapy *(76)*. Docetaxel, paclitaxel, gemcitabine, vinorelbine, and vindesine are commonly used as the second agent in such protocols. Direct comparison of several such doublet combinations (cisplatin and paclitaxel, as the standard, compared to cisplatin and gemcitabine, cisplatin and docetaxel, or carboplatin and paclitaxel) in a large, randomized trial of over 1200 chemotherapy-naïve patients (ECOG 1594) showed a disappointingly similar response rate and median overall survival in each of the four arms *(77)*. The lack of major differences in outcome between arms has meant that selection of a specific doublet pairing for newly diagnosed patients of adequate performance status is influenced by toxicity profile, patient comorbidities, and cost *(78)*. There is little doubt that chemotherapy in this setting has two major clinical benefits compared to best supportive care; prolongation of survival and improvement in quality of life *(79,80)*.

The use of docetaxel-based doublet chemotherapy is associated with a response rate of approx 25–35% and a median overall survival of 8–11 mo *(81,82)*. The toxicity profile of the cisplatin–docetaxel combination includes hematological toxicity, edema, skin and nail changes, and hypersensitivity reactions in addition to the platinum-associated neurotoxicity and nephrotoxicity. Phase I studies of docetaxel in combination with cisplatin established that 75 mg/m^2 of each agent could be administered with reasonable safety and appeared to be active in metastatic NSCLC, a regimen that was validated in phase III trials *(82)*.

Table 3
Randomized Phase III Clinical Trials for Locally Advanced (Stage IIIB) or Metastatic (Stage IV) NSCLC

No. of patients	Treatment (dose mg/m²/schedule)	Efficacy (p-value)			Main trial results of docetaxel or docetaxel-containing regime	Reference
		% Overall RR (CR + PR)	Median TTP	Median OS		
Single Agent, First Line						
207; no prior CT	Docetaxel (100/q3w) + best supportive care	13.1%	12.6 w (<0.001)	6.0 m (0.026)	Longer TTP; improves quality of life for pain, dyspnea, emotional functioning and clinical symptoms	Roszkowski et al., 2000 (84)
	Best supportive care	—	8.9 w	5.7 m		
Single Agent, Second Line						
373; failed platinum -containing CT	Docetaxel (100/q3w)	10.8 (0.001 v V/I)	8.4 w (0.044 v V/I)	5.5 m (NS)	Higher RR; higher TTP; greater than 1 yr survival for Docetaxel 75 mg/m² q3w	Fossella et al., 2000 (TAX 320 Study Group) (90)
	Docetaxel (75/q3w)	6.7 (036 v V/I)	8.5 w (0.093 v V/I)	5.7 m (0.025 v V/I)		
	Vinorelbine (30 iv infusion on d 1,8, 15 q3w) or Ifosfamide (2g/m² /d 1–3 /q3w)	0.8	7.9 w	5.6 m		

Patients	Regimen	RR	TTP	OS	Comments	Reference
103; failed platinum-containing CT	Docetaxel (100/q3w)	6.3	10.6 w (<0.001)	5.9 m (0.78)	Prolonged survival at 75 mg/m^2	Shepherd et al., 2000 (TAX 317 Group) (88)
	Docetaxel (75/q3w)	5.5		7.5 m (0.01)		
246; as second line treatment	Best supportive care	—	6.7 w	4.6 m	Preliminary results on 170 pts: similar RR and MS triweekly and weekly equivalent dose	Camps et al., 2003 (The Spanish Lung Group) (99)
	Docetaxel (75/q3w)	11.0	3.4 m	6.3 m		
	Docetaxel (36/q1w)	8.9	3.5 m	6.1 m		
571; previously treated with CT	Docetaxel (75/q3w)	8.8	2.9 m	7.9 m	Similar RR, TTP, and OS; higher toxicity profile with neutropenic fever	Shepherd et al., 2003 (91)
	Pemetrexed (500/q3w)	9.1	2.9 m	8.3 m		

First-Line
Doublet Combinations

Patients	Regimen	RR	TTP	OS	Comments	Reference
441; phase IIb	Docetaxel (100) + cisplatin (80 d 2) q3w	34.6	8 m	10 m	Similar RR, TTP, OS; superior toxicity profile	Georgoulias, 2001 (Greek Oncology Cooperative Group) (100)
	Docetaxel (100 d8) + gemcitabine (1100 d 1,8/q3w	33.3	9 m (0.778)	9.5 m (0.98)		
251; no prior CT	Docetaxel (100 d8) + gemcitabine (1000 d 1,8) q3w	29	8	9 (survival)	Preliminary results indicate comparable activity	Kakolyris et al, 2002 (The Greek Cooperative Group for Lung Cancer) (101)
	Vinorelbine (30 d 1,8) + cisplatin (80 d8) q3w	36	8.5	11.5		

(Continued)

Table 3 (continued)

No. of patients	Treatment (dose mg/m² /schedule)	Efficacy (p-value)				Main trial results of docetaxel or docetaxel-containing regime	Reference
		% Overall RR (CR + PR)	Median TTP	Median OS			
1207; no prior CT	Paclitaxel (135/d 1) + cisplatin (75/d 2) q3w	21	3.4 m	7.8 m	No arm showed statistical superiority or inferiority in terms of response, median survival	Schiller et al., 2002 (77)
	Gemcitabine (1000/d 1,8,15) + cisplatin, (100 d 1) q4w	22	4.2 m	8.1 m		
	Docetaxel (75) + cisplatin (75) q3w	17	3.7 m	7.4 m		
	Paclitaxel (225) + carboplatin (AUC 6.0 mg/mL/min)q3w	17	3.1 m	8.1 m		
1218; no prior CT	A: Docetaxel (75) + c isplatin (75)/q3w	31.6 (0.029 v C)	NR	11.3 m v 10.1 m (0.044)	Higher RR, OS; improved quality of life	Fossella et al., 2003 (TAX 326 Study Group) (102)
	B: Docetaxel (75) + carboplatin (AUC 6 mg/mL min)/q3w v C)	23.9 (0.870	NR (0.657)	9.4 m v 9.9 m	Similar RR, OS with Arm C	
	C: Vinorelbine (25) + cisplatin (100) d 1, 8, 15, 22/q4w	24.5				
311; CT naive	Docetaxel (60/d1) + cisplatin (80)/ q3–4w	37.1	10.0 w (median duration of response)	11.3 m	Higher RR, OS; better quality of life	Kubota et al., 2004 (Japanese Taxotere Lung Cancer Study Group) (81)
	Cisplatin (80) + vindesine (3)/d 1, 8,15)/q4w	21.2 (<0.01)	8.4 w (0.20)	9.6 m (0.014)		

Abbreviations: RR, response rate; TTP, time to progression; w, weeks; mo, months; pt, patient; OS, overall survival; q3w, every three weeks; d1, day 1.

As with other chemotherapy protocols, performance status appears to be a particularly important determinant of outcome for docetaxel-based chemotherapy in patients with NSCLC *(83)*. Consequently, frail elderly patients and those with poor performance status might not obtain significant benefit from platinum-based doublet chemotherapy. Interest has been renewed in finding tolerable and beneficial treatments specifically for this group of patients. Recent trials have shown docetaxel to be effective as a single agent at several doses: 100 mg/m^2 every 3 wk, 75 mg/m^2 every 3 wk, and weekly at 35 mg/m^2 *(84)*. Administering docetaxel weekly at the 35-mg/m^2 dose improves the toxicity profile significantly minimizing myelosuppression and reducing nonhematologic side effects. At this dose, response rates of up to 20% have been described, making this regimen an option for the frailer or more elderly patient *(85)*.

The use of docetaxel in combination with agents other than cisplatin is also the subject of investigation. A phase II trial of docetaxel and gemcitabine was explored as first-line therapy for NSCLC patients. Patients were randomized to one of the two drugs, followed by the other after tumor progression. Patients who received gemcitabine followed by docetaxel fared best, with a median survival of 8 mo and 1-yr survival of 31% *(79)*. The reason for this schedule dependency has not yet been determined. Docetaxel has also been used in combination with irinotecan *(86)* and with vinorelbine *(87)* in small phase I studies with promising results. Further work will undoubtedly explore several other possible combinations as new antineoplastic drugs are introduced.

Another recent development is the use of second-line chemotherapy in advanced NSCLC (e.g., in patients refractory to cisplatin). After promising phase II data, a pivotal study by Shepherd demonstrated the utility of single agent docetaxel in this second line setting. A dose of 75 mg/m^2 docetaxel every 21 d in 105 patients previously treated with cisplatin yielded a median survival of 7.5 mo, compared to 4.6 mo, for best supportive care *(88)*. Patients in the 75-mg/m^2 arm had fewer episodes of febrile neutropenia (8 vs 22%) and a significantly lower risk of weight loss of greater than 10% (reviewed by Lynch [89]). A second phase III trial replicated this finding while also demonstrating that 75 mg/m^2 generated superior quality of life and lower toxicity than 100 mg/m^2 *(90)*. On the basis of these data, docetaxel became the first drug approved for this use in North America and Europe *(79)*. Some practitioners have exhibited hesitancy in choosing the cisplatin/docetaxel combination as first-line treatment for advanced NSCLC knowing that docetaxel is the only approved second-line drug. However, the recent demonstration that pemetrexed (Alimta), an antifolate antimetabolite, is also effective as a single agent in the second-line setting might allay such concerns *(91)*. A large phase III trial is ongoing to compare the activity of pemetrexed vs docetaxel in the second-line treatment of NSCLC *(92)*.

Although traditional cytotoxic agents remain the mainstay of treatment of NSCLC, newer molecularly targeted therapy is slowly showing promise in this disease. Several ongoing and recently completed trials have investigated the role of docetaxel in combination with such agents. Gefitinib, an EGFR tyrosine kinase inhibitor, demonstrated dramatic antitumor activity with little toxicity as a single agent in phase II trials in refractory, advanced NSCLC *(93)*. However, in phase III trials in combination with cisplatin and another taxane paclitaxel, gefitinib provided no benefit in terms of improved quality of life, increased response rate, or prolonged median survival *(94)*. The reason for this disappointing result remains unclear. Another potential target is Her2/neu which is expressed in about 20% of NSCLC tumors. Experience in combining Her2/neu-targeted therapy with traditional chemotherapy in breast cancer suggests that a similar approach would be useful in NSCLC. However, in a phase II trial in which docetaxel was used after cisplatin-based therapy in combination with trastuzumab in those tumors overexpressing HER2/neu, no clinical benefit was demonstrated (95). A proportion of NSCLC express the antiapoptotic protein Bcl-2 (96), which is thought to result in increased chemo-resistance and interest is growing in therapeutic approaches aimed at downregulating Bcl-2 expression in several different cancers. The combination of docetaxel and the Bcl-2 antisense oligonucleotide G3139 (Genasense®, Genta, Inc.) has shown some promise in phase I trials in the setting of advanced NSCLC (97) and has now been taken to phases II and III. Overall, combinations of docetaxel and other traditional cytotoxic agents with targeted therapies have shown inconsistent results. Clearly, a greater understanding of the mechanism of action is required before the dosing and sequencing of such combinations can be optimized for advanced NSCLC.

Finally, ongoing clinical trials are investigating how best to combine docetaxel with radiotherapy in NSCLC. Docetaxel is believed to be a radiosensitizing agent, but its role in combination with radiation in either the palliative setting or in locally advanced disease remains ill-defined at present (reviewed by Gandara [98]). Ongoing studies are focused on confirming the results observed with consolidation docetaxel in locally advanced NSCLC (SWOG 9504) and docetaxel in combination with molecularly targeted agents (99–102).

3.3. Docetaxel in Other Solid Tumors

A phase II trial of docetaxel 100 mg/m^2 every 3 wk was carried out in previously treated small cell lung cancer (SCLC) patients with progressive disease. Seven of 34 patients experienced a partial response. After 2 cycles, the response rate was 25% for the eligible 28 patients, with duration of response up to 12 mo. Toxicities were similar to other phase II trials with docetaxel at this dose (103). Refractory solid tumors in pediatric patients have also been treated with docetaxel as a single agent in combination with G-CSF (104) as a supportive measure to minimize neutropenia and allow dose escalation with or without G-CSF (105). In the absence of G-CSF, 44 pediatric patients were treated with docetaxel 50–150 mg/m^2 every 3 wk. They were able to tolerate 65 mg/m^2 if they were heavily pretreated (>2 other chemotherapy regimens) or 125 mg/m^2 if not so heavily pretreated. Neutropenia was dose limiting. For five patients receiving three cycles of docetaxel, only two had peripheral edema. One partial response and one complete response were observed. When GCSF (5 μg/kg/d) was administered with docetaxel in the second trial (17 patients), doses up to 185 mg/m^2 were well tolerated. One minor response was achieved. Dose-limiting toxicities at 235 mg/m^2 were desquamating skin rash and myalgias. Neutropenia was not dose limiting in the trial utilizing G-CSF. In both trials, adverse reactions were similar to those in the adult population.

Docetaxel has also been used in a variety of other metastatic diseases: ovarian cancer (reviewed by Kavanagh [106]), gastric carcinoma in combination with cisplatin (107) or 5-FU (108), malignant melanoma (109) squamous cell head and neck, urothelial, pancreatic adenocarcinoma, renal carcinoma, and cancers with an unknown primary site (Table 4) (110–119).

4. DOCETAXEL IN HORMONE-REFRACTORY AND METASTATIC PROSTATE CANCER

Prostate cancer is the most common cancer diagnosed and the second most common cause of cancer death in men in North America (120). Many patients with localized

Table 4
Clinical Trials With Docetaxel in Other Solid Tumors

	Trial type	No. of patients	Treatment mg/m^2/schedule	% Overall RR (CR + PR)	Median TTP	Median OS	Main results
Locally advanced or metastic urothelial/t transitional cell	**Single-Agent**						
	Phase II	30; previously treated with cisplatin-based chemotherapy	Docetaxel 100 mg/m^2 q3wk	13.3%			
	Phase II	29; no prior chemotherapy	100 mg/m^2 q3wk	31%			
	Phase II	11 100 mg/m^2 q3wk	45%				
	Combinations						
	Phase II	32; No prior chemotherapy (prior adjuvant chemotherapy > 6 m allowed)	Repeat every 3 w: epirubicin 40 mg/m^2 iv push, docetaxel 75 mg/m^2 1h infusion (with premedication) and cisplatin 75 mg/m^2 w/prehydration and posthydration	66.7%	Not reported	14.5 m	RR and toxicity were comparable with methotrexate, vinblastine, doxorubicin, displatin) regimen. No cardiac problems, no drug-related death
	Phase II	25; previously untreated	Docetaxel 75 mg/m^2, cisplatin 75 mg/m^2, every 3 w	60%		13.6 m	
	Phase II	66; 2 treated with MVAC (methotrexate, vinblastin, doxorubicin, cisplatin)	Docetaxel 75 mg/m^2, cisplatin 75 mg/m^2, every 3 w	52%		8 m	
	Phase II	19; previously untreated	Docetaxel 75 mg/m^2, cisplatin 75 mg/m^2, every 3 w	53%			
Recurrent or metastatic squamous cell carcinoma of the head and neck	All phase II						
Ovarian cancer	All phase II						
Malignant pleural mesothelioma	Phase II	30, chemotherapy naive		10% (PR)			Mildly effective

Abbreviations: RR, response rate; TTP, time to progression; w, weeks; mo, months; OS, overall survival; CR, complete response; PR, panal response.

disease have an excellent long-term survival and high cure rates with standard approaches *(121)*. However, patients with high-risk, locally advanced and metastatic disease have a poor prognosis, and although hormonal therapy in the form of medical or surgical castration can induce significant long-term remissions, development of androgen-independent disease is inevitable. Androgen-independent (AI) disease, also termed hormone-refractory prostate cancer (HRPC), is clinically detected by a rise in prostate-specific antigen (PSA) and/or worsening of symptoms. The current standard of care for HRPC is palliative in its intent and includes analgesia, radiation, and chemotherapy such as mitoxantrone *(122,123)* or docetaxel *(124,125)*. Docetaxel was first used in advanced prostate cancer as a single-agent treatment in phase I trials in 1994. Docetaxel has been used in a number of combinations, and phase II trials have reported biochemical PSA response rates in the 40% range as a single agent *(124–127)* (Table 5). PSA response rates exceeding 60% have been reported for docetaxel in combination with a number of other agents, including estramustine *(128–133)*. The results of two large phase III studies evaluating the efficacy of docetaxel in patients with metastatic HRPC were first reported in June 2004 at the American Society of Clinical Oncology's Annual Meeting. Both were powered to detect a difference of docetaxel on overall survival, with one comparing docetaxel and prednisone against mitoxantrone and prednisone and sponsored by Aventis, and the other a comparison of docetaxel and estramustine with mitoxantrone and prednisone that was run through the Southwest Oncology Group (SWOG). In the Aventis trial, 1006 men from Europe and North America with metastatic HRPC were randomized to three arms, receiving either standard therapy with mitoxantrone chemotherapy, or docetaxel administered once every 3 wk, or docetaxel administered weekly. Treatment on all three arms was generally well tolerated with a relatively low incidence of serious side effects. The men treated with docetaxel had improved responses to treatment in terms of PSA decreases, pain control, and enhancement in quality of life. Importantly, men treated with docetaxel every 3 wk also had a better survival overall. Median survival was 16.5 mo for patients treated with mitoxantrone, 18.9 mo ($p = 0.009$) for patients treated with docetaxel every 3 wk, 17.4 mo ($p = 0.36$) for patients treated with weekly docetaxel, and 18.3 mo for the combined docetaxel groups ($p = 0.04$). The SWOG trial confirms the overall survival benefit of docetaxel-based chemotherapy in men with HRPC. In this trial, 770 men with metastatic HRPC were randomized to receive either standard chemotherapy with mitoxantrone or to treatment with docetaxel in combination with estramustine. Similar to the Aventis trial, those men treated with the docetaxel combination had an improved PSA response rate and a better overall survival than those men treated with mitoxantrone. For men treated with the docetaxel-estramustine combination, median duration of survival was 18 mo, and 16 mo for those men treated with mitoxantrone. Unfortunately however, there were some serious side effects likely associated with the estramustine, including nausea and vomiting and thrombo-embolic complications. The results of these two landmark trials demonstrate for the first time that overall survival for patients with metastatic HRPC can be improved with a systemic therapy.

4.1. Preclinical Models and Treatment
of Prostate Cancer Metastatic to Bone

Advanced prostate cancer typically metastasizes to bone, resulting in significant pain and loss of quality of life. The reasons why prostate cancer metastasizes to bone are

Table 5
Phase II Trials With Docetaxel in Hormone-Refractory Prostate Cancer

Phase	No. of patients	Treatment (mg/m²/schedule)	Measurable disease RR (%)	Median time to disease progression	PSA RR (%)	Median survival	Ref.
Single-Agent							
II	21; 11 prior CT; 10 no prior CT	Docetaxel (75/q3w)	29 (1/6)		38 (6/16)		(126)
II	35; no prior CT	Docetaxel (75/q3w)	28 (7/25)		46		(125)
II	25; no prior CT	Docetaxel (36/d1,8,15,22,29, 36 q8w)	48 (2/5)	20 w	46 (11/24)		(124)
II	60; 25% received prior CT;	Docetaxel (36/d1,8,15,22,29, 36 q8w)	NR	5.1 m	41	9.4 m	(2)
II	20; 85% no prior CT	Docetaxel (25/w)	NR	5.6 m	61	NR	(132)
	19; 47% no prior CT	Docetaxel (70/q3w)	NR	6.8 m	60	NR	
Combination							
II	35; CT naive	Docetaxel (70/d2) + estramustine (280 mg × 3/d1–5) q3w	57 (4/7)	18 w	66	NR	(129)
II	46; no prior CT; metastatic	Docetaxel (70 d1) + estramustine (10 mg/kg d1–5) + hydrocortisone (40 mg/d) q3w	50 (12/24)	8 m	68	20 m	(128)
II	75; no prior CT	Docetaxel (30/w, 3/4w)+ thalidomide (200 mg/d)			51 (25/49)		(133)
		Docetaxel (30/w, 3/4w)			37 (9/24)		
		Docetaxel (70) + estramustine (280 mg × 5 doses) q3w	20 (4/20)	4 m	45	13.5 m	
		Docetaxel (36/d2) + calcitriol (0.5 µg/kg/d1) for 6 w of 8 w cycle	53 (8/15)	11.4 m	81	19.5 m	
		Docetaxel (75 iv d6) + G3139 (bcl-2 antisense oligonucleotide) (7 mg/kg/d) d1–8) /q3w	27		48		
		Docetaxel (36 mg/m² per week, 3 wk out of 4) + dexamethasone (0.75 mg po BID)3/4w		143 d			
		Docetaxel (70/d1) + estramustine (280 mg × 3/d1–3) q3w					
		Vinorelbine + docetaxel	60 (3/5)	NR	52	NR	
		Docetaxel (70/d1) + estramustine (240 mg × 3/d1–5) + hydrocortisone 40 mg/d) q3w	52	8.1	68	19.0 m	
		Docetaxel (70/d1)+ estramustine (600/d1–5) + vinblastine (5/d1) q3w		6 m		NR	
		Docetaxel (30/q1w)+ estramustine (280 mg × 2/5d)	NR	NR	NR	> 8 m	

NR, not yet reported.

rooted in the environmental milieu of the bone and of prostate stroma. Animal models to study the biology and treatment of bony metastases have been developed in several centers. For example, intravenous injection of metastatic prostate cancer cells into severe combined immune deficient (SCID) mice previously implanted with human adult bone results in metastases specifically to the human bone *(134)*. There have been some well-described orthotopic models of prostate cancer, where cells are injected into the prostate and metastases to the bone were observed *(135)*. Alternatively, intrafemur injections of prostate cancer cells results in tumor growth associated with osteoblastic and osteolytic changes that are comparable to those seen in humans *(136)*. Another approach involves coinoculation of bone fibroblasts with prostate cancer LNCaP cells to study paracrine factors facilitating osseous site-specific metastases *(137,138)*. Finally, the laboratory of Fidler and researchers at MD Anderson Cancer Center used a selection approach to isolate prostate cancer cells that can localize in the bone following intravenous or intracardiac injection *(139)*. Serial monitoring of the bony metastases can be performed to assess the effect of various in vivo treatments.

A strong case for stroma–prostate interactions in the growth of prostate cancer cells has been developed. Stromal factors mimic the microenvironment of bone in many aspects, thereby establishing the predilection for prostate cancer–bone interactions (seed and soil hypothesis) that promote the growth of bony metastases in prostate cancer in preference to other tissues. The prostate cancer cells also cause increased growth of fibromuscular stomal cells and increased production of extracellular matrix and growth factors. Stromal factors from bone aid prostate cancer growth and metastasis, and the prostate carcinoma cells begin behaving more like bone in that environment, producing osteoblast-type proteins such as RANKL (ligand for the transcription factor NF-κB), transcription factor Runx2, alkaline phosphatase, and bone matrix proteins such as osteopontin, osteocalcin, osteonectin, and bone sialoprotein. Bone minerals can be formed in prostate carcinoma cells in mineralizing media as well. A vicious cycle is set up in which the tumor cells produce factors that encourage bone remodeling (osteoblastic primarily, but also osteolytic reactions), which, in turn, causes the production of factors that promote tumor cell proliferation and metastasis (Fig. 3). For example, prostate tumor cells produce inflammatory mediators, such as IL-1β, TNF-α, and transforming growth factor-β (TGF-β). TGF-β, in turn promotes the production of parathyroid hormone (PTH) in bone, which promotes osteolytic reactions in bone. This bone turnover produces more TGF-β to perpetuate the cycle. The breakdown of bone generates hydrogen peroxide (H_2O_2), which induces formation of vascular endothelial growth factor (VEGF). VEGF then induces production of more H_2O_2 from tumor and bone cells and another vicious cycle is set up *(140)*.

Vascular endothelial growth factor is pro-angiogenic, thereby supporting the vascularization and growth of bony metastases. Prostate tumor cells also induce osteoblast growth via the endothelin-1 pathway (ET-1) *(141)*, making this pathway a very attractive target for treating metastases *(139)*, although this topic will not be addressed further here. In addition, osteoblast-derived factors have been demonstrated to promote the growth of prostate cancer cells. In media conditioned with primary bone tissue, lymph node cancer of the prostate (LNCaP) cells proliferate more rapidly than in regular media. IL-6 is one of the factors implicated, which has also been demonstrated to induce expression of PSA in hormone-refractory prostate cancer cells *(142)* via the androgen receptor, yet independent of androgen itself *(143)*.

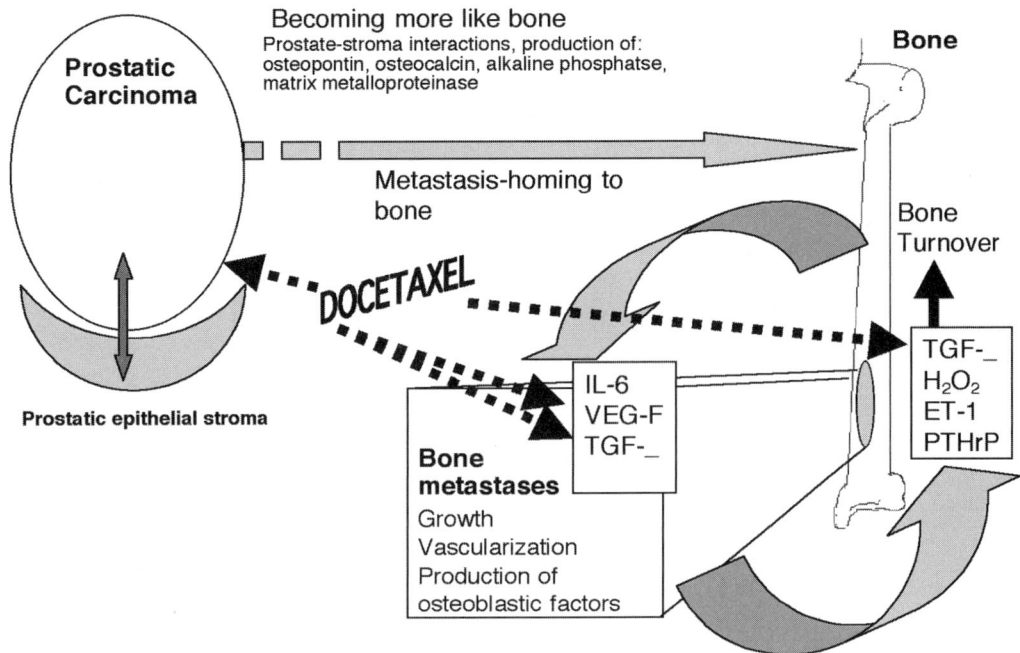

Fig. 3. Interactions between prostate carcinoma and bone promote the growth of bony metastasis of prostate cancer.

Treatment of bone metastases remains a challenge. Standard first-line therapy for metastatic HRPC is androgen ablation. Current additional modalities for the treatment of prostate bone metastases include spot radiation or strontium, hormonal therapy, mitoxantrone with prednisone, docetaxel with estramustine, and bisphosphonates (Table 6) *(144–147)*. Docetaxel can be particularly suited for the treatment of the bony metastases of prostate cancer not only via its effects on microtubules but also via its effects on angiogenesis and immune modulators (Fig. 3). A phase III clinical trial is completed in 740 patients with stage D1 prostate cancer to compare docetaxel/ estramustine with the standard of mitoxantrone/prednisone *(148)* as discussed above.

Basic research into the mechanisms of bone tropism for prostate cancer has led to additional ideas about novel targets for metastatic prostate cancer beyond conventional chemotherapy and radiation. As representative examples, novel targets under consideration that will be discussed here include Bcl-2, clusterin, IGFBP-2, and IGFs.

4.2. Novel Therapies for Advanced Prostate Cancer in Combination With Docetaxel

The high activity rate of docetaxel reported in phase II trials has lead to a number of novel combinations being evaluated clinically. Randomized studies in patients with prostate cancer have been planned or are underway with docetaxel in combination with an antisense to Bcl-2 *(149)*, high-dose calcitriol *(150)* (1,25-dihydroxyvitamin D; a therapeutically active metabolite of vitamin D), and bevacizumab (an anti-VEGF antibody)

Table 6
Randomized Phase III Trials for Hormone-Refractory Prostate Cancer

| No. of patients | Treatment | Efficacy (p-value) | | | | Ref. |
		RR	TTP	≥50% PSA decline (%)	Median survival	
162	Doxorubicin + diethylstilbestrol diphosphate	63				(144)
	Doxorubicin	27 (0.04)				
120	Mitoxantrone + prednisone		8.1 m	50	23 m	(2)
	Prednisone		4.1 m	24	19 m	
	Suramin + hydrocortisone			33		(145)
	Hydrocortisone			16 (0.01)		
201	Vinblastine + estramustine		3.7 m	25.2	11.9 m	(146)
	Vinblastine		2.2 m	3.2	9.2 m	
			(<0.001)	(<0.0001)		
103	Cyclophosphamide + doxorubicin + methotrexate		6.2 m		9.5 m	(147)
	Cyclophosphamide		4.4 m		9.0 m	

(42). In addition, earlier-phase clinical studies with docetaxel combinations, such as with an antisense oligonucleotide against clusterin (OGX-011), are also ongoing. It is hoped that readers understand that although there is a great deal of excitement about these new treatment modalities, their value has yet to be proven in large, multicenter phase III clinical studies.

4.3. Antisense Molecules for BCL-2

The Bcl-2 pathway is an obvious target for therapy in prostate cancer. The rationale for development of preclinical and clinical studies combining cytotoxic agents with inhibitors of Bcl-2 is summarized in a recent review by Gleave *(151)*. In brief, Bcl-2 expression, typically determined by immunohistochemistry, is low or absent in normal prostate epithelial cells, but it is highly upregulated in prostate cancer cells in direct relation to its grade and stage *(152,153)*. Bcl-2 levels also increase after androgen withdrawal (e.g., after androgen depletion in mouse xenograft models) *(154)*. Studies have shown that Bcl-2 levels in human prostate cancer are closely associated with the transition from androgen-dependent to the more aggressive androgen-independent tumors, with stage and grade of prostate tumors, and the tendency to produce metastases. Bcl-2 levels rise in prostate tumors after castration in patients *(155)* and during progression to androgen-independence in patients with advancing disease *(156,157)*.

Increased levels of Bcl-2 have also been noted after external-beam radiation treatment in localized prostate cancers *(158)* and in untreated hormone-refractory cancers *(157)*. Elevated levels of this antiapoptotic protein have been associated with radiation treatment failure *(158)*. Expression of Bcl-2 in prostate cancers has been used as a clinical prognostic marker *(159,160)*.

In vitro experiments suggested that Bcl-2 played a major role in the response of malignant cells to a variety of stresses that produce cellular damage, including chemotherapy. Additionally, cell lines overexpressing Bcl-2 were rendered more sensitive to chemotherapeutic agents either with the introduction of antisense oligonucleotides directed at the *bcl-2* message into the culture or upon transfection of the cells with a vector bearing the antisense sequence. The preclinical and clinical research exploring the use of anti-Bcl-2 therapies was fostered by the pharmaceutical development of stable and therapeutically effective antisense oligonucleotides targeting Bcl-2. Appropriately designed synthetic antisense oligonucleotides (ASOs) bind RNA molecules in a sequence-specific manner and either directly impair interaction with factors in the cytoplasm that are required for its translation into a protein or recruit endogenous RNaseH to cleave the RNA backbone. An 18-mer phosphorothioated oligonucleotide, Genasense (formerly known as G3139), directed against the first six codons of the open reading frame of the *bcl-2* gene message has been developed by Genta, Inc. The availability of the sequence made it possible to pursue a number of preclinical studies that provided compelling evidence for the development of clinical trials. The preclinical studies suggested that Bcl-2 inhibition alone delayed progression to androgen independence *(161)* and could increase sensitivity to cytotoxic agents such as paclitaxel *(162)*. Phase I clinical studies assessing Bcl-2 antisense oligonucleotide therapy in combination with docetaxel *(163)* or with mitoxantrone *(164)* in HRPC have been reported. Larger, randomized phase III clinical studies are currently underway to assess the therapeutic potential for improved survival with docetaxel treatment in combination with Genasense in prostate cancer.

4.4. Antisense Oligonucleotides Targeting Clusterin

Clusterin, also known as TRPM-2 (testosterone-repressed prostate message 2), apolipoprotein J, and sulfated glycoprotein (SGP)-2, is a cytoprotective inhibitor of protein precipitation and has been implicated as a player in the early development of prostate cancer and in resistance to hormone therapy, chemotherapy, and radiotherapy. Levels of clusterin might have prognostic value, as it has been correlated to prostate tumor grade *(165)*. Clusterin, like Bcl-2, is upregulated after androgen ablation therapy or castration in prostate cancer and contributes to the development of a chemo- and radiation-resistant phenotype. Thus, treatment targeted at clusterin activity has the potential to be a part of multimodality strategies aimed at treating advanced, poorly responsive prostate cancer *(166,167)*.

The clusterin gene is translated into several glycoprotein isoforms that differ in posttranslational modifications and in function. It has a variety of biological roles in normal tissues, including the male reproductive tract, breast, ovary, kidney, brain, cartilage, the eye, and the blood *(167)*. Its role in natural aging has also been investigated. Some members of the clusterin protein family are pro-apoptotic, whereas others are antiapoptotic/antiproliferative *(168,169)*, based on studies assessing the level of clusterin expression in tumors or tumor cells undergoing apoptosis or during cellular proliferation *(170,171)* as well as examination of clusterin's role in progression to HRPC *(172,173)*. In a study of clusterin levels in patients with advanced prostate cancer, clusterin levels were elevated in 80% of radical prostatectomy specimens after hormone ablation therapy, but in only 20% of prostate cancer cells in the specimens from untreated patients *(174)*.

In the PC-3 and LNCaP prostate cancer models, transduced cell lines overexpressing clusterin resulted in chemoresistance *(174–176)* and radiation resistance *(177)* compared to wild-type cells. Inhibition of clusterin with phosphorothioate oligodeoxynucleotides targeting clusterin expression resulted in chemosensitization in vitro and in vivo to mitoxantrone and paclitaxel in the PC-3 model, which expresses high levels of clusterin *(175)*. Interestingly, addition of the clusterin antisense by itself did not affect PC-3 cell proliferation in vitro in the absence of cytotoxic agents in this study, although clusterin mRNA was clearly downregulated. Inhibition of clusterin expression with antisense also was shown to sensitize PC-3 and LNCaP cells approx twofold to radiation-induced apoptosis compared to mismatch antisense controls, consistent with an anti-apoptotic role for clusterin in these prostate cancer cells *(177)*. Clusterin antisense has also been shown to sensitize renal cell carcinoma cells in vitro *(176)* and NSCLC to paclitaxel both in vitro and in vivo *(178)*.

Antisense oligonucleotides to clusterin have been developed and a second-generation phosphorothioate antisense is currently in clinical testing (OGX-011, OncoGenex) and phase I clinical trials began in late 2002. This single-agent study has a novel design in evaluating the biologic effect of OGX-011 in inhibiting clusterin expression in prostate cancer when given to men with localized prostate cancer prior to radical prostatectomy. This will allow the establishment of a phase II dose that incorporates optimal biological effectiveness. In a second trial, which started in March 2003, OGX-011 is being evaluated in combination with docetaxel in patients with cancers that potentially overexpress clusterin (breast, prostate, renal cell, bladder, breast, ovarian, non-small-cell lung cancers). Phase II trials of OGX-011 in combination with chemotherapy in patients with prostate cancer, lung cancer, and breast cancer are scheduled to start in mid-2004 to late 2004. Results of these trials are eagerly awaited.

4.5. Insulin-Like Growth Factor and Its Binding Proteins as Targets: Potential for Combination Therapies With Docetaxel for Advanced Disease

The insulin-like growth factor (IGF) system is involved in the progression and metastases of several cancers, including breast and prostate. IGF is another potentially interesting target in the treatment of metastatic cancer, although, presently, only in the preclinical testing stage. The system is comprised of two growth factors (IGF-1 and IGF-2), two receptor types (IGFR-1, IGFR-2), and six binding proteins (IGFBP-1 through IGFBP-6). The function of the binding proteins is generally to downregulate the activity mediated through the IGF receptors by binding to the IGFs. IGFBP-2 can be inhibitory for prostate cell growth in early, premalignant stages, but stimulates prostate cancer cell growth *(179,180)*. IGFBPs 2, 3, and 5 have been implicated in prostate cancer. IGFBP-2 increases significantly in HRPC and has been shown recently to enhance IGF-1 signaling and PI3-K activity after androgen ablation, thereby contributing to the development of androgen-independent growth *(181)*.

Both IGFBP-2 and IGFBP-3 are inversely related to disease progression *(182,183)*. In a study examining preoperative IGF-1, IGFBP-2, and IGFBP-3 levels in the plasma of men undergoing radical prostatectomy, it was found that men with higher levels of IGFBP-2 or IGFBP-3 showed a longer time to progression to advanced disease. Patients with metastases to lymph nodes or to bone had significantly lower plasma IGFBP-3 levels than patients with localized disease *(184)*. The role of IGFs is important in metastatic prostate cancer because IGFBP-5 is one of the most abundant stromal growth factors in bone. IGFBP-3 from bone reduces osteoblastic activity induced by IGFs and has been associated with development of bony metastases. Its action is thought to be dependent on PSA-related mechanisms, because IGFBP-3 levels are lower in prostate cancer bony metastases (PSA positive) than breast cancer bony metastases (PSA negative). Thus the IGF system is under intense study in hopes of uncovering a novel target for metastatic disease. At this time, however, there is sufficient rationale to consider the development of antisense oligonucleotides targeting IGFBP-2 and IGFBP-5 and this has recently been reviewed by Gleave *(185)*.

5. TARGETED DRUG DELIVERY TO BONE METASTASES

In the context of this chapter, which evaluates the use of docetaxel for treatment of advanced metastatic prostate cancer, it has been important to consider how systemic treatment strategies using approved cytotoxic agents in combination with emerging agents targeting specific molecular defects could achieve improved therapeutic results. It can be argued that one of the key elements in the development of better treatments for advanced metastatic disease will be based on the use of targeted drugs for management of cancer growth within the milieu of the bone. As mentioned in Section 1, targeted drug delivery for bony metastases involves three distinct approaches: (1) targeting molecular defects, which lead to the survival and progression of metastatic cancer cells in the bone, (2) targeting normal bone structural elements and growth or maintenance processes, which includes bone formation and resorption homeostasis, in order to improve delivery of drugs to bone, and (3) targeting to tumor-specific changes in bone structure, which might also aid in reducing toxicity to healthy bone. At the moment the first approach assumes that molecular defects existing in the primary tumor might still exist in cells that have metastasized to the bone. This provides the rationale for some of the emerging clinical studies summarized in this chapter, where agents targeting specific molecular targets believed to play a role in tumor cell survival and metastasis are being combined with conventional cytotoxic agents, such as docetaxel, in an attempt to prolong patient survival. Tumor-cell-specific agents being tested in clinical settings include the antisense oligonucleotides discussed here as well as agents targeting endothelial cell proliferation and migration (e.g. Avastin [bevacizumab]) *(186)* and those tumor-cell-derived targeting signals involved in bone remodeling (e.g., TGF-α, IL-1, IL-6, and TNF-α, etc.).

In the future, because genomic, proteomic, and functional molecular assays define features about cancer cells that survive and proliferate within the unique environment that exists within the bone, it is anticipated that unique combinations of drugs will be selected in order to treat the bone-localized disease. Although there is not sufficient space in this review to consider this topic, investigators are evaluating primary tumors by expression analysis with cDNA arrays to help identify molecular signatures associated with disease that has a propensity to metastasize *(187,188)*. Alternatively, cancer cells that have already metastasized to sites such as the bone might have a unique molecular signature. Obviously, these molecular signatures can be use in a predictive manner, but knowledge of these signatures will also be critical for making better decisions on the selection of therapeutic agents that will be used to treat the patient.

The above-outlined approaches contrast with efforts directed to provide palliative care for those patients with metastatic disease involving the bone, an effort focused on reducing the pain and morbidity associated with progressive disease development in the bone. The impact of cancer-mediated bone pain is substantial, and efforts to develop therapeutic approaches to improve the quality of life of patients suffering from this pain are warranted *(189)*. However, it would be preferential to implement therapeutic strategies prior to the observation of bone pain. What is interesting is that these efforts at palliative care are being used to design better targeted therapies effective in treating cancer progression. This leads to the second targeted therapeutic approach, which is centered on normal processes of bone-forming and bone-destroying events that are well regulated in unaffected bones, but can become highly dysregulated when cancer has spread to the bone. In most simplistic terms, bone homeostasis is controlled by osteoblasts, cells that synthesize collagen and control its subsequent mineralization, and osteoclasts, large multinucleated cells that play an active role in bone resorption. In an effort to control cancer-mediated osteolysis, osteoclast-inhibiting agents have been employed with some success. This effort was initiated based on the belief that bone metastasis and subsequent bone erosion requires, in part, recruitment of osteoclasts and agents such as the bisphosphonates (e.g., etidronate, pamidronate, clodronate) can inhibit the activity of these cells. Pamidronate frequently has been used for palliative treatment of patients with advanced cancer and the use of bisphosphonates and aminobisphosphonate (e.g., Fosamax®) has provided effective amelioration of pain in patients with bone lesions *(190)*. More recently, studies completed with zoledronic acid have suggested that this bisphosphonate can reduce skeletal complications such as bone fracture as well as pain *(191)*. The use of bisphosphonates for treatment of bone metastasis has been covered elsewhere in this book; however, as indicated in the following, bisphosphonates also have "bone-seeking" attributes because of their strong affinity for hydroxyapatite.

Mineralization of bone (i.e., bone forming activity) occurs by deposition of carbonated hydroxyapatite in a collagen matrix. Thus, bisphosphonates have direct targeting attributes, which leads to approaches where targeting to bone metastases is based on bone-remodeling activity that could be enhanced in regions where tumor growth is occurring. For example, bisphosphonates have been used in conjugates to direct agents such as methotrexate into bone, thereby altering its pharmacokinetic and toxicological profiles as well as achieving more specific drug targeting (osteotropic drug delivery systems [ODDs]) (reviewed by Stepensky [192]). The disadvantage of this targeting method, however, is the need for parenteral administration and, more importantly, there is a lack of control over where the drug is delivered in the skeleton. The entire skeleton becomes the likely recipient of such ODDs and, therefore, can result in new dose-limiting toxicities.

The third approach combines elements of the strategies outlined earlier and will result in therapeutic combinations of agents that target changes that occur as a consequence of the association between tumor cells and bone stromal elements. In one form, the specificity of bisphosphonate-conjugated drugs could be increased if the conjugated therapeutic agent exerted its activity primarily on unique features expressed in cancer cells growing within this site. Thus, delivery might occur throughout the skeleton, but the agent delivered would exert its therapeutic impact more selectively on cancer cells as opposed to normal cells with the bone. Efforts have been directed toward the development and preclinical evaluation of bisphosphonates conjugated to estrogen as well as bisphosphonates conjugated to proteins/peptides (193,194), and it is not unreasonable to assume that bone-specific delivery of small-molecule kinase inhibitors and/or antisense oligonucleotides will also be achievable using similar strategies. The former is exemplified by a recent report by Wang et al. that described the development of a Src tyrosine kinase inhibitor synthesize with covalently attached bisphosphonate (195). The Scr kinase inhibitor retained activity and exhibited affinity to hydroxyapatite. The company developing this technology (ARIAD Pharmaceuticals, Inc.) argues that they are designing small-molecule inhibitors that inhibit bone breakdown while blocking the growth of cancer cells that have spread to bone.

A fourth approach used to achieve targeted delivery to bone metastases takes advantage of the unique microenvironment that exists when tumor cells proliferate in bone. This is not dissimilar from strategies targeting neovasculature and vascular endothelium damage associated with tumor growth. Investigators have developed methods to target endothelial cells, but the value of these approaches for cancer is only realized if the targeting strategies consider changes in the endothelial cells that are uniquely associated with tumor growth. Tumor growth changes the surrounding endothelium in a manner that makes the associated endothelial cells a unique target, distinct from normal endothelial cells throughout the body. In the case of prostate cancer, investigators have shown that prostate cancer cells bind preferentially to human bone marrow endothelial cells (196–198). Thus one can consider targeting strategies that recognize the unique attributes of these bone marrow endothelial cells. Similar to other sites of tumor growth, changes in bone marrow blood vessels induced by tumor growth could also be used to achieve targeting. A greater understanding of the microenvironment and the host–tumor cell interface in the bone will be required in order to develop such strategies.

Further opportunities arise for targeting bone when one considers that the targeting strategies described earlier might involve intravenous administration of the selected drug combinations. In consideration of the blood vessel structure of bone marrow, investigators have pursued development of injectable colloidal drug carriers to improve the delivery of drugs for treatment of bone disease. Capillaries in the bone marrow are described as either fenestrated or discontinuous. Fenestrated capillaries exhibit large (60–100 nm in diameter) fenestrae or "openings," which have an underlying thin diaphragm that lacks the typical structure of blood vessels. These capillaries have a continuous basal lamina and are typically associated with regions where rapid exchanges between blood and tissue spaces are required. This type of capillary is found in the kidney, intestine, and endocrine organs but has also been shown to be present in bone. Discontinuous or sinusoidal capillaries possess open fenestrations through their endothelium. This type of capillary normally is associated with tissues rich in tissue macrophages such as the liver, spleen, and bone marrow. Because of the open blood vessel structure in bone marrow, small (<200 nm) drug carrier systems can be used to achieve improved, and more selective, delivery to the bone. This was recognized more than 15 yr ago by Illum and Davies, who demonstrated polymer-coated microspheres deposited in the bone marrow (198). More recently, the laboratory of Couvreur has pursued polymer-based nanoparticles to deliver agents to the bone (199–201). In the case of the anticancer drug doxorubicin, marrow toxicity, as judged by myelosuppression, was increased as a result of increased drug delivery and prolonged exposure achieved by associating this cytotoxic drug with a nanoparticle (199). Our research laboratory obtained similar results when delivering doxorubicin in liposomal drug carriers (202). These negative results are not surprising when one considers that these nano-drug delivery systems enhanced the delivery of a drug active against proliferating bone marrow hemopoietic cells. The advent of more selective, molecularly targeted drugs makes it interesting to consider application of drug carrier technology to improve delivery of these agents. Couvreur's laboratory, for example, has used nanoparticles as carriers for human recombinant granulocyte colony-stimulating factor with the aim of developing a formulation that exhibits improved therapeutic effects when used to treat neutropenia (203).

In the case of treating bony metastases, a more specific delivery of the pharmacologic agent is desired and, as implied earlier, this might require a combination of approaches. For example, the pairing of focused radiation therapy with drug delivery systems that release their contents upon irradiation would be a sophisticated approach. Liposomes that are lysed or disrupted by radiation energy (204) such that permeability changes occur resulting in drug release (205) could possibly be designed to incorporate docetaxel and/or the novel biological response modifiers, providing site-specific therapy and minimizing exposure at nontarget sites. These ideas have yet to be tested in vivo.

Characterization of the uptake of systemically administered drug delivery systems, such as liposomes, into bony metastases of human patients has not been studied sufficiently to know whether carriers can actually improve delivery. One study of the bone metastases of two patients who received a long circulating formulation (PEGylated) liposomal doxorubicin (Caelyx®, Schering-Plough) indicated a 10-fold greater drug level in bone compared to muscle after receiving the drug (206). Presently, local delivery (without systemic administration) of anticancer drugs to bony metastases is also under investigation using various implantable devices such as bone cement containing anticancer drugs (207,208), calcium phosphate matrix implants for methotrexate release in bone (209) or controlled release pastes or polymeric delivery systems (210), which might be suitable for the delivery of docetaxel as well.

6. CONCLUSIONS

In this chapter, we have reviewed the pharmacology and the major clinical applications of docetaxel for advanced metastatic cancer, particularly HRPC. The multiple mechanisms of action of docetaxel and its wide range of single-agent activity in first- and second-line therapies make docetaxel particularly valuable when devising combination strategies to combat metastatic disease. In June 2004, the results of critically important phase III clinical trials of combination chemotherapy with docetaxel released. These positive results will guide the further development of docetaxel in advanced prostate cancer. Novel, molecularly targeted therapies, including antisense oligonucleotides against targets such as Bcl-2 and clusterin, will provide further opportunities to expand and define the most valuable roles of docetaxel. Finally, as drug delivery strategies are developed to target these optimized therapies directly to the sites of bony metastasis, we anticipate that in the near future, bone metastases will not be considered untreatable disease.

REFERENCES

1. Jewett MA, Khakpour G, Moore MJ. Supportive care is not the only option in prostate cancer patients resistant to hormone therapy: the argument against. *Eur Urol* 1996; 29(Suppl 2):45–48.
2. Berry W, Dakhil S, Modiano M, Gregurich M, Asmar L. Phase III study of mitoxantrone plus low dose prednisone versus low dose prednisone alone in patients with asymptomatic hormone refractory prostate cancer. *J Urol* 2002; 168(6):2439–2443.
3. Oh WK, Halabi S, Kelly WK, Werner C, Godley PA, Vogelzang NJ, et al. Cancer and Leukemia Group B 99813. A phase II study of estramustine, docetaxel, and carboplatin with granulocyte-colony-stimulating factor support in patients with hormone-refractory prostate carcinoma: Cancer and Leukemia Group B 99813. *Cancer* 2003; 98(12):2592–2598.
4. Petrylak DP, Macarthur R, O'Connor J, Shelton G, Weitzman A, Judge T, et al. Phase I/II studies of docetaxel (Taxotere) combined with estramustine in men with hormone-refractory prostate cancer. *Semin Oncol* 1999; 26(5 Suppl 17):28–33.
5. Herbst RS, Khuri FR. Mode of action of docetaxel - a basis for combination with novel anticancer agents. *Cancer Treat Rev* 2003; 29:407–415.
6. Schimming, R, Mason KA, Hunter N, Weil M, Kishi K, Milas L. Lack of correlation between mitotic arrest or apoptosis and antitumor effect of docetaxel. *Cancer Chemother Pharmacol* 1999; 43(2):165–172.
7. Lavelle F, Bissery MC, Combeau C, Riou JF, Vrignaud P, Andre S. Preclinical evaluation of docetaxel (Taxotere). *Semin Oncol* 1995; 22(2 Suppl 4):3–16.
8. Cory S. Regulation of lymphocyte survival by the Bcl-2 gene family. *Ann Rev Immunol* 1995; 13:513–543.
9. Kroemer G. The proto-oncogene Bcl-2 and its role in regulating apoptosis. *Nat Med* 1997; 3(6):614–620.
10. Reed JC. Bcl-2 and the regulation of programmed cell death. *J Cell Biol* 1994; 124:1–6.
11. Reed JC. Bcl-2 family proteins: strategies for overcoming chemoresistance in cancer. *Adv Pharmacol* 1997; 41:501–532.
12. Thompson CB. Apoptosis in the pathogenesis and treatment of disease. *Science* 1995; 267:1456–1462.
13. Yang E, Korsmeyer SJ. Molecular thanatopsis: a discourse on the Bcl-2 family and cell death. *Blood* 1996; 88:386–401.
14. Vander Heiden MG, Thompson CB. Bcl-2 proteins: regulators of apoptosis or of mitochondrial homeostasis? *Nat Cell Biol* 1999;1:E209–E216.
15. Hsu Y-T, Wolter KG, Youle RJ. Cytosol-to-membrane redistribution of Bax and Bcl-XL during apoptosis. *Proc Nat Acad Sci USA* 1997; 94:3668–3672.
16. Wolter KG. Hsu Y-T, Smith CL, Nechushtan A, Xi X-G, Youle RJ Movement of Bax from the cytosol to mitochondria during apoptosis. *J Cell Biol* 1997; 139:1281–1292.
17. Gross A, Jockel J, Wei MC, Korsmeyer SJ. Enforced dimerization of Bax results in its translocation, mitochondrial dysfunction and apoptosis. *EMBO J* 1998; 17:3878–3885.

18. Nechushtan A, Smith CL, Hsu Y-T, Youle RJ Conformation of the Bax C-terminus regulates subcellular location and cell death. *EMBO J* 1999; 18:2330–2341.

19. Manon S, Chaudhuri B, Guerin M. Release of cytochrome c and decrease of cytochrome c oxidase in Bax-expressing yeast cells and prevention of these effects by coexpression of Bcl-XL. *FEBS Lett* 1997; 415:29–32.

20. Antonsson B, Montessuit S, Sanchez B, Martinou JC. Bax is present as a high molecular weight oligomer-complex in the mitochondrial membrane of apoptotic cells. *J Biol Chem* 2001; 2765: 11,615–11,623.

21. Mikhailov V, Mikhailova M, Pulkrabek DJ, Dong Z, Venkatachalam MA, Saikumar P. Bcl-2 prevents Bax oligomerization in the mitochondrial outer membrane. *J Biol Chem* 2001; 276:18,361– 18,374.

22. Li P, Nijhawan D, Budihardjo I, Srinivasula SM, Manzoor A, Emad S, et al. Cell Cytochrome c and dATP-dependent formation of Apaf-1/caspase-9 complex initiates an apoptotic protease cascade. *Cell* 1997; 91:479–489.

23. Oltval ZN, Milliman CL, Korsmeyer SJ. Bcl-2 heterodimerizes in vivo with a conserved homolog, Bax, that accelerates programmed cell death. *Cell* 1993; 74:609–619.

24. Hou Q, Cymbalyuk E, Hsu S-C, Xu M, Hsu Y-T. Apoptosis modulatory activities of transiently expressed Bcl-2: Roles in cytochrome c release and Bax regulation. *Apoptosis* 2003; 8:617–629.

25. Yang E, Zha J, Jockel J, Boise LH, Thompson CB, Korsmeyer SJ. Bad, a heterodimeric partner for Bcl-XL and Bcl-2, displaces Bax and promotes cell death. *Cell* 1995; 80:285–291.

26. Shitashige M, Toi M, Yano T, Shibata M, Matsuo Y, Shibasaki F. Dissociation of Bax from a BCl-2/ Bax heterodimer triggered by phosphorylation of serine 70 of Bcl-2. *J Biochemistry* (Tokyo) 2001; 130(6):741–748.

27. Wang Q, Weider R. All-trans retinoic acid potentiates Taxotere-induced cell death mediated by Jun N-terminal kinase in breast cancer cells. *Oncogene* 2004; 23(2):426–433.

28. Schimming R, Mason KA, Hunter N, Weil M, Kishi K, Milas L. Lack of correlation between mitotic arrest or apoptosis and antitumor effect of docetaxel. *Cancer Chemother Pharmacol* 1999; 43(2): 165–172.

29. Hartley-Asp B, Kruse E. Nuclear protein matrix as a target for estramustine-induced cell death. *Prostate* 1986; 9:387–395.

30. Pienta KJ, Lehr JE. Inhibition of prostate cancer growth by estramustine and etoposide: evidence for interaction at the nuclear matrix. *J Urol* 1993; 149:1622–1625.

31. Hartley-Asp, B. Estramustine-induced mitotic arrest in two human prostatic carcinoma cell lines DU-145 and PC-3. *Prostate* 1984; 5:93–100.

32. Kraus LA, Samuel SK, Schmid SM, Dykes DJ, Waud WR, Bissery MC. The mechanism of action of docetaxel (Taxotere) in xenograft models is not limited to bcl-2 phosphorylation. *Investigational New Drugs* 2003; 21(3): 259–268.

33. Maestre N, Bezombes C, Plo I, Levied T, Lavelle F, Laurent G, Jaffrezou JP. Phosphatidylcholine-derived phosphatidic acid and diacylglycerol are involved in the signaling pathways activated by docetaxel. *J Exp Ther Oncol* 2003; 3(1):36–46.

34. Sweeney CJ, Miller KD, Sissons SE, Nozaki S, Heilman DK, Shen J, Sledge GW Jr. The antiangiogenic property of docetaxel is synergistic with a recombinant humanized monoclonal antibody against vascular endothelial growth factor or 2-methoxyestradiol but antagonized by endothelial growth factors. *Cancer Res* 2001; 61(8):3369–3372.

35. Vacca A, Ribatti D, Iurlaro M, Merchionne F, Nico B, Ria R, Dammacco F. Docetaxel versus paclitaxel for antiangiogenesis. *J Hematother Stem Cell Res* 2002; 11(1):103–118.

36. Avramis IA, Kwock R, Avramis VI. Taxotere and vincristine inhibit the secretion of the angiogenesis inducing vascular endothelial growth factor (VEGF) by wild-type and drug-resistant human leukemia T-cell lines. *Anticancer Res* 2001; 21(4A):2281–2286.

37. Guo XL, Lin GJ, Zhao H, Gao Y, Qian LP, Xu SR, et al. Inhibitory effects of docetaxel on expression of VEGF, bFGF and MMPs of LS174T cell. *World J Gastroenterol* 2003; 9(9):1995–1998.

38. Bertolini F, Paul S, Mancuso P, Monestiroli S, Gobbi A, Shaked Y, et al. Maximum tolerable dose and low-dose metronomic chemotherapy have opposite effects on the mobilization and viability of circulating endothelial progenitor cells. *Cancer Res* 2003; 63(15):4342–4346.

39. Man S, Bocci G, Francia G, Green SK, Jothy S, Hanahan D, et al. Antitumor effects in mice of low-dose (metronomic) cyclophosphamide administered continuously through the drinking water. *Cancer Res* 2002; 62(10):2731–2735.

40. Inoue K, Chikazawa M, Fukata S, Yoshikawa C, Shuin T. Docetaxel enhances the therapeutic effect of the angiogenesis inhibitor TNP-470 (AGM-1470) in metastatic human transitional cell carcinoma. *Clin Cancer Res* 2003; 9(2):886–899.

41. Koukourakis MI, Simopoulos C, Polychronidis A, Perente S, Botaitis S, Giatromanolaki A, et al. The effect of trastuzumab/docatexel combination on breast cancer angiogenesis: dichotomus effect predictable by the HIFI alpha/VEGF pre-treatment status? *Anticancer Res* 2003; 23(2C):1673–1680.

42. Salimichokami M. Combining angiogenesis inhibitors with cytotoxic chemotherapy enhances PSA response in hormone refractory prostate cancer (HRPC), a randomized study of weekly docetaxel alone or in combination with thalidomide. *Proc Am Soc Clin Oncol* 2003; 22:429 (abstract no. 1725).

43. Dai J, Kitagawa Y, Zhang J, Yao Z, Mizokami A, Cheng S, et al. Vascular endothelial growth factor contributes to the prostate cancer-induced osteoblast differentiation mediated by bone morphogenetic protein. *Cancer Res* 2004; 64(3):994–999.

44. Cassidy PB, Moos PJ Kelly RC, Fitzpatrick FA. Cyclooxygenase-2 induction by paclitaxel, docetaxel and taxane analogues in human monocytes and murine macrophages: structure-activity relationships and their implications. *Clinical Cancer Res* 2002; 8(3):846–855.

45. Tsavaris N, Kosmas C, Vadiaka M, Kanelopoulos, Boulamatsis D. Immune changes in patients with advanced breast cancer undergoing chemotherapy with taxanes. *Br J Cancer* 2002; 87(1):21–27.

46. Tong AW, Seamour B, Lawson JM, Ordonez G, Vukelja S, Hyman W, et al. Cellular immune profile of patients with advanced cancer before and after taxane treatment. *Am J Clin Oncol* 2000; 23(5):463–472.

47. Chan OT, Yang LX. The immunological effects of taxanes. *Cancer Immunol Immunother* 2000; 49 (4–5):181–185.

48. Rosing H, Lustig V, van Warmerdam LJ, Huizing MT, ten Bokkel Huinink WW, Schellens JH, et al. Pharmacokinetics and metabolism of docetaxel administered as a 1-h intravenous infusion. *Cancer Chemother Pharmacol* 2000; 45(3):213–218.

49. Bruno R, Riva D, Hille A, Lebecq A, Thomas L. Pharmacokinetic and pharmacodynamic properties of docetaxel: Results of phase I and phase II trials. *Am J Health-Syst Pharm* 54 1997; (Suppl. 2):S16–S19.

50. Bruno R, Mille D, Riva A, Vivier N, ten Bokkel Huinink WW, van Oosterom AT, et al. Population pharmacokinetics/pharmacodynamics of docetaxel in phase II studies in patients with cancer. *J Clin Oncol* 1998; 16:187–196.

51. Hirth J, Watkins PB, Strawderman M, et al. The effect of an individual's cytochrome CYP3A4 activity on docetaxel clearance. *Clin Cancer Res* 2000; 6(4):1255–1258.

52. Sparreboom A, van Tellingen O, Nooijen WJ, Beijnen JH. Preclinical pharmacokinetics of paclitaxel and docetaxel. *Anticancer Drugs* 1998; 9(1):1–17.

53. Aventis Pharmaceuticals, Inc. Taxotere® package insert. 2003.

54. Ramos M, Gonzalez-Ageitos A, Amenedo M, Gonzalez-Quintas A, Gamazo JL, Togores P, et al. Weekly docetaxel as second-line therapy for patients with advanced breast cancer resistant to previous anthracycline treatment. *J Chemother* 2003; 15(2):192–197.

55. Mey U, Gorschluter M, Ziske C, Kleinschmidt R, Glasmacher A, Schmidt-Wolf IG. Weekly docetaxel in patients with pretreated metastatic breast cancer: a phase II trial. *Anticancer Drugs* 2003; 14(3):233–238.

56. Masters GA, Brockstein BE, Mani S, Ratain MJ. Phase 1 dose escalation study of docetaxel with filgrastim support in patients with advanced solid tumors. *Med Oncol* 2003; 20(1):7–12.

57. Kuroi K, Shimozuma K. Neurotoxicity of taxanes: symptoms and quality of life assessment. *Breast Cancer* 2004; 11(1):92–99.

58. Pronk LC, Hilkens PH, van den Bent MJ, van Putten WL, Stoter G, Verweij J. Corticosteroid co-medication does not reduce the incidence and severity of neurotoxicity induced by docetaxel. *Anticancer Drugs* 1998; 9(9):759–764.

59. Wasner G, Hilpert F, Schattschneider J, Binder A, Pfisterer J, Baron R. Docetaxel-induced nail changes—a neurogenic mechanism: a case report. *J Neurooncol* 2002; 58(2):167–174.

60. Peccart, M. The role of taxanes in the adjuvant treatment of early stage breast cancer. *Breast Cancer Res Treat* 2003; 79(Suppl 1):S25–34.

61. Hutcheon AW, Heys SD, Sarkar TK, Aberdeen Breast Group. Neoadjuvant docetaxel in locally advanced breast cancer. *Breast Cancer Res Treat* 2003; 79(Suppl 1):S19–24.

62. Fumoleau, P. Efficacy and safety of docetaxel in clinical trials. *Am J Health-Syst Pharm* 1997; 54 (Suppl 2):S19–24.

63. Nabholtz JM, Falkson C, Campos D, Szanto J, Martin M, Chan S, et al. Docetaxel and doxorubicin compared with doxorubicin and cyclophosphamide as first-line chemotherapy for metastatic breast cancer: results of a randomized, multicenter, phase III trial. *J Clin Oncol* 2003; 21(6):968–975.

64. Chan S, Friedrichs K, Noel D, Pinter T, Van Belle S, Vorobiof D, et al. Prospective randomized trial of docetaxel versus doxorubicin in patients with metastatic breast cancer. *J Clin Oncol* 1999; 17(8): 2341–2354.

65. Nabholtz JM, Senn HJ, Bezwoda WR, Melnychuk D, Deschenes L, Douma J, et al. Prospective randomized trial of docetaxel versus mitomycin plus vinblastine in patients with metastatic breast cancer progressing despite previous anthracycline-containing chemotherapy. *J Clin Oncol* 1999; 17(5): 1413–1424.

66. Sjöström J, Blomqvist C, Mouridsen H, Pluzanska A, Ottosson-Lönn S, Bengtsson NO, et al. Docetaxel compared with sequential methotrexate and 5-fluorouracil in patients with advanced breast cancer after anthracycline failure: a randomised phase III study with crossover on progression by the Scandinavian Breast Group. *Eur J Cancer* 1999; 35(8):1194–1201.

67. Bonneterre J, Roche H, Monnier A, Guastalla JP, Namer M, Fargeot P, et al. Docetaxel vs 5-fluorouracil plus vinorelbine in metastatic breast cancer after anthracycline therapy failure. *Br J Cancer* 2002; 87: 1210–1215.

68. Mackey JR, Paterson A, Dirix LY, Dewar J, Chap L, Miguel M, et al. Final results of the phase III randomized trial comparing docetaxel (T), doxorubicin (A) and cyclophosphamide (C) to FAC as first line chemotherapy (CT) to patients (pts) with metastatic breast cancer (MBC). *American Society of Clinical Oncology* Annual Meeting, 2002 (abstract 137).

69. O'Shaughnessy J, Miles D, Vukelja S, Moiseyenko V, Ayoub JP, Cervantes G, et al. Superior survival with capecitabine plus docetaxel combination therapy in anthracycline-pretreated patients with advanced breast cancer: phase III trial results. *J Clin Oncol* 2002; 20(12):2812–2823.

70. Nabholtz JM. Docetaxel-anthracycline combinations in metastatic breast cancer. *Breast Cancer Res Treat* 2003; 79(Suppl 1):S3–9.

71. Goble S, Bear HD. Emerging role of taxanes in adjuvant and neoadjuvant therapy for breast cancer: the potential and the questions. *Surg Clin North Am* 2003; 83(4):943–971.

72. Perotti A, Cresta S, Grasselli G, Capri G, Minotti G, Gianni L. Cardiotoxic effects of anthracycline-taxane combinations. *Expert Opin Drug Saf* 2003; 2(1):59–71.

73. Fumoleau P. Gemcitabine combined with docetaxel in metastatic breast cancer. *Semin Oncol* 2003; 30(2 Suppl 3):15–18.

74. Non-small Cell Lung Cancer Collaborative Group. Chemotherapy in non-small cell lung cancer: a meta-analysis using updated data on individual patients form 52 randomised clinical trials. *BMJ* 1995; 311:899–909.

75. Rapp E, Pater JL, Willan A, et al. Chemotherapy can prolong survival in patients with advanced non-small cell lung cancer-report of a Canadian multicenter randomized trial. *J Clin Oncol* 1988; 6: 633–641.

76. ASCO Special Article. Clinical practice guidelines for the treatment of unresectable non-small-cell lung cancer. *J Clin Oncol* 1997; 15:2996–3018.

77. Schiller JH, Harrington D, Belani CP, Langer C, Sandler A, Krook J, et al. Comparison of four chemotherapy regimens for advanced non-small-cell lung cancer. *N Engl J Med* 2002; 346(2):92–98.

78. Belani CP. Chemotherapy regimens in advanced non small-cell lung cancer: recent randomized trials. *Clin Lung Cancer* 2000; 2(Suppl 1):S7–S10.

79. Manegold C, Pilz L, Koschel G, Schott K, Hruska D, Mezger J. Single agent gemcitabine and docetaxel given sequentially in various doses and schedules are effective in advanced NSCLC: survival data from two randomized phase II studies. *American Society of Clinical Oncology* Annual Meeting, 2001; 337a, abstract 1346.

80. Simon GR, Bunn PA Jr. Taxanes in the treatment of advanced (stage III and IV) non-small cell lung cancer (NSCLC): recent developments. *Cancer Invest* 2003; 21(1):87–104.

81. Kubota K, Watanabe K, Kunitoh H, Noda K, Ichinose Y, Katakami N, et al. Phase III randomized trial of docetaxel plus cisplatin versus vindesine plus cisplatin in patients with stage IV non-small-cell lung cancer: the Japanese Taxotere Lung Cancer Study Group. *J Clin Oncol* 2004; 22(2):254–261.

82. Fossella F. Docetaxel + Cisplatin (DC) and Docetaxel + Carboplatin (DCCb) vs Vinorelbine + Cisplatin (VC) in chemotherapy–naïve patients with advanced and metastatic non-small cell lung cancer (NSCLC): results of a multicenter, randomized phase III study. *Eur J Cancer* 2001; 37(Suppl.6):154.

83. Gralla RJ. Docetaxel trials in non-small-cell carcinoma of the lung, In: Johnson DH, Klastersky J, eds. *Taxanes in Lung Cancer Therapy*. New York: Marcel Dekker, 1998:103–116.

84. Roszkowski K, Pluzanska A, Krzakowski M, Smith AP, Saigi E, Aasebo U, et al. A multicenter, randomized, phase III study of docetaxel plus best supportive care versus best supportive care in

chemotherapy-naive patients with metastatic or non-resectable localized non-small cell lung cancer (NSCLC). *Lung Cancer* 2000; 27(3):145–57.

85. Hainsworth JD, Burris HA 3rd, Greco FA. Weekly docetaxel as a single agent and in combination with gemcitabine in elderly and poor performance status patients with advanced non-small cell lung cancer. *Semin Oncol* 2001; 28(3 Suppl 9):21–25.

86. Murren JR, Davies M. Irinotecan and taxane combinations for non small-cell lung cancer. *Clin Lung Cancer* 2001; 2(Suppl 2):S20–25.

87. Miller VA. Trials of vinorelbine and docetaxel in the treatment of advanced non small-cell lung cancer. *Clin Lung Cancer* 2000; 1(Suppl 1):S24–26.

88. Shepherd FA, Dancey J, Ramlau R, Mattson K, Gralla R, O'Rourke M, et al. Prospective randomized trial of docetaxel versus best supportive care in patients with non-small-cell lung cancer previously treated with platinum-based chemotherapy. *J Clin Oncol* 2000; 18(10):2095–2103.

89. Lynch TJ Jr. Review of two phase II randomized trials of single-agent docetaxel in previously treated advanced non-small cell lung cancer. *Semin Oncol* 2001; 28(3 Suppl 9):5–9.

90. Fossella FV, DeVore R, Kerr RN, Crawford J, Natale RR, Dunphy F, et al. Randomized phase III trial of docetaxel versus vinorelbine or ifosfamide in patients with advanced non-small-cell lung cancer previously treated with platinum-containing chemotherapy regimens. The TAX 320 Non-Small Cell Lung Cancer Study Group. *J Clin Oncol* 2000; 18(12):2354–2362.

91. Hanna NH, Shepherd FA, Rosell JR, Pereira F, et al. A phase III study of permetrexed vs. docetraxel in patients with recurrent non-small cell lung cancer (NSCLC) who were previously treated with chemotherapy. *Proc Am Soc Clin Oncol* 2003; 22:622.

92. Fossella, FV. Pemetrexed for treatment of advanced non-small cell lung cancer. *Semin Oncol* 2004; 31(1 Suppl 1):100–105.

93. Johnson DH. Gefitinib (Iressa) trials in non-small cell lung cancer. *Lung Cancer* 2003; 41(Suppl 1): S23–28.

94. Herbst RS, Giaccone G, Schiller JH, Natale RB, Miller V, Manegold C, et al. Gefitinib in combination with paclitaxel and carboplatin in advanced non-small-cell lung cancer: a phase III trial—INTACT 2. *J Clin Oncol* 2004; 22(5):785–794.

95. Lara PN Jr, Laptalo L, Longmate J, Lau DH, Gandour-Edwards R, Gumerlock PH, et al. Trastuzumab plus docetaxel in HER2/neu-positive non-small-cell lung cancer: a California Cancer Consortium screening and phase II trial. *Clin Lung Cancer* 2004; 5(4):231–236.

96. Au NHC, Cheang M, Huntsman DG, Yorida E, Coldman A, Elliott WM, et al. Evaluation of immunohistochemical markers in non-small cell lung cancer by unsupervised hierarchical clustering analysis: a tissue microarray study of 284 cases and 18 markers. *Br J Pathol* 2004; in press.

97. Rudin CM, Otterson GA, Mauer AM, Villalona-Calero MA, Tomek R, Prange B, et al. A pilot trial of G3139, a bcl-2 antisense oligonucleotide, and paclitaxel in patients with chemorefractory small-cell lung cancer. *Ann Oncol* 2002; 13(4):539–545.

98. Gandara DR, Lara PN Jr, Goldberg Z, Lau DH. Integration of new chemotherapeutic agents into chemoradiotherapy for stage III non-small cell lung cancer: focus on docetaxel. *Semin Oncol* 2001; 28(3 Suppl 9):26–32.

99. Camps C, Massuti A, Jimenez AM, Maestu I, Almenar D, Garcia R, et al. Second-line docetaxel administrated every 3 weeks versus weekly in advanced non-small-cell lung cancer (NSCLC): a Spanish Lung Cancer Group (SLCG) phase III trial. *Proc of Am Soc Clin Oncol* 2003; 22:625, (abstract no. 2514).

100. Georgoulias V, Papadakis E, Alexopoulos A, Tsiafaki X, Rapti A, Veslemes M, et al. Platinum-based and non-platinum-based chemotherapy in advanced non-small-cell lung cancer: a randomised multicentre trial. *Lancet* 2001; 357(9267):1478-1484.

101. Kakolyris X, Tsiafaki A, Agelidou J, Arapis J, Boukovinas N, Samaras P, et al. Preliminary results of a multicenter randomized phase III trial of docetaxel plus gemcitabine (DG) versus vinorelbine plus cisplatin (VC) in patients with advanced non-small cell lung cancer. *American Society of Clinical Oncology* Annual Meeting, 2002 (abstract 1182).

102. Fossella F, Pereira JR, von Pawel J, Pluzanska A, Gorbounova V, Kaukel E, et al. Randomized, multinational, phase III study of docetaxel plus platinum combinations versus vinorelbine plus cisplatin for advanced non-small-cell lung cancer: the TAX 326 study group. *J Clin Oncol* 2003; 21 (16):3016–3024.

103. Smyth JF, Smith IE, Sessa C, et al. Activity of docetaxel (Taxotere) in small cell lung cancer. The Early Clinical Trials Group of the EORTC. *Eur J Cancer* 1994;30A(8):1058–1060.

104. Seibel NL, Blaney SM, O'Brien M, Krailo M, Hutchinson R, Mosher RB, et al. Phase I trial of docetaxel with filgrastim support in pediatric patients with refractory solid tumors: a collaborative Pediatric Oncology Branch, National Cancer Institute and Children's Cancer Group trial. *Clin Cancer Res* 1999; 5(4):733–737.

105. Blaney SM, Seibel NL, O'Brien M, Reaman GH, Berg SL, Adamson PC, et al. Phase I trial of docetaxel administered as a 1-hour infusion in children with refractory solid tumors: a collaborative pediatric branch, National Cancer Institute and Children's Cancer Group trial. *J Clin Oncol* 1997; 15(4):1538–1543.

106. Kavanagh JJ. Docetaxel in the treatment of ovarian cancer. *Oncology* 2002; 16 (6 Suppl):73–82.

107. Schull B, Kornek GV, Schmid K, Raderer M, Hejna M, Lenauer A, et al. Effective combination chemotherapy with bimonthly docetaxel and cisplatin with or without hematopoietic growth factor support in patients with advanced gastroesophageal cancer. *Oncology* 2003; 65(3):211–217.

108. Haller DG, Misset JL. Docetaxel in advanced gastric cancer. *Anticancer Drugs* 2002; 13(5):451–460.

109. Einzig AI, Schuchter LM, Recio A, Coatsworth S, Rodriquez R, Wiernik PH. Phase II trial of docetaxel (Taxotere) in patients with metastatic melanoma previously untreated with cytotoxic chemotherapy. *Med Oncol* 1996; 13(2):111–117.

110. McCaffrey JA, Hilton S, Mazumdar M, Sadan S, Kelly WK, Scher HI, et al. Phase II trial of docetaxel in patients with advanced or metastatic transitional-cell carcinoma. *J Clin Oncol* 1997; 15(5):1853–1857.

111. de Wit R, Kruit WH, Stoter G, de Boer M, Kerger J, Verweij J. Docetaxel (Taxotere): an active agent in metastatic urothelial cancer; results of a phase II study in non-chemotherapy-pretreated patients. *Br J Cancer* 1998; 78(10):1342–1345.

112. Dimopoulos MA, Deliveliotis C, Moulopoulos LA, Papadimitriou C, Mitropoulos D, Anagnostopoulos A, et al. Treatment of patients with metastatic urothelial carcinoma and impaired renal function with single-agent docetaxel. *Urology* 1998; 52(1):56–60.

113. Pectasides D, Visvikis A, Aspropotamitis A, et al. Chemotherapy with cisplatin, epirubicin and docetaxel in transitional cell urothelial cancer. Phase II trial. *Eur J Cancer* 2000; 36(1):74–79.

114. Sengelov L, Kamby C, Lund B, Engelholm SA. Docetaxel and cisplatin in metastatic urothelial cancer: a phase II study. *J Clin Oncol* 1998; 16(10):3392–3397.

115. Dimopoulos MA, Bakoyannis C, Georgoulias V, et al. Docetaxel and cisplatin combination chemotherapy in advanced carcinoma of the urothelium: a multicenter phase II study of the Hellenic Cooperative Oncology Group. *Ann Oncol* 1999; 10(11):1385–1388.

116. De Muro XG, Marcuello E, Climent MA, Paz-Ares L, Parra S, Guma J, et al. Phase II study of docetaxel and cisplatin in advanced urothelial cancer: preliminary results. *Proceedings of American Society of Clinical Oncology*, 1999 (abstract no. 1306).

117. Couteau C, Chouaki N, Leyvraz S, et al. A phase II study of docetaxel in patients with metastatic squamous cell carcinoma of the head and neck. *Br J Cancer* 1999; 81(3):457–462.

118. Kaye SB, Piccart M, Aapro M, et al. Phase II trials of docetaxel (Taxotere) in advanced ovarian cancer—an updated overview. *Eur J Cancer* 1997; 33(13):2167–2170.

119. Vorobiof DA, Chasen MR, Abratt RP, et al. Phase II trial of single agent taxotere (T) in malignant pleural mesothelioma (MPM) (meeting abstract). *Proc Am Soc Clin Oncol* 2000; 19:578a.

120. Jemal A, Murray T, Samuels A, Ghafoor A, Ward E, Thun MJ. Cancer statistics, 2003. *Cancer J Clin* 2003; 53(1):5–26.

121. D'amico AV, Whittington R, Malkowicz SB, Schultz D, Blank K, Broderick GA, et al. Biochemical outcome after radical prostatectomy, external beam radiation therapy, or interstitial radiation therapy for clinically localized prostate cancer. *JAMA* 1998; 280(11): 969–974.

122. Tannock IF, Osobad D, Stockler MR, et al. Chemotherapy with mitoxantrone plus prednisone or prednisone alone for symptomatic hormone-resistant prostate cancer: a Canadian randomized trial with palliative end points. *J Clin Oncol* 1996; 14(6):1756–1764.

123. Kantoff PW, Halabi S, Conaway M, et al. Hydrocortisone with or without mitoxantrone in men with hormone-refractory prostate cancer: results of the cancer and leukemia group B 9182 study. *J Clin Oncol* 1999; 17(8):2506–2513.

124. Beer TM, Pierce WC, Lowe BA, et al. Phase II study of weekly docetaxel in symptomatic androgen-independent prostate cancer. *Ann Oncol* 2001; 12(9):1273–1279.

125. Picus J, Schultz M. Docetaxel (Taxotere) as monotherapy in the treatment of hormone-refractory prostate cancer: preliminary results. *Semin Oncol* 1999; 26(5 Suppl 17):14–18.

126. Friedland D, Cohen J, Miller R Jr, Voloshin M, Gluckman R, Lembersky B, et al. A phase II trial of docetaxel (Taxotere) in hormone-refractory prostate cancer: correlation of antitumor effect to phosphorylation of Bcl-2. *Semin Oncol* 1999; 26(5 Suppl 17):19–23.

127. Berry W, Dakhil S, Gregurich MA, Asmar L. Phase II trial of single-agent weekly docetaxel in hormone-refractory, symptomatic, metastatic carcinoma of the prostate. *Semin Oncol* 2001; 28(4 Suppl 15): 8–15.

128. Savarese DM, Halabi S, Hars V, Akerley WL, Taplin ME, Godley PA, et al. Phase II study of docetaxel, estramustine, and low-dose hydrocortisone in men with hormone-refractory prostate cancer: a final report of CALGB 9780. Cancer and Leukemia Group B. *J Clin Oncol* 2001; 19(9):2509–2516

129. Petrylak DP, Macarthur R, O'Connor J, Shelton G, Weitzman A, Judge T, et al. Phase I/II studies of docetaxel (Taxotere) combined with estramustine in men with hormone-refractory prostate cancer. *Semin Oncol* 1999; 26(5 Suppl 17):28–33.

130. Natale R, Zarestsky S. Phase I/II trial of estramustine (E) and taxotere (T) in patients with metastatic hormone-refractory prostate cancer (HRPC). (Meeting abstract). *American Society of Clinical Oncology* Annual Meeting, 1999 (abstract no. 1343).

131. Kosty MP, Ferreira A, Bryntesen A. Weekly docetaxel and low-dose estramustine phosphate in hormone refractory prostate cancer: a phase II study. *Amercan Society of Clinical Oncology* Annual Meeting, 2001 (abstract no. 2360).

132. Scholz MC, Guess B, Barrios F, Strum S, Leibowitz R. Low-dose single-agent weekly docetaxel (taxotere) is effective and well tolerated in elderly men with prostate cancer. *American Society of Clinical Oncology* Annual Meeting, 2001 (abstract no. 2441).

133. Gulley J, Dahut W. Novel clinical trials in androgen-independent prostate cancer. *Clin Prostate Cancer* 2002; 1(1):51–57.

134. Yonou H, Yokose T, Kamijo T, Kanomata N, Hasebe T, Nagai K, et al. Establishment of a novel species- and tissue-specific metastasis model of human prostate cancer in humanized non-obese diabetic/severe combined immunodeficient mice engrafted with human adult lung and bone. *Cancer Res* 2001; 61(5):2177–2182.

135. Thalmann GN, Anezinis PE, Chang SM, Zhau HE, Kim EE, Hopwood VL, et al. Androgen-independent cancer progression and bone metastasis in the LNCaP model of human prostate cancer. *Cancer Res* 1994; 54(10):2577–2581.

136. Soos G, Jones RF, Haas GP, Wang CY. Comparative intraosseal growth of human prostate cancer cell lines LNCaP and PC-3 in the nude mouse. *Anticancer Res* 1997; 17(6D):4253–4258.

137. Gleave ME, Hsieh JT, Gao C, von Eschenbach AC, Chung LWK. Acceleration of human prostate carcinoma growth in vivo by factors produced by prostate and bone fibroblasts. *Cancer Res* 1991; 51: 375–3761.

138. Gleave ME, Hsieh JT, von Eschenbach AC, Chung LWK. Prostate and bone fibroblasts induce human prostate cancer growth in vivo: Implications for bidirectional stromal-epithelial interaction in prostate carcinoma growth and metastasis. *J Urol* 1992; 147:1151–1159.

139. Pettaway CA, Pathak S, Greene G, Ramirez E, Wilson MR, Killion JJ, et al. Selection of highly metastatic variants of different human prostatic carcinomas using orthotopic implantation in nude mice. *Clin Cancer Res* 1996; 2(9):1627–1636.

140. Chung LWK. Prostate carcinoma bone-stroma interaction and its biologic and therapeutic implications. *Cancer* 2003; 97(Suppl. 3):772–778.

141. Nelson JB, Carducci MA. The role of endothelin-1 and endothelin receptor antiagonists in prostate cancer. *BJU Int.* 2000; 85(Suppl 2):45–48.

142. Hobisch A, Eder IE, Putz T, Horninger W, Bartsch G, Klocker H, et al. Interleukin-6 regulates prostate-specific protein expression in prostate carcinoma cells by activation of the androgen receptor. *Cancer Res* 1998; 58:4640–4645.

143. Blaszczyk N, Masri BA, Mawji NR, Ueda T, McAlinden G, Duncan CP, et al. Osteoblast-derived factors induce androgen-independent proliferation and expression of prostate-specific antigen in human prostate cancer cells. *Clin Cancer Res* 2004; 10(5):1860–1869.

144. Leaf AN, Propert K, Corcoran C, Catalano PJ, Trump DL, Harris JE, et al. Phase III study of combined chemohormonal therapy in metastatic prostate cancer (ECOG 3882): an Eastern Cooperative Oncology Group study. *Med Oncol* 2003; 20(2):137–146.

145. Small EJ, Bok R, Reese DM, Sudilovsky D, Frohlich M. Docetaxel, estramustine, plus trastuzumab in patients with metastatic androgen-independent prostate cancer. *Semin Oncol* 2001; 28(4 Suppl 15): 71–76.

146. Hudes G, Einhorn L, Ross E, Balsham A, Loehrer P, Ramsey H, et al. Vinblastine versus vinblastine plus oral estramustine phosphate for patients with hormone-refractory prostate cancer: a Hoosier Oncology Group and Fox Chase Network phase III trial. *J Clin Oncol* 1999; 17(10):3160–3166.

147. Saxman S, Ansarai R, Drasga R, et al. Phase III trial of cyclophosphamide versus cyclophosphamide, doxorubicin, and methotrexate in hormone-refractory prostatic cancer. A Hoosier Oncology Group study. *Cancer* 1992; 70:2488–2492.

148. Hussain M, Petrylak D, Fisher E, Tangen C, Crawford D. Docetaxel (Taxotere) and estramustine versus mitoxantrone and prednisone for hormone-refractory prostate cancer: scientific basis and design of Southwest Oncology Group Study 9916. *Semin Oncol* 1999; 26(5 Suppl 17):55–60.

149. Chi KN, Murray RN, Gleave ME, Kuhn J, Izbicka E, Berg K, et al. A phase II study of oblimersen sodium (G3139) and docetaxel (D) in patients (pts) with metastatic hormone-refractory prostate cancer (HRPC). *Proc Am Soc Clin Oncol* 2001; 22:393 (abstract no. 1580).

150. Beer TM, Hough KM, Garzotto M, Pierce WC, Lowe BA, Henner D. Treatment of Androgen-Independent Prostate Cancer with Weekly High-Dose Calcitriol and Docetaxel. *Proc Am Soc Clin Oncol* 2001 (abstract no. 2369).

151. Gleave M, Nelson C, Chi K. Antisense targets to enhance hormone and cytotoxic therapies in advanced prostate cancer. *Curr Drug Targets* 2003; 4(3):209–221.

152. Krajewska M, Krajewski S, Epstein JI, Shabaik A, Sauvageot J, Song K, et al. Immunohistochemical analysis of bcl-2, bax, bcl-X, and mcl-1 expression in prostate cancers. *Am J Pathol* 1996; 148(5): 1567–1576.

153. Bubendorf L, Sauter G, Moch H, Jordan P, Blochlinger A, Gasser TC, et al. *Am J Pathol* 1996; 148(5): 1557–1565.

154. Raffo AJ, Perlman H, Chen MW, Day ML, Steitman JS, Buttyan R. Overexpression of bcl-2 protects prostate cancer cells from apoptosis in vitro and confers resistance to androgen depletion in vivo. *Cancer Res* 1995; 55(19):4438–4445.

155. Stattin P, Damber JE, Karlberg L, Nordgren H, Bergh A. Bcl-2 immunoreactivity in prostate tumorigenesis in relation to prostatic intraepithelial neoplasia, grade, hormonal status, metastatic growth and survival. *Urol Res* 1996; 24(5):257–264.

156. McDonnell TJ, Troncoso P, Brisbay SM, Logothetis C, Chung LW, Hsiesh JT, et al. Expression of the protooncogene bcl-2 in the prostate and its association with emergence of androgen-independent prostate cancer. *Cancer Res* 1992; 52(24):6940–6944.

157. Colombel M, Symmans F, Gil S, O'Toole KM, Chopin D, Benson M, et al. Detection of the apoptosis-suppressing oncoprotein bcl-2 in hormone-refractory human prostate cancers. *Am J Pathol* 1993; 143(2):390–400.

158. Rosser CJ, Reyes A O, Vakar-Lopez F, Levy LB, Kuban DA, Hoover DC, et al. Bcl-2 is significantly overexpressed in localized radio-recurrent prostate carcinoma, compared with localized radio-naïve prostate carcinoma. *Int J Radiation Oncol Biol Phys* 2003; 56(1):1–6.

159. Pollack A, Cowen D, Troncoso P, Zagars GK, von Eschenbach AC, Meistrich ML, et al. Molecular markers of outcome after radiotherapy in patients with prostate carcinoma: Ki-67, bcl-2, bax, and bcl-x. *Cancer* 2003; 97(1):1630–1638.

160. Bauer JJ, Sesterhenn IA, Mostofi FK, McLeod DG, Srivastava S, Moul JW. Elevated levels of apoptosis regulator proteins p53 and bcl-2 are independent prognostic biomarkers in surgically treated clinically localized prostate cancer. *J Urol* 1996; 156(4):1511–1516.

161. Gleave M, Tolcher A, Miyake H, Nelson C, Brown B, Beraldi E, Goldie J. Progression to androgen independence is delayed by adjuvant treatment with antisense Bcl-2 oligodeoxynucleotides after castration in the LNCaP prostate tumor model. *Clin Cancer Res* 1999; 5(10): 2891–2898.

162. Miayake H, Tolcher A, Gleave ME. Chemosensitization and delayed androgen-independent recurrence of prostate cancer with the use of antisense Bcl-2 oligodeoxynucleotides. *J Natl Cancer Inst* 2000; 92(1):34–41.

163. Tolcher AW. Preliminary phase I results of G3139 (bcl-2 antisense oligonucleotide) therapy in combination with docetaxel in hormone-refractory prostate cancer. *Semin Oncol* 2001; 28(4 Suppl 15):67–70.

164. Chi KN, Gleave ME, Klasa R, Murray N, Bryce C, Lopes de Menezes, DE, et al. A phase I dose-finding study of combined treatment with an antisense Bcl-2 oligonucleotide (Genasense) and mitoxantrone in patients with metastatic hormone-refractory prostate cancer. *Clin Cancer Res* 2001; 7(12):3920–3927.

165. Steinberg J, Oyasu R, Lang S, Sintich S, Rademaker A, Lee C, et al. Intracellular levels of SGP-2 (clusterin) correlate with tumor grade in prostate cancer. *Clin Cancer Res* 1997; 3:1807–1811

166. Gleave ME, Zellweger T, Chi K, Miyake H, Kiyama S, July L, et al. Targeting anti-apoptotic genes upregulated by androgen withdrawal using antisense oligonucleotides to enhance androgen- and chemo-sensitivity in prostate cancer. *Invest New Drugs* 2002; 20(2):145–158.

167. Gleave M, Miyake H, Zangemeister-Wittke U, Jansen B. Antisense therapy: current status in prostate cancer and other malignancies. *Cancer Metastasis Rev* 2002; 21(1):79–92.

168. Jenne DE, Tschopp J. Clusterin: the intriguing guises of a widely expressed glycoprotein. *Trends Biochem Sci* 1992; 17(4):154–159.

169. Sensibar JA, Sutkowski DM, Raffo A, Buttyan R, Griswold MD, Sylvester SR, et al. Prevention of cell death induced by tumor necrosis factor alpha in LNCaP cells by overexpression of sulfated glycoprotein-2 (clusterin). *Cancer Res* 1995; 55:2431–2437.

170. Zhou W, Janulis L, Park II, Lee C. A novel anti-proliferative property of clusterin in prostate cancer cells. *Life Sci* 2002; 72(1):11–21.

171. Bettuzzi S, Hiipakka RA, Gilna P, Liao ST. Identification of an androgen-repressed mRNA ventral prostate as coding for mulphated glycoprotein 2 by cDNA cloning and sequence analysis. *Biochem J* 1989; 257:293–296.

172. Scaltriti M, Brausi M, Amorosi A, Caporali A, D'Arca D, Astancolle S, et al. Clusterin (SGP-2, ApoJ) expression is downregulated in low- and high-grade human prostate cancer. *Int J Cancer* 2004; 108:23–30.

173. Miyake H, Nelson C. Rennie PS, Gleave ME. Testosterone-repressed prostate message-2 is an antiapoptotic gene involved in progression to androgen-independence in prostate cancer. *Cancer Res* 2000; 60(1):170–176.

174. Gleave ME, Miyake H, Zellweger T, Chi K, July L, Nelson C, et al. Use of antisense oligonucleotides targeting the antiapoptotic gene, clusterin/testosterone-repressed prostate message 2, to enhance androgen sensitivity and chemosensitivity in prostate cancer. *Urology* 2001; 58(2 Suppl 1):39–49.

175. Miyake H, Nelson C, Rennie PS, Gleave ME. Acquisition of chemoresistant phenotype by overexpression of the antiapoptotic gene testosterone-repressed prostate message-2 in prostate cancer xenograft models. *Cancer Res* 2000; 60(9):2547–2554.

176. Zellweger T, Miyake H, July LV, Akbari M, Kiyama S, Gleave ME. Chemosensitization of human renal cell cancer using antisense oligonucleotides targeting the antiapoptotic gene clusterin. *Neoplasia* 2001; 3(4):360–367.

177. Zellweger T, Kiyama S, Chi K, Miyake H, Adomat H, Skov K, et al. Overexpression of the cytoprotective protein clusterin decreases radiosensitivity in the human LNCaP prostate tumour model. *BJU Int* 2003; 92(4):463–469.

178. July LV, Beraldi E, So AI, Evans K, English J, Fazli L, Gleave ME. Nucleotide-based therapies targeting clusterin chemosensitizes human lung adenocarcinoma cells both in vitro and in vivo. *Molec Cancer Ther* 2004; 3:223–232.

179. Moschos SJ, Mantzoros CS. The role of the IGF system in cancer: from basic to clinical studies and clinical applications. *Oncology* 2002; 63(4):317–332.

180. Moore MG, Wetterau LA, Francis MJ, Peehl DM, Cohen P. Novel stimulatory role for insulin-like growth factor binding protein-2 in prostate cancer cells. *Int J Cancer* 2003; 105(1):14–19.

181. Kiyama S, Morrison K, Zellweger T, Akbari M, Cox M, Yu D, et al. Castration-induced increases in insulinlike growth factor-binding protein-2 promotes proliferation of androgen-independent human prostate LNCaP tumors. *Cancer Res* 2003; 63:3575–3584.

182. Yu H, Nicar MR, Shi R, Berkel HJ, Nam R, Trachtenberg J, et al. Levels of insulin-like growth factor (IGF-1) and IGF binding proteins 2 and 3 in serial postoperative serum samples and riskof prostate cancer recurrence. *Urology* 2001; 57(3):471–475.

183. Mita K, Nakahara M, Usui T. Expression of the insulin-like growth factor system and cancer progression in hormone-treated prostate cancer patients. *Int J Urology* 2000; 7(9):321–329.

184. Shariat SF, Lamb DJ, Kattan MW, Nguyen C, Kim J, Beck J, et al. Association of preoperative plasma levels of insulin-like growth factor I and insulin-like growth factor binding proteins-2 and -3 with prostate cancer invasion, progression, and metastasis. *J Clin Oncol* 2002; 20(3):833–841.

185. Gleave M, Jansen B. Clusterin and IGFBPs as antisense targets in prostate cancer. *Ann NY Acad Sci* 2003; 1002:95–104.

186. Sweeney P, Karashima T, Kim SJ, Kedar D, Mian B, Huang S, et al. Anti-vascular endothelial growth factor receptor 2 antibody reduces tumorigenicity and metastasis in orthotopic prostate cancer xenografts via induction of endothelial cell apoptosis and reduction of endothelial cell matrix metalloproteinase type 9 production. *Clin Cancer Res* 2002; 8:2714–2724.

187. Woelfle U, Cloos J, Sauter G, Riethdorf L, Janicke F, van Diest P, et al. Molecular signature associated with bone marrow micrometastasis in human breast cancer. *Cancer Res* 2003; 63(18):5679–5684.

188. Kang Y, Siegel PM, Shu W, Drobnjak M, Kakonen SM, Cordon-Cardo C, et al. A multigenic program mediating breast cancer metastasis to bone. *Cancer Cell* 2003; 3(6):537-549.

189. Mantyh PW, Clohisy DR, Koltzenburg M, Hunt SP. Molecular Mechanisms of Cancer Pain. *Nature Rev Cancer* 2002; 2:201–209.

190. Body JJ, Mancini I. Bisphosphonates for cancer patients: why, how, and when? *Support Care Cancer* 2002; 10(5):399–407.

191. Saad F, Schulman CC. Role of bisphosphonates in prostate cancer. *Eur Urol* 2004; 45:26–34.

192. Stepensky D, Kleinberg L, Hoffman A. Bone as an effect compartment: models for uptake and release of drugs. *Clin Pharmacokinet* 2003; 42(10):863–881.

193. Tsushima N, Yabuki M, Harada H, Katsumata T, Kanamaru H, Nakatsuka I, et al. Tissue distribution and pharmacological potential of SM-16896, a novel oestrogen-bisphosphonate hybrid compound. *J Pharm Pharmacol* 2000; 52:27–37

194. Hirabayashi H, Fujisaki J. Bone-specific drug delivery systems: approaches via chemical modification of bone-seeking agents. *Clin Pharmacokinet* 2003; 42:1319–1330.

195. Wang Y, Metcalf CA 3rd, Shakespeare WC, Sundaramoorthi R, Keenan TP, Bohacek RS, et al. Bone-targeted 2,6,9-trisubstituted purines: novel inhibitors of Src tyrosine kinase for the treatment of bone diseases. *Bioorg Med Chem Lett* 2003; 13:3067–3070.

196. Cooper CR, McLean L, Walsh M, Taylor J, Hayasaka S, Bhatia J, et al. Preferential adhesion of prostate cancer cells to bone is mediated by binding to bone marrow endothelial cells as compared to extracellular matrix components in vitro. *Clin Cancer Res* 2000; 6:4839–4847.

197. Nemeth JA, Roberts JW, Mullins CM, Cher ML. Persistence of human vascular endothelium in experimental human prostate cancer bone tumors. *Clin Exp Metastasis* 2000; 18:231–237.

198. Illum L, Davis SS. Targeting of colloidal particles to the bone marrow. *Life Sci* 1987; 40:1553–1560.

199. Gibaud S, Andreux JP, Weingarten C, Renard M, Couvreur P. Increased bone marrow toxicity of doxorubicin bound to nanoparticles. *Eur J Cancer* 1994; 30A(6):820–826.

200. Gibaud S, Demoy M, Andreux JP, Weingarten C, Gouritin B, Couvreur P. Cells involved in the capture of nanoparticles in hematopoietic organs. *J Pharm Sci* 1996; 85(9):944–950.

201. Gibaud S, Weingarten C, Andreux JP, Couvreur P. Targeting bone marrow with the help of polyalkylcyanoacrylate nanoparticles. *Ann Pharm Fr* 1999; 57(4):324–231.

202. Bally MB, Nayar R, Masin D, Cullis PR, Mayer LD. Studies on the Myelosuppressive Activity of Doxorubicin Entrapped in Liposomes. *Cancer Chemother Pharmacol* 1990; 27:13–19.

203. Gibaud S, Rousseau C, Weingarten C, Favier R, Douay L, Andreux JP, et al. Polyalkylcyanoacrylate nanoparticles as carriers for granulocyte-colony stimulating factor (G-CSF). *J Control Release* 1998; 52(1-2):131–139.

204. Shadyro OI, Yurkova IL, Kisel MA. Radiation-induced peroxidation and fragmentation of lipids in a model membrane. *Int J Radiat Biol* 2002; 78(3):211–217.

205. Marathe D, Mishra KP. Radiation-induced changes in permeability in unilamellar phospholipid liposomes. *Radiat Res* 2002; 157(6):685–692.

206. Symon Z, Peyser A, Tzemach D, Lyass O, Sucher E, Shezen E, et al. Selective delivery of doxorubicin to patients with breast carcinoma metastases by stealth liposomes. *Cancer* 1999; 86(1):72–78.

207. Guan WY, Yi WT, Zhi MY, Zhen SS. Experimental research on the use of an antineoplastic drug with a bone implant. *Int Orthop* 1990; 14(4):387–391.

208. Katagiri H, Sato K, Takahashi M, Sugiura H, Yamamura S, Iwata H. Use of adriamycin-impregnated methylmethacrylate in the treatment of tumor metastases in the long bones. *Arch Orthop Trauma Surg* 1997; 116(6–7):329–333.

209. Lebugle A, Rodrigues A, Bonnevialle P, Voigt JJ, Canal P, Rodriguez F. Study of implantable calcium phosphate systems for the slow release of methotrexate. *Biomaterials* 2002; 23(16):3517–3522.

210. Froschle G, Zieron JO, Carl UM, Beck-Bornholdt HP. Combined modality treatment of bone metastases: response of the rhabdomyosarcoma R1H of the rat to postoperative irradiation combined with local release of daunorubicin from acrylic cement. *Radiother Oncol* 1998; 46(3):317–320.

17

Use of Tetracyclines for Bone Metastases

Eric Seidlitz, MSc, Zeina Saikali, PhD, and Gurmit Singh, PhD

1. INTRODUCTION

Tetracyclines are a class of related antibiotic compounds first discovered by retired American botanist Benjamin Duggar (1) in the late 1940s. Duggar extracted a yellowish crystalline compound with unique antibacterial properties, called aureomycin (7-chlortetracycline), from soil found near cemeteries containing *Streptomyces aureofaciens*, a fungallike bacteria of the *Actinomycetales* order. The parent compound, tetracycline, was subsequently produced by the removal of the chlorine atom from aureomycin by catalytic hydrogenation *(2)*. Tetracycline and its semisynthetic derivatives are active against a wide variety of Gram-positive and Gram-negative bacteria, chlamydiae, mycoplasmas, rickettsiae, and protozoan parasites. Although tetracyclines have been used commercially only since the 1950s, earlier civilizations might have unknowingly benefited from their antibiotic properties. Bone samples from 1600-yr-old Nubian (northern Sudanese) mummies have shown evidence of intermittent tetracycline incorporation, apparently from Streptomycetes contamination of grains used to make bread and beer *(3)*. More than

From: *Cancer Drug Discovery and Development*
Bone Metastasis: Experimental and Clinical Therapeutics
Edited by: G. Singh and S. A. Rabbani © Humana Press Inc., Totowa, NJ

50 different antibiotics have been isolated from *Streptomycetes* species, including streptomycin, neomycin, chloramphenicol, and tetracyclines.

2. STRUCTURE–ACTIVITY RELATIONSHIP AND MODE OF ACTION OF TETRACYCLINES

Tetracyclines comprised a linear series of four fused six-member rings to which functional groups are attached *(4)*. The pharmacokinetic properties of tetracyclines are related to the identity of these functional groups. Figure 1 demonstrates the conserved common structure for tetracyclines, and Table 1 lists several functional side-group combinations at the four most common substitution sites. Mainly the result of the oxygen atoms in the B- and C-rings, tetracyclines possess a great tendency toward the formation of complexes with a number of different chemical species. Particularly favorable are interactions with iron, copper, zinc, magnesium, and calcium ions—with the latter thought to be responsible for their strong affinity for localizing to the calcium-rich hydroxyapatite structure of bone *(5–7)*. This osteotropism is so pronounced that tetracyclines have long been used as bone markers in imaging analysis. Semisynthetic derivatives of tetracyclines (e.g., doxycycline and minocycline) were developed primarily to improve water solubility, thus allowing for parenteral administration or to enhance oral absorption *(4)*. More recently, other side-group substitutions have eliminated their antibiotic capabilities altogether *(4,8)*, yet these tetracyclines maintain their characteristic bone-targeting/chelating activities while developing other interesting pharmacologic features *(9–11)*. Table 2 identifies the structural alterations found in several of these chemically modified tetracyclines.

The application and modes of action of tetracyclines as antibiotics have been extensively reviewed *(4,12)*. Their bacteriostatic properties result from the inhibition of protein synthesis in bacterial cells by preventing the attachment of aminoacyl-tRNA to the ribosomal acceptor (A) site *(13–16)*. In recent years, tetracyclines and their derivatives have attracted significant interest in the scientific communitybecause of the discovery of biological activities independent of their antimicrobial properties, many of which are directly relevant to cancer research. These numerous effects include inhibition of tumor cell progression *(17)*, matrix metalloproteinases (MMPs) *(18)*, osteoclast functions *(19)*, inflammation *(20)*, nitric oxide synthase (NOS) expression *(9,21)*, superoxide production *(22–24)* (possibly with increased free-radical scavenging *[25]*), and angiogenesis *(26–28)*, in addition to various effects on neural cells *(29–31)*. Tetracyclines have been used in the treatment of periodontal diseases, but their efficacy in that setting is thought to be related more to anti-inflammatory *(32)* and MMP-inhibitory properties *(33,34)*.

3. EFFECT OF TETRACYCLINES ON TUMOR CELLS

Tetracyclines have shown cytostatic and cytotoxic capacities on tumor cells of many different origins, both in vitro and in animal models. They inhibit the growth of carcinogen-induced tumors *(35)* and T-cell leukemia in rats *(36)*. Doxycycline has been found to be cytostatic to human renal and prostate carcinoma cells, and cytotoxic after prolonged treatment *(37)*. In vitro studies have now confirmed the cytotoxic effects of tetracyclines on a variety of cultured human tumor cell lines, including prostate cancer, breast cancer, osteosarcoma, leukemia, and mesothelioma cells *(38–42)*. Whenever ana-

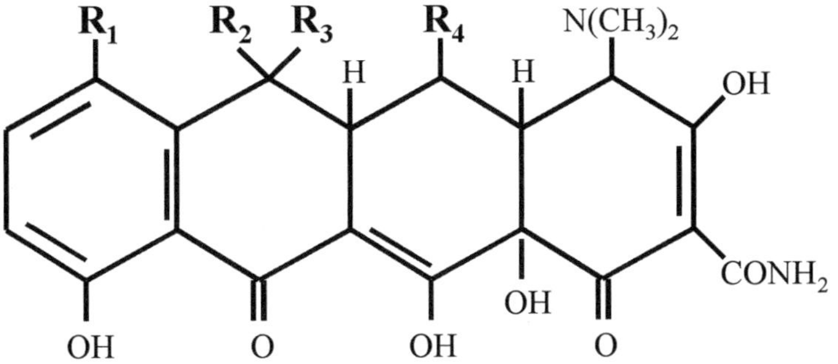

Fig. 1. Conserved chemical structure of tetracyclines (the four rings are identified as A through D, from the right to left).

Table 1
Tetracycline Functional Side Groups

Compound	Trade names	R_1	R_2	R_3	R_4
Tetracycline	Achromycin, Sumycin, Panmycin	H	CH_3	OH	H
Chlortetracycline	Aureomycin, Lymecycline	Cl	CH_3	OH	H
Oxytetracycline	Terramycin, Oxacycline, Clinimycin	H	CH_3	OH	H
Minocycline	Minocin, Vectrin, Klinomycin	$N(CH_3)_2$	H	H	H
Doxycycline	Vibramycin, Hydramycin, Vivox	H	CH_3	H	OH

Table 2
Chemically-Modified Tetracyclines

Compound	R_1	R_2	R_3	R_4	Additional modifications
Tetracycline	H	CH_3	OH	H	
CMT-1	H	CH_3	OH	H	A-ring $N(CH_3)_2$ replaced by H
CMT-2	H	CH_3	OH	H	A-ring $N(CH_3)_2$ replaced by $N(CH_3)_2$ and CONH2 replaced by N
CMT-3 (COL-3)	H	H	H	H	A-ring $N(CH_3)_2$ replaced by H
CMT-4	Cl	CH_3	OH	H	
CMT-5	H	CH_3	OH	H	Nitrogen between C and D rings
CMT-6	H	CH_3	OH	H	A-ring $N(CH_3)_2$ replaced by OH
CMT-7	H	CH_3	OH	H	A-ring $N(CH_3)_2$ replaced by H; C-ring O replaced by OH
CMT-8	H	CH_3	H	OH	A-ring $N(CH_3)_2$ replaced by H

lyzed, apoptosis was observed to be occurring in these cells after doxycycline cytotoxic treatment *(39,40)*, and caspase-3 activation has been implicated as the mechanism of induction of apoptosis in a leukemia cell line *(43)*. Doxycycline inhibited the migration of MDA-MB-435 breast adenocarcinoma cells through Matrigel (an invasion assay) *(44)*, whereas CMT-3 inhibits colon cancer cell invasiveness *(17)*. Several tetracyclines have been shown to reduce tumor burden and growth in a nude mouse model of human metastatic breast cancer (45) and in a rat prostate cancer model (Dunning MATLyLu) (8). In an experimental mouse model, malignant cell growth in pleural effusions was suppressed significantly by doxycycline (46). These effects of tetracyclines on tumor cells are usually observed at supra-antimicrobial doses, which may be in part responsible for the adverse effects observed in clinical trials when tetracyclines have been tested as anticancer agents (47–50). In the bone, however, the natural osteotropism of tetracyclines leads to a much higher concentration of the drug than in the circulation, making these cytotoxic doses of tetracyclines easy to achieve in bone tissue while avoiding unwanted side effects.

4. EFFECT OF TETRACYCLINES ON MMPS

The role of MMPs and their inhibitors in bone and in cancer therapy have been extensively reviewed (51–55), including in Chapter 6 in this book. The importance of these enzymes in cancer progression and metastasis is now well established (56). The first documented evidence of MMP inhibition by tetracyclines, specifically minocycline, was of gingival collagenase in diabetic rats (57) and this finding was later confirmed in synovial tissue or fluid of patients treated with minocycline (58). Since then, many groups have found most tetracyclines to inhibit a variety of MMPs. Most interesting in this context is the inhibition by tetracyclines of MMPs produced by tumor cell lines, such as breast and prostate carcinoma cells, osteosarcoma cells, and mesothelioma cells (38–41,59). Several individual MMPs have thus been documented to be affected, including MMP-8 (60) and MMP-1 (61) by doxycycline treatment, MMP-14 by CMT-3 (62) and MMP-2 and MMP-9 by a variety of tetracyclines, including doxycycline and minocycline (38). With regard to the potential mechanism of these effects, it is considered that the chelation of metal ions such as zinc results in the inhibition by tetracyclines of MMPs (14,38).

The inhibition of MMPs by tetracyclines is doubly important for the potential treatment of bone metastases, because MMPs are used by both tumor cells (63,64) and osteoclasts (65) for bone resorption. Similarly to the dose needed for a cytotoxic effect, the inhibitory effect of tetracyclines on MMPs is usually observed at levels higher than can be achieved with standard antibiotic doses. Once again, in the context of bone pathologies such as bone metastases, the necessary concentrations would be easy to achieve because of the osteotropism of tetracyclines.

5. EFFECTS OF TETRACYCLINES ON OSTEOCLASTS AND OSTEOBLASTS

Many effects of tetracyclines on osteoclast function can be explained by their MMP inhibitory activity; however, evidence is accumulating that tetracyclines have other effects on these cells that are independent of MMP inhibition. Additionally, some evidence is also available to show that tetracyclines can modulate some functions in osteoblasts. This literature enhances the potential that tetracyclines have with regard to treatment of bone pathologies such as metastases, but needs to be analyzed with care because of some differences in the effects of various members of the tetracycline family.

The observed effect of tetracyclines on osteoclasts in culture is most often inhibitory, but there are variations depending on the conditions of the experiment, the source of cells, and the type of tetracycline. Chick embryo osteoclasts cultured on devitalized cortical bone are inhibited from exhibiting pit formation by doxycycline and CMT-1 *(66)*. In similar experiments, CMT-8 dose-dependently inhibited mouse osteoclast pit formation *(67)*. These observations could be the result of either inhibition of MMP activity or other effects on these cells such as reduction of osteoclast viability. Effectively, both CMT-3 and doxycycline have been reported to reduce spreading and induce apoptosis in mature rabbit osteoclasts cultured in vitro, whereas CMT-2 and CMT-5 did not have similar effects *(68)*. CMT-1 and minocycline also reduce osteoclast spreading or induce retraction *(69)*. In addition, doxycycline and CMT-3 inhibited the formation of tartrate-resistant acid phosphatase (TRAP)-positive multinuclear cells from osteoblast/bone marrow cocultures, indicative of an inhibition of osteoclastogenesis *(68)*. Similar to the effect observed for CMT-8 *(67)*, both of these agents inhibited the formation of resorption lacunae *(68)*. This indicates that although the inhibition of pit formation by tetracyclines could be the result of the inhibition of MMPs, it could also be the result of the inhibition of osteoclast maturation and/or cell death and of a combination of these multiple effects. The potential mechanism of action of tetracyclines on osteoclasts is not yet clear, although there is the possibility that at least part of their effects might be at the level of calcium signaling *(70,71)*, known to be important in osteoclast function. Although less research on tetracyclines has been done with osteoblasts than with osteoclasts in culture, minocycline has been shown to stimulate the colony-forming efficiency of marrow stromal cells, indicating that this particular tetracycline may aid osteoblast differentiation *(72)*.

These observations from in vitro work with osteoclasts and osteoblasts are backed up by much more data from in vivo work with animal models of osteoclast and osteoblast recruitment and function. An experimental model for postmenopausal osteoporosis is often used in these studies, that of aged rats that have been ovariectomized to induce loss of trabecular bone. Using this model, Williams et al. *(73,74)* have shown that minocycline was able to both increase bone formation and decrease bone loss in trabecular bone. CMT-8 also has this ability in the same rat model, and ultrastructural analysis shows reduced ruffled border formation in osteoclasts in the affected bones *(67)*. Other in vivo models, in particular surgical inducement of bone injury, have shown similar results. Surgery to the maxillary molars, an experimental model of periodontitis, induces osteoclast recruitment to the affected bone areas as part of the repair process. Doxycycline significantly inhibits mononuclear cell influx and the number of osteoclasts colonizing the area of repair in such a model *(75,76)*. This was also observed with minocycline in a similar surgical inducement of bone remodeling, and in addition to the effect of inhibition of osteoclast recruitment, the osteoclasts recruited were also significantly smaller *(77)*. Streptozotocin-induced diabetes in rats leads to osteopenia, and both minocycline and CMT-1 were found to restore osteoblast structure and function in the affected bones *(78,79)*.

Some of these observed in vivo effects might be occurring by a lack of stimulation of osteoclasts by osteoblasts. Effectively, minocycline treatment leads to a decrease in IL-6 expression, the latter being a stimulator of osteoclast differentiation and activation *(72)*. Similarly, CMT-8 has been shown to inhibit IL-6 secretion in a murine osteoblastic cell line, likely by decreasing mRNA stability *(80,81)*. Another possibility discussed earlier is that tetracyclines might be turning off the signaling for recruitment and differentiation of osteoclasts. Knowing that monocytes are the precursor cells of osteoclasts, this possibility is defended by the observation that CMT-3 and doxycycline are cytotoxic toward cells of the monocytic pathway *(82)*.

6. ANTI-INFLAMMATORY EFFECTS OF TETRACYCLINES

The anti-inflammatory effects of tetracyclines are likely mediated through a prostaglandin-based mechanism. Tetracyclines are known to directly inhibit cyclooxygenase-2 (COX-2) production *(10,83)*, and this COX-2 inhibition should theoretically reduce PGE2 levels because the COX-2 enzyme is involved in the synthesis of prostaglandins from arachidonic acid *(84)*. One report, however, indicated that low doses of tetracycline in vitro augmented PGE2 production *(85)* (although high tetracycline levels resulted in no effect on PGE2 levels). Because PGE2 is known to trigger osteoclastic bone resorption *(86)*, this might be one of the mechanisms through which tetracyclines might be able to reduce the destructive effects of prostate and breast cancer metastasis *(75,86-88)*. Further to this, the COX-2 enzyme itself is implicated in enhancing the metastatic spread of colon cancer *(89)* and the promotion of tumor angiogenesis *(90,91)*. Colon cancer cells modified to express high levels of COX-2 also possessed potent matrix-degrading activity, likely the result of increased MMP-2 *(89)*. The combination of a selective COX-2 inhibitor and doxycycline (employed as an MMP-2 inhibitor) produced significant antitumor effects in a human osteosarcoma model *(92)*.

7. EFFECT OF TETRACYCLINES ON NEURAL TISSUE

Tetracyclines also have demonstrated effects on neural cells. Minocycline inhibited the activation of microglia resulting from an induced inflammatory process *(29,30)*. Glial cells are known to be involved in the neurostructural responses to pain stimuli, and although they are also involved to some extent in chronic neuropathic pain, these cells are particularly relevant to advanced bone cancer pain. The number of astroglia found in the spinal cord of rats as a result of chronic pain was found to be dramatically higher when bone degradation was the source of the stimulus *(93)*. A measurable increase in the expression of glial fibrillary acidic protein (a marker for astroglia) in the spinal nerves is thought to be a unique feature of bone pain *(94,95)*. Minocycline has been shown to prevent neuropathic pain, via a glial activation mechanism, but it was unable to reverse the pain after it had been established (31).

8. COMBINED EFFECTS OF TETRACYCLINES IN THE BONE ENVIRONMENT AND FUTURE TREATMENT POSSIBILITIES

As we have seen, tetracyclines not only target themselves specifically to the mineral structures of bone, but they also produce various effects on the cellular components present in the bone microenvironment under normal or pathological conditions. Tetracyclines are bacteriostatic, are tumour cytotoxic, inhibit MMPs, inflammation, and bone degradation, and reduce pain. These effects together provide members of the tetracycline family with the potential for useful activity in a variety of bone-related pathologies. Low-dose doxycycline has already been approved by the Food and Drug Administration for the treatment of adult periodontitis. Our studies in a mouse model of metastatic breast cancer have shown that doxycycline has the potential to reduce tumor burden in the bone *(87)*. This encouraging result has paved the way for a phase II trial of doxycycline in bone metastases prevention in breast and prostate cancer patients at our institute.

An important issue not often addressed is the specificity of some effects to certain members of the tetracycline family and not others. This means that a good delineation of the mechanisms involved in particular pathologies might provide researchers with a better idea as to which tetracycline to select for studies, based on the particular effects of each specific tetracycline. In this regard, comparative analysis of different members of the tetracycline family for variation of effects in the same model system is not always performed but might eventually be required when selecting a drug to use.

Doxycycline is used extensively as a transcriptional activator to provide on/off control over the expression of a wide variety of desired transgenes both in vitro and in vivo *(96)*. Although it has been recently applied in this manner to inhibit angiogenesis in a model of bone cancer metastasis *(97)*, another report demonstrated a significant upregulation of thrombospondin-1 (an endogenous angiogenesis inhibitor) by doxycycline itself *(98)*, suggesting caution when applying tetracyclines to control gene expression in bone- and angiogenesis-related model systems.

REFERENCES

1. Duggar BM. Aureomycin: a product of the continuing search for new antibiotics. *Ann NY Acad Sci* 1948; 51:177–181.
2. Boothe JH, Morton J, Petisi JP, Wilkinson RG, Williams JH. Tetracycline. *J Am Chem Soc* 1953; 75:4621.
3. Bassett EJ, Keith MS, Armelagos GJ, Martin DL, Villanueva AR. Tetracycline-labeled human bone from ancient Sudanese Nubia (A.D. 350). *Science* 1980; 209:1532–1534.
4. Chopra I, Roberts M. Tetracycline antibiotics:mode of action, applications, molecular biology, and epidemiology of bacterial resistance. *Microbiol Mol Biol Rev* 2001; 65:232–260.
5. Lambs L, Venturini M, Decock-Le Reverend B, Kozlowski H, Berthon G. Metal ion-tetracycline interactions in biological fluids. Part 8. Potentiometric and spectroscopic studies on the formation of Ca(II) and Mg(II) complexes with 4-dedimethylamino-tetracycline and 6-desoxy-6-demethyl-tetracycline. *J Inorg Biochem* 1988; 33:193–210.
6. Myers HM, Tochon-Danguy HJ, Baud CA. IR absorption spectrophotometric analysis of the complex formed by tetracycline and synthetic hydroxyapatite. *Calcif Tissue Int* 1983; 35:745–749.
7. Stepensky D, Kleinberg L, Hoffman A. Bone as an effect compartment: models for uptake and release of drugs. *Clin Pharmacokinet* 2003; 42:863–881.
8. Lokeshwar BL, Selzer MG, Zhu BQ, Block NL, Golub LM. Inhibition of cell proliferation, invasion, tumor growth and metastasis by an oral non-antimicrobial tetracycline analog (COL-3) in a metastatic prostate cancer model. *Int J Cancer* 2002; 98:297–309.
9. Amin AR, Attur MG, Thakker GD, Patel PD, Vyas PR, Patel RN, et al. A novel mechanism of action of tetracyclines:effects on nitric oxide synthases. *Proc Natl Acad Sci USA* 1996; 93:14,014–14,019.
10. Patel RN, Attur MG, Dave MN, Patel IV, Stuchin SA, Abramson SB, et al. A novel mechanism of action of chemically modified tetracyclines: inhibition of COX-2-mediated prostaglandin E2 production. *J Immunol* 1999; 163:3459–3467.
11. Ramamurthy NS, Rifkin BR, Greenwald RA, Xu JW, Liu Y, Turner G, et al. Inhibition of matrix metalloproteinase-mediated periodontal bone loss in rats: a comparison of 6 chemically modified tetracyclines. *J Periodontol* 2002; 73:726–734.
12. Cunha BA. New uses for older antibiotics. The 'rediscovery' of four beneficial and cost-effective antimicrobials. *Postgrad Med* 1997; 101(4):68–79.
13. Clark JMJ, Chang AY. Inhibitors of the transfer of amino acids from aminoacyl soluble ribonucleic acid to proteins. *J Biol Chem* 1965; 240:4734–4739.
14. Chopra I, Hawkey PM, Hinton M. Tetracyclines, molecular and clinical aspects. *J Antimicrob Chemother* 1992; 29:245–277.
15. Schnappinger D, Hillen W. Tetracyclines:antibiotic action, uptake, and resistance mechanisms. *Arch Microbiol* 1996; 165:359–369.
16. Brodersen DE, Clemons WM, Jr, Carter AP, Morgan-Warren RJ, Wimberly BT, Ramakrishnan V. The structural basis for the action of the antibiotics tetracycline, pactamycin, and hygromycin B on the 30S ribosomal subunit. *Cell* 2000; 103:1143–1154.
17. Gu Y, Lee HM, Roemer EJ, Musacchia L, Golub LM, Simon SR. Inhibition of tumor cell invasiveness by chemically modified tetracyclines. *Curr Med Chem* 2001; 8:261–270.

18. Uitto VJ, Firth JD, Nip L, Golub LM. Doxycycline and chemically modified tetracyclines inhibit gelatinase A (MMP-2) gene expression in human skin keratinocytes. *Ann NY Acad Sci* 1994; 732: 140–151.

19. Vernillo AT, Rifkin BR. Effects of tetracyclines on bone metabolism. *Adv Dent Res* 1998; 12:56–62.

20. Popovic N, Schubart A, Goetz BD, Zhang SC, Linington C, Duncan ID. Inhibition of autoimmune encephalomyelitis by a tetracycline. *Ann Neurol* 2002; 51:215–223.

21. Trachtman H, Futterweit S, Greenwald R, Moak S, Singhal P, Franki N, et al. Chemically modified tetracyclines inhibit inducible nitric oxide synthase expression and nitric oxide production in cultured rat mesangial cells. *Biochem Biophys Res Commun* 1996; 229:243–248.

22. Gabler WL, Creamer HR. Suppression of human neutrophil functions by tetracyclines. *J Periodontal Res* 1991; 26:52–58.

23. Akamatsu H, Asada M, Komura J, Asada Y, Niwa Y. Effect of doxycycline on the generation of reactive oxygen species: a possible mechanism of action of acne therapy with doxycycline. *Acta Derm Venereol* 1992; 72:178,179.

24. Miyachi Y, Yoshioka A, Imamura S, Niwa Y. Effect of antibiotics on the generation of reactive oxygen species. *J Invest Dermatol* 1986; 86:449–453.

25. van Barr HM, van de Kerkhof PC, Mier PD, Happle R. Tetracyclines are potent scavengers of the superoxide radical. *Br J Dermatol* 1987; 117:131,132.

26. Fife RS, Sledge GW, Jr, Sissons S, Zerler B. Effects of tetracyclines on angiogenesis in vitro. *Cancer Lett* 2000; 153:75–78.

27. Sipos EP, Tamargo RJ, Weingart JD, Brem H. Inhibition of tumor angiogenesis. *Ann NY Acad Sci* 1994; 732:263–272.

28. Tamargo RJ, Bok RA, Brem H. Angiogenesis inhibition by minocycline. *Cancer Res* 1991; 51:672–675.

29. Kempermann G, Neumann H. Neuroscience. Microglia: the enemy within? *Science* 2003; 302:1689,1690.

30. Ekdahl CT, Claasen JH, Bonde S, Kokaia Z, Lindvall O. Inflammation is detrimental for neurogenesis in adult brain. *Proc Natl Acad Sci USA* 2003; 100:13,632–13,637.

31. Raghavendra V, Tanga F, DeLeo JA. Inhibition of microglial activation attenuates the development but not existing hypersensitivity in a rat model of neuropathy. *J Pharmacol Exp Ther* 2003; 306:624–630.

32. Walker C, Thomas J, Nango S, Lennon J, Wetzel J, Powala C. Long-term treatment with subantimicrobial dose doxycycline exerts no antibacterial effect on the subgingival microflora associated with adult periodontitis. *J Periodontol* 2000; 71:1465–1471.

33. Golub LM, Lee HM, Greenwald RA, Ryan ME, Sorsa T, Salo T, et al. A matrix metalloproteinase inhibitor reduces bone-type collagen degradation fragments and specific collagenases in gingival crevicular fluid during adult periodontitis. *Inflamm Res* 1997; 46:310–319.

34. Caton JG, Ciancio SG, Blieden TM, Bradshaw M, Crout RJ, Hefti AF, et al. Treatment with subantimicrobial dose doxycycline improves the efficacy of scaling and root planing in patients with adult periodontitis. *J Periodontol* 2000; 71:521–532.

35. Kroon AM, Dontje BH, Holtrop M, Van den BC. The mitochondrial genetic system as a target for chemotherapy: tetracyclines as cytostatics. *Cancer Lett* 1984; 25:33–40.

36. Van den Bogert C, Dontje BH, Kroon AM. The antitumour effect of doxycycline on a T-cell leukaemia in the rat. *Leuk Res* 1985; 9:617–623.

37. Van den Bogert C, Dontje BH, Holtrop M, Melis TE, Romijn JC, van Dongen JW, et al. Arrest of the proliferation of renal and prostate carcinomas of human origin by inhibition of mitochondrial protein synthesis. *Cancer Res* 1986; 46:3283–3289.

38. Duivenvoorden WC, Hirte HW, Singh G. Use of tetracycline as an inhibitor of matrix metalloproteinase activity secreted by human bone-metastasizing cancer cells. *Invasion Metastasis* 1997; 17:312–322.

39. Fife RS, Rougraff BT, Proctor C, Sledge GWJ. Inhibition of proliferation and induction of apoptosis by doxycycline in cultured human osteosarcoma cells. *J Lab Clin Med* 1997; 130:530–534.

40. Fife RS, Sledge GWJ, Roth BJ, Proctor C. Effects of doxycycline on human prostate cancer cells in vitro. *Cancer Lett* 1998; 127:37–41.

41. Rubins JB, Charboneau D, Alter MD, Bitterman PB, Kratzke RA. Inhibition of mesothelioma cell growth in vitro by doxycycline. *J Lab Clin Med* 2001; 138:101–106.

42. Tolomeo M, Grimaudo S, Milano S, La Rosa M, Ferlazzo V, Di Bella G, et al. Effects of chemically modified tetracyclines (CMTs) in sensitive, multidrug resistant and apoptosis resistant leukaemia cell lines. *Br J Pharmacol* 2001; 133:306–314.

43. Iwasaki H, Inoue H, Mitsuke Y, Badran A, Ikegaya S, Ueda T. Doxycycline induces apoptosis by way of caspase-3 activation with inhibition of matrix metalloproteinase in human T-lymphoblastic leukemia CCRF-CEM cells. *J Lab Clin Med* 2002; 140:382–386.
44. Fife RS, Sledge GW, Jr. Effects of doxycycline on in vitro growth, migration, and gelatinase activity of breast carcinoma cells. *J Lab Clin Med* 1995; 125:407–411.
45. Duivenvoorden WC, Popovic SV, Lhotak S, Seidlitz E, Hirte H. W, Tozer RG, et al. Doxycycline decreases tumor burden in a bone metastasis model of human breast cancer. *Cancer Res* 2002; 62:1588–1591.
46. Wakai K, Ohmura E, Satoh T, Murakami H, Isozaki O, Emoto N, et al. Mechanism of inhibitory actions of minocycline and doxycycline on ascitic fluid production induced by mouse fibrosarcoma cells. *Life Sci* 1994; 54:703–709.
47. Cianfrocca M, Cooley TP, Lee JY, Rudek MA, Scadden DT, Ratner L, et al. Matrix metalloproteinase inhibitor COL-3 in the treatment of AIDS-related Kaposi's sarcoma: a phase I AIDS malignancy consortium study. *J Clin Oncol* 2002; 20:153–159.
48. Ghate JV, Turner ML, Rudek MA, Figg WD, Dahut W, Dyer V, et al. Drug-induced lupus associated with COL-3: report of 3 cases. *Arch Dermatol* 2001; 137:471–474.
49. Rudek MA, Figg WD, Dyer V, Dahut W, Turner ML, Steinberg SM, et al. Phase I clinical trial of oral COL-3, a matrix metalloproteinase inhibitor, in patients with refractory metastatic cancer. *J Clin Oncol* 2001; 19:584–592.
50. Rudek MA, Horne M, Figg WD, Dahut W, Dyer V, Pluda JM, et al. Reversible sideroblastic anemia associated with the tetracycline analogue COL-3. *Am J Hematol* 2001; 67:51–53.
51. Kahari VM, Saarialho-Kere U. Matrix metalloproteinases and their inhibitors in tumour growth and invasion. *Ann Med* 1999; 31:34–45.
52. Hidalgo M, Eckhardt SG. Development of matrix metalloproteinase inhibitors in cancer therapy. *J Natl Cancer Inst* 2001; 93:178–193.
53. Chambers AF, Matrisian LM. Changing views of the role of matrix metalloproteinases in metastasis. *J Natl Cancer Inst* 1997; 89:1260–1270.
54. Yoon SO, Park SJ, Yun CH, Chung AS. Roles of matrix metalloproteinases in tumor metastasis and angiogenesis. *J Biochem Mol Biol* 2003; 36:128–137.
55. Rudek MA, Venitz J, Figg WD. Matrix metalloproteinase inhibitors: do they have a place in anticancer therapy? *Pharmacotherapy* 2002; 22:705–720.
56. Vihinen P, Kahari VM. Matrix metalloproteinases in cancer:prognostic markers and therapeutic targets. *Int J Cancer* 2002; 99:157–166.
57. Golub LM, Lee HM, Lehrer G, Nemiroff A, McNamara TF, Kaplan R, et al. Minocycline reduces gingival collagenolytic activity during diabetes. Preliminary observations and a proposed new mechanism of action. *J Periodontal Res* 1983; 18:516–526.
58. Greenwald RA, Golub LM, Lavietes B, Ramamurthy NS, Gruber B, Laskin RS, et al. Tetracyclines inhibit human synovial collagenase in vivo and in vitro. *J Rheumatol* 1987; 14:28–32.
59. Fife RS, Sledge GW, Jr. Effects of doxycycline on in vitro growth, migration, and gelatinase activity of breast carcinoma cells. *J Lab Clin Med* 1995; 125:407–411.
60. Hanemaaijer R, Sorsa T, Konttinen YT, Ding Y, Sutinen M, Visser H, et al. Matrix metalloproteinase-8 is expressed in rheumatoid synovial fibroblasts and endothelial cells. Regulation by tumor necrosis factor-alpha and doxycycline. *J Biol Chem* 1997; 272:31,504–31,509.
61. Cakir Y, Hahn KA. Direct action by doxycycline against canine osteosarcoma cell proliferation and collagenase (MMP-1) activity in vitro. *In Vivo* 1999; 13:327–331.
62. Lee HM, Golub LM, Cao J, Teronen O, Laitinen M, Salo T, et al. CMT-3, a non-antimicrobial tetracycline (TC), inhibits MT1-MMP activity: relevance to cancer. *Curr Med Chem* 2001; 8:257–260.
63. Sanchez-Sweatman OH, Lee J, Orr FW, Singh G. Direct osteolysis induced by metastatic murine melanoma cells: role of matrix metalloproteinases. *Eur J Cancer* 1997; 33:918–925.
64. Sanchez-Sweatman OH, Orr FW, Singh G. Human metastatic prostate PC3 cell lines degrade bone using matrix metalloproteinases. *Invasion Metastasis* 1998; 18:297–305.
65. Duivenvoorden WC, Lhotak S, Lee F, Tozer RG, Hirte HW, Singh G. Bone metastasis in human breast and prostate cancer: involvement of matrix metalloproteinases. *Recent Res Devel Cancer* 2000; 2:115–141.
66. Chowdhury MH, Moak SA, Rifkin BR, Greenwald RA. Effect of tetracyclines which have metalloproteinase inhibitory capacity on basal and heparin-stimulated bone resorption by chick osteoclasts. *Agents Actions* 1993; 40:124–128.

67. Sasaki T, Ohyori N, Debari K, Ramamurthy NS, Golub LM. Effects of chemically modified tetracycline, CMT-8, on bone loss and osteoclast structure and function in osteoporotic states. *Ann NY Acad Sci* 1999; 878:347–360.
68. Bettany JT, Peet NM, Wolowacz RG, Skerry TM, Grabowski PS. Tetracyclines induce apoptosis in osteoclasts. *Bone* 2000; 27:75–80.
69. Zaidi M, Moonga BS, Huang CL, Towhidul Alam AS, Shankar VS, Pazianas M, et al. The effect of tetracyclines on quantitative measures of osteoclast morphology. *Biosci Rep* 1993; 13:175–182.
70. Bax CM, Shankar VS, Towhidul Alam AS, Bax BE, Moonga BS, Huang CL, et al. Tetracyclines modulate cytosolic Ca2+ responses in the osteoclast associated with "Ca2+ receptor" activation. *Biosci Rep* 1993; 13:169–174.
71. Donahue HJ, Iijima K, Goligorsky MS, Rubin CT, Rifkin BR. Regulation of cytoplasmic calcium concentration in tetracycline-treated osteoclasts. *J Bone Miner Res* 1992; 7:1313–1318.
72. Williams S, Barnes J, Wakisaka A, Ogasa H, Liang CT. Treatment of osteoporosis with MMP inhibitors. *Ann NY Acad Sci* 1999; 878:191–200.
73. Williams S, Wakisaka A, Zeng QQ, Barnes J, Martin G, Wechter WJ, et al. Minocycline prevents the decrease in bone mineral density and trabecular bone in ovariectomized aged rats. *Bone* 1996; 19: 637–644.
74. Williams S, Wakisaka A, Zeng QQ, Barnes J, Seyedin S, Martin G, et al. Effect of minocycline on osteoporosis. *Adv Dent Res* 1998; 12:71–75.
75. Bezerra MM, Brito GA, Ribeiro RA, Rocha FA. Low-dose doxycycline prevents inflammatory bone resorption in rats. *Braz J Med Biol Res* 2002; 35:613–616.
76. Grevstad HJ, Boe OE. Effect of doxycycline on surgically induced osteoclast recruitment in the rat. *Eur J Oral Sci* 1995; 103:156–159.
77. Klapisz-Wolikow M, Saffar JL. Minocycline impairment of both osteoid tissue removal and osteoclastic resorption in a synchronized model of remodeling in the rat. *J Cell Physiol* 1996; 167:359–368.
78. Sasaki T, Kaneko H, Ramamurthy NS, Golub LM. Tetracycline administration restores osteoblast structure and function during experimental diabetes. *Anat Rec* 1991; 231:25–34.
79. Sasaki T, Ramamurthy NS, Golub LM. Tetracycline administration increases collagen synthesis in osteoblasts of streptozotocin-induced diabetic rats: a quantitative autoradiographic study. *Calcif Tissue Int* 1992; 50:411–419.
80. Kirkwood K, Martin T, Andreadis ST, Kim YJ. Chemically modified tetracyclines selectively inhibit IL-6 expression in osteoblasts by decreasing mRNA stability. *Biochem Pharmacol* 2003; 66:1809–1819.
81. Kirkwood KL, Golub LM, Bradford PG. Non-antimicrobial and antimicrobial tetracyclines inhibit IL-6 expression in murine osteoblasts. *Ann NY Acad Sci* 1999; 878:667–670.
82. Bettany JT, Wolowacz RG. Tetracycline derivatives induce apoptosis selectively in cultured monocytes and macrophages but not in mesenchymal cells. *Adv Dent Res* 1998; 12:136–143.
83. Yrjanheikki J, Tikka T, Keinanen R, Goldsteins G, Chan PH, Koistinaho J. A tetracycline derivative, minocycline, reduces inflammation and protects against focal cerebral ischemia with a wide therapeutic window. *Proc Natl Acad Sci USA* 1999; 96:13,496–13,500.
84. Garavito RM, Mulichak AM. The structure of mammalian cyclooxygenases. *Annu Rev Biophys Biomol Struct* 2003; 32:183–206.
85. Attur MG, Patel RN, Patel PD, Abramson SB, Amin AR. Tetracycline up-regulates COX-2 expression and prostaglandin E2 production independent of its effect on nitric oxide. *J Immunol* 1999; 162: 3160–3167.
86. Robinson DR, Tashjian AH, Jr, Levine L. Prostaglandin-stimulated bone resorption by rheumatoid synovia. A possible mechanism for bone destruction in rheumatoid arthritis. *J Clin Invest* 1975; 56: 1181–1188.
87. Duivenvoorden WC, Popovic SV, Lhotak S, Seidlitz E, Hirte HW, Tozer RG, et al. Doxycycline decreases tumor burden in a bone metastasis model of human breast cancer. *Cancer Res* 2002; 62: 1588–1591.
88. Saikali Z, Singh G. Doxycycline and other tetracyclines in the treatment of bone metastasis. *Anticancer Drugs* 2003; 14:773–778.
89. Tsujii M, Kawano S, DuBois RN. Cyclooxygenase-2 expression in human colon cancer cells increases metastatic potential. *Proc Natl Acad Sci USA* 1997; 94:3336–3340.
90. Tsujii M, Kawano S, Tsuji S, Sawaoka H, Hori M, DuBois RN. Cyclooxygenase regulates angiogenesis induced by colon cancer cells. *Cell* 1998; 93:705–716.

91. Kawai N, Tsujii M, Tsuji S. Cyclooxygenases and colon cancer. *Prostaglandins Other Lipid Mediat* 2002; 68–69:187–196.

92. Dickens DS, Cripe TP. Effect of combined cyclooxygenase-2 and matrix metalloproteinase inhibition on human sarcoma xenografts. *J Pediatr Hematol Oncol* 2003; 25:709–714.

93. Garber K. Why it hurts: researchers seek mechanisms of cancer pain. *J Natl Cancer Inst* 2003; 95: 770–772.

94. Sabino MA, Ghilardi JR, Jongen JL, Keyser CP, Luger NM, Mach DB, et al. Simultaneous reduction in cancer pain, bone destruction, and tumor growth by selective inhibition of cyclooxygenase-2. *Cancer Res* 2002; 62:7343–7349.

95. Medhurst SJ, Walker K, Bowes M, Kidd BL, Glatt M, Muller M, et al. A rat model of bone cancer pain. *Pain* 2002; 96:129–140.

96. Zhu Z, Zheng T, Lee CG, Homer RJ, Elias JA. Tetracycline-controlled transcriptional regulation systems: advances and application in transgenic animal modeling. *Semin Cell Dev Biol* 2002; 13:121–128.

97. Peyruchaud O, Serre CM, NicAmhlaoibh R, Fournier P, Clezardin P. Angiostatin inhibits bone metastasis formation in nude mice through a direct anti-osteoclastic activity. *J Biol Chem* 2003; 278: 45,826–45,832.

98. Kalas W, Gilpin S, Yu JL, May L, Krchnakova H, Bornstein P, et al. Restoration of thrombospondin 1 expression in tumor cells harbouring mutant ras oncogene by treatment with low doses of doxycycline. *Biochem Biophys Res Commun* 2003; 310:109–114.

18 Role of Bisphosphonates in Skeletal Metastases

Arif Hussain, MD, and Fred Saad, MD, FRCS

CONTENTS

1. INTRODUCTION

The clinical usefulness of bisphosphonates lie in their ability to inhibit bone resorption, which underlies various pathological conditions ranging from osteoporosis and Paget's disease to hypercalcemia of malignancy and complications associated with cancer metastasis to bone.

Bisphosphonates are analogs of pyrophosphates (P-O-P) in which the central oxygen atom is replaced by a carbon atom, resulting in a P-C-P backbone. Because of this modification, the resulting molecule resists degradation by endogenous phosphatases (such as alkaline phosphatase which, at neutral pH, can hydrolyze inorganic pyrophosphates). Two additional side chains (R1, R2) attach to the central carbon atom, resulting in a number of bisphosphonate derivatives with varying potencies *(1)*.

2. MECHANISMS UNDERLYING BONE METASTASIS

The human skeleton is a dynamic organ, with the dry skeleton (excluding water and fat) representing about 10% of the total body weight. The extracellular component includes an organic phase and a mineral phase; 90–95% of the organic matrix is made up of type I collagen and the mineral component is made up of poorly crystallized hydroxyapatite. Some of the noncollagenous proteins within the organic phase might be involved in mediating bone mineralization. Central to both bone physiology and bone pathology

From: *Cancer Drug Discovery and Development*
Bone Metastasis: Experimental and Clinical Therapeutics
Edited by: G. Singh and S. A. Rabbani © Humana Press Inc., Totowa, NJ

are two cells: the osteoblast and the osteoclast. The osteoblast is of mesenchymal origin, synthesizes the organ matrix, and has receptors for parathyroid hormone (PTH) and 1,25(OH)$_2$ vitamin D. Osteoclasts are derived from granulocyte-macrophage colony-forming units (GM-CFUs) and have receptors for calcitonin. Upon activation, osteoclasts secrete carbonic anhydrase-generated acid via a proton pump. The acid results in dissolution of the mineral component, followed by protease-mediated degradation of the organic matrix. The balance between formation and resorption of bone that normally occurs under physiological conditions is disrupted when the tumor invades and establishes metastatic lesions in the bone.

Because of its vascular supply and rich mileau of bone marrow cell-derived and osteoblast-derived growth factors and cytokines, the bone is a fertile soil for invasion and establishment of metastasis from a variety of tumors. However, not all tumors have a predilection for bone, suggesting that properties inherent to tumors of specific lineages are also important for establishing bone metastasis. Clinically, metastatic bone lesions are considered osteolytic, osteoblastic, or a combination of both, with mixed lesions being the most common. Regardless of the type of lesion seen, activation of osteoclasts is a key feature of bone metastasis. Tumors can secrete certain cytokines, growth factors, or hormones that directly or indirectly stimulate osteoclastic activity by modulating osteoblast to osteoclast signaling. Osteoclast-mediated bone resorption leads to the release of various bone-marrow-derived growth factors (e.g., transforming growth factor [TGF-β], platelet derived growth factor [PDGF], insulin-like growth factors [IGF], bone morphogenetic proteins [BMP]) that, in turn, stimulate the tumor cells. Thus, a feed-forward cycle is created in which the osteoclast plays a central role.

Some of the signaling networks between tumor cells and the cellular components of the bone are being elucidated, potentially providing additional therapeutic opportunities for treating bone metastasis. Several key regulators of osteoclast activity are members of the tumor necrosis factor (TNF)-related family. Receptor activator of NF-κB (RANK), its ligand (RANKL), and osteoprotegerin (OPG, a soluble decoy receptor for RANKL) *(2–6)* are expressed and secreted by bone marrow stromal cells and osteoblasts. RANKL binds to its receptor RANK on osteoclasts, leading to osteoclast activation. On the other hand, OPG inhibits RANKL binding to RANK, thus downmodulating osteoclast activity. Certain tumors can also express RANKL under appropriate conditions. For instance, myeloma cells express RANKL when cocultured with bone marrow stromal cells *(7)*. Bone-derived growth factors such as transforming growth factor (TGF)-β can stimulate tumor cells to secrete parathyroid hormone-related protein (PTHrP), which, in turn, induces osteoblasts to increase secretion of RANKL, resulting in osteoclast activation *(8–11)*. Other tumor-derived and/or host bone marrow cell-derived factors such as macrophage inflammatory protein 1α (MIP1α), interleukin-11 (IL-11), IL-6, and TNF can directly or indirectly enhance osteoclast activity *(12–18)*. These factors can enhance osteoclast activity indirectly by modulating osteoblast function. Another important pathway recently identified in multiple myeloma relates to Wnt signaling *(19)*. Both the Wnt receptor and the low-density lipoprotein receptor-related protein 5 (LRP5) or LRP6 coreceptors are engaged by the Wnt growth factor for cell signaling to occur *(20–22)*. Myeloma cells can secrete molecules like dickkopf 1 (DKK1), which bind to the LRP5 coreceptor, resulting in inhibition of Wnt signaling and osteoblast differentiation *(19)*. Thus, the characteristic osteolytic lesions in multiple myeloma are a consequence of both enhanced osteoclast activation and decreased osteoblast function.

Although bone metastases in multiple myeloma are dominated by osteolytic lesions, most tumors lead to a mixed skeletal response. Prostate cancer is characterized primarily by osteoblastic skeletal lesions. The mechanism(s) of enhanced osteoblast activity in bone metastasis have not been as clearly defined as that for osteoclasts. Several tumor-derived growth factors, such endothelin-1 (ET-1) and certain proteases such as uroki-nase-type plasminogen activator (uPA) and prostate-specific antigen (PSA) have been implicated as direct or indirect stimulators of osteoblasts (23–29). Other studies have suggested that gene expression patterns of prostate cancer cells with a predilection for bone can mimic that of osteoblasts, including expression of an important osteoblast-specific transcription factor Runx2 (Cbfa1) (30). Remarkably, under appropriate conditions, prostate cancer cells in culture can also direct bone mineralization (31). Taken together, these studies reveal that several properties inherent to prostate cancer lead to an osteoblastic response in the skeleton. However, bone-resorption markers are also significantly elevated in metastatic prostate cancer, consistent with prominent osteoclast activity in this disease as well (32–35). Thus, osteoclast activation underlies the pathogenesis of metastatic bone lesions irrespective of their clinical appearance.

3. MECHANISMS OF BISPHOSPHONATE ACTION

By substituting different moieties in the R1 and R2 positions of the P-C-P backbone, a series of bisphosphonates have been developed over the last few decades. In most bisphosphonates, a hydroxyl group (OH) is present in the R1 position (some exceptions include clodronate with chloride [Cl] in the R1 position, and tiludronate with hydrogen [H] in the R1 position). Substitutions in the R2 position have yielded a series of compounds with varying potencies in terms of their antiresorptive activity. First-generation bisphosphonates have simple substitutions in the R2 position (e.g., CH_3 in etidronate, Cl in clodronate). The second-generation bisphosphonates (e.g., pamidronate, alendronate, ibandronate) have different nitrogen (N)-containing alkyl groups in the R2 position, whereas the more recent third-generation compounds (e.g., risedronate, zoledronic acid) have N-containing heterocyclic rings in this position. Introduction of nitrogen into the R2 position has increased the antiresorptive potency of the newer bisphosphonates. Activity was determined by assays of relative inhibition of vitamin D-induced hypercalcemia in thyroparathyroidectomized rats or inhibition of stimulator-induced calcium release from mouse calvaria in culture. The second-generation bisphosphonates are approximately two orders of magnitude more potent than the first-generation compounds, whereas the third-generation bisphosphonates are about two orders more potent than the second-generation derivatives (36,37).

Because of the phosphonic acid groups, the bisphosphonates bind with high affinity to the calcium-containing hydroxyapatite in mineralized bone; this binding is further enhanced by the OH substitution in the R1 position (37–39). High doses of bisphosphonates can cause defects in bone mineralization. With the newer more potent bisphosphonates, effective antiresorption can be achieved with lower doses and they are less likely to cause mineralization defects.

Studies are beginning to shed light on the antiresorptive properties of the bisphosphonates. By binding to mineralized bone, bisphosphonates make osteolysis of bone more difficult by the bone-resorbing osteoclasts. Bisphosphonates also have direct antiosteoclast activities. After initial binding to bone, bisphosphonates are released in the local microenvironment upon osteoclast-mediated resorption and taken up by these cells. The non-nitrogen bisphosphonates (e.g., etidronate, clodronate) form ATP analogs, which are potentially toxic to cells *(40)*. The N-containing bisphosphonates, on the other hand, appear to have a different mechanism of action. These bisphosphonates inhibit the mevalonate pathway, which is involved in the synthesis of sterols like cholesterol and isoprenoids, in a number of cell types *(41)*. The isoprenoids are necessary for the post-translational modification or prenylation of small G-proteins, such as members of the Ras family. Prenylation of the G-proteins is important for their function, including cell localization and integration of extracellular signals to downstream signaling pathways. The N-containing bisphosphonates inhibit a key enzyme called farnesyl pyrophosphate synthase in the complex mevalonate biosynthetic pathway, resulting in decreased farnesylation of Ras *(41,42)*. Regardless of their molecular mechanisms of action, the rapid accumulation of bisphosphonates into the skeleton minimizes their exposure to nonskeletal tissues. Hence, their effects are essentially skeletal-specific, with relatively minimal toxicity to the other tissues.

Bisphosphonates can also inhibit secretion of certain osteoclastogenic growth factors and cytokines (like IL-6) by bone marrow stromal cells, osteoblasts, and host immune cells *(43,44)*. Inhibition of osteoclast-mediated bone resorption prevents release of bone-bound tumor-stimulatory factors such as TGF-β. Because tumors in turn secrete osteoclastogenic factors (e.g., PTHrP, RANKL), inhibition of osteoclast function can break this vicious cycle.

In addition to modulating either directly or indirectly osteoclastic function recent studies, particularly with the newer-generation bisphosphonates, are beginning to demonstrate that they have several other biological effects, at least in vitro and in cell culture systems. For instance, the N-containing bisphosphonates are antiproliferative (causing G_1- or S-phase arrest) or proapoptotic for several tumor types, including myeloma, breast, prostate, and others *(45–47)*. These effects might be further enhanced when they are used in combination with certain anticancer drugs *(48,49)*. Bisphosphonates can also inhibit adhesion of tumor cells to the bone matrix *(50)*. By chelating zinc, which is necessary for the activity of matrix metalloproteases (MMPs), bisphosphonates can block the function of these enzymes and, hence, potentially inhibit extracellular matrix breakdown and tumor invasion *(51)*. Recent data also suggest that the most potent bisphosphonate (i.e., zoledronic acid) has antiangiogenic properties because it can inhibit endothelial cell proliferation and adhesion *(52)*. Furthermore, the N-containing bisphosphonates might have immunomodulatory activity in that they stimulate antitumor cytotoxic T-cells and affect antigen-presenting cell function *(53–55)*. Although many of the pleiotropic effects of the bisphosphonates occur in the micromolar or millimolar range, such concentrations are potentially achievable locally in the bone microenvironment in which they are preferentially concentrated *(56)*. However, at present, it is not clear whether these additional mechanisms of action contribute to the overall activity of the bisphosphonates in the clinical setting.

4. CLINICAL USES OF BISPHOSPHONATES

Several consequences, resulting in significant morbidity, can occur as a result of skeletal metastasis, including pain, hypercalcemia (which might or might not be associated with actual tumor invasion of bone), and other skeletal-related events such as pathological fractures, spinal cord compression, need for surgery to stabilize bone, or radiation to palliate pain or prevent bone-related complications. Also, osteopenia/osteoporosis, which is often induced or exacerbated by some of the anticancer treatments, is being recognized as a potentially important source of morbidity in cancer patients. An important role for the bisphosphonates is being defined in the management of some of these skeletal-related complications.

4.1. Hypercalcemia of Malignancy

Hypercalcemia of malignancy (HCM) is a serious complication associated with advanced stages of malignancy, occurring in 10–20% of cancer patients. As with other malignancy-related skeletal complications, osteoclast activation is a common underlying pathophysiologic mechanism of HCM irrespective of whether or not clinically evident bone metastasis is present. In the absence of clinical metastasis, HCM can occur as a result of the release of soluble factors (e.g., parathyroid hormone-related protein [PTHrP], cytokines) in the circulation by tumor cells that activate osteoclasts. At the other end of the spectrum, enhanced osteoclast-mediated resorption as a result of the local presence of tumor cells in the bone can lead to HCM. Multiple myeloma (MM) is the most common hematologic malignancy associated with hypercalcemia, and breast and lung cancer account for a majority of the nonhematologic HCM cases. Interestingly, although most advanced prostate cancer patients have bone metastasis, hypercalcemia is rare in these men.

In addition to the standard therapies for hypercalcemia, bisphosphonates have become an important component of managing HCM. Etidronate was the first bisphosphonate approved for HCM and is given at 7.5 mg/kg/d over 4 h intravenously for 3 consecutive days *(57)*. Studies comparing pamidronate to etidronate or pamidronate to etidronate or clodronate demonstrated that pamidronate given intravenously was more effective in lowering serum calcium levels than the first-generation compounds *(58,59)*. This, coupled with the more convenient 1-d dosing schedule and less inhibitory effects on bone mineralization, made pamidronate the bisphosphonate of choice for treating HCM *(60,61)*. More recently, zoledronic acid has been compared to pamidronate in HCM in two double-blind, double-dummy controlled trials, and the pooled results reported *(62)*. Two hundred eighty-seven patients with HCM were randomized to one of three arms: 4mg or 8 mg zoledronic acid via 5 min intravenous infusion or pamidronate 90 mg given intravenously over 2 h. By d 10, the proportion of patients achieving normalization of corrected serum calcium (CSC; the primary end point of the study) were 88.4%, 86.7%, and 69.7% for 4 mg and 8 mg zoledronic acid and 90 mg pamidronate, respectively. A greater proportion of patients normalized CSC by d 4 in the zoledronic acid arm than the pamidronate arm (50% vs 33%). The median duration of complete response was 32, 43, and 18 d for 4 mg and 8 mg zoledronic acid and 90 mg pamidronate, respectively *(62)*. Thus, with zoledronic acid, more patients achieved normal serum calcium levels faster and for longer duration than with pamidronate. Based on these results, zoledronic acid was approved for HCM by the US Food and Drug Administration (FDA) in 2001. Although the studies were done with zoledronic acid given at 4 or 8 mg over 5 min, current guidelines for HCM are zoledronic acid 4 mg infused over 15 min. No specific minimal interval between repeat doses has been established, but, if necessary, doses can be repeated; it is generally recommended to wait a minimum of 7 d before giving a repeat dose.

4.2. Other Complications of Bone Metastasis

Although the incidence of HCM is decreasing, other serious complications from tumor invasion to bone often occur. Pain from skeletal metastasis can be a significant problem. Such events as vertebral and nonvertebral pathological fractures (that might or might not require surgical intervention), impending fractures requiring surgical stabilization or radiation, spinal cord compression, and radiotherapy to palliate pain represent a spectrum of potential complications that can occur as a consequence of bone metastasis. Although there have been some variations in the primary and secondary end points used to assess efficacy, in the more recently completed larger-scale randomized trials the impact of bisphosphonates on skeletal-related events (SREs) (pathologic fracture, cord compression, surgery, radiation because of bone metastasis) has been the primary criteria for evaluating their relative effectiveness clinically.

There are several parameters regarding the use of SREs as an end point in evaluating response. For instance, one end point is the proportion of patients experiencing at least one SRE during the period of observation. Using this criterion, a patient experiencing two or more SREs during the observation period would count the same as a patient having only one SRE in the same time period. On the other hand, the skeletal morbidity rate (SMR), defined as the number of SREs per patient per unit time, does not provide information in terms of numbers of patients experiencing SRE, but, rather, indicates the number of SREs experienced by an individual patient over time. Another end point that is often used is the time to first occurrence of an SRE. In addition, a statistical analytic tool, the so-called multiple event analysis that looks at several chosen variables related to the event, can provide a composite view of the event and its risk of occurrence in an individual patient treated on one arm of a trial relative to a control arm (hazard ratio). As an example, some of the bisphosphonate trials have incorporated the total number of SREs, time to first SRE, and interval between SREs into deriving hazard ratios that describe the risk of developing a skeletal complication with respect to the bisphosphonate being tested.

The most common hematologic malignancy associated with bone involvement is multiple myeloma. Of the nonhematologic malignancies, breast and prostate cancer account for the majority (up to 80%) of the tumors metastasizing to bone, with other solid tumors making up the rest. In the following subsections, an overview of the role of bisphosphonates in these malignancies is presented.

4.2.1. Multiple Myeloma

Studies done with oral etidronate have shown that it does not impact the skeletal complications of MM *(63)*. On the other hand, oral clodronate has shown more promise *(64,65)*. In one trial, newly diagnosed myeloma patients were randomized to receive 2400 mg clodronate orally or placebo daily for 2 yr, in addition to standard chemotherapy *(64)*. A significant reduction in the proportion of patients experiencing progression of bone lesions in favor of the clodronate arm was found, although there was essentially no impact on other parameters, such as incidence of fracture, hypercalcemia or analgesia use. In a second randomized trial, newly diagnosed patients received 1600 mg/d clodronate or placebo along with their chemotherapy *(65)*. The incidence of pathologic fracture was decreased with clodronate but no significant differences in terms of performance status or pain were noted between the clodronate and placebo arms.

Oral pamidronate has not proven to be effective in MM *(66)*. By contrast, intravenous pamidronate, given at 90 mg over 4 h every 4 wk, has had a positive impact *(67,68)*. In the pivotal trial, 392 patients with stage III myeloma and at least 1 lytic bone lesion were enrolled *(67)*. About two-thirds of the patients were receiving first-line antimyeloma chemotherapy (stratum 1) and one-third were receiving second-line therapy (stratum 2) at the time of enrollment. Results after 9 mo and 21 mo of treatment have been reported *(67,68)*. At 9 mo, the primary end point of mean number of SREs/yr (i.e., SMR) was 1.1 in the pamidronate arm vs 2.1 in the placebo arm ($p = 0.0006$) *(67)*. Bone pain and analgesic use were also decreased in the pamidronate arm. At 21 mo, the SMR was 1.3 vs 2.2 ($p = 0.008$), proportion of patients with at least one SRE was 38% vs 51% ($p = 0.015$), and median time to first SRE 21 mo vs 10 mo, all in favor of pamidronate over placebo *(68)*. Although overall survival (OS) was not different between the two arms, OS for stratum 2 patients was 21 mo in the pamidronate group compared to 14 mo for placebo ($p = 0.041$), suggesting that in subgroups of patients pamidronate might also impact survival. Based on the above data, intravenous pamidronate received approval by the FDA for use in stage III MM with bone metastasis. Of note is that pamidronate has not been tested directly against clodronate in MM. On the other hand, intravenous pamidronate has recently been compared to zoledronic acid in MM in a randomized trial designed to show equivalence between the two drugs *(69,70)*. At 12 mo and 24 mo of treatment, 4 mg zoledronic acid given intravenously over 15 min decreased the proportion of patients experiencing an SRE and reduced the mean SMR to the same extent as 90 mg pamidronate given intravenously over 2 h *(69,70)*. Further, no differences between the two drugs were found on multiple event analysis *(70)*. Although the two drugs appear equivalent in MM, the shorter infusion time of zoledronic acid offers a potential advantage. Guidelines for the use of bisphosphonates in MM have been published *(71)*.

4.2.2. BREAST CANCER

Many trials with first- and second-generation bisphosphonates have been reported in breast cancer. Here, some of the relevant phase III trials in advanced breast cancer will be reviewed. Oral clodronate at 1600 mg/d has been compared to placebo in patients with advanced breast cancer receiving systemic therapy *(72)*. A significant decrease in skeletal morbidity from 3.05 events/yr to 2.19 events/yr was found. Two separate, placebo-controlled trials of intravenous pamidronate given at 90 mg every 3–4 wk for up to 2 yr have been conducted in women with metastatic breast cancer having at least one untreated bone lesion. In one trial, women were treated with chemotherapy ± pamidronate, and in the second trial women received endocrine therapy with or without pamidronate *(73,74)*. Data from these trials have been reported separately (at 12 and 24 mo of treatment), and after pooling both studies together *(73–76)*. The combined analysis provides an overall picture of the role of intravenous pamidronate in women with breast cancer having bone involvement and receiving standard systemic anticancer therapies *(76)*. The pooled data at 24 mo demonstrates the following: (1) The proportion of women experiencing at least one SRE (excluding HCM) is 51% vs 64% ($p = 0.001$), (2) mean SMR is 2.4 vs 3.7 events/yr, and (3) median time to first SRE is 12.7 mo vs 7 mo for pamidronate vs placebo, respectively *(76)*. Thus, pamidronate has clearly been shown to decrease complications associated with bone metastasis in breast cancer. Guidelines for use of bisphosphonates in breast cancer have been published, and pamidronate as an adjunct to systemic therapies in patients with breast cancer and bone metastasis has become standard *(77)*.

Zoledronic acid has also been evaluated in breast cancer. In particular, 4 mg zoledronic acid given intravenously over 15 min was compared to 90 mg pamidronate given intravenously over 2 h every 3–4 wk in a trial designed to show noninferiority of the former with respect to the latter in women with stage IV breast cancer and at least one skeletal lesion. In both arms, women also received standard systemic therapy for breast cancer. Results have been reported at 12 and 24 mo of treatment *(69,70)*. At 12 mo, zoledronic acid was found to be equivalent to pamidronate in terms of percentage of patients with at least one SRE, median time to first SRE, mean SMR, and relative reduction in pain/analgesic use *(69)*. Interestingly, in the subgroup of women treated with hormone therapy, the mean SMR for radiation to bone decreased significantly in the zoledronic acid group compared to pamidronate (0.33 vs 0.58 events/yr, $p = 0.015$). The extension study demonstrated that zoledronic acid maintained its equivalence to pamidronate at 24 mo of treatment, whereas the multiple-event analysis showed that in the subgroup of women treated with hormone therapy zoledronic acid decreased the individual risk of developing a skeletal complication by 30% (hazard ratio = 0.693, $p = 0.009$) *(70)*. Based on the current data, either pamidronate or zoledronic acid can be used in breast cancer patients with bone metastasis.

4.2.3. PROSTATE CANCER

In contrast to MM and breast cancer, the role of bisphosphonates in metastatic prostate cancer has been less well defined. Small, randomized, placebo-controlled trials failed to show a benefit for etidronate or clodronate in terms of palliating pain in metastatic disease *(78–82)*. A recent study reported on 311 men with hormone-sensitive metastatic prostate cancer randomized to oral clodronate vs placebo for 3 yr *(83)*. A nonsignificant reduction in symptomatic bone progression-free survival in the clodronate group was observed. Subgroup analysis appears to indicate that patients who began bisphosphonate therapy at an earlier stage of the metastatic state did better.

Pooled data from two randomized trials comparing pamidronate (90 mg every 3 wk for a total of 27 wk) to placebo has been presented recently. This study failed to show a benefit for the second-generation bisphosphonate in palliating pain or decreasing analgesic use in men with painful bone metastasis *(84)*. The secondary end points looked at SREs in the pooled study; again, no differences were found between the pamidronate and placebo groups even though bone resorption markers were decreased by pamidronate *(84)*. On the other hand, 4 mg zoledronic acid over 15 min every 3 wk for 15 mo has shown a benefit over placebo in advanced prostate cancer progressing on hormone ablation therapy *(85)*. In this study, the primary endpoint was the proportion of men experiencing SREs (a change in antineoplastic therapy to treat bone pain was also included in the definition of SRE in this trial), whereas evaluation of pain was one of the secondary end points *(85)*. At 15 mo, 33% of the patients on the zoledronic acid arm had at least one SRE compared to 44% on the placebo arm ($p = 0.021$), and this difference was maintained in the extension phase of the study to 24 mo. A statistically significant difference was also noted for the time to first SRE (488 vs 321 d) and the mean SMR favoring zoledronic acid over placebo. Further, patients on the zoledronic acid arm experienced less pain compared to those in the placebo arm throughout the course of the study, and this relative reduction in pain reached statistical significance at several time-points of evaluation (3, 9, 21, and 24 mo) *(86)*. Overall, zoledronic acid reduced the risk of developing a skeletal complication by 36%, with a hazard ratio of 0.640 (95% confidence interval = 0.485–0.845; $p = 0.002$).

Zoledronic acid is the first bisphosphonate approved by the FDA for the treatment of men with prostate cancer and bone metastasis progressing on hormone ablation therapy. A somewhat puzzling aspect of the zoledronic acid trial relates to dosing. Originally, in this trial (and other randomized zoledronic acid trials in bone metastasis) there were two dose levels of zoledronic acid (i.e., 4 mg and 8 mg). However, because of concerns for renal toxicity, the 8-mg dose was decreased to 4 mg in mid-trial and, hence, this arm became a composite of 8-mg and 4-mg doses. The proportion of patients experiencing an SRE in the 8/4-mg arm was lower than in the 4-mg arm and not statistically different compared to placebo *(85)*. This is unexpected in view of the favorable outcome in the 4-mg arm, where men received less total zoledronic acid.

4.2.4. OTHER SOLID TUMORS

Of all the bisphosphonates, zoledronic acid is the only one that has been tested for relative efficacy in bone metastasis from a variety of solid tumors other than breast cancer and prostate cancer in a randomized placebo-controlled fashion *(87,88)*. Patients were treated with zoledronic acid every 3 wk for 9 mo in the core portion of the trial, with an additional 12-mo extension phase. Approximately 50% of the enrolled patients had non-small-cell lung cancer. The median survival of the enrolled group was 6 mo, reflecting the advanced stages of cancer in the trial. Initial efficacy analysis of the 4-mg zoledronic acid arm (257 patients) vs placebo (250 patients) at 9 mo of treatment has been presented *(87)*. The proportion of patients with at least one SRE (excluding HCM) was lower in the zoledronic acid group than in the placebo group (38% vs 44%) but did not reach statistical significance ($p = 0.127$). If HCM is included, then the difference between the two groups did reach statistical significance (38% vs 47%, $p = 0.039$). Zoledronic acid also extended the median time to first SRE (excluding HCM) by 2 mo compared to placebo ($p = 0.023$). From this trial, interesting data in the subgroup of patients with renal cell cancer (RCC) are also emerging *(89)*. Although the total number of patients with RCC enrolled in the trial was small, the time to first SRE was 72 d for the placebo arm and was not reached at 9 mo for the 4-mg zoledronic acid arm ($p = 0.006$). Further, the time to first pathologic fracture was 168 d for the placebo arm, but a fracture event had not yet been reached at 9 mo for 4-mg zoledronic acid ($p = 0.003$). Seventy-four RCC patients, representing about 10% of the total, entered the trial; 26 patients received 4 mg zoledronic acid, 19 received placebo, and the rest were in the 8/4-mg group. These data suggest that zoledronic acid might be particularly beneficial in RCC patients with bone metastasis.

4.3. Side Effects and Adverse Reactions of Bisphosphonates

Gastrointestinal intolerance occurs primarily with oral formulations of bisphosphonates. Nausea and vomiting can also occur with intravenous administration but occurs less frequently. Because of rapid clearance from the circulation after intravenous infusion as a result of uptake by the bone and excretion by the kidneys, exposure to other tissues is limited, which minimizes potential toxicity. The bulk of the excretion by the kidneys occurs within 24 h of drug administration. Both glomerular and tubular mechanisms might be involved in excretion of bisphosphonates by the kidneys. Although the mechanisms are not clearly defined, renal toxicity is a potential concern, possibly because of the rate of intravenous infusion. Flulike symptoms (including fever, chills, arthralgias, myalgias) can occur in a proportion of patients, particularly after the initial dose. However, these symptoms tend to subside with subsequent administration. The levels of certain cytokines such as TNF-α and IL-6 (but not IL-1) can increase in the serum of patients within 24 to 72 h of IV administration *(90)*. The significance of this in the context of the acute phase reaction, however, is not clear because there might be no correlation between serum cytokine levels and the acute symptoms *(90)*. The possibility of metabolic abnormalities, particularly with hypocalcemia and hypophosphatemia, also exists with bisphosphonate use. To minimize this, both calcium and vitamin D supplements were used in the recently conducted large-scale zoledronic acid trials for bone metastasis.

The duration of bisphosphonate therapy for skeletal metastasis has not been clearly defined, although once initiated, patients are generally maintained on it through the course of their disease. Experience suggests that bisphosphonates can be administered to patients for up to 2 yr safely. However, a theoretical concern is that because bisphosphonates become incorporated into bone with very slow turnover, continued accumulation with prolonged use could make the bone less "malleable" and compromise its ability to sustain/respond to stress and strain *(91)*. Further, defects in bone mineralization can occur with continued use, particularly with the earlier generation bisphosphonates.

5. OTHER ISSUES REGARDING BISPHOSPHONATES IN CANCER PATIENTS

Two emerging issues in the context of cancer and bisphosphonates are prevention of bone metastasis in high-risk patients and risk of osteoporosis as a consequence of anticancer therapies. Several recent reviews on bisphosphonates have highlighted these clinically important issues *(92–95)*.

5.1. Prevention Studies

A body of preclinical cell culture and animal data suggests that bisphosphonates could have a role in preventing metastasis to bone *(50,51,96–100)*. Several recent clinical trials in women with breast cancer have begun to address this issue. Despite some differences in the patient populations studied, a common feature of these trials is that the enrolled patients were given the first-generation bisphosphonate clodronate orally for 2–3 yr. In the largest trial of its kind so far, more than 1000 women with operable breast cancer undergoing standard adjuvant therapy received 1600 mg/d clodronate or placebo for 2 yr *(101)*. At a median follow-up of 5 yr there were no statistical differences in the incidence of skeletal or extra-skeletal metastasis, although overall survival appeared to favor the clodronate arm ($p = 0.047$). A smaller randomized trial ($n = 302$) in a more selected population of women with $T_{1-4}N_{0-2}$ breast cancer and tumor cells in the bone marrow (as determined by immunohistochemistry), but without overt skeletal metastasis, has also been reported *(102)*. After initial local therapy (mastectomy or breast-conserving surgery with radiation), women received appropriate adjuvant therapy with or without clodronate at 1600 mg/d for 2 yr *(102)*. Approximately 50% of the enrolled women had no axillary node involvement. At a median follow-up of 3 yr, the incidence of distant metastasis was 50% lower in the clodronate group compared to the nonclodronate group, with a significant decrease in both skeletal and extraskeletal lesions. Further, overall survival favored the clodronate group ($p = 0.001$). In an updated follow-up of the trial, although the statistical difference in visceral metastasis disappeared between the two groups, both the lower incidence of bone metastasis and overall increased survival were maintained in the clodronate group *(103)*. In contrast to this study, another trial of similar size (*n* = 299) in women with breast cancer receiving adjuvant therapy (all had node-positive disease but were not selected for study enrollment according to bone marrow status) ± clodronate (3 yr at 1600 mg/d) showed no benefit to using clodronate *(104)*. Similar rates of skeletal metastasis were found between the clodronate and control groups, whereas the incidence of extra-skeletal metastasis was significantly higher in the clodronate group, which also had poorer overall survival. With the contradictory outcomes of these two trials, the role of clodronate in the adjuvant setting in high-risk breast cancer remains unresolved. Hopefully, the results will be clarified in an ongoing, much larger NSABP–sponsored trial in this patient population.

With the availability of more potent bisphosphonates, it is apparent that much work remains to be done in the area of prevention of skeletal metastasis, not only in breast cancer but also other malignancies. A potential role for zoledronic acid in men with prostate cancer showing elevated PSA levels and undergoing androgen deprivation without overt bone metastasis has been addressed in a randomized trial (primary end point being bone-metastasis-free survival). This trial has since been closed prematurely for a variety of reasons, including issues related to zoledronic acid dosing as well as lower than expected event rates. This underscores the importance of carefully defining the appropriate risk groups and end points in prevention trials.

5.2. Osteoporosis in Cancer

Osteoporosis is being recognized as an increasingly significant problem in patients with cancer, particularly breast and prostate cancer, predisposing them to increased risk of fractures. In premenopausal women with breast cancer, purposeful suppression of ovarian function as part of endocrine therapy, or ovarian dysfunction as a result of systemic chemotherapy, can lead to a decrease in bone mineral density (BMD) and increased risk of osteoporosis. Tamoxifen can also decrease BMD in premenopausal women and can actually increase bone density in postmenopausal women. In postmenopausal women, the basal loss in bone density can be aggravated with use of aromatase inhibitors that further decrease any residual estrogens. Both oral clodronate and risedronate have been shown to decrease the chemotherapy-induced loss in BMD in women with breast cancer *(105,106)*. Several doses and schedules of zoledronic acid have been evaluated in a study of postmenopausal women with low BMD *(107)*. Even with once-a-year dosing, zoledronic acid (4 mg intravenous) was found to increase BMD to levels seen with daily oral bisphosphonate therapy. Potentially, this study provides background data for designing osteoporosis prevention/treatment trials with zoledronic acid in cancer patients.

Significant losses in bone density occur in men with prostate cancer undergoing androgen deprivation. Although oral alendronate has shown efficacy in treating men with osteoporosis from a variety of causes, it has yet to be tested in prostate cancer patients *(108)*. On the other hand, the effects of intravenous pamidronate have been determined in men with prostate cancer and established bone metastasis, as well as in men with locally advanced/recurrent prostate cancer but without bone metastasis *(109,110)*. In the former trial, men had to be on androgen deprivation for at least 6 mo prior to trial entry, whereas in the latter study, men were assigned prospectively to androgen deprivation ± pamidronate. In the former trial, BMD increased when patients received pamidronate and decreased when on placebo *(109)*. The latter trial demonstrated that pamidronate administered at the start of androgen deprivation therapy, and given periodically thereafter (every 3 mo), can prevent androgen-deprivation–induced osteoporosis *(110)*. In a more recent trial in men with MO prostate cancer starting androgen-deprivation therapy, zoledronic acid (4 mg intravenous every 3 mo for 1 yr) was compared to placebo *(111)*. The primary end point of the trial was percentage change in BMD from baseline to the end of study at 1 yr. This study demonstrated that zoledronic acid actually increased BMD during androgen ablation. Although pamidronate and zoledronic acid have not been compared directly, data from the last trial would suggest that zoledronic acid is more effective in that it not only prevents but also increases BMD in the setting of concurrent androgen ablation.

6. CONCLUSIONS

An increasingly greater role for bisphosphonates is being defined in the overall management of patients with advanced cancers. Bisphosphonates are part of the standard therapies used to treat malignancy-associated hypercalcemia. In patients with bone lesions from solid tumors and multiple myeloma, bisphosphonates have become an important adjunct to systemic therapies for treating these malignancies. Randomized trials have demonstrated that this class of compounds can decrease complications, termed SREs, and pain from bone metastases. Recently, more potent bisphosphonate derivatives have been developed and tested. Although recent studies have expanded the use of the most potent bisphosphonates (zoledronic acid) to all solid tumors, their clinical effects are modest. It could be that therapeutic limits have been reached with these compounds. With greater understanding of the pathophysiologic mechanisms underlying bone metastasis, additional targets for treatment are being identified. Conceivably, agents such as anti-PTHrP antibodies, recombinant osteoprotegerin (OPG), MMP, and angiogenesis inhibitors aimed at modifying these additional targets can be integrated with the bisphosphonates for greater clinical benefit in patients with bone metastases. Integrating radiopharmaceuticals with bisphosphonates in the appropriate clinical setting needs to be explored. Further optimization of bisphosphonate use and prediction of treatment outcome, based on their effects on bone-resorption and bone-formation markers, also requires additional study. As more data are obtained from ongoing and future studies, a greater role for bisphosphonates might be established, such as in prevention of bone metastasis and iatrogenically induced osteoporosis.

ACKNOWLEDGMENTS

This work was in part supported by a Merit Review Award from the Medical Research Service of the Department of Veteran Affairs (A.H.). We would like to thank Florence Wade, Helen Spiker, and Joan Wertz for typing the manuscript.

REFERENCES

1. Shinoda H, Adamek G, Felix R, et al. Structure-activity relationships of various bisphosphonates. *Calcif Tiss Int* 1983; 35:887–899.
2. Lacey DL, Timms E, Tan HL, et al. Osteoprotegerin ligand is a cytokine that regulates osteoclast differentiation and activation. *Cell* 1998; 93:165–176.

3. Burgess TL, Qian YX, Kaufman S, et al. The ligand for osteoprotegerin (OPGL) directly activates mature osteoclasts. *J Cell Biol* 1999; 145:527–538.

4. Simonet WS, Lacey DL, Dunstan CR, et al. Osteoprotegerin: a novel secreted protein involved in the regulation of bone density. *Cell* 1997; 89:309–319.

5. Roodman GD. Biology of osteoclast activation in cancer. *J Clin Oncol* 2001; 19:3562–5571.

6. Theill LE, Boyle WJ, Penninger JM. RANK-L and RANK. T cells, bone loss, and mammalian evolution. *Annu Rev Immunol* 2002; 20:795–823.

7. Michigami T, Shimizu N, Williams PJ, et al. Cell-cell contact between marrow stromal cells and myeloma cells via VCAM-1 and α4β1-integrin enhances production of osteoclast-stimulating activity. *Blood* 2000; 96:1953–1960.

8. Guise TA, Yin JJ, Taylor SD, et al. Evidence for a casual role of parathyroid hormone-related protein in breast cancer-mediated osteolysis. *J Clin Invest* 1996; 98:1544–1548.

9. Pfeilschifter J, Mundy GR. Modulation of transforming growth factor beta activity in bone cultures by osteotropic hormones. *Proc Natl Acad Sci USA* 1987; 84:2024–2028.

10. Yin JJ, Selander K, Chirgwin JM, et al. TGF-β signaling blockade inhibits PTHrP secretion by breast cancer cells and bone metastases development. *J Clin Invest* 1999; 103:197–206.

11. Lee SK, Lorenzo JA. Parathyroid hormones stimulates TRANCE and inhibits osteoprotegerin messenger ribonucleic acid expression in murine bone marrow cultures: correlation with osteoclast-like cell formation. *Endocrinology* 1999; 140:3552–3561.

12. Choi S, Cruz JC, Craig J, et al. Macrophage inflammatory protein (MIP)-1α is a potential osteoclast stimulatory factor in myeloma. *Blood* 2000; 96:671–675.

13. Han JH, Choi SJ, Kurihara N, et al. Macrophage inflammatory protein-1 alpha is an osteoclastogenic factor in myeloma that is independent of receptor activator of nuclear factor KappaB ligand. *Blood* 2001; 97:3349–3353.

14. Choi SJ, Oba Y, Gazitt Y, et al. Antisense inhibition of macrophage inflammatory protein 1-alpha blocks bone destruction in a model of myeloma bone disease. *J Clin Invest* 2001; 108:1833–1841.

15. Hughes FJ, Howells GJ. Interleukin-11 inhibits bone formation in vitro. *Calcif Tissue Int* 1993; 53: 362–364.

16. Morinaga Y, Fujita N, Ohishi K, Tsuruo T. Stimulation of interleukin-11 production from osteoblast-like cells by transforming growth factor-beta and tumor cell factors. *Int J Cancer* 1997; 71: 422–428.

17. Kurihara N, Bertolini D, Suda T, et al. Interleukin-6 stimulates osteoclast-like multinucleated cell formation in long term human marrow cultures by inducing interleukin-1. *J Immunol* 1990; 144: 4226–4230.

18. Tamura T, Udagawa N, Takahashi N, et al. Soluble interleukin-6 receptor triggers osteoclast formation by interleukin-6. *Proc Natl Acad Sci USA* 1993; 90:11,924–11,928.

19. Tian E, Zhan F, Walker R, et al. The role of the Wnt-signaling antagonist DKK1 in the development of osteolytic lesions in multiple myeloma. *N Engl J Med* 2003; 349:2483–2494.

20. Gong Y, Slee RB, Fukai N, et al. LDL receptor-related protein 5 (LRP5) affects bone accrual and eye development. *Cell* 2001; 107:513–523.

21. Boyden LM, Mao J, Belsky J, et al. High bone density due to a mutation in LDL-receptor-related protein 5. *N Engl J Med* 2002; 346:1513–1521.

22. Glass DA, Patel MS, Karsenty G. A new insight into the formation of osteolytic lesions in multiple myeloma. *N Engl J Med* 2003; 349:2479,2480.

23. Guise TA, Mundy GR. Cancer and bone. *Endocr Rev* 1998; 19:18–55.

24. Nelson JB, Hedican SP, George DJ, et al Identification of endothelin-1 in the pathophysiology of metastatic adenocarcinoma of the prostate. *Nature Med* 1995; 1:944–949.

25. Chiao JW, Moonga BS, Yang YM, et al. Endothelin-1 from prostate cancer cells is enhanced by bone contact which blocks osteoclastic bone resorption. *Br J Cancer* 2000; 83:360–365.

26. Guise TA, Yin JJ, Mohammad KS. Role of endothelin-1 in osteoblastic bone metastases. *Cancer* 2003; 97(3 Suppl):779–784.

27. Koutsillieris M, Frenette G, Lazure C, et al. Urokinase-type plasminogen activator: a paracrine factor regulating the bioavailability of IGFs in PA-III cell-induced osteoblastic metastases. *Anticancer Res* 1993; 13:481–486.

28. Kanety H, Madjar Y, Dagan Y, et al. Serum insulin-like growth factor-binding protein-2 (IGFBP-2) is increased and IGFBP-3 is decreased in patients with prostate cancer: correlation with serum prostate-specific antigen. *J Clin Endocrin Metab* 1993; 77:229–233.

29. Koutsillieris M, Polychronakos C. Proteinolytic activity against IGF-binding proteins involved in the paracrine interactions between prostate adenocarcinoma cells and osteoblasts. *Anticancer Res* 1992; 12:905–910.

30. Koeneman KS, Yeung F, Chung LW. Osteomimetic properties of prostate cancer cells: a hypothesis supporting the predilection of prostate cancer metastasis and growth in the bone environment. *Prostate* 1999; 39:246–261.

31. Lin DL, Tarnowski CP, Zhang J, et al. Bone metastatic LNCaP-derivative C4-2B prostate cancer cell line mineralizes in vitro. *Prostate* 2001; 47:212–221.

32. Percival RC, Urwin GH, Harris S, et al. Biochemical and histological evidence that carcinoma of the prostate is associated with increased bone resorption. *Eur J Surg Oncol* 1987; 13:41–49.

33. Clark NW, McClure J, George NJR. Disodium pamidronate identifies differential osteoclastic bone resorption in metastatic prostate cancer. *Br J Urol* 1992; 69:64–70.

34. Takeuchi S-I, Arai K, Saitoh H, et al. Urinary pyridinoline and deoxypyridinoline as potential markers of bone metastasis in patients with prostate cancer. *J Urol* 1996; 156:1691–1695.

35. Ikeda I, Miura T, Kondo I. Pyridinium cross-links as urinary markers of bone metastases in patients with prostate cancer. *Br J Urol* 1996; 77:102–106.

36. Green JR, Mgller K, Jaeggi KA. Preclinical pharmacology of CGP 42' 446, a new potent, heterocyclic bisphosphonate compound. *J Bone Miner Res* 1994; 9:745–751.

37. Green JR. Chemical and biological prerequisites for novel bisphosphonate molecules: results of comparative preclinical studies. *Semin Oncol* 2001; 28(6 Suppl):4–10.

38. Osterman T, Lauren L. Level of clodronate in bone after single and repeated subcutaneous infections in rats. *Pharmacol Toxicol* 1991; 69:369–371.

39. Jung A, Bisaz S, Fleisch H. The binding of pyrophosphate and two diphosphonate by hydroxyapatite crystals. *Calif Tissue Res* 1973; 11:269–280.

40. Frith JC, Monkkonen J, Blackburn GM, et al. Clodronate and liposome-encapsulated clodronate are metabolized to a toxic ATP analog, adenosine 5'-(beta, gamma-dichloromethylene) triphosphate, by mammalian cells in vitro. *J Bone Min Res* 1997; 12:1358–1367.

41. Luckman SP, Hughes DE, Coxon FP, et al. Nitrogen-containing bisphosphonates inhibit the mevalonate pathway and prevent post-translational prenylation of GTP-binding proteins, including Ras. *J Bone Miner Res* 1998; 13:581–589.

42. van Beek E, Pieterman E, Cohen L, et al. Nitrogen-containing bisphosphonates inhibit isopentenyl pyrophosphate isomerase/farnesyl pyrophosphate synthase activity with relative potencies corresponding to their antiresorptive potencies in vitro and in vivo. *Biochem Biophys Res Commun* 1999; 255:491–494.

43. Savage AD, Belson DJ, Vescio RA, et al. Pamidronate reduces IL-6 production by bone marrow stroma from multiple myeloma patients. *Blood* 1996; 88(1 suppl):105a.

44. Pennanen N, Lapinjoki S, Urtti A, Monkkonen J. Effect of liposomal and free bisphosphonates on the IL-1 beta, IL-6 and TNF alpha secretion from RAW264 cells in vitro. *Pharm Res* 1995; 12:916–922.

45. Lee MV, Fong EM, Singer FR, Guenette RS. Bisphosphonate treatment inhibits the growth of prostate cancer cells. *Cancer Res* 2001; 61:2602–2608.

46. Shipman CM, Rogers MJ, Apperlay JF, et al. Bisphosphonates induce apoptosis in human myeloma cell lines: a novel anti-tumor activity. *Br J Haematol* 1997; 98:665–672.

47. Fromigue O, Lagneaux L, Body JJ. Bisphosphonates induce breast cancer cell death in vitro. *J Bone Miner Res* 2000; 15:2211–2221.

48. Jagdev SP, Coleman RE, Shipman CM, et al. This bisphosphonate, zoledronic acid induces apoptosis of breast cancer cells: evidence for synergy with paclitaxel. *Br J Cancer* 2001; 84:1126–1134.

49. Tassone P, Forciniti S, Galea E, et al. Growth inhibition and synergistic induction of apoptosis by zoledronate and dexamethasone in human myeloma cell lines. *Leukemia* 2000; 14:841–844.

50. Boissier S, Magnetto S, Frappert L, et al. Bisphosphonates inhibit prostate and breast carcinoma cell adhesion to unmineralized and mineralized bone extracellular matrices. *Cancer Res* 1997; 57:3890–3894.

51. Teronen O, Heikkilo P, Konttinen YT, et al. MMP inhibition and down-regulation by bisphosphonates. *Ann NY Acad Sci* 1999; 878:453–465.

52. Wood J, Bonjean K, Ruetz S, et al. Novel anti-angiogenic effects of the bisphosphonate compound zoledronic acid, a potent inhibitor of bone resorption. *J Pharmacol Exp Ther* 2002; 302:1055–1061.

53. Kunzmann V, Bauer E, Feurle J, et al. Stimulation of gamma delta T cells by aminobisphosphonates and induction of antiplasma cell activity in multiple myeloma. *Blood* 2000; 96:384–392.

54. Sansoni P, Passeri G, Fagnoni F, et al. Inhibition of antigen presenting cell function by alendronate in vitro. *J Bone Miner Res* 1995; 10:1719–1725.

55. Cuenca AG, Cheng FD, Wang HW, et al Modulation of antigen-presenting cells (ACP) function by aminobisphosphonates enhances T-cell priming and prevents tumor-induced T-cell tolerance. *Blood* 2001; 98:235a.

56. Sato M, Grasser W, Endo N, et al. Bisphosphonate action. Alendronate localization in rat bone and effects on osteoclast ultrastructure. *J Clin Invest* 1991; 88:2095–2105.

57. Singer FR, Ritch PS, Lad TE, et al. Treatment of hypercalcemia of malignancy with intravenous etidronate: a controlled multi-center study. *Arch Intern Med* 1991; 151:471–476.

58. Ralston SH, Gallacher SJ, Patel V, et al. Comparison of three intravenous bisphosphonates in cancer-associated hypercalcemia. *Lancet* 1989; 2:1180–1182.

59. Gucalp R, Ritch P, Wiernick PH, et al. Comparative study of pamidronate disodium and etidronate disodium in the treatment of cancer-related hypercalcemia. *J Clin Oncol* 1992; 10:134–142.

60. Sawyer N, Newstead C, Drummond A, et al. Fast (4h) or slow (24h) infusions of pamidronate disodium (aminohydroxypropylidene diphosphonate [APD]) as single shot treatment of hypercalcemia. *Bone Miner* 1990; 9:121–128.

61. Nussbaum SR, Younger J, Vandepol CJ, et al. Single-dose intravenous therapy with pamidronate for the treatment of hypercalcemia of malignancy: comparison of 30, 60, 90 mg dosages. *Am J Med* 1993; 95:297–304.

62. Major P, Lortholary A, Hon J, et al. Zoledronic acid is superior to pamidronate in the treatment of hypercalcemia of malignancy: a pooled analysis of two randomized, controlled clinical trials. *J Clin Oncol* 2001; 19:558–567.

63. Belch AR, Bergsagel DE, Wilson K, et al. Effect of daily etidronate on the osteolysis of multiple myeloma. *J Clin Oncol* 1991; 9:1397–1402.

64. Lahtinen R, Laakso M, Palva I, et al. Randomized placebo-controlled multicentre trial of clodronate in multiple myeloma. Finnish Leukemia Group. *Lancet* 1992; 340:1049–1052.

65. McCloskey EV, MacLennan IC, Drayson MT, et al. A randomized trial of the effect of clodronate on skeletal morbidity in multiple myeloma. MRC Working Party on Leukemia in Adults. *Br J Haematol* 1998; 100:317–325.

66. Brincker H, Westin J, Abildgaard N, et al. Failure of oral pamidronate to reduce skeletal morbidity in multiple myeloma: a double-blind placebo-controlled trial. Danish-Swedish Co-Operative Study Group. *Br J Haematol* 1998; 101:280–286.

67. Berenson JR, Lichtenstein A, Porter L, et al. Efficacy of pamidronate in reducing the skeletal events in patients with advanced multiple myeloma. *N Engl J Med* 1996; 334:488–493.

68. Berenson JR, Lichtenstein A, Porter L, et al. Long-term pamidronate treatment of advanced multiple myeloma reduces skeletal events. *J Clin Oncol* 1998; 16:593–602.

69. Rosen LS, Gordon D, Kaminski M, et al. Zoledronic acid versus pamidronate in the treatment of skeletal metastases in patients with breast cancer or osteolytic lesions of multiple myeloma: a phase III, double-blind, comparative trial. *Cancer J* 2001; 7:377–387.

70. Rosen LS, Gordon D, Kaminski M, et al. Long-term efficacy and safety of zoledronic acid compared with pamidronate disodium in the treatment of skeletal complications in patients with advanced multiple myeloma or breast carcinoma: a randomized, double-blind, multicenter, comparative trial. *Cancer* 2003; 98:1735–1744.

71. Berenson JR, Hillner BE, Kyle RA, et al. American Society of Clinical Oncology clinical practice guidelines: the role of bisphosphonates in multiple myeloma. *J Clin Oncol* 2002; 20:3719–3736.

72. Paterson AHG, Powles TJ, Kanis TA, et al. Double-blind controlled trial of oral clodronate in patients with bone metastases from breast cancer. *J Clin Oncol* 1993; 11:59–65.

73. Hortobagyi GN, Theriault RL, Porter L, et al. Efficacy of pamidronate in reducing skeletal complications in patients with breast cancer and lytic bone metastases. Protocol 19 Aredia Breast Cancer Study Group. *N Engl J Med* 1996; 335:1785–1791.

74. Theriault RL, Lipton A, Hortobagyi GN, et al. Pamidronate reduces skeletal morbidity in women with advanced breast cancer and lytic bone lesions: a randomized, placebo-controlled trial. Protocol 18 Aredia Breast Cancer Study Group. *J Clin Oncol* 1999; 17:846–854.

75. Hortobagyi GN, Theriault RL, Lipton A, et al. Long-term prevention of skeletal complications of metastatic breast cancer with pamidronate. *J Clin Oncol* 1998; 16:2038–2044.

76. Lipton A, Theriault RL, Hortobagyi GN, et al. Pamidronate prevents skeletal complications and is effective palliative treatment in women with breast carcinoma and osteolytic bone metastases: long term follow-up of two randomized, placebo-controlled trials. *Cancer* 2000; 88:1082–1090.

77. Hillner BE, Ingle JN, Berenson JR, et al. American Cancer Society of Clinical Oncology guidelines on the role of bisphosphonates in breast cancer. *J Clin Oncol* 2000; 18:1378–1391.

78. Smith JA Jr. Palliation of painful bone metastases from prostate cancer using sodium etidronate: results of a randomized, prospective, double-blind, placebo-controlled study. *J Urol* 1989; 141:85–87.

79. Elomaa I, Kylmala T, Tammela T, et al. Effect of oral clodronate on bone pain: a controlled study in patients with metastatic prostate cancer. *Int Urol Nephrol* 1992; 24:159–166.

80. Kylmala T, Taube T, Tammela T, et al. Concomitant I.V. and oral clodronate in the relief of bone pain: a double-blind placebo-controlled study in patients with prostate cancer. *Br J Cancer* 1997; 76:939–942.

81. Strang P, Nilsson S, Brandstedt S, et al. The analgesic efficacy of clodronate compared with placebo in patients with painful bone metastases from prostate cancer. *Anticancer Res* 1997; 17:4717–4721.

82. Ernst DS, Tannock IF, Winquist EW, et al. Randomized double-blind controlled trial of mitoxantrone/ prednisone and clodronate versus mitoxantrone/prednisone and placebo in patients with hormone refractory prostate cancer and pain. *J Clin Oncol* 2003; 21:3335–3342.

83. Dearnaley DP, Sydes MR, Mason MD, et al. A double-blind placebo controlled randomized trial of oral sodium clodronate for metastatic prostate cancer (MRC PR05 trial). *J Natl Cancer Inst* 2003; 95: 1300–1311.

84. Small EJ, Smith MR, Seamon JJ, et al. Combined analysis of two multicenter, randomized, placebo-controlled studies of pamidronate disodium for the palliation of bone pain in men with metastatic prostate cancer. *J Clin Oncol* 2003; 21:4277–4284.

85. Saad F, Gleason DM, Murray R, et al. A randomized, placebo-controlled trial of zoledronic acid in patients with hormone-refractory metastatic prostate carcinoma. *J Natl Cancer Inst* 2002; 94:1458–1468.

86. Saad F, Gleason DM, Murray R, et al. Long-term efficacy of zoledronic acid or the prevention of skeletal complications in patients with metastatic hormone refractory prostate cancer. *J Natl Cancer Inst* 2004; 96:879–883.

87. Rosen L, Gordon D, Tcheckmedyian S, et al. Zoledronic acid significantly reduces skeletal related events in patients with bone metastasis form solid tumors. *Proc Am Soc Clin* 2002; 21:295a.

88. Rosen L, Harland SJ, Ooserlinck W. Broad clinical activity of zoledronic acid in osteolytic to osteoblastic bone lesions in patients with a broad range of solid tumors. *AM J Clin Oncol* (CCT) 2002; 25 (6 Suppl):S19–S24.

89. Lipton A, Zheng M, Seaman J. Zoledronic acid delays the onset of skeletal-related events and progression of skeletal disease in patients with advanced renal cell carcinoma. *Cancer* 2003; 98:962–969.

90. Thiebaud D, Sauty A, Burckhardt P, et al. An in vitro and in vivo study of cytokines in the acute-phase response associated with bisphosphonates. *Calcif Tissue Int* 1997; 61:386–392.

91. Mashiba T, Hirano T, Turner CH, et al. Suppressed bone marrow turnover by bisphosphonates increases microdamage accumulation and reduces some biomechanical properties in dog rib. *J Bone Miner Res* 2000; 15:613–620.

92. Coleman RE. Current and future status of adjuvant therapy for breast cancer. *Cancer* 2003; 97 (3 Suppl):880–886.

93. Ramaswamy B, Shapiro CL. Bisphosphonates in the prevention and treatment of bone metastasis. *Oncology* 2003; 17:1261–1270.

94. Dawson NA. Bisphosphonates: their evolving role in the management of prostate cancer-related bone disease. *Curr Opin Urol* 2002; 12:413–418.

95. Smith MR. Diagnosis and management of treatment-related osteoporosis in men with prostate cancer-related bone disease. *Cancer* 2003; 97(3 Suppl):789–795.

96. Nemoto R, Satou S, Miyagawa I, Koiso K Inhibition by a new bisphosphonate (AHBuBP) of bone resorption induced by the MBT-2 tumor. *Cancer* 1991; 67:643–648.

97. Yu-Cheng S, Geldof AA, Newling DW, Rao BR. Progression delay of prostate tumor skeletal metastasis effects by bisphosphonates. *J Urol* 1992; 148:1270–1273.

98. Sasaki A, Boye BF, Story B, et al. Bisphosphonate risedronate reduces metastatic human breast cancer burden in bone in nude mice. *Cancer Res* 1995; 55:3551–3557.

99. Dallas SL, Garrett IR, Oyajobi BO, et al. Ibandronate reduces osteolytic lesions but not tumor burden in a murine model of myeloma bone disease. *Blood* 1999; 93:1697–1706.

100. Nobuyuki H, Hiraga T, Williams PJ, et al. The bisphosphonate zoledronic acid inhibits metastasis to bone and liver with suppression of osteopontin production in mouse mammary tumor. *J Bone Miner Res* 2000; 16(1 Suppl):S191.

101. Powles T, Paterson S, Kanis JA, et al. Randomized, placebo-controlled trial of clodronate in patients with primary operable breast cancer. *J Clin Oncol* 2002; 20:3219–3224.

102. Diel IJ, Solomayer EF, Costa SD, et al. Reduction in new metastases in breast cancer with adjuvant clodronate treatment. *N Engl J Med* 1998; 339:357–363.

103. Diel IJ, Solomayer E, Gollan C, et al. Bisphosphonates in the reduction of metastasis in breast cancer: results of the extended follow-up of the first study population. *Proc Am Soc Clin Oncol* 2000; 19:314.

104. Saarto T, Blomquist C, Virkkunen P, Elomaa I. Adjuvant clodronate treatment does not reduce the frequency of skeletal metastasis in node-positive breast cancer patients: 5 year results of randomized controlled trial. *J Clin Oncol* 2001; 19:10–17.

105. Powles TJ, McCloskey E, Paterson AH, et al. Oral clodronate and reduction in loss of bone mineral density in women with operable primary breast cancer. *J Natl Cancer Inst* 1998; 90:704–708.

106. Delmas PD, Balena R, Confravreaux E, et al. Bisphosphonate risedronate prevents bone loss in women with artificial menopause due to chemotherapy of breast cancer: a double-blind, placebo-controlled study. *J Clin Oncol* 1997; 15:955–962.

107. Reid IR, Brown JP, Burckhardt P, et al. Intravenous zoledronic acid in postmenopausal women with low bone mineral density. *N Engl J Med* 2002; 346:653–661.

108. Orwoll E, Ettinger M, Weiss S, et al. Alendronate for the treatment of osteoporosis in men. *N Engl J Med* 2000; 343:604–610.

109. Diamond TH, Winters J, Smith A, et al. The antiosteoporotic efficacy of intravenous pamidronate in men with prostate carcinoma receiving combined androgen blockade: a double blind, randomized, placebo-controlled cross-over study. *Cancer* 2001; 92:1444–1450.

110. Smith MR, McGovern FJ, Zietman AL, et al. Pamidronate to prevent bone loss in men receiving gonadotropin releasing hormone agonist therapy for prostate cancer. *N Engl J Med* 2001; 345:948–955.

111. Smith MR, Eastham J, Gleason DM, et al. Randomized controlled trial of zoledronic acid to prevent bone loss in men receiving androgen deprivation therapy for nonmetastatic prostate cancer. *J Urol* 2003; 169:2008–2012.

19 Radiation Treatment of Bone Metastases

Edward Chow, MBBS, FRCPC, *Jackson Wu,* MD, FRCPC, *and Elizabeth Toni Barnes,* MD, FRCPC

CONTENTS

1. INTRODUCTION

Radiation is used to treat cancer with ionizing radiation resulting in damage to cellular DNA. When radiation passes through a living cell, it can damage the reproductive material in the cell directly and indirectly. Direct damage includes base deletions and single- and double-strand breaks in the DNA chain. Indirect damage occurs when radiation interacts with water molecules in the cell, releasing toxic free radicals. Repair of the damage is possible both in normal cells and cancer cells, although it is thought that cancer cells have less capacity to repair damaged DNA and, hence, a therapeutic ratio can be exploited.

The radiation dose is measured in Gray (Gy), which is 1 joule of absorbed energy per kilogram of mass. Another unit used to describe radiation dose is centigray (cGy), which is equivalent to 0.01 Gy. When radiation is given with a palliative intent, the most common treatment schema, or dose-fractionation schedules, are an 8 Gy as a single treatment, 20 Gy in five daily treatments (4 Gy per treatment), and 30 Gy in 10 daily treatments (3 Gy per treatment).

From: *Cancer Drug Discovery and Development*
Bone Metastasis: Experimental and Clinical Therapeutics
Edited by: G. Singh and S. A. Rabbani © Humana Press Inc., Totowa, NJ

Radiation can be delivered by an external beam of radiation directed at the site of interest, by brachytherapy, in which a radioactive source is applied into or around the tumor site, or in the form of radionuclide given intravenously as an inorganic soluble compound.

External beam radiation is generated from a machine called a linear accelerator or a cobalt machine. The linear accelerator generates high-energy X-ray or electron beams, whereas the cobalt machine utilizes a radioactive element (Co-60) that generates high-energy γ-rays through radioactive decay. X-rays and γ-rays are used to treat tumors located deep in the body, whereas electron beam radiation treats superficial cancers.

For superficial lesions that are visible or palpable, the area to be radiated can be easily delineated on clinical examination. Deep-seated tumors will require radiographic localization using a treatment simulator. The conventional simulator is a specialized fluoroscopic unit completely identical to a therapy machine in its geometric specifications and movements. The difference is the former emits a diagnostic X-ray beam, producing an image of the proposed therapy beam. Modern radiographic visualization and localization of deep-seated tumors can be achieved with computer-tomography-based simulator (i.e., CT simulation).

In brachytherapy, radioactive sources can be permanently implanted in a tumor or placed temporarily near the tumor location. Permanently implanted radiation sources are used, for example, to treat prostate cancer. The radiation source gradually decays until no further radiation is emitted. Radioactive sources that are placed in a catheter are temporarily adjacent to the lung cancer, blocking the bronchus for a prescribed amount of time to deliver a specific radiation dose. The radiation dose in brachytherapy is extremely localized because of the inverse square law (radiation dose proportional to $1/d^2$). The radiation dose drops off rapidly as the distance from radiation source increases. Because radiation is well localized, brachytherapy can be used to reirradiate tissues that have been previously irradiated and treatment side effects with brachytherapy are usually limited.

The inorganic forms of radionuclides (radioactive isotopes) have affinity to bone and thyroid gland. They can be injected into the bloodstream. Although acting as a systemic agent, the effects of radiation are localized to the site of deposition, and little radiation is administered to adjacent tissues. Radionuclides, like brachytherapy, are ideal in cases of retreatment of previously irradiated areas and are effective in alleviating pain from multiple sites of bone metastases.

2. CLINICAL TRIALS ON LOCALIZED EXTERNAL BEAM RADIATION

About 50% of cancer patients will receive palliative radiation therapy during the course of their disease. Palliation of bone metastases comprises a significant workload in the specialty of radiation oncology. Radiation therapy has been long employed in the management of bone metastases. Radiotherapy is effective in relieving bone pain, preventing impending fractures, and promoting healing in pathological fractures. Stabilization of bony destruction occurs in 80% and reossification takes place in varying degrees after radiotherapy.

External beam radiation therapy is effective and cost-efficient in palliation of symptomatic bone metastases. Retrospective series have documented pain improvement in 80–90% of patients with bone metastases treated with radiotherapy of various dose fractionations. Hematological or gastrointestinal side effects were usually mild and transient.

Numerous randomized trials have been conducted on dose-fractionation schedules of palliative radiotherapy. Despite that, there is still no uniform consensus on the optimal dose-fractionation scheme. One of the first randomized studies on bone metastases was conducted by the Radiation Therapy Oncology Group (RTOG 74-02) *(1)*. Ninety percent of patients experienced some relief of pain and 54% achieved eventual complete pain relief. The initial analysis of this trial concluded that the low-dose, short-course schedules were as effective as the high-dose, protracted programs. However, this study was criticized for using physician-based pain assessment. A reanalysis of the same set of data, grouping solitary and multiple bone metastases, using the end point of pain relief and taking into account analgesic intake and retreatment, concluded that the number of radiation fractions was statistically significant related to complete combined relief (i.e., absence of pain and cessation of the use of narcotics). The conclusion was that protracted dose-fractionation schedules were most effective than short-course schedules *(2)*. This re-analysis was contrary to the initial report, highlighting that the choice of end points is very important in defining the outcomes of clinical trials *(3)*.

Several prospective randomized trials that compared the efficacy of different dose-fractionation schedules were subsequently performed. The UK Bone Pain Trial Working Party randomized 765 patients with bone metastases to receive either a 8-Gy single fraction or a multifraction regimen (20 Gy/5 fractions or 30 Gy/10 fractions) *(4)*. There were no differences in the time to first improvement in pain, time to complete pain relief, or in time to first increase in pain at any time up to 12 mo from randomization. Retreatment was twice as common after 8 Gy than after multifraction radiotherapy. There were no significant differences in the incidence of nausea, vomiting, spinal cord compression, or pathological fracture between the two groups. The authors concluded that a single fraction of 8 Gy is as safe and effective as a multifraction regimen for the palliation of metastatic bone pain for at least 12 mo. The greater convenience and lower cost make 8 Gy single fraction the treatment of choice for the majority of patients.

The Dutch Bone Metastases Study included 1171 patients and found no difference in pain relief or the quality of life following a single 8-Gy or 24-Gy dose in six daily radiation treatments *(5)*. However, the retreatment rates were 25% in the single 8-Gy arm and 7% in the multiple-treatment arm, respectively. More pathological fractures were observed in the single-fraction group, but the absolute percentage was low. In their cost–utility analysis of this randomized trial, there was no difference in life expectancy or quality-adjusted life expectancy. The estimated cost of radiotherapy, including retreatments and nonmedical costs, was statistically significantly lower for the single-fraction schedule than for the multiple-fraction schedule. Single-fraction radiotherapy provides equal palliation and quality of life and has lower medical and societal costs in The Netherlands *(6)*.

One critical review on the subject of radiation dose-fractionation included a systematic search for randomized trials of localized radiotherapy of bone metastases employing different dose fractionations *(7)*. The primary outcomes of interest were complete and overall pain relief. The authors suggested that protracted fractionated radiotherapy, given over 2–4 wk, results in more complete and durable pain relief. It was unclear if higher radiation doses would be called for to maintain durable pain relief in patients who survived longer.

A recent meta-analysis has a different conclusion *(8)*. There was no significant difference in complete and overall pain relief between single-fraction and multifraction palliative radiotherapy for bone metastases. There was no dose–response relationship that could be detected by including data from trials that evaluated several different radiation schedules. The meta-analysis reported that the complete response rates (absence of pain after radiotherapy) were 33.4% and 32.3% after single-fraction and multifraction radiation treatment, respectively, whereas the overall response rates were 62.1% and 58.7%, respectively. The latter became 72.7% and 72.5%, respectively, when the analysis was restricted to evaluated patients solely. Most patients will experience pain relief in the first 2–4 wk after radiotherapy, be it single or multiple fractionations.

In view of the differing conclusions from the previous trial, RTOG has repeated a phase III randomized trial of 8 Gy in 1 fraction versus 30 Gy in 10 fractions for palliation of painful bone metastases from breast or prostate cancers *(9)*. A total of 949 patients were enrolled in the study, of whom 897 were eligible and analyzable. Complete or partial improvement in pain was seen in 66% of patients. Pain and narcotic relief was equivalent for both arms. At 3 mo follow-up, there was no difference between the two treatment arms. Again, the treatment was well tolerated with few adverse effects.

What should be an optimal dose for single-fraction treatment then? A prospective randomized trial on 270 patients with painful bone metastases compared 4-Gy and 8-Gy single doses in its efficacy *(10)*. At 4 wk, the actual response rates were 69% for 8 Gy and 44% for 4 Gy ($p < 0.001$), but there was no difference in complete response (no pain) rates at 4 wk or duration of response between the two arms. It is concluded that 8 Gy gives a higher probability of pain relief than 4 Gy, but that 4 Gy can be an effective alternative in situations of reduced tolerance. Another randomized trial of three single-dose radiation therapy regimens in the treatment of metastatic bone pain consisted of a single 4-Gy, 6-Gy, or 8-Gy dose *(11)*. The authors confirmed that 8 Gy could be considered as probably "lowest" optimal single-fraction radiation treatment for painful bone metastases, although single-fraction 4 Gy should not be easily discarded because of its applicability in specific cases. In their study, single-fraction 6 Gy achieved results not different from that obtained with 8 Gy, they recommend further studies to define the "lowest" optimal single-fraction radiation in the treatment of painful bone metastases.

Despite the equivalence of single and multiple fractionations, recent surveys on the patterns of practice of radiation oncologists do not suggest the implementation of employing single fractionation in daily practice *(12–14)*.

How, then, are radiation oncologists to prescribe treatment? The answer most likely resides within the clinical circumstances and individual wishes of each patient. There is no doubt that in patients with short life expectancy, protracted schedules are a burden. However, in patients with a longer expected survival, such as breast and prostate cancer patients with bone metastases only, other parameters need to be taken into account. Because retreatment rates are known to be higher following single vs multiple fractions, about 25% vs 10%, respectively, patients with good performance status might wish to share decision-making process. A recent survey of patients with bone metastases has suggested that patients are not prepared to trade off long-term outcomes in favor of a shorter treatment course. Durability of pain relief was more important than short-term "convenience" factors. Patients prefer multiple treatments upfront in hopes of avoiding retreatment *(15,16)*. However, they need to be aware of the potential physician bias of more readiness to retreat after single fraction, accounting for the difference in retreatment rates in the trials.

3. CLINICAL TRIALS ON WIDE-FIELD
OR HALF-BODY EXTERNAL BEAM RADIATION

Wide-field or half-body irradiation (HBI) differs from localized external beam radiation mainly in the volume of tissues and bone metastases covered as a single-treatment field. It is more useful for patients with multiple painful bone metastases. HBI is usually delivered either to the upper half or to the lower half of the body.

Single-fraction HBI has been shown in retrospective and prospective phase I and II studies to provide pain relief in 70 to 80% of patients *(17–20)*. Pain relief is apparent within 24–48 h *(20,21)*, suggesting that cells of the inflammatory response pathway might be the initial target tissue, because tumor cell activities are unlikely to be halted so quickly. Toxicities include minor bone marrow suppression and gastrointestinal side effects such as nausea and vomiting in upper-abdominal radiation and might be controlled with Ondansetron or dexamethasone *(21–23)*. Pulmonary toxicity is minimal, provided the lung dose is limited to 6 Gy *(24)*.

Fractionated HBI was investigated in a randomized phase II study involving 29 patients, comparing a single fraction with fractionated HBI (25–30 Gy in 9–10 fractions). Pain relief was achieved in over 94% of patients. At 1 yr, 70% in the fractionated and 15% in the single-fraction group had pain control, and repeat radiation was required in 71% and 13% for the single-dose and fractionated group *(25)*. Poulter and colleagues reported results of a randomized trial of 499 patients comparing local radiation alone vs local radiation plus a single fraction of HBI. The study documented a lower incidence of new bone metastases (50% vs 68%) and fewer patients requiring further local radiotherapy at 1 yr after HBI (60% vs 76%) *(26)*.

The choice of dose-fractionation schedule for HBI was explored by Salazar et al. *(27)* among 156 randomized patients from 6 countries. Among the three trial arms of 15 Gy in five fractions over 5 d, 8 Gy in two fractions over 1 d, and 12 Gy in four fractions over 2 d, the 15 Gy/5 fractions/5 d regimen not only provided pain relief as much as the other regimens but also a longer survival duration in prostate cancer patients. More prostate cancer patients are planned to be entered into another study to confirm this unexpected finding.

4. REIRRADIATION

Because effective systemic treatment and better supportive care result in improved survival, certain subsets of patients with bone metastases have longer life expectancies than before. An increasing number of patients outlive the duration of the benefits of initial palliative radiotherapy for symptomatic bone metastases, requiring reirradiation of the previously treated sites. Additionally, some patients fail to respond initially but could benefit from reirradiation.

Among the radiation trials comparing single- vs multiple-fraction schemes, reirradiation rates varied from 11% to 42% following single fraction and from 0% to 24% following multiple-fraction schedules. There are at least three scenarios of "failure" where reirradiation might be considered. Response to reirradiation might be different for each of these scenarios:

1. No pain relief or pain progression after initial radiotherapy.
2. Partial response with initial radiotherapy and the hope to achieve further pain reduction with more radiotherapy.

3. Partial or complete response with initial radiotherapy but subsequent recurrence of pain.

Mithal et al. *(28)* reported a retrospective analysis of 105 consecutive patients treated with palliative radiotherapy for painful bone metastases. A total of 280 individual treatment sites were identified, of which 57 were retreated once and 8 were retreated twice. The overall response rate to initial treatment was 84% for pain relief, and at first retreatment, this was 87%. Seven out of eight (88%) patients retreated a second time also achieved pain relief. A total of 17/23 (74%) patients responded (complete response and partial response) to second radiation that used a number of single-fraction regimens, which was not significantly inferior to 31/34 (91%) obtained with more protracted regimens. No relationships to radiation dose, primary tumour type, or site was seen *(28)*.

Jeremic et al. *(29)* investigated the effectiveness of a single fraction of 4 Gy given for retreatment of bone metastasis after previous single-fraction radiotherapy. Of 135 patients retreated, 109 patients were retreated because of pain relapsing and 26 patients were reirradiated after initial nonresponse. Of the 109 patients who were reirradiated for pain relapse, 80 (74%) patients responded (complete response [CR] = 31%; partial response [PR] = 42%). Among the 26 patients who initially did not respond, there were 12 (46%) responses. The authors concluded that the lack of response to the initial single-fraction radiotherapy should not deter repeat irradiation. Toxicity in their series was low and only gastrointestinal. Grade 1 or 2 diarrhea (RTOG acute toxicity criteria) was observed in 25/135 (19%) patients. No acute toxicity ≥ grade 3 was reported. Pathological fractures were reported in 3/135 (2%) patients and spinal cord compression was reported in 3/135 (2%) patients in their series *(29)*.

The same group recently reported the efficacy of the second single 4-Gy reirradiation for painful bone metastases following the previous two single fractions. The overall response rate of the 25 patients (19 responders and 6 nonresponders to the 2 prior single fractions) was 80%, with both complete response and partial response being 40%. No acute or late high-grade toxicity (≥3) was observed in their study. No pathological fracture or spinal cord compression was seen in any of these patients during the follow-up *(30)*.

The Dutch Bone Metastases Study Group recently presented the efficacy of reirradiation of painful bone metastases *(31)*. For patients not responding to the initial radiation who were reirradiated, 66% of patients who initially received a single 8 Gy dose (SF) responded to the retreatment vs 33% of patients who received the initial multifraction regimens (MF). Retreatment for patients with progression was successful in 70% SF patients vs 57% MF patients. In general, retreatment was effective in 63% of all retreated patients.

In summary, available data support the reirradiation of sites of metastatic bone pain following initial irradiation, particularly where this follows an initial period of response. There is also limited evidence that a proportion of nonresponders would respond to reirradiation. However, there remains a small group of patients who appear to be nonresponsive to any amount of palliative radiotherapy. Although the data do support the clinical practice of reirradiation, the preferred dose fractionation at time of reirradiation is unknown. A phase III international randomized trial of single vs multiple fractions for reirradiation of painful bone metastases is ongoing and will help address the practical questions facing radiation oncologists when providing palliative radiation services.

5. SYSTEMIC RADIONUCLIDES

Patients with bone metastases often have diffuse bony disease. Administration of a systemic radionuclide has the advantage of targeting all bony lesions simultaneously and can be given as a single administration on an outpatient basis. Osteoblastic bone metastases can be detected by a technetium-99m methylenediphosphonate (MDP) bone scan. Radionuclides react with bone mineral (hydroxyapatite), and the pattern of uptake mirrors that seen on the bone scan. Strontium-89 and samarium-153 are the agents most commonly utilized in clinical practice. Phosphorus-32, rhenium-186, tin-117m have also been used *(32)*. These radionuclides emit β-particles with a mean range between 0.2 and 3 mm, thereby minimizing toxicity to surrounding tissue. Retention in the areas of bone metastases is greater than in the normal bone marrow, with a tumor-to-marrow ratio of 10:1. The average time to clinical response is 7–14 d, with a median duration of action of 18 wk. Retreatment is possible, with an interval of 10–12 wk for strontium-89 and 6–10 wk for samarium-153, although a nonresponder is unlikely to respond to subsequent administration *(33)*. The mechanism of pain reduction is unclear but might include radiation-induced apoptosis of lymphocyte-secreting cytokines and direct cell kill and reduction of mass effect *(32)*.

Treatment-related toxicity consists mainly of reversible myelosuppression, especially thrombocytopenia. The nadir is 4–6 wk after injection, recovery completed by 6–10 wk, with severity related to disease burden. Bone marrow toxicity is, therefore, of concern with the use of systemic chemotherapy. A small percentage of patients (10–20%) may experience a pain flare shortly after administration. Contraindications to the use of radionuclides include poor performance status, <2 mo projected survival, extensive soft tissue metastases, platelet count $<60 \times 10^9$/L, recent rapid fall in platelet count even if $>60 \times 10^9$/L, white count $<2.5 \times 10^9$/L, disseminated intravascular coagulation, within 1 mo of myelosuppressive chemotherapy, and within 2 mo of hemibody radiotherapy. Impending or actual pathologic fracture and cord compression are also contraindications for use *(33)*.

The evidence for use of radionuclides has been reported in several phase II and III trials. Overall pain-reduction rates for the various radionuclides are comparable and similar to localized and hemibody external beam radiotherapy, with an overall response rate of 80% and complete response rate of 20% *(33)*. The "Trans Canada" study reported on 126 patients with metastatic prostate cancer randomized to strontium-89 or placebo in addition to external beam radiotherapy *(34)*. Patients receiving strontium showed a significant improvement at 3 mo in analgesic use and an improved quality of life. Reduced lifetime requirements for radiotherapy and reduction in development of new painful bone metastases were seen. Hematologic toxicity was acceptable. A lifetime management cost savings of $5800 in the group receiving strontium-89 was found *(35)*. A second multicenter trial in prostate cancer patients compared strontium-89 with either local-field or wide-field radiotherapy and found no significant difference in analgesic efficacy, with a significant increase in time for further radiotherapy and development of new pain sites *(36)*. Samarium-153 is also licensed for use in the United States and has shown similar efficacy to strontium although no head-to-head comparative trials have been performed. Patients with a variety of primary malignancies had an 85% pain response rate, with breast cancer patients achieving the best palliation *(37,38)*.

Radionuclides offer a method of delivering localized radiation to osteoblastic metastasis with response rates similar to external beam radiotherapy. Advantages lie in the ability to treat all metastatic lesions simultaneously with a single injection administered on an outpatient basis. A reduction in the management costs has been found. Myelosuppression is the major toxicity and might limit the use of radionuclides in patients managed with systemic chemotherapy.

6. MECHANISMS OF ACTIONS OF RADIOTHERAPY

Palliative radiotherapy is well established for the treatment of symptomatic bone metastases. Exact mechanism of its action is still uncertain, although tumor cell kill might be an important reason. However, the absence of a dose–response relationship, rapid responses, and poor correlation of symptomatic relief with radiosensitivity suggest that an effect on host mechanisms of pain could also be important.

Markers of bone remodeling have been shown to be suppressed by antiresorptive therapy, and the response of these bone markers has been applied to monitoring therapy for bone metastases. In the recent UK Bone Pain Radiotherapy Trial *(4)*, 22 patients were entered into a supplementary study to establish the effects of local radiotherapy for metastatic bone pain on markers of osteoclast activity, particularly the pyridinium crosslinks pyridinoline and deoxypyridinoline, the latter being specific for bone turnover. Urine samples were collected before and 1 mo after radiotherapy. Patients were treated with either a single 8-Gy or 20-Gy dose in five daily fractions. Pain response was scored with validated pain charts completed by patients.

Urinary pyridinium concentrations were correlated with pain response. In patients who did not respond to palliative radiation (nonresponders), baseline concentrations of both pyridinoline and deoxypyridinoline were higher than those who responded (responders) and rose further after treatment, whereas in responders, the mean values remained unchanged. This resulted in significant differences between responders and nonresponders for both indices after treatment ($p = 0.027$). The authors conclude that radiotherapy-mediated inhibition of bone resorption and, thus, osteoclastic activity could be a predictor for pain response. They also propose that tumor cell killing reduces the production of osteoclast-activating factors, or there is a direct effect on osteoclasts within the radiation volume, distinct from tumor shrinkage. Their study supports the results from randomized trials that high-dose radiotherapy is not necessary for pain relief and that single low doses of treatment are more than adequate for most patients *(39)*.

7. CONTROLLING SIDE EFFECTS OF TREATMENT

Radiation treatment planning is the most critical aspect of reducing radiation side effects. Management of the acute effects of radiotherapy requires attentive medical management that prevents the expected side effect. Radiation side effects are specific to the area treated. No side effects are anticipated when a femoral bone metastasis is treated by radiation. Careful radiation treatment planning that avoids critical structures like mucosal surfaces can prevent most side effects.

Patients should be reassured that the unavoidable side effects that they experience will resolve following the completion of radiotherapy. Skin reactions are usually minimal during radiotherapy for bone metastases and are limited only to the radiation portal. Nausea and vomiting, resulting from a radiation portal that includes the abdomen, will usually respond to antiemetic therapy, but Ondansetron or dexamethasone also is commonly used, especially if patients have recently received emetogenic chemotherapy.

Diarrhea, resulting from abdominopelvic radiation, will respond to antidiarrhea medications such as Loperamide. Local irritation from mucositis of the oropharyngeal region might be relieved by soluble aspirin, analgesics, or benzydamine mouthwashes. Secondary infections, like candida, should be treated.

The side effects of electron beam radiation are more limited because they only treat superficial structures like the ribs, skin lesions, and superficial lymph nodes. Underlying structures are spared with the selection of the proper electron beam energy. This characteristic is especially important with reirradiation to avoid injury to critical structures like the spinal cord. The most prominent side effect of electron beam radiation is an erythematous skin reaction. Other side effects listed earlier do not occur with electron beam radiation because the radiation beam does not penetrate to these structures.

No side effects, other than a possible flare of pain in the first 2 wk after administration, are observed with systemic radioisotope therapy because all of the radiation is localized to the bone. This is a significant consideration for patients who have significant symptoms of the disease or other treatments. Side effects from external beam radiation also are more severe when the radiation fields are large because more normal tissues are treated. Systemic radioisotopes can have significant advantage over large external beam radiation fields by reducing risk for side effects like nausea and diarrhea.

8. PATHOLOGICAL AND IMPENDING FRACTURES

Pathological fractures are handled with orthopedic stabilization whenever possible. Surgery rapidly controls pain and returns that patient to mobility. Elective orthopedic stabilization has reportedly resulted in good pain relief and sustained mobility in up to 90% of patients. Early identification of patients with a high risk of fracture is especially important. A fracture of the weight-bearing long bones can be a devastating event even in a healthy person. Prophylactic orthopedic fixation is often advised to avoid the trauma of a pathological fracture. The operative procedure has fewer complications and less impact on functional outcome.

The criteria often used to determine fracture risk in long bones include the following:

- Persistent or increasing local pain despite radiotherapy, particularly when aggravated by functional loading
- A solitary, well-defined lytic lesion greater than 2.5 cm
- A solitary, well-defined lesion circumferentially involving more than 50% of the cortical bone
- Metastatic involvement of the proximal femur associated with a fracture of the lesser trochanter

In the randomized Dutch Bone Metastasis Study on the palliative effect of a single fraction of 8 Gy vs six fractions of 4 Gy on painful bone metastases, 14 fractures occurred in 102 patients with femoral metastases. The authors analyzed the pretreatment radiographs of femoral metastases and concluded that fracturing of the femur primarily depended on the amount of axial cortical involvement of the metastases. They recommended treating femoral metastases with an axial cortical involvement of 30 mm or less with a single fraction of 8 Gy for relief of pain. If the axial cortical involvement is greater than 30 mm, prophylactic surgery should be considered to minimize the risk of pathological fracturing or, if the patient's condition is limited, irradiation to a higher total dose *(40)*.

Although radiotherapy provides pain relief and tumor control, it does not restore bone stability. Postoperative radiotherapy is usually recommended after surgical stabilization of a pathologic fracture. Patients who are without visceral metastases and who have a relatively long survival (e.g., > 3 mo) are more likely to benefit from postoperative radiotherapy. Because the entire bone is at risk for microscopic involvement and the procedure involved in rod placement might seed the bone at other sites, the length of the entire rod used for bone stabilization should be included in the radiation field. When the radiation fields are more limited, instability of the rod, resulting in pain and need for reoperation, can result from recurrent osteolytic metastases outside the radiation portal.

9. SPINAL CORD COMPRESSION

Spinal cord compression (SCC) involves compression of the dural sac and contents (spinal cord and/or cauda equina) by an extradural tumor mass *(41)*. A recent population-based study in Ontario found that in the 5 yr preceding death, 2.5% of all cancer patients had at least one hospital admission for SCC, ranging from 0.2% in pancreatic cancer to 7.9% in myeloma *(42)*. At presentation, 90% of patients had back pain, 50% were unable to walk, and 10–15% had paraplegia *(43)*. The strongest prognostic factor for overall survival and ambulation posttreatment is pretreatment neurological status *(44)*. If left untreated, progressive pain, motor, and sensory loss, and sphincter dysfunction result. To minimize treatment delays, once SCC is clinically suspected, an urgent whole-spine magnetic resonance imaging (MRI) scan needs to be performed. The benefits of MRI vs myelography include being noninvasive, imaging the entire length of the spinal column to identify possible compression at multiple levels, multiplanar imaging, high-contrast signal among cord, cerebral spinal fluid, and tumor, and identifying spinal instability or bone retroplusion and paraspinal masses. Disadvantages for the patient include claustrophobia and the length of time to acquire images *(41)*.

Management of SCC consists of corticosteriods, surgery, and/or radiotherapy. Corticosteriods are routinely used to decrease peritumoral edema. One randomized trial of 57 patients showed a significant improvement in ambulation after radiotherapy with high-dose steroids vs placebo; however, this use of steroids was associated with an increase in serious toxicity *(45)*. Given the lack of evidence for the use of high-dose over moderate-dose steroids, many physicians dose empirically with 4 mg qid decadron *(43)*. The choice between surgery and radiotherapy should be individualized, taking into consideration the patient's general performance status, medical comorbidities, neurological function, and patient preference. If surgically feasible and medically acceptable, patients with spinal instability or bone compression are better treated surgically, as neurological outcomes are thought to be improved *(44)*. Radiotherapy is given post-operatively to impede tumor regrowth. Other indications for surgery might include neurological deterioration during or after radiotherapy and the absence of a tissue diagnosis. A recent randomized trial, presented in abstract form, compared decompressive surgery followed by radiotherapy to radiotherapy alone *(46)*. The trial accrued 101 patients before meeting early stopping criteria because of surgical patients being more likely to retain/maintain ambulatory status compared to patients in the radiotherapy-alone arm. They found that 58% (9/16) of nonambulatory patients in the surgery arm retained the ability to walk after treatment, compared to 19% (3/16) in the radiotherapy-alone arm. However, 35% of patients in the radiotherapy arm had spinal instability, usually considered an indication for primary surgical management.

Neurological status after treatment is dictated by pretreatment function. A pooled analysis found that after radiotherapy, 95% of patients ambulatory pretreatment retained ambulation, compared with 63% of patients requiring ambulation assistance, 36% of paraparetic patients, and 13% of paraplegic patients *(41)*. There are no randomized controlled trials investigating the optimal radiotherapy regime. A recent retrospective review of 102 patients found no difference in motor and sphincter function or pain control for patients treated with one or two fractions vs a longer fractionation schedule *(47)*. Early detection and prompt treatment of SCC remains vital to preserve neurological outcomes. Future research efforts might examine the use of neuroprotectants and prophylactic spinal radiotherapy.

10. FUTURE DIRECTIONS

Clinical experience supports the continuing role of radiation as an independent modality able to offer palliation (pain relief and treatment of bone complications) and disease modification (prevention of new pain), depending on the volume of radiation given. Localized external beam treatment is well tolerated with little known impact on bone marrow functions, but its is unlikely to have clinically meaningful impact on the overall disease process. Wide-field, hemibody irradiation and intravenous radionuclide treatments offer benefits in a systemic level beyond that of localized radiation, but they have greater short- and long-term morbidity, particularly interference on bone marrow functions in the setting of regular administration of palliative chemotherapy. Novel local physical treatment modalities involving image-guided injection of polymethylmethacralate (percutaneous vertebroplasty) *(48)* and percutaneous radio-frequency ablation *(49)* are new treatment options that show promising results in selected patients. Their role as local palliative therapy for bone metastases awaits confirmation by other investigators.

With advances in chemotherapeutics and new, potent bisphosphonates having different molecular and tissue targets, and therefore different toxicities, new combinations or sequencing of modalities might be explored for additive and/or synergistic effects to improve clinical outcomes. Kouloulias et al. recently demonstrated excellent radiographic results of lytic bone lesions treated with palliative radiotherapy followed by 24 mo of intravenous pamidronate in breast cancer patients *(50)*. Wong et al. conducted a randomized study of radiation alone vs radiation + pamidronate in breast cancer patients *(51)*. Although no difference in overall pain response was observed, patients receiving both radiotherapy and pamidronate experienced significantly less pain flare in the first week of treatment than those receiving radiation alone. For metastatic prostate cancer, Scuito et al. reported improved pain response in a small randomized trial comparing strontium-89 alone against strontium-89 with low-dose concurrent cisplatin *(52)*. Hamdy et al. on the other hand, proposed combining radionucludes such as strontium-89 with bisphosphonates to alter the disease course of hormone refractory metastatic prostate cancer *(53,54)*. However, no clinical evidence is yet available for this postulate.

These examples illustrate an exciting time of clinical research into disease modification and symptom palliation in patients with advanced metastatic cancers. Collaboration among investigators of various clinical disciplines and basic sciences will hopefully translate into measurable and meaningful improvements in clinical outcomes.

REFERENCES

1. Tong D, Gillick L, Hendrickson F. The palliation of symptomatic osseous metastases: final results of the study by the Radiation Therapy Oncology Group. *Cancer* 1982; 50:893–899.
2. Blitzer P. Reanalysis of the RTOG study of the palliation of symptomatic osseous metastases. *Cancer* 1985; 55:1468–1472.
3. Chow E, Wu JS, Hoskin P, et al. International consensus on palliative radiotherapy endpoints for future clinical trials in bone metastases. *Radiother Oncol* 2002; 64(3):275–280.
4. Bone Pain Trial Working Party. 8 Gy single fraction radiotherapy for the treatment of metastatic skeletal pain:randomized comparison with multi-fraction schedule over 12 months of patient follow-up. *Radiother Oncol* 1999; 52:111–121.
5. Steenland E, Leer J, van Houwelingen H, et al. The effect of a single fraction compared to multiple fractions on painful bone metastases:a global analysis of the Dutch Bone Metastasis Study. *Radiother Oncol* 1999; 52:101–109.
6. Van den Hout WB, van der Linden YM, Steenland E, et al. Single- versus multiple-fraction radiotherapy in patients with painful bone metastases:cost-utility analysis based on a randomized trial. *J Natl Cancer Inst* 2003; 95(3):222–229
7. Ratanatharathorn V, Powers W, Moss W, et al. Bone metastasis: review and critical analysis of random allocation trials of local field treatment. *Int J Radiat Oncol Biol Phys* 1999; 44:1–18.
8. Wu J, Wong R, Johnston M, et al. Meta-analysis of dose-fractionation radiotherapy trials for the palliation of painful bone metastases. *Int J Radiat Oncol Biol Phys* 2002; 55(3):594–605.
9. Hartsell WF, Scott C, Bruner DW, et al. Phase III randomized trial of 8 Gy in 1 fraction vs 30 Gy in 10 fractions for palliation of painful bone metastases: preliminary results of RTOG 97-14. *Int J Radiat Onocol Biol Phys* 2003; 57(Suppl):S124.
10. Hoskin PJ, Price P, Easton D, et al. A prospective randomized trial of 4 Gy or 8 Gy single doses in the treatment of metastatic bone pain. *Radiother Oncol* 1992; 23(2):74–78.
11. Jeremic B, Shibamoto Y, Acimovic L, et al. A randomized trial of three single-dose radiation therapy regimens in the treatment of metastatic bone pain. *Int J Radiat Oncol Biol Phys* 1998; 41(1):161–167.
12. Ben-Josef E, Shamsa F, Williams A, et al. Radiotherapeutic management of osseous metastases: a survey of current patterns of care. *Int J Radiat Oncol Phys* 1998; 40:915–921.
13. Chow E, Danjoux C, Wong R, et al. Palliation of bone metastases: a survey of patterns of practice among Canadian radiation oncologists. *Radiother Oncol* 2000; 56:305–314.
14. Roos D. Continuing reluctance to use single fractions of radiotherapy for metastatic bone pain: an Australian and New Zealand practice survey and literature review. *Radiother Oncol* 2000; 56:315–322.
15. Barton MB, Dawson R, Jacob S, et al. Palliative radiotherapy of bone metastases: an evaluation of outcome measures. *J Eval Clin Pract* 2001; 7(1):47–64.
16. Shakespeare TP, Lu JJ, Back MF, et al. Patient preference for radiotherapy fractionation schedule in the palliation of painful bone metastases. *J Clin Oncol* 2003; 21(11):2156–2162.
17. Fitzpatrick PJ, Rider WD. Half body radiotherapy. *Int J Radiat Oncol Biol Phys* 1976; 1(3-4):197–207.
18. Hoskin PJ, Ford HT, Harmer CL. Hemibody irradiation (HBI) for metastatic bone pain in two histologically distinct groups of patients. *Clin Oncol* (R Coll Radiol) 1989; 1(2):67–69.
19. Kuban DA, Delbridge T, el-Mahdi AM, Schellhammer PF. Half-body irradiation for treatment of widely metastatic adenocarcinoma of the prostate. *J Urol* 1989; 141(3):572–574.
20. Salazar OM, Rubin P, Hendrickson FR, et al. Single-dose half-body irradiation for palliation of multiple bone metastases from solid tumors. Final Radiation therapy Oncology Group report. *Cancer* 1986; 58(1):29–36.
21. Dearnaley DP, Bayly RJ, A'Hern RP, Gadd J, Zivanovic MM, Lewington VJ. Palliation of bone metastases in prostate cancer. Hemibody irradiation or strontium-89? *Clin Oncol* (R Coll Radiol); 1992; 4(2):101–107.
22. Priestman TJ, Roberts JT, Lucraft H, et al. Results of a randomized, double-blind comparative study of ondansetron and metoclopramide in the prevention of nausea and vomiting following high-dose upper abdominal irradiation. *Clin Oncol (R Coll Radiol)* 1990; 2(2):71–75.
23. Quilty PM, Kirk D, Bolger JJ, et al. A comparison of the palliative effects of strontium-89 and external beam radiotherapy in metastatic prostate cancer. *Radiother Oncol* 1994; 31(1):33–40.
24. Van Dyk J, Keane TJ, Kan S, Rider WD, Fryer CJ. Radiation pneumonitis following large single dose irradiation: a re-evaluation based on absolute dose to lung. *Int J Radiat Oncol Biol Phys* 1981; 7(4): 461–467.

25. Zelefsky MJ, Scher HI, Forman JD, Linares LA, Curley T, Fuks Z. Palliative hemiskeletal irradiation for widespread metastatic prostate cancer: a comparison of single dose and fractionated regimens. *Int J Radiat Oncol Biol Phys* 1989; 7(6):1281–1285.

26. Poulter CA, Cosmatos D, Rubin P, et al. A report of RTOG 8206: a phase III study of whether the addition of single dose hemibody irradiation to standard fractionated local field irradiation is more effective than local field irradiation alone in the treatment of symptomatic osseous metastases. *Int J Radiat Oncol Biol Phys* 1992; 23(1):207–214.

27. Salazar OM, Sandhu T, da Motta NW, et al. Fractionated half-body irradiation (HBI) for the rapid palliation of widespread, symptomatic, metastatic bone disease: a randomized Phase III trial of the International Atomic Energy Agency (IAEA). *Int J Radiat Oncol Biol Phys* 2001; 50(3):765–775.

28. Mithal N, Needham P, Hoskin P. Retreatment with radiotherapy for painful bone metastases. *Int J Radiat Oncol Biol Phys* 1994; 29:1011–1014.

29. Jeremic B, Shibamoto Y, Igrutinovic I. Single 4 Gy re-irradiation for painful bone metastases following single fraction radiotherapy. *Radiother Oncol* 1999; 52:123–127.

30. Jeremic B, Shibamoto Y, Igrutinovic I. Second single 4 Gy reirradiation for painful bone metastasis. *J Pain Symptom Manage* 2002; 23:26–30.

31. van der Linden Y, Lok J, Steenland E, et al. Re-irradiation of painful bone metastases:a further analysis of the Dutch Bone Metastasis Study. *Int J Radiat Oncol Biol Phys* 2003; 57(Suppl):S222.

32. Silberstein EB. Systemic radiopharmaceutical therapy of painful osteoblastic metastases. *Semin Radiat Oncol* 2000; 10:240–249.

33. McEwan AJB. Use of radionuclides for the palliation of bone metastases. *Semin Radiat Oncol* 2000; 10:103–114.

34. Porter AT, McEwan AJB, Powe JE, et al. Results of a randomized phase-III trial to evaluate the efficacy of strontium-89 adjuvant to local field external beam irradiation in the management of endocrine resistant metastatic prostate cancer. *Int J Radiat Oncol Biol Phys* 1993; 25:805–813.

35. McEwan AJB, Amoytte GA, McGowan DG, et al. A retrospective analysis of the cost effectiveness of treatment with Metastron (89Sr-chloride) in patients with prostate cancer metastatic to bone. *Nucl Med Commun* 1994; 15:499–504.

36. Quilty PM, Kirk D, Bolger JJ, et al. A comparison of the palliative effects of strontium-89 and external beam radiotherapy in metastatic prostate cancer. *Radiother Oncol* 1994; 31:33–40.

37. Resche I, Chatal J-F, Pecking A, et al. A dose-controlled study of 153 Sm-ethylenediaminsetetramethylene phosphonate (EDTMP) in the treatment of patients with painful bone metastases. *Eur J Cancer* 1997; 33:1583–1591.

38. Tian JH, Zhang JM, Hou QT, et al. Multicenter trial on the efficacy and toxicity of single-dose samarium-153-ethylene diamine tetramethylene phosphonate as a palliative treatment for painful skeletal metastases in China. *Eur J Nucl Med* 1999; 26:2–7.

39. Hoskin PJ, Stratford MRL, Folkes LK, et al. Effect of local radiotherapy for bone pain on urinary markers of osteoclast activity. *Lancet* 2000; 355:1428–1429.

40. Van der Linden YM, Kroon HM, Dijkstra SPDS, et al. Simple radiographic parameter predicts fracturing in metastatic femoral bone lesions: results from a randomised trial. *Radiother Oncol* 2003; 69(1):21–31.

41. Loblaw DA, Laperriere NJ, Chambers A, Perry J, Group at CCOPGIN-ODS (2003) Diagnosis and management of malignant epidural spinal cord compression (evidence summary Report no. 9-9). *Cancer Care Ontario*, http://www.ccopebc.ca./neucpg.html.

42. Loblaw DA, Laperriere NJ, Mackillop WJ. A population-based study of malignant spinal cord compression in Ontario. *Clin Oncol* (R Coll Radiol). 2003; 15:211–217.

43. Sundaresan N, Galicich JH. Treatment of spinal metastases by vertebral body resection. *Cancer Invest* 1984; 2:383–397.

44. Talcott JA, Stomper PC, Drislane FW, Wen PY, Block CC, Humphrey CC, et al. Assessing suspected spinal cord compression:a multidisciplinary outcomes analysis of 342 episodes. *Support Care Cancer* 1999; 7:31–38.

45. Sorensen S, Helweg-Larsen S, Mouridsen H, Hansen HH. Effect of high-dose dexamethasone in carcinomatous metastatic spinal cord compression treated with radiotherapy: a randomised trial. *Eur J Cancer* 1994; 30A:22–27.

46. Patchell R, Tibbs PA, Regine F, Payne R, Saris S, Kryscio RJ, et al. A randomized trial of direct decompressive surgical resection in the treatment of spinal cord compression caused by metastasis [abstract]. *Proceedings American Society of Clinical Oncology Annual* 2003; 22:1.

47. Hoskin PJ, Grover A, Bhana R. Metastatic spinal cord compression: radiotherapy outcome and dose fractionation. *Radiother Oncol* 2003; 68:175–180.

48. Fourney DR, Schomer DF, Nader R, et al. Percutaneous vertebroplasty and kyphoplasty for painful vertebral body fractures in cancer patients. *J Neurosurg* 2003; 98(1 Suppl):21–30.

49. Callstrom MR, Charboneau JW, Goetz MP, et al. Painful metastases involving bone: feasibility of percutaneous CT- and US-guided radio-frequency ablation. *Radiology* 2002 ; 224(1):87–97.

50. Kouloulias V, Matsopoulos G, Kouvaris J, et al. Radiotherapy in conjunction with intravenous infusion of 180 mg of disodium pamidronate in management of osteolytic metastases from breast cancer: clinical evaluation, biochemical markers, quality of life, and monitoring of recalcification using assessments of gray-level histogram in plain radiographs. *Int J Radiat Oncol Biol Phys* 2003; 57(1):143–157.

51. Wong KSR, Franssen E, Danjoux C, Bezjak A. On behalf of the Rapid Response Radiotherapy Program and Palliative Radiation Oncology Program. A randomized double blind placebo controlled trial of radiotherapy (XRT) ± single dose pamidronate (PAM) for pain relief in patients with painful bone metastases. [abstract]. *Proceedings American Society of Clinical Oncology Annual* 2003; 22:771.

52. Sciuto R, Festa A, Rea S, et al. Effects of low-dose cisplatin on 89Sr therapy for painful bone metastases from prostate cancer: a randomized clinical trial. *J Nucl Med* 2002; 43(1):79–86.

53. Hamdy NA, Papapoulos SE. The palliative management of skeletal metastases in prostate cancer:use of bone-seeking radionuclides and bisphosphonates. *Semin Nucl Med* 2001; 31(1):62–68.

54. Soerdjbalie-Maikoe V, Pelger RC, Lycklama a Nijeholt GA, et al. Strontium-89 (Metastron) and the bisphosphonate olpadronate reduce the incidence of spinal cord compression in patients with hormone-refractory prostate cancer metastatic to the skeleton. *Eur J Nucl Med Mol Imaging* 2002; 29(4):494–498.

Index